Thieme

Essentials of Audiology

Fourth Edition

Stanley A. Gelfand, PhD
Professor
Department of Linguistics and Communication Disorders
Queens College of The City University of New York
Flushing, New York
PhD Program in Speech-Language-Hearing Sciences and AuD Program
Graduate Center of The City University of New York
New York, New York

290 illustrations

Thieme
New York • Stuttgart • Delhi • Rio de Janeiro

Executive Editor: Anne Sydor
Managing Editor: Elizabeth Palumbo
Director, Editorial Services: Mary Jo Casey
Editorial Assistant: Natascha Morris
Production Editor: Kenneth L. Chumbley
International Production Director: Andreas Schabert
Senior Vice President, Editorial and E-Product Development:
    Vera Spillner
International Marketing Director: Fiona Henderson
International Sales Director: Louisa Turrell
Director of Sales, North America: Mike Roseman
Senior Vice President and Chief Operating Officer: Sarah Vanderbilt
President: Brian D. Scanlan

Library of Congress Cataloging-in-Publication Data
Names: Gelfand, Stanley A., 1948- , author.
Title: Essentials of audiology / Stanley A. Gelfand.
Description: Fourth edition. | New York : Thieme, [2016] |
    Includes bibliographical references and index.
Identifiers: LCCN 2015041466| ISBN 9781604068610 (hardback :
    alk. paper) | ISBN 9781604068627 (e-book)
Subjects: | MESH: Audiology.
Classification: LCC RF290 | NLM WV 270 | DDC 617.8—dc23
    LC record available at http://lccn.loc.gov/2015041466

© 2016 Thieme Medical Publishers, Inc.
Thieme Publishers New York
333 Seventh Avenue, New York, NY 10001 USA
+1 800 782 3488, customerservice@thieme.com

Thieme Publishers Stuttgart
Rüdigerstrasse 14, 70469 Stuttgart, Germany
+49 [0]711 8931 421, customerservice@thieme.de

Thieme Publishers Delhi
A-12, Second Floor, Sector-2, Noida-201301
Uttar Pradesh, India
+91 120 45 566 00, customerservice@thieme.in

Thieme Publishers Rio de Janeiro, Thieme Publicações Ltda.
Edifício Rodolpho de Paoli, 25º andar
Av. Nilo Peçanha, 50 – Sala 2508
Rio de Janeiro 20020-906, Brasil
+55 21 3172 2297

Cover design: Thieme Publishing Group
Typesetting by Prairie Papers

Printed in China by Asia Pacific Offset Ltd   5 4 3 2 1

ISBN 978-1-60406-861-0

Also available as an eBook:
eISBN 978-1-60406-862-7

Important note: Medicine is an ever-changing science undergoing continual development. Research and clinical experience are continually expanding our knowledge, in particular our knowledge of proper treatment and drug therapy. Insofar as this book mentions any dosage or application, readers may rest assured that the authors, editors, and publishers have made every effort to ensure that such references are in accordance with **the state of knowledge at the time of production of the book.**

Nevertheless, this does not involve, imply, or express any guarantee or responsibility on the part of the publishers in respect to any dosage instructions and forms of applications stated in the book. **Every user is requested to examine carefully** the manufacturers' leaflets accompanying each drug and to check, if necessary in consultation with a physician or specialist, whether the dosage schedules mentioned therein or the contraindications stated by the manufacturers differ from the statements made in the present book. Such examination is particularly important with drugs that are either rarely used or have been newly released on the market. Every dosage schedule or every form of application used is entirely at the user's own risk and responsibility. The authors and publishers request every user to report to the publishers any discrepancies or inaccuracies noticed. If errors in this work are found after publication, errata will be posted at www.thieme.com on the product description page.

Some of the product names, patents, and registered designs referred to in this book are in fact registered trademarks or proprietary names even though specific reference to this fact is not always made in the text. Therefore, the appearance of a name without designation as proprietary is not to be construed as a representation by the publisher that it is in the public domain.

To Janice

In loving memory

Contents

Preface

What is audiology? *Audiology* is the clinical profession that deals with hearing and balance disorders. It is also the scientific study of normal and abnormal audition and related areas in the broadest sense.

What is an audiologist? An *audiologist* is a practitioner of audiology as a clinical profession. Audiologists are principally concerned with the identification, evaluation and management of patients with auditory and balance disorders, as well as with the prevention of hearing impairment. The scope of audiological practice also includes such diverse areas as the evaluation of the vestibular system, noise assessment, and hearing conservation, as well as the physiological monitoring of various neurological functions during surgical procedures. As a result, audiologists possess a broad scope of knowledge and skills, and often have interests in common with a variety of other disciplines such as speech-language pathology; speech and hearing science; education of the deaf and hearing impaired; engineering; acoustics; industrial hygiene; musicology; medicine; physiology; psychology; linguistics; and vocational counseling.

Much like many other scholarly professions, pursuing a career in audiology involves a rigorous course of doctoral education and training. Most audiologists earn the Doctor of Audiology (Au.D.) degree, while others with research and academic as well as clinical interests obtain a Ph.D. Some pursue both. In addition, those qualified to practice audiology are usually certified by the American Speech-Language-Hearing Association (ASHA) and/ or the American Academy of Audiology (AAA), as well as possessing professional licenses from the states in which they practice.

So who is this book for? Introductory audiology is an essential and fundamental aspect of the education of all students who are interested in the two related professions of Speech-Language Pathology and Audiology. This book is primarily intended to serve as a comprehensive introductory text for students who are preparing to enter both of these fields. As such, it tries to address the needs of two rather different groups of students. Those planning a career in audiology need a broad overview of the field and a firm understanding of its many basic principles so that they have a solid foundation for futures as doctors of audiology in clinical practice. The audiological needs of future speech-language pathologists are just as important, and go well beyond knowing the auditory implications of speech, language and related disorders, and being able to understand audiological reports. Speech-language pathologists often find themselves working hand-in-hand with their audiological colleagues. They also need to perform certain audiological procedures themselves when these fall within the speech-language pathology scope of practice, especially when screening is involved; and they regularly make interpretations and referrals that are of audiological relevance. Moreover, speech-language pathologists often work with patients who have hearing losses and auditory processing disorders directly and on an ongoing basis. They frequently must explain the nature and management of auditory disorders to family members, teachers and other professionals. This is especially true in school settings and long-term care facilities. What's more, cochlear implant and other multidisciplinary programs are enhancing the scope and depth of interactions among speech-language pathologists and audiologists, and are making a knowledge and understanding of audiology all the more important for budding speech-language pathologists. With considerations like these in mind, I hope that students who become speech-language pathologists will find this text useful as a reference source long after their audiology courses have been completed. (Of course, I do admit hoping that at least a few speech-language pathology students will be attracted to a career in audiology by what they read here.)

This textbook attempts to provide a comprehensive overview of audiology at the introductory level; including such topics as acoustics, anatomy and physiology, sound perception, auditory disorders and the nature of hearing impairment, methods of measurement, screening, clinical assessment and clinical management. It is intended to serve as the core text for undergraduate students in speech, language and hearing, and might also serve the needs of beginning-level graduate students who need to learn or review the fundamentals of audiology. It is anticipated that the material will be covered in a one-, two- or three-term undergraduate sequence, depending on the organization of the communication sciences and disorders curriculum at a given college or university. For example, the first three chapters are often used the text for an undergraduate hearing science course, while selections from the other chapters might be used in one or two audiology courses.

With these considerations in mind, I have tried to prepare a textbook that is extensive enough for professors pick and choose material that provides the right depth and scope of coverage for a particular course. For example, text readings can be assigned to cover clinical masking at almost any level from simple to complex by selecting various sections of Chapter 9. It is unlikely that all of that chapter will be assigned in a single undergraduate class. However, the material is there if needed for further study, to provide the groundwork for a term-paper or independent study report, or for future reference. I have tried to provide relatively extensive reference lists are provided for similar reasons.

This fourth edition was undertaken to provide the beginning student with an up-to-date coverage of a field that is steadily developing, as well as to take advantage of accumulating experience to improve upon what is included and how it is presented. Many developments and changes have taken place since the third edition was published. Some of them are in areas of rapidly unfolding development like cochlear implants and related technologies and in electrophysiological assessment. But most of them are the slow, methodical and often subtle—albeit important—advances that unfold over time in an active clinical science. Others changes reflect the influence of systematic reviews, changes in guidelines, expert position papers, standards and regulations which affect clinical practices and technical matters. Of course, there are always a few developments that surfaced the day *after* the prior edition was printed—a frustration to the textbook author, but the kind of thing that makes audiology such an exciting and interesting field.

As with the prior editions, this one was influenced by the input graciously provided by of many audiologists involved in clinical practice, research, and teaching and student supervision. In addition, considerable attention was given to the comments and insights of students who were taking or recently completed introductory audiology courses, including those who used the third edition of this text as well as other books. The content and especially the style of the text were substantially influenced by their advice. As a result of their insights, the current edition retains a writing style that has been kept as conversational and informal as possible; and only classroom-proven examples and drawings are included. Similarly, clinical masking, acoustic immittance and screening have been kept in separate chapters; the material on audiological management continues to be spread over two chapters;

and the history of audiology has been omitted. The use of gender-specific pronouns (*he, she, him, her,* etc.)—originally undertaken with great trepidation—was very well received in all three prior editions, and has been continued in this one. Its purpose is to maximize clarity for the benefit of the reader. The alternative would have resulted in longer phrases and a more formal style, and would have detracted from the goal of providing the student with text that is maximally reader-friendly (or at least minimally unfriendly). This style also makes the material considerably easier to follow by using different genders for the clinician and patient when describing clinical procedures and interactions. Gender fairness is maintained by referring to both genders in both roles more-or-less equally throughout the text.

This book would not exist without the influence of many very special people. I am particularly grateful to my colleagues and students in the Department of Linguistics and Communication Disorders at Queens College, and in the Au.D. Program and the Ph.D. Program in Speech Language and Hearing Sciences at the City University of New York Graduate Center. I would also like to express my appreciation to the extraordinary, talented and dedicated professionals at Thieme Medical Publishers, who have been so helpful, cooperative and supportive throughout the process of preparing this book, in spite of its demanding and dyslexic author. With sincere apologies to anyone inadvertently omitted, I would like to extend my heartfelt thanks to the following individuals for their influence, insights, advice, encouragement, assistance, support, and friendship: Moe Bergman, Arthur Boothroyd, Lauren Calandruccio, Kenny Chumbley, Joseph Danto, Becky Dille, Lillian and Sol Gelfand, Irving Hochberg, Gertrude and Oscar Katzen, Arlene Kraat, William Lamsbeck, Harry Levitt, John Lutolf, Dave Mason, Maurice Miller, Natascha Morris, Elizabeth Palumbo, Neil Piper, John Preece, Brian Scanlan, Teresa Schwander, Shlomo Silman, Carol Silverman, Anne Sydor, Helen and Harris Topel, Barbara Weinstein, and Mark Weiss.

Finally, my greatest appreciation is expressed to Janice, whose memory will always be a blessing and inspiration; and to my wonderful children, Michael, Joshua and Erin, and Jessica and Robert for their love, encouragement, support, insight and unimaginable patience.

Stanley A. Gelfand

1 Acoustics and Sound Measurement

We begin our study of audiology by reviewing the nature of sound because, after all, sound is what we hear. The science of sound is called acoustics, which is a branch of physics, and relies on several basic physical principles. Many useful sources are available for students wishing to pursue the areas covered in this chapter in greater detail (e.g., Beranek 1986; Gelfand 2010; Hewitt 1974; Kinsler, Frey, Coppens, & Sanders 1982; Peterson & Gross 1972; Sears, Zemansky, & Young 1982).

■ Physical Quantities

The basic physical quantities are mass, time, and length (or distance). All other physical quantities are derived by combining these three basic ones, as well as other derived quantities, in a variety of ways. The principal basic and derived quantities are summarized in **Table 1.1**. These basic quantities are expressed in terms of conventional units that are measurable and repeatable. The unit of **mass (M)** is the **kilogram (kg)** or the **gram (g)**; the unit of **length (L)** is the **meter (m)** or the **centimeter (cm)**; and the unit of **time (t)** is the **second (s)**. Mass is not really synonymous with weight even though we express its magnitude in kilograms. The mass of a body is related to its density, but its weight is related to the force of gravity. If two objects are the same size, the one with greater density will weigh more. However, even though an object's mass would be identical on the earth and the moon, it would weigh less on the moon, where there is less gravity.

When we express mass in kilograms and length in meters, we are using the meter–kilogram-second or **MKS** system. Expressing mass in grams and length in centimeters constitutes the centimeter-gram-second or **cgs** system. These two systems also have different derived quantities. For example, the units of force and work are called newtons and joules in the MKS system, and dynes and ergs in the cgs system, respectively. We will emphasize the use of MKS units because this is the internationally accepted standard in the scientific community, known as the **Systeme Internationale (SI)**. Equivalent cgs values will often be given as well because the audiology profession has traditionally worked in cgs units, and the death of old habits is slow and labored. These quantities are summarized with equivalent values in MKS and cgs units in **Table 1.1**. In addition, the correspondence between scientific notation and conventional numbers, and the meanings of prefixes used to describe the sizes of metric units are shown for convenience and ready reference in **Table 1.2** and **Table 1.3**.

Quantities may be scalars or vectors. A **scalar** can be fully described by its magnitude (amount or size), but a **vector** has both direction and magnitude. For example, length is a scalar because an object that is one meter long is always one meter long. However, we are dealing with a vector when we measure the distance between two coins that are one meter apart because their relationship has both magnitude and direction (from point x_1 to point x_2). This quantity is called **displacement (d)**. Derived quantities will be vectors if they have one or more components that are vectors; for example, velocity is a vector because it is derived from displacement, and acceleration is a vector because it involves velocity. We distinguish between scalars and vectors because they are handled differently when calculations are being made.

Velocity Everyone knows that "55 miles per hour" refers to the speed of a car that causes it to travel a distance of 55 miles in a one-hour period of time. This is an example of **velocity (v)**, which is equal to the amount of displacement (d) that occurs over time (t):

$$v = \frac{d}{t}$$

Table 1.1 Principal physical quantities

Quantity	Formula	MKS (SI) units	cgs units	Comments
Mass (M)	M	kilogram (kg)	gram (g)	1 kg = 10^3 g
Time (t)	t	second (s)	s	
Area (A)	A	m^2	cm^2	1 m^2 = 10^4 cm^2
Displacement (d)	d	meter (m)	centimeter (cm)	1 m = 10^2 cm
Velocity (v)	v = d/t	m/s	cm/s	1 m/s = 10^2 cm/s
Acceleration (a)	a = v/t	m/s^2	cm/s^2	1 m/s^2 = 10^2 cm/s^2
Force (F)	F = Ma = Mv/t	kg • m/s^2 newton (N)	g • cm/s^2 dyne	1 N = 10^5 dyne
Pressure (p)	p = F/A	N/m^2 pascal (Pa)	$dyne/cm^2$ microbar (μbar)	2×10^{-5} N/m^2 or 20 μPa (reference value) 2×10^{-4} $dyne/cm^2$ or μbar (reference value)
Work (W)	W = Fd	N • m joule (J)	dyne • cm erg	1 J = 10^7 erg
Power (P)	P = W/t = Fd/t = Fv	joule/s watt (w)	erg/s watt (w)	1 w = 1 J/s = 10^7 erg/s
Intensity (I)	I = P/A	w/m^2	w/cm^2	10^{-12} w/m^2 (reference value) 10^{-16} w/cm^2 (reference value)

Displacement is measured in meters and time is measured in seconds (sec); thus, velocity is expressed in meters per second (m/s). Velocity is the vector equivalent of speed because it is based on displacement, which has both magnitude and direction. When we take a trip we usually figure out the distance traveled by making a mental note of the starting odometer reading and then subtracting it from the odometer reading at the destination (e.g., if we start at 10,422 miles and arrive at 10,443 miles, then the distance must have been 10,443 – 10,422 = 21 miles). We do the same thing to calculate the time it took to make the trip (e.g., if we left at 1:30 and arrived at 2:10, then the trip must have taken 2:10 – 1:30 = 40 minutes). Physical calculations involve the same straightforward approach. When an object is displaced, it starts at point x_1 and time t_1 and arrives at point x_2 and time t_2. Its *average velocity* is simply the distance traveled ($x_2 - x_1$) divided by the time it took to make the trip ($t_2 - t_1$):

$$v = \frac{x_2 - x_1}{t_2 - t_1}$$

The term *instantaneous velocity* describes the velocity of a body at a *particular moment* in time. For the math-minded, it refers to the velocity when the displacement and time between one point and the next one approach zero, that is, the derivative of displacement with respect to time:

$$v = \frac{dx}{dt}$$

Acceleration Driving experience has taught us all that a car increases its speed to get onto a highway, slows down when exiting, and also slows down while making a turn. "Speeding up" and "slowing down" mean that the velocity is changing over time. The change of velocity over time is **acceleration (a)**. Suppose a body is moving between two points. Its velocity at the first point is v_1, and the time at that point is t_1. Similarly, its velocity at the second point is v_2 and the time at that point is t_2. *Average accelera-*

Table 1.2 Expressing numbers in standard notation and scientific notation

Standard notation	Scientific notation
0.000001	10^{-6}
0.00001	10^{-5}
0.0001	10^{-4}
0.001	10^{-3}
0.01	10^{-2}
0.1	10^{-1}
1	10^{0}
10	10^{1}
100	10^{2}
1,000	10^{3}
10,000	10^{4}
100,000	10^{5}
1,000,000	10^{6}
3600	3.6×10^{3}
0.036	3.6×10^{-2}
0.0002	2×10^{-4}
0.00002	2×10^{-5}

tion is the difference between the two velocities ($v_2 - v_1$) divided by the time interval ($t_2 - t_1$):

$$a = \frac{v_2 - v_1}{t_2 - t_1}$$

In more general terms, acceleration is written simply as

$$a = \frac{v}{t}$$

Because velocity is the same as displacement divided by time, we can replace v with d/t, so that

$$a = \frac{d/t}{t}$$

which can be simplified to

$$a = \frac{d}{t^2}$$

Consequently, acceleration is expressed in units of *meters per second squared (m/s²)* in the MKS system. When measurements are made in cgs units, acceleration is expressed in centimeters per second squared (cm/s²).

Acceleration at a given moment is called *instantaneous acceleration*, and quantitatively oriented readers should note it is equal to the derivative of velocity with respect to time, or

$$a = \frac{dv}{dt}$$

Table 1.3 Examples of prefixes used to express metric units

Prefix	Symbol	Definition	Multiply by	
			Standard notation	Scientific notation
micro	μ	millionths	1/1,000,000 *or* 0.000001	10^{-6}
milli	m	thousanths	1/1000 *or* 0.001	10^{-3}
cent	c	hundredths	1/100 *or* 0.01	10^{-2}
deci	d	tenths	1/10 *or* 0.1	10^{-1}
deka	da	tens	10	10^{1}
hecto	h	hundreds	100	10^{2}
kilo	k	thousands	1000	10^{3}
mega	M	millions	1,000,000	10^{6}

Because velocity is the first derivative of displacement, we find that acceleration is the second derivative of displacement:

$$a = \frac{d^2 x}{dt^2}$$

Force An object that is sitting still will not move unless some outside influence causes it to do so, and an object that is moving will continue moving at the same speed unless some outside influence does something to change it. This commonsense statement is Newton's first law of motion. It describes the attribute of **inertia**, which is the property of mass to continue doing what it is already doing. The "outside influence" that makes a stationary object move, or causes a moving object to change its speed or direction, is called **force (F)**. Notice that force causes the moving object to change velocity or the motionless object to move, which is also a change in velocity (from zero to some amount). Recall that a change of velocity is acceleration. Hence, force is that influence (conceptually a "push" or "pull") that causes a mass to be accelerated. In effect, the amount of "push" or "pull" needed depends on how much mass you want to influence and the amount of acceleration you are trying to produce. In other words, force is equal to the product of mass times acceleration:

$$F = Ma$$

Since acceleration is velocity over time (v/t), we can also specify force in the form

$$F = \frac{Mv}{t}$$

The quantity Mv is called **momentum**, so we may also say that force equals momentum over time.

The amount of force is measured in kg • m/s^2 because force is equal to the product of mass (measured in kg) and acceleration (measured in m/s^2). The *unit of force* is the **newton (N)**, where one newton is the amount of force needed to cause a 1 kg mass to be accelerated by 1 m/s^2; hence, 1 N = 1 kg • 1 m/s^2. (This might seem very technical, but it really simplifies matters; after all, it is easier to say "one newton" than "one kg • m/s^2.".) It would take a 2 N force to cause a 1 kg mass to be accelerated by 2 m/s^2, or a 2 kg mass to be accelerated by 1 m/s^2. A 4 N force is needed to accelerate a 2 kg mass by 2 m/s^2, and a 63 N force is needed to accelerate a 9 kg mass by 7 m/s^2. In the cgs system, the unit of force is called the **dyne**, which is the force needed to accelerate a 1 g mass by 1 cm/s^2; that is, 1 dyne = 1 g • cm/s^2. It takes 10^5 dynes to equal 1 N.

Many different forces are usually acting upon an object at the same time. Hence, the force we have been referring to so far is actually the **net** or **resultant force**, that is, the "bottom line" effect of all the forces that act upon an object. If a force of 3 N is pushing an object toward the right and a second force of 8 N is also pushing that object toward the right, then the net force would be 3 + 8 = 11 N toward the right. In other words, if two forces push a body in the same direction, then the net force would be the sum of those two forces. Conversely, if a 4 N force pushes an object toward the right at the same time that a 9 N force pushes it toward the left, then the net force is 9 – 4 = 5 N toward the left. Thus, if two forces push an object in opposite directions, then the net force is the difference between the two opposing forces, and it causes the object to accelerate in the direction of the greater force. If two *equal* forces push in *opposite* directions, then the net force is zero. Because the net force is zero it will not cause the motion of the object to change. The situation in which net force is zero is called **equilibrium**. In this case, a moving object will continue moving and an object that is **at rest** (i.e., not moving) will continue to remain still.

Friction When an object is moving in the real world, it tends to slow down and eventually comes to a halt. This happens because anything that is moving in the real world is always in contact with other bodies or mediums. The sliding of one body on the other constitutes a force that opposes the motion, called **resistance** or **friction**.

The opposing force of friction or resistance depends on two parameters. The first factor is that the amount of friction depends on the nature of the materials that are sliding on one another. Simply stated, the amount of friction between two given objects is greater for "rough" materials than for "smooth" or "slick" ones, and is expressed as a quantity called the *coefficient of friction*. The second factor that determines how much friction occurs is easily appreciated by rubbing the palms of your hands back and forth on each other. First rub slowly and then more rapidly. The rubbing will produce heat, which occurs because friction causes some of the mechanical energy to be converted into heat. This notion will be revisited later, but for now we will use the amount of heat as an indicator of the amount of resistance. Your hands become hotter when they are rubbed together more quickly. This illustrates the notion that the amount of friction depends on the *velocity* of motion. In quantitative terms,

$$F = Rv$$

where F is the force of friction, R is the coefficient of friction between the materials, and v is the velocity of the motion.

Elasticity and restoring force It takes some effort (an outside force) to compress or expand a spring; and the compressed or expanded spring will bounce back to its original shape after it is released. Compressing or expanding the spring is an example of deforming an object. The spring bouncing back to its prior shape is an example of elasticity. More formally, we can say that **elasticity** is the property whereby a deformed object returns to its original form. Notice the distinction between deformation and elasticity. A rubber band and saltwater taffy can both be stretched (deformed), but only the rubber band bounces back. In other words, what makes a rubber band *elastic* is not that it stretches, but rather that it bounces back. The more readily a deformed object returns to its original form, the more elastic (or stiff) it is.

We know from common experiences, such as using simple exercise equipment, that it is relatively easy to *begin* compressing a spring (e.g., a "grip exerciser"), but that it gets progressively harder to *continue* compressing it. Similarly, it is easier to *begin* expanding a spring (e.g., pulling apart the springs on a "chest exerciser") than it is to *continue* expanding it. In other words, the more a spring-like material (an elastic element) is deformed, the more it *opposes* the applied force. The force that opposes the deformation of an elastic or spring-like material is known as the **restoring force**. If we think of deformation in terms of how far the spring has been compressed or expanded from its original position, we could also say that the restoring force increases with displacement. Quantitatively, then, restoring force (F_R) depends on the stiffness (S) of the material and the amount of its displacement as follows:

$$F_R = Sd$$

Pressure Very few people can push a straight pin into a piece of wood, yet almost anyone can push a thumbtack into the same piece of wood. This is possible because a thumbtack is really a simple machine that concentrates the amount of force being exerted over a larger area (the head) down to a very tiny area (the point). In other words, force is affected by the size of the area over which it is applied in a way that constitutes a new quantity. This quantity, which is equal to force divided by area (A), is called **pressure (p)**, so

$$p = \frac{F}{A}$$

Because force is measured in newtons and area is measured in square meters in MKS units, pressure is measured in newtons per square meter (N/m^2).

The unit of pressure is the **Pascal (Pa)**, so that 1 Pa = 1 N/m^2. In the cgs system, pressure is measured in dynes per square centimeter (dynes/cm^2), occasionally referred to as **microbars (μbars)**.

Work and energy As a physical concept, **work (W)** occurs when the force applied to a body results in its displacement, and the amount of work is equal to the product of the force and the displacement, or

$$W = Fd$$

Because force is measured in newtons and displacement is measured in meters, work itself is quantified in newton-meters (N • m). For example, if a force of 2 N displaces a body by 3 m, then the amount of work is 2 × 3 = 6 N. There can only be work if there is displacement. There cannot be work if there is no displacement (i.e., if d = 0) because work is the product of force and displacement, and zero times anything is zero. The MKS unit of work is the **joule (J)**. One joule is the amount of work that occurs when one newton of force effects one meter of displacement, or 1 J = 1 N • m. In the cgs system, the unit of work is called the erg, where 1 erg = 1 dyne • cm. One joule corresponds to 10^7 ergs.

Energy is usually defined as the capability to do work. The energy of a body at rest is **potential** energy and the energy of an object that is in motion is **kinetic** energy. The total energy of a body is the sum of its potential energy plus its kinetic energy, and work corresponds to the exchange between these two forms of energy. In other words, energy is not consumed when work is accomplished; it is converted from one form to the other. This principle is illustrated by the simple example of a swinging pendulum. The pendulum's potential energy is greatest when it reaches the extreme of its swing, where its motion is momentarily zero. On the other hand, the pendulum's kinetic energy is greatest when it passes through the midpoint of its swing because this is where it is moving the fastest. Between these two extremes, energy is being converted from potential to kinetic as the pendulum speeds up (on each down swing), and from kinetic to potential as the pendulum slows down (on each up swing).

Power The rate at which work is done is called **power (P)**, so that power can be defined as work divided by time,

$$P = \frac{W}{t}$$

The unit of power is called the **watt (w)**. One unit of power corresponds to one unit of work divided by one unit of time. Hence, one watt is equal to one joule divided by one second, or 1 w = 1 J/s. Power is also expressed in watts in the cgs system, where work is measured in ergs. Since 1 J = 10^7 erg, we can also say that 1 w = 107 erg/s.

Power can also be expressed in other terms. For example, because W = Fd, we can substitute Fd for W in the power formula, to arrive at

$$P = \frac{Fd}{t}$$

We know that v = d/t, so we can substitute v for d/t and rewrite this formula as

$$P = Fv$$

In other words, power is also equal to force times velocity.

Intensity Consider a hypothetical demonstration in which one tablespoonful of oil is placed on the surface of a still pond. At that instant the entire amount of oil will occupy the space of a tablespoon. As time passes, the oil spreads out over an expanding area on the surface of the pond, and it therefore also thins out so that much less than all the oil will occupy the space of a tablespoon. The wider the oil spreads the more it thins out, and the proportion of the oil covering any given area gets smaller and smaller, even though the total amount of oil is the same. Clearly, there is a difference between the amount of oil, per se, and the concentration of the oil as it is distributed across (i.e., divided by) the surface area of the pond.

An analogous phenomenon occurs with sound. It is common knowledge that sound radiates outward in every direction from its source, constituting a sphere that gets bigger and bigger with increasing distance from the source, as illustrated by the concentric circles in **Fig. 1.1**. Let us imagine that the sound source is a tiny pulsating object (at the center of the concentric circles in the figure), and that it produces a finite amount of power, analogous to the fixed amount of oil in the prior example. Consequently, the sound power will be divided over the ever-expanding surface as distance increases from the source, analogous to the thinning out of the widening oil slick. This notion is represented in the figure by the thinning of the lines at greater distances from the source. Suppose we measure how much power registers on a certain fixed amount of surface area (e.g., a square inch). As a result, a progressively smaller proportion of the original power falls onto a square inch as the distance from the source increases, represented in the figure by the lighter shading of the same-size ovals at increasing distances from the source.

The examples just described reveal that a new quantity, called **intensity (I),** develops when power

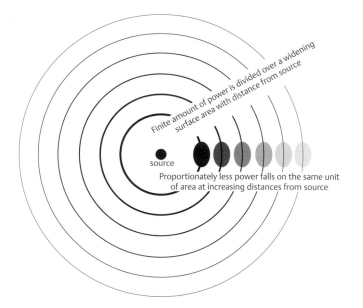

Fig. 1.1 Intensity (power divided by area) decreases with distance from the sound source because a fixed amount of power is spread over an increasing area, represented by the thinning of the lines. Proportionately less power falls on the same unit area (represented by the lighter shading of the ovals) with increasing distance from the source.

is distributed over area. Specifically, intensity is equal to power per unit area, or power divided by area, or

$$I = \frac{P}{A}$$

Because power is measured in watts and area is measured in square meters in the MKS system, intensity is expressed in watts per square meter (w/m²). Intensity is expressed in watts per square centimeter (w/cm²) in the cgs system.

Intensity decreases with increasing distance from a sound source according to a rule called the **inverse square law**. It states that the amount of intensity drops by 1 over the square of the change in distance. Two examples are illustrated in **Fig. 1.2**. Frame **a** shows that when the distance from a loudspeaker is doubled from 5 m to 10 m, the amount of intensity at 10 m will be one quarter of what it was at 5 m (because $1/2^2$ = 1/4). Similarly, frame **b** shows that tripling the distance from 5 m to 15 m causes the intensity to fall to one ninth of its value at the closer point because $1/3^2$ = 1/9.

An important relationship to be aware of is that power is equal to pressure squared,

$$P = p^2$$

Fig. 1.2 Illustrations of the inverse square law. **(a)** Doubling of distance: The intensity at 10 m away from a loudspeaker is one quarter of its intensity at 5 m because $1/2^2 = 1/4$. **(b)** Tripling of distance: The intensity at 15 m away from the sources is one ninth of its intensity at 5 m because $1/3^2 = 1/9$.

and pressure is equal to the square root of power,

$$p = \sqrt{P}$$

In addition, intensity is proportional to pressure squared,

$$I \propto p^2$$

and pressure is proportional to the square root of intensity,

$$p \propto \sqrt{I}$$

This simple relationship makes it easy to convert between sound intensity and sound pressure.

■ The Nature of Sound

Sound is often defined as a form of vibration that propagates through the air in the form of a wave. **Vibration** is nothing more than the to-and-fro motion (oscillation) of an object. Some examples include a playground swing, a pendulum, the floorboards under a washing machine, a guitar string, a tuning fork prong, and air molecules. The vibration is usually called **sound** when it is transferred from air particle to air particle (we will see how this happens later). The vibration of air particles might have a simple pattern such as the tone produced by a tuning fork, or a very complex pattern such as the din heard in a school cafeteria. Most naturally occurring sounds are very complex, but the easiest way to understand sound is to concentrate on the simplest ones.

Simple Harmonic Motion

A vibrating tuning fork is illustrated in **Fig. 1.3**. The initial force that was applied by striking the tuning fork is represented by the green arrow in frame 1. The progression of the drawings represents the motion of the prongs at selected points in time after the fork has been activated. The two prongs vibrate as mirror images of each other, so that we can describe what is happening in terms of just one prong. The *insert* highlights the motion of the right prong. Here the center position is where the prong would be at rest. When the fork is struck the prong is forced inward as shown by arrow **a**. After reaching the leftmost position it bounces back (arrow **b**), accelerating along the way. The rapidly moving prong overshoots the center and continues rightward (arrow **c**). It slows down along the way until it stops for an instant at the extreme right, where it reverses direction again and starts moving toward the left (arrow **d**) at an ever-increasing speed. It overshoots the center again, and as before, the prong now follows arrow **a**, slowing down until it stops momentarily at the extreme left. Here it reverses direction again and repeats the same process over and over again. One complete round trip (or replication) of an oscillating motion is called a **cycle**. The number of cycles that occur in one second is called **frequency**.

This form of motion occurs when a force is applied to an object having the properties of inertia and elasticity. Due to its elasticity, the deformation of the fork caused by the applied force is opposed by a restoring force. In the figure the initial leftward force is opposed by a restoring force in the opposite direction, that is, toward the right. The rightward restoring force increases as the prong is pushed progressively toward the left. As a result, the movement of the prong slows down and eventually stops. Under the influence of its elasticity the prong now reverses direction and starts moving rightward. As the restoring force brings the prong back toward the center, we must also consider its mass. Because the prong has mass, inertia causes it to accelerate as it moves back

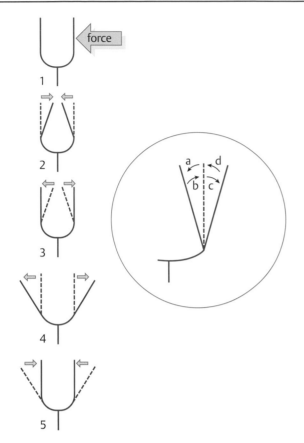

Fig. 1.3   After being struck, a tuning fork vibrates or oscillates with a simple pattern that repeats itself over time. One replication (cycle) of this motion is illustrated going from frames 1 to 5. The arrows in the insert highlight the motion of one of the prongs.

toward its center resting position. In fact, the prong is moving at its maximum speed as it passes through the resting position. The force of inertia causes the prong to overshoot the center and continue moving rightward. The deformation process begins again once the prong overshoots its resting position. As a result, opposing elastic restoring forces start building up again, now in the leftward direction. Just as before, the increasing (leftward) restoring force eventually overcomes the rightward inertial force, thereby stopping the prong's displacement at the rightmost point, and causing a reversal in the direction of its movement. Hence, the same course of events is repeated again, this time in the leftward direction; then rightward, then leftward, etc., over and over again. This kind of vibration is called **simple harmonic motion (SHM)** because the oscillations repeat themselves at the same rate over and over again.

We know from experience that the oscillations just described do not continue forever. Instead, they dissipate over time and eventually die out com-

pletely. The dying out of vibrations over time is called **damping**, and it occurs due to resistance or friction. Resistance occurs because the vibrating prong is always in contact with the surrounding air. As a result, there will be friction between the oscillating metal and the surrounding air molecules. This friction causes some of the mechanical energy that has been supporting the motion of the tuning fork to be converted into heat. In turn, the energy that has been converted into heat is no longer available to maintain the vibration of the tuning fork. Consequently, the sizes of the oscillations dissipate and eventually die out altogether.

A diagram summarizing the concepts just described is shown in **Fig. 1.4**. The curve in the figure represents the tuning fork's motion. The amount of displacement of the tuning fork prong around its resting (or center) position is represented by distance above and below the horizontal line. These events are occurring over time, which is represented by horizontal distance (from left to right). The initial displacement of the prong due to the original applied force is represented by the dotted segment of the curve. Inertial forces due to the prong's mass and elastic restoring forces due to the elasticity of the prong are represented by labeled arrows. Damping of the oscillations due to friction is shown by the decline in the displacement of the curve as time goes on. The curve in this diagram is an example of a **waveform**, which is a graph that shows displacement (or another measure of magnitude) as a function of time.

Sound Waves

Tuning fork vibrations produce sound because the oscillations of the prongs are transmitted to the surrounding air particles. When the tuning fork prong moves to the right, it displaces air molecules to its right in the same direction. These molecules are thus displaced to the right of their own resting positions. Displacing air molecules toward the right pushes them closer to the air particles to their right. The pressure that exists among air molecules that are not being disturbed by a driving force (like the tuning fork) is known as *ambient or atmospheric pressure.* We can say that the rightward motion of the tuning fork prong exerts a force on the air molecules that pushes them together relative to their undisturbed, resting situation. In other words, forcing the air molecules together causes an increase in air pressure relative to the ambient pressure that existed among the undisturbed molecules. This state of positive air pressure is called **compression**. The amount of compression increases as the prong continues displacing

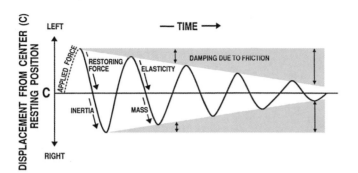

Fig. 1.4 Diagrammatic representation of tuning fork oscillations over time. Vertical displacement represents the amount of the tuning fork prong displacement around its resting position. Distance from left to right represents the progression of time. (From Gelfand 2010, courtesy of Informa.)

the air molecules rightward. A maximum amount of positive pressure occurs when the prong and air molecules reach their greatest rightward displacement.

The tuning fork prong then reverses direction, overshoots its resting position, and proceeds to its leftmost position. The compressed air molecules reverse direction along with the prong. This occurs because air is an elastic medium, so the particles compressed to the right develop a leftward restoring force. Small as they are, air particles do have mass. Therefore, inertia causes the rebounding air particles to overshoot their resting positions and to continue toward their extreme leftward positions. As the particles move leftward, the amount of compression decreases and is momentarily zero as they pass through their resting positions. As they continue to move to the left of their resting positions, the particles are now becoming increasingly farther from the molecules to their right (compared with when they are in their resting positions). We now say that the air particles are rarefied compared with their resting states, so that the air pressure is now below atmospheric pressure. This state of lower than ambient pressure is called **rarefaction**. When the air particles reach the leftmost position they are maximally rarefied, which means that the pressure is maximally negative. At this point, the restoring force instigates a rightward movement of the air molecules. This movement is enhanced by the push of the tuning fork prongs that have also reversed direction. The air molecules now accelerate rightward (so that the amount of rarefaction decreases), overshoot their resting positions, and continue to the right, and so on. The tuning fork vibrations have now been transmitted to the surrounding particles, which are now also oscillating in simple harmonic motion. Sounds

that are associated with simple harmonic motion are called **pure tones**.

Let us consider one of the air molecules that has already been set into harmonic motion by the tuning fork. This air particle now vibrates to-and-fro in the same direction that was originally imposed by the vibrating prong. When this particle moves toward its right it will cause a similar displacement of the particle that is located there. The subsequent leftward motion is also transmitted to the next particle, etc. Thus, the oscillations of one air particle are transmitted to the molecule next to it. The second particle is therefore set into oscillation, which in turn initiates oscillation of the next one, and so forth down the line. In other words, each particle vibrates back and forth around its own resting point, and causes successive molecules to vibrate back and forth around their own resting points, as shown schematically in **Fig. 1.5**. Notice that each molecule vibrates "in place" around its own average position; it is the vibratory pattern that is transmitted through the air.

This propagation of vibratory motion from particle to particle constitutes the sound wave. This wave appears as alternating compressions and rarefactions radiating from the sound source in all directions, as already suggested in **Fig. 1.1**. The transmission of particle motion along with the

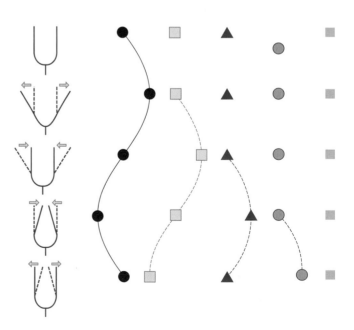

Fig. 1.5 Sound is initiated by transmitting the vibratory pattern of the sound source to nearby air particles, and then the vibratory pattern is passed from particle to particle as a wave. Notice how it is the pattern of vibration that is being transmitted, whereas each particle oscillates around its own average location.

resulting variations in air pressure with distance from the source are represented in **Fig. 1.6**. Most people are more familiar with the kinds of waves that develop on the surface of a pond when a pebble is dropped into the water. These are **transverse waves** because the particles are moving at right angles to the direction that the wave is propagating. That is, the water particles oscillate up and down (vertically) even though the wave moves out horizontally from the spot where the pebble hit the water. This principle can be demonstrated by floating a cork in a pool, and then dropping a pebble in the water to start a wave. The floating cork reflects the motions of the water particles. The wave will move out horizontally, but the floating cork bobs up and down (vertically) at right angles to the wave. In contrast, sound waves are **longitudinal waves** because each air particle oscillates in the same direction in which the wave is propagating (**Fig. 1.6**). Although sound waves are longitudinal, it is more convenient to draw them with a transverse representation, as in **Fig. 1.6**. In such a diagram the vertical dimension represents some measure of the size of the signal (e.g., displacement, pressure, etc.), and left to right distance represents time (or distance). For example, the waveform in **Fig. 1.6** shows the amount of positive pressure (compression) above the baseline, negative pressure (rarefaction) below the baseline, and distance horizontally going from left to right.

The Sinusoidal Function

Simple harmonic motion is also known as **sinusoidal motion**, and has a waveform that is called a **sinusoidal wave** or a **sine wave**. Let us see why. **Fig. 1.7** shows one cycle of a sine wave in the center, surrounded by circles labeled to correspond to points on the wave. Each circle shows a horizontal line corresponding to the horizontal baseline on the sine wave, as well as a radius line (r) that will move around the circle at a fixed speed, much like a clock hand but in a counterclockwise direction.

Point **a** on the waveform in the center of the figure can be viewed as the "starting point" of the cycle. The displacement here is zero because this point is *on* the horizontal line. The radius appears as shown in circle **b** when it reaches 45° of rotation, which corresponds to point **b** on the sine wave. The angle between the radius and the horizontal is called the **phase angle** (θ) and is a handy way to tell location going around the circle and on the sine wave. In other words, we consider one cycle (one "round trip" of oscillation) to be the same as going around a circle one time. Just as a circle has 360°, we also

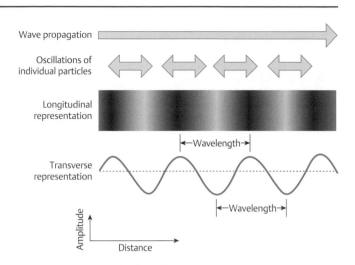

Fig. 1.6 Longitudinal and transverse representations of a sound wave. Wavelength (λ) is the distance covered by one replication (cycle) of a wave, and is most easily visualized as the distance from one peak to the next.

consider one cycle to have 360°. Since 45/360 = ⅛, a phase angle (θ) of 45° is the same as one eighth of the way around a circle or one eighth of the way into a sine wave. Returning to the circle, the vertical displacement from the horizontal to the point where r intersects the circle is represented by a vertical line labeled **d**. This vertical line corresponds to the displacement of point **b** on the sine wave, where the displacement of the air particle is represented by the height of the point above the baseline. Notice that we now have a right triangle in the circle, where r is the

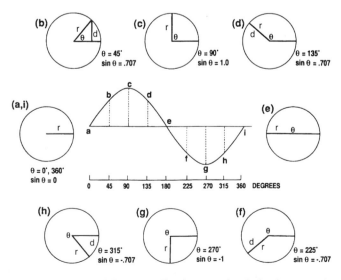

Fig. 1.7 Sinusoidal motion (θ, phase angle; d, displacement). (Adapted from Gelfand 2010, courtesy of Informa.)

hypotenuse, θ is an angle, and d is the leg opposite that angle. Recall from high school math that the sine of an angle equals the length of the opposite leg over the length of the hypotenuse. Here, sin θ = d/r. If we conveniently assume that the length of r is 1, then displacement d becomes the sine of angle θ, which happens to be 0.707. In other words, displacement is determined by the sine of the phase angle, and displacement at any point on the sine wave corresponds to the sine of θ. This is why it is called a sine wave.

The peak labeled **c** on the sine wave corresponds to circle **c**, where the rotating radius has reached the straight-up position. We are now one fourth of the way into the wave and one fourth of the way around the circle. Here, θ = 90° and the displacement is the largest it can be (notice that d = r on the circle). Continuing the counterclockwise rotation of r causes the amount of displacement from the horizontal to decrease, exemplified by point **d** on the sine wave and circle **d**, where θ is 135°. The oscillating air particle has already reversed direction and is now moving back toward the resting position. When it reaches the resting position there is again no displacement, as shown by point **e** on the sine wave and by the fact that r is now superimposed on the horizontal at θ = 180° in circle **e**. Notice that 180° is one half of the 360° round trip, so we are now halfway around the circle and halfway into the cycle of SHM. In addition, displacement is zero at this location (180°).

Continuing the rotation of r places it in the lower left quadrant of circle **f**, corresponding to point **f** on the wave, where θ = 225°. The oscillating particle has overshot its resting position and the displacement is now increasing in the other direction, so that we are in the rarefaction part of the wave. Hence, displacement is now drawn in the negative direction, indicating rarefaction. The largest negative displacement is reached at point **g** on the wave, where θ = 270°, corresponding to circle **g**, in which r points straight down.

The air particle now begins moving in the positive direction again on its way back toward the resting position. At point **h** and circle **h** the displacement in the negative direction has become smaller as the rotating radius passes through the point where θ = 315° (point **h** on the wave and circle **h**). The air particle is again passing through its resting position at point **i**, having completed one round trip or 360° of rotation. Here, displacement is again zero. Having completed exactly one cycle, 360° corresponds to 0°, and circle **i** is the same one previously used as circle **a**.

Recall that r rotates around the circle at a fixed speed. Hence, how fast r is moving will determine how many degrees are covered in a given amount of time. For example, if one complete cycle of rotation takes 1 second, then 360° is covered in 1 second;

180° is covered in ½ second; 90° takes ¼ second; 270° takes ¾ second; etc. Hence, the phase angle also reflects the elapsed time from the onset of rotation. This is why the horizontal axis in **Fig. 1.8** can be labeled in terms of phase. As such, the phase of the wave at each of the points indicated in **Fig. 1.7** is 0° at **a**, 45° at **b**, 90° at **c**, 135° at **d**, 180° at **e**, 225° at **f**, 270° at **g**, 315° at **h**, and 360° at **i**, which is also 0° for the next cycle.

Phase is often used to express relationships between two waves that are displaced relative to each other, as in **Fig. 1.8**. Each frame in the figure shows two waves that are identical to each other except that they do not line up exactly along the horizontal (time) axis. The top panel shows two waves that are 45° apart. Here, the wave represented by the thicker line is at 45° at the same time that the other wave (shown by the thinner line) is at 0°. The phase displacement is highlighted by the shaded area and the dotted vertical guideline in the figure. This is analogous to two radii that are always 45° apart as they move around a circle. In other words, these two waves are 45° apart or *out-of-phase*. The second panel shows the two waves displaced from each another by 90°, so that one wave is at 90° when other one is at 0°. Hence, these waves are 90° out-of-phase, analogous to two radii that are always 90° apart as they move around a circle. The third panel shows two waves that are 180° out-of-phase, Here, one wave it at its 90° (positive) peak at the same time that the other one is at its 270° (negative) peak, which is analogous to two radii that are always 180° apart as they move around a circle. Notice that these two otherwise identical waves are exact mirror images of each other when they are 180° out-of-phase, just as the two radii are always pointing in opposite directions. The last example in the bottom panel shows the two waves 270° out-of-phase.

Parameters of Sound Waves

We already know that a **cycle** is one complete replication of a vibratory pattern. For example, two cycles are shown for each sine wave in the upper frame of **Fig. 1.9**, and four cycles are shown for each sine wave in the lower frame. Each of the sine waves in this figure is said to be **periodic** because it repeats itself exactly over time. Sine waves are the simplest kind of periodic wave because simple harmonic motion is the simplest form of vibration. Later we will address complex periodic waves.

The duration of one cycle is called its **period**. The period is expressed in time (t) because it refers to the amount of time that it takes to complete one cycle (i.e., how long it takes for one round trip). For

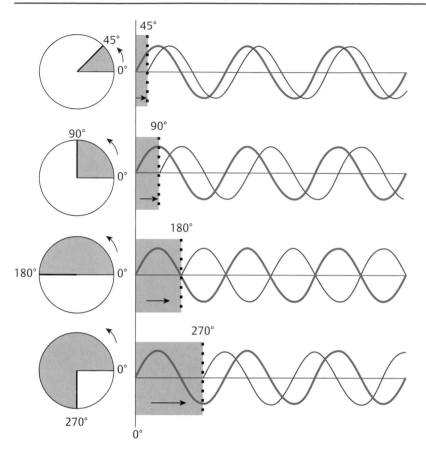

Fig. 1.8   Each panel shows two waves that are identical in every way except they are displaced from one another in terms of phase, highlighted by the shaded areas and the dotted vertical guidelines. Analogous examples of two radii moving around a circle are shown to the left of the waveforms. Top panel: Two waves that are 45° out-of-phase, analogous to two radii that are always 45° apart as they move around a circle. Second panel: Waves that are 90° out-of-phase, analogous to two radii moving around a circle 90° apart. Third panel: Waves that are 180° out-of phase, analogous to two radii that are always 180° apart (pointing in opposite directions) moving around a circle. Bottom panel: Two waves (and analogous radii moving around a circle) that are 270° out-of-phase.

example, a periodic wave that repeats itself every one hundredth of a second has a period of 1/100 second, or t = 0.01 second. One hundredth of a second is also 10 thousandths of a second (milliseconds), so we could also say that the period of this wave is 10 milliseconds.

Similarly, a wave that repeats itself every one thousandth of a second has a period of 1 millisecond or 0.001 second; and the period would be 2 milliseconds or 0.002 second if the duration of one cycle is two thousandths of a second.

The number of times a waveform repeats itself in one second is its frequency (f), or the number of **cycles per second (cps)**. We could say that frequency is the number of cycles that can fit into one second. Frequency is expressed in units called **hertz (Hz)**, which means the same thing as cycles per second. For example, a wave that is repeated 100 times per second has a frequency of 100 Hz; the frequency of a wave that has 500 cycles per second is 500 Hz; and a 1000 Hz wave has 1000 cycles in one second.

If frequency is the number of cycles that occur each second, and period is how much time it takes to complete one cycle, then frequency and period must be related in a very straightforward way. Let us consider the three examples that were just used to illustrate the relationship of period and frequency:

- A period of 0.01 second goes with a frequency (f) of 100 Hz.
- A period of 0.002 second goes with a frequency of 500 Hz.
- A period of 0.001 second goes with a frequency of 1000 Hz.

Now, notice the following relationships among these numbers:

- 1/100 = 0.01 and 1/0.01 = 100.
- 1/500 = 0.002 and 1/0.002 = 500.
- 1/1000 = 0.001 and 1/0.001 = 1000.

In each case the period corresponds to 1 over the frequency, and the frequency corresponds to 1 over the period. In formal terms, frequency equals the reciprocal of period,

$$f = \frac{1}{t}$$

and period equals the reciprocal of frequency,

$$t = \frac{1}{f}$$

Each wave in the upper frame of **Fig. 1.9** contains two cycles in 4 milliseconds, and each wave in the lower frame contains four cycles in the 4 milliseconds. If two cycles in the upper frame last 4 milliseconds, then the duration of one cycle is 2 milliseconds. Hence, the period of each wave in the upper frame is 2 milliseconds (t = 0.002 second), and the frequency is 1/0.002, or 500 Hz. Similarly, if four cycles last 4 milliseconds in the lower frame, then one cycle has a period of 1 millisecond (t = 0.001), and the frequency is 1/0.001, or 1000 Hz.

Fig. 1.9 also illustrates differences in the amplitude between waves. **Amplitude** denotes size or magnitude, such as the amount of displacement, power, pressure, etc. The larger the amplitude at some point along the horizontal (time) axis, the greater its distance from zero on the vertical axis. With respect to the figure, each frame shows one wave that has a smaller amplitude and an otherwise identical wave that has a larger amplitude.

As illustrated in **Fig. 1.10**, the **peak-to-peak amplitude** of a wave is the total vertical distance between its negative and positive peaks, and **peak amplitude** is the distance from the baseline to one peak. However, neither of these values reflects the overall, ongoing size of the wave because the amplitude is constantly changing. At any instant an oscillating particle may be at its most positive or most negative displacement from the resting position, or anywhere between these two extremes, including

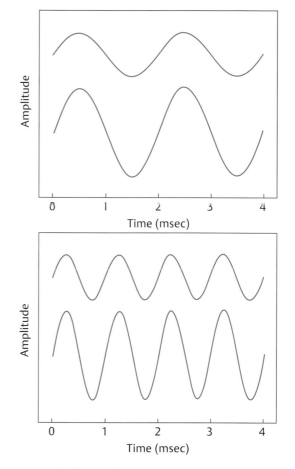

Fig. 1.9 Each frame shows two sine waves that have the same frequency but different amplitudes. Compared with the upper frame, twice as many cycles occur in the same amount of time in the lower frame; thus the period is half as long and the frequency is twice as high.

Fig. 1.10 Peak, peak-to-peak, and root-mean-square (RMS) amplitude.

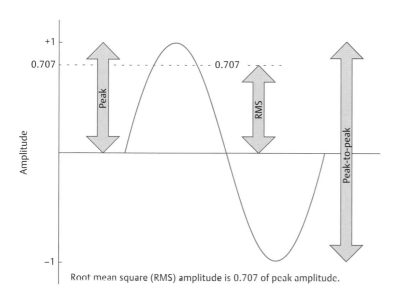

Root mean square (RMS) amplitude is 0.707 of peak amplitude.

the resting position itself, where the displacement is zero. The magnitude of a sound at a given instant (**instantaneous amplitude**) is applicable only for that moment, and will be different at the next moment. Yet we are usually interested in a kind of "overall average" amplitude that reveals the magnitude of a sound wave throughout its cycles. A simple average of the positive and negative instantaneous amplitudes will not work because it will always be equal to zero. A different kind of overall measure is therefore used, called the **root-mean-square (RMS) amplitude**. Even though measurement instruments provide us with RMS amplitudes automatically, we can understand RMS by briefly reviewing the steps that would be used to calculate it manually: (1) All of the positive and negative values on the wave are squared, so that all values are positive (or zero for values on the resting position itself). (2) A mean (average) is calculated for the squared values. (3) This average of the squared values is then rescaled back to the "right size" by taking its square root. This is the RMS value. The RMS amplitude is numerically equal to 70.7% of (or 0.707 times) the peak amplitude (or 0.354 times the peak-to-peak amplitude). Even though these values technically apply only to sinusoids, for practical purposes RMS values are used with all kinds of waveforms.

Referring back to **Fig. 1.6**, we see that the distance covered by one cycle of a propagating wave is called its **wavelength (λ)**. We have all seen water waves, which literally appear as alternating crests and troughs on the surface of the water. Using this common experience as an example, wavelength is simply the distance between the crest of one wave and the crest of the next one. For sound, wavelength is the distance between one compression peak and the next one, or one rarefaction peak and the next one, that is, the distance between any two successive peaks in **Fig. 1.6**. It is just as correct to use any other point, as long as we measure the distance between the same point on two successive replications of the wave. The formula for wavelength is

$$\lambda = \frac{c}{f}$$

where f is the frequency of the sound and c is the speed of sound (~ 344 m/s in air). This formula indicates that wavelength is inversely proportional to frequency. Similarly, frequency is inversely proportional to wavelength:

$$f = \frac{c}{\lambda}$$

These formulas show that wavelength and frequency are inversely proportional to each other. In other words, low frequencies have long wavelengths and high frequencies have short wavelengths.

Complex Waves

When two or more pure tones are combined, the result is called a complex wave. Complex waves may contain any number of frequencies from as few as two up to an infinite number of them. **Complex periodic waves** have waveforms that repeat themselves over time. If the waveform does not repeat itself over time, then it is an **aperiodic wave**.

Combining Sinusoids

The manner in which waveforms combine into more complex waveforms involves algebraically adding the amplitudes of the two waves at every point along the horizontal (time) axis. Consider two sine waves that are to be added. Imagine that they are drawn one above the other on a piece of graph paper so that the gridlines can be used to identify similar moments in time (horizontally) for the two waves, and their amplitudes can be determined by simply counting boxes vertically. The following exercise is done at every point along the horizontal time axis: (1) Determine the amplitude of each wave at that point by counting the boxes in the positive and/or negative direction. (2) Add these two amplitudes *algebraically* (e.g., +2 plus +2 is +4; –3 plus –3 is –6; and +4 plus –1 is +3; etc.). (3) Plot the algebraic sum just obtained on the graph paper at the same point along the horizontal time axis. After doing this for many points, drawing a smooth line through these points will reveal the combined wave.

Several examples of combining two sinusoids are illustrated in **Fig. 1.11**. This figure shows what occurs when two sinusoids being combined have exactly the same frequencies and amplitudes. The two sinusoids being combined in **Fig. 1.11a** are in phase with each other. Here, the combined wave looks like the two identical components, but has an amplitude twice as large. This case is often called complete **reinforcement** for obvious reasons. The addition of two otherwise identical waves that are 180° out-of-phase is illustrated in **Fig. 1.11b**. In this case, the first wave is equal and opposite to the second wave at every moment in time, so that algebraic addition causes the resulting amplitude to be zero at every point along the horizontal (time) axis. The result is complete **cancellation**.

When the sinusoids being combined are identical but have a phase relationship that is any value other than 0° (in-phase) or 180° (opposite phase), then the appearance of the resulting wave will depend on

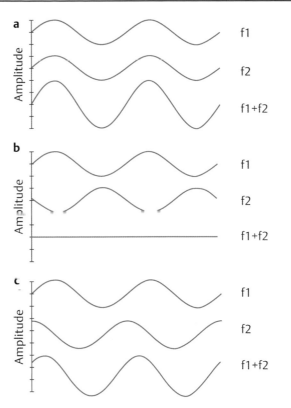

Fig. 1.11 Combining sinusoids that have the same frequency and amplitude when they are **(a)** in-phase (showing complete reinforcement); **(b)** 180° out-of-phase (showing cancellation); **(c)** 90° out-of-phase.

how the two components happen to line up in time. **Fig. 1.11c** shows what happens when the two otherwise identical sinusoids are 90° out-of-phase. The result is a sinusoid with the same frequency as the two (similar) original waves but that differs in phase and amplitude.

Complex Periodic Waves

The principles used to combine any number of similar or dissimilar waves are basically the same as those just described for two similar waves: Their amplitudes are algebraically summed on a point-by-point basis along the horizontal (time) axis, regardless of their individual frequencies and amplitudes or their phase relationships. However, combining unequal frequencies will not produce a sinusoidal result. Instead, the combined waveform depends on the nature of the particular sounds being combined. For example, consider the three different sine waves labeled f1, f2, and f3 in **Fig. 1.12**. Wave f1 has a frequency of 1000 Hz, f2 is 2000 Hz, and f3 is 3000 Hz. The lower waveforms show various combinations of these sinusoids. The combined waves (f1 + f2, f1 + f3, and f1 + f2 + f3) are not longer sinusoids, but they are periodic because they repeat themselves at regular intervals over time. In other words, they are all complex periodic waves.

Notice that the periods of the complex periodic waves in **Fig. 1.12** are the same as the period of f1,

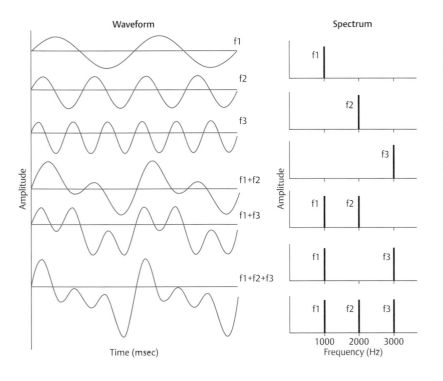

Fig. 1.12 Waveforms (*left*) and corresponding spectra (*right*) for three harmonically related sine waves (pure tones) of frequencies f1, f2, and f3; and complex periodic waves resulting from the in-phase addition of f1 + f2, f1 + f3, and f1 + f2 + f3. Notice that the fundamental frequency is f1 for all of the complex waves. Also notice that each pure tone spectrum has one vertical line, while the spectrum of each complex periodic sound has a separate vertical line for each of its components.

which is the lowest component for each of them. The lowest frequency component of a complex periodic wave is called its **fundamental frequency**. The fundamental frequency of each of the complex periodic waves in the figure is 1000 Hz because f1 is the lowest component in each of them. The period (or the time needed for one complete replication) of a complex periodic wave is the same as the period of its fundamental frequency. **Harmonics** are whole number or integral multiples of the fundamental frequency. In other words, the fundamental is the largest whole number common denominator of a wave's harmonics, and the harmonics are integral multiples of the fundamental frequency. In fact, the fundamental is also a harmonic because it is equal to 1 times itself. In the case of wave f1 + f2 + f3, 1000 Hz is the fundamental (first harmonic), 2000 Hz is the second harmonic, and 3000 Hz is the third harmonic.

Another example of combining sinusoids into a complex periodic wave is given in **Fig. 1.13**. Here, the sine waves being added are odd harmonics of the fundamental (1000 Hz, 3000 Hz, 5000 Hz, etc.), and their amplitudes get smaller with increasing frequency. The resulting complex periodic wave becomes squared off as the number of odd harmonics is increased, and is called a **square wave** for this reason.

Waveforms show how amplitude changes with time. However, the frequency of a pure tone (sine wave) is not directly provided by its waveform, and the frequencies in a complex sound cannot be determined by examining its waveform. In fact, the same

frequencies can result in dramatically different-looking complex waveforms if their phase relationships are changed. Hence, another kind of graph is needed when we want to know what frequencies are present. This kind of graph is a **spectrum**, which shows amplitude on the y-axis as a function of frequency along the x-axis. Several examples are given in **Fig. 1.12** and **Fig. 1.13**. The frequency of the pure tone is given by the location of a vertical line along the horizontal (frequency) axis, and the amplitude of the tone is represented by the height of the line. According to Fourier's **theorem** complex sounds can be mathematically dissected into their constituent pure tone components. The process of doing so is called **Fourier analysis**, which results in the information needed to plot the spectrum of a complex sound. The spectrum of a complex periodic sound has as many vertical lines as there are component frequencies. The locations of the lines show their frequencies, and their heights show their amplitudes, as illustrated in **Fig. 1.13**.

Aperiodic Waves

Aperiodic sounds are made up of components that are not harmonically related and have waveforms that do not repeat themselves over time, which is why they are called aperiodic. The extreme cases of aperiodic sounds are transients and random noise. A **transient** is an abrupt sound that is extremely brief

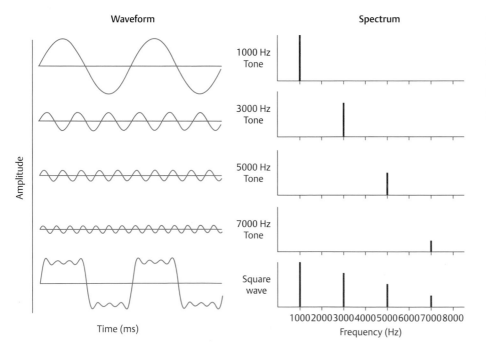

Fig. 1.13 Waveforms (*left*) and corresponding spectra (*right*) of odd harmonics combined to form a square wave (bottom). Notice that the spectrum of a pure tone has one vertical line, whereas the spectrum of a complex periodic sound has a separate vertical line for each of its components.

in duration. It is aperiodic by definition because its waveform is not repeated (**Fig. 1.14a**). **Random noise** has a completely random waveform (**Fig. 1.14b**) so that it contains all possible frequencies at the same average amplitude over the long run. Random noise is also called **white noise** in analogy to white light because all possible frequencies are represented.

The spectrum of white noise is depicted in **Fig. 1.15a**. Individual vertical lines are not drawn because there would be an infinite number of them. It is more convenient to draw a continuous line over their tops and leave out the vertical lines themselves. This kind of spectrum is used for most aperiodic sounds and is called a **continuous spectrum**. *Random noise* has a *flat* continuous spectrum because the amplitudes are the same, on average, for all frequencies. An ideal *transient* also has a *flat spectrum*.

Most aperiodic sounds do not have flat spectra because they have more amplitude concentrated in one frequency range or the other. This notion is demonstrated by a simple experiment: Tap or scratch several different objects. The resulting noises will sound different from one another because they have energy concentrations in different frequency ranges. This is exactly what is represented on the spectrum. For example, different continuous spectra might show concentrations of aperiodic sounds with greater amounts of amplitude at higher frequencies (**Fig. 1.15b**), at lower frequencies (**Fig. 1.15c**), or within a particular band (range) of frequencies (**Fig. 1.15d**).

Standing Waves and Resonance

The frequency(ies) at which a body or medium vibrates most readily is (are) called its **natural** or **resonant frequency(ies)**. Differences in resonant frequency ranges enable different devices or other objects to act as filters by transmitting energy more readily for certain frequency ranges than for others. Examples of the frequency ranges that are transmitted by high-, low-, and band-pass filters are illustrated in **Fig. 1.15b–d**.

Vibrating strings Consider what happens when you pluck a guitar string. The waves initiated by the pluck move outward toward the two tied ends of the string. The waves are then reflected back and they propagate in opposite directions. The result is a set of waves that are moving toward each other, a situation that is sustained by continuing reflections from the two ends. Being reflections of one another, all of these waves will have the same frequency, and they will, of course, be propagating at the same velocity. Recall that waves interact with one another so that their instantaneous displacements add algebraically. As a result, the net displacement of the string at any

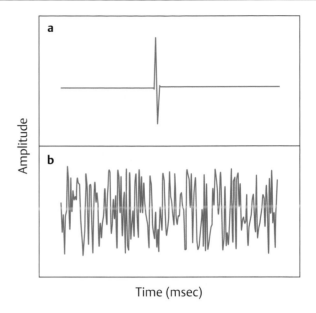

Fig. 1.14 Artist's conceptions of the waveforms of **(a)** a transient and **(b)** random or white noise.

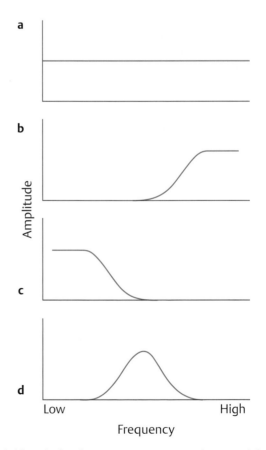

Fig. 1.15 Idealized continuous spectra showing **(a)** equal amplitude at all frequencies for a transient or white noise; **(b)** greater amplitude in the higher frequencies (also a high-pass filter); **(c)** greater amplitude in the lower frequencies (also a low-pass filter); **(d)** amplitude concentrated within a certain band of frequencies (also a band-pass filter).

point along its length will be due to the way in which the superimposed waves interact. The resulting combined wave appears as a pattern that is standing still even though it is derived from the interaction of waves, which themselves are propagating. Consequently, the points of maximum displacement (peaks of the combined wave pattern) and no displacement (baseline crossings of the combined wave pattern) will occur at fixed locations along the string. This pattern is called a **standing wave**.

Places along the string where there is zero displacement in the standing wave pattern are called **nodes**, and the locations where maximum displacement occurs are called **antinodes**. The string is tied down at its two ends so that it cannot move at these locations. In other words, the displacement must always be zero at the two ends of the string. This means that the standing wave pattern must have nodes that occur at the two ends of the string. Just as no displacement occurs at each end of the string because it is most constrained at these points, the greatest displacement occurs in the middle of the string, where it is least constrained and therefore has the most freedom of motion. In other words, the standing wave pattern will have a node at each end of the string and an antinode at the center of the string. This pattern is illustrated in **Fig. 1.16a**. Notice that the antinode occurs halfway between the nodes just as peaks (at 90° and 270°) alternate with zero displacements (at 0° and 180°) in a cycle of a sine wave.

The standing wave pattern that has a node at each end and an antinode in the center is not the only one that can occur on a given string; rather, it is just the *longest* one. This longest standing wave pattern is called the **first mode** of vibration. This standing wave pattern goes from no displacement to a peak and back to no displacement, which is analogous to going from 0° to 180° on a wave cycle. In other words, the pattern comprises exactly half of a cycle. Because we are dealing with displacement as a function of *distance* along the string (rather than over time), the parameter of the cycle with which we are dealing here is its wavelength (λ). In other words, the length of the longest standing wave pattern is the length of the whole string, and this length corresponds to one half of a wavelength ($\lambda/2$). Of course, if we know $\lambda/2$, then we can easily figure out λ. Now, a given wavelength is associated with a particular frequency because f = c/λ (recall that c is the speed of sound). Consequently, the first mode of vibration is equal to half the wavelength ($\lambda/2$) of some frequency, which will, in turn, be its frequency of vibration. This will be the lowest **resonant frequency** of the string, which is its *fundamental frequency*. Finding this frequency is a matter of substituting what we know into the formula f = c/λ. We know the length of the

string (L), and we also know that L = $\lambda/2$. Therefore, λ = 2L. Substituting 2L for λ, the string's lowest resonant frequency is found with the formula f = c/2L. [In reality, the speed of sound (c) is different for a vibrating string than it is for air. For the benefit of the math-minded student, the value of c for a string equals the square root of the ratio of its tension (T) to its mass (M), so that the real formula for the string's resonant frequency F_0 is

$$F_0 = \frac{1}{2L} \cdot \sqrt{\frac{T}{M}}$$

Other standing waves can also develop, provided they meet the requirement that there must be a node at each end of the string. For this criterion to be met, the string must be divided into exact halves, thirds, fourths, etc., as illustrated in **Fig. 1.16**. These standing wave patterns are called the second, third, fourth, etc., modes of vibration. Because the segments of the second mode are exactly half of the length of first mode, they produce a frequency that is exactly twice the fundamental. If we call the fundamental the first harmonic, then the second mode produces the second harmonic. Similarly, the segments of the third mode are exactly one-third the length of the first mode, so that they produce a third harmonic that is exactly three times the fundamental. The same principles apply to the fourth mode and harmonic, and beyond.

Vibrations in tubes The column of air inside a tube can be set into vibration by various means, such as blowing across the tube's open end. If this is done with different-size tubes we would find that (1) shorter tubes are associated with higher pitches than longer ones, and (2) the same tube produces a higher pitch when it is open at both ends compared with when it is open at one end and closed at the other.

When a column of air is vibrating in a tube that is open at both ends, the least amount of particle displacement occurs in the center of the tube, where the pressure is greatest. The greatest amount of displacement occurs at the two open ends, where the pressure is lowest. Hence, there will be a standing wave that has a displacement node in the middle of the tube and antinodes at the two ends, as illustrated in **Fig. 1.17a**. This standing wave pattern involves one half of a cycle in the sense that going from one end of the tube to the other end involves going from a displacement peak to a zero crossing to another peak. This trip would cover 180° (half of a cycle) on a sine wave, and thus a distance corresponding to half of a wavelength. Because this longest standing wave involves half of a wavelength ($\lambda/2$), the tube's lowest resonant (fundamental) frequency must have a wavelength that is twice the length of the tube (where λ = 2L). For this reason, tubes open at both ends are **half-**

a

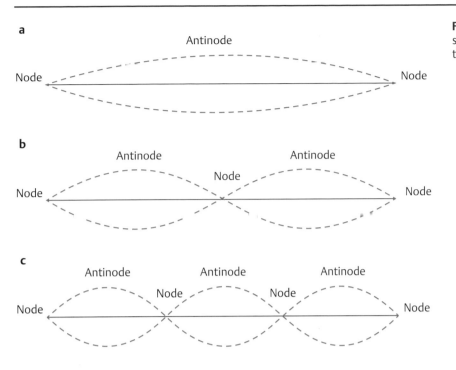

Fig. 1.16 Standing wave patterns corresponding to the **(a)** first, **(b)** second, and **(c)** third modes of a vibrating string.

b

c

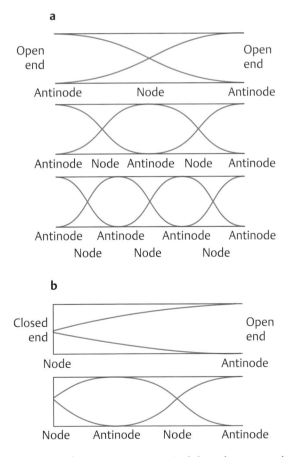

Fig. 1.17 Standing waves patterns in **(a)** a tube open at both ends (a half-wavelength resonator), and **(b)** a tube open at one end and closed at the other end (a quarter-wavelength resonator).

wavelength resonators. In other words, the lowest resonant frequency of a tube open at both ends is determined by the familiar formula f = c/2L. We could also say that the longest standing wave pattern is the first mode of vibration for the tube and that it is related to its fundamental frequency (lowest harmonic). As for the vibrating string, each successive higher mode corresponds to exact halves, thirds, etc., of the tube length, as illustrated in **Fig. 1.17a**. In turn, these modes produce harmonics that are exact multiples of the fundamental frequency. Harmonics will occur at each multiple of the fundamental frequency for a tube open at both ends.

Air particles vibrating in a tube that is closed at one end and open at the other end are restricted most at the closed end. As a result, their displacement will be least at the closed end, where the pressure is the greatest. Thus, in terms of displacement, there must be a node at the closed end and an antinode at the open end, as illustrated in **Fig. 1.17b**. This pattern is analogous to the distance from a zero crossing to a peak, which corresponds to one quarter of a cycle (0° to 90°), and a distance of one quarter of a wavelength (λ/4). Because the length of the tube corresponds to λ/4, its lowest resonant frequency has a wavelength that is four times the length of the tube (4L). Hence, f = c/4L. For this reason, a tube that is open at one end and closed at the other end is a **quarter-wavelength resonator**. Because a node can occur at only one end, these tubes have only odd modes of vibration and produce only odd harmonics of the fundamental frequency (e.g., f1, f3, f5, f7, etc.), as illustrated in the figure.

Immittance

Immittance is the general term used to describe how well energy flows through a system. The *opposition* to the flow of energy is called **impedance (Z)**. The inverse of impedance is called **admittance (Y)**, which is the *ease* with which energy flows through a system.

The concept of impedance may be understood in terms of the following example. (Although this example only considers mass, we will see that immittance actually involves several components.) Imagine two metal blocks weighing different amounts. Suppose you repetitively push and pull the lighter block back and forth across a smooth table top with a certain amount of effort. This is a mechanical system in which a sinusoidally alternating force (the pushing and pulling) is being applied to a mass (the block). The effort with which you are pushing (and pulling) the block is the amount of applied force, and the velocity of the block reflects how well energy flows through this system to effect motion. A particular block will move at a certain velocity given the amount of effort you are using to push (and pull) it. If the *same* amount of *effort* was used to push and pull the *heavier* block, then it would move slower than the first one. In other words, the heavier block (greater mass) moves with less velocity than the lighter block (smaller mass) in response to the same amount of applied force. We can say that the flow of energy is opposed more by the heavier block than by the lighter one. For this reason, the heavier block (greater mass) has more impedance and less admittance than the lighter block (smaller mass).

This example shows that impedance and admittance are viewed in terms of the relationship between an applied force and the resulting amount of velocity. In effect, higher impedance means that more force must be applied to result in a given amount of velocity, and lower impedance means that less force is needed to result in a given amount of velocity. For the mathematically oriented, we might say that impedance (Z) is the ratio of force to velocity:

$$Z = \frac{F}{v}$$

The amount of impedance is expressed in **ohms**. The larger the number of ohms, the greater the opposition to the flow of energy.

Admittance (Y) is the reciprocal of impedance:

$$Y = \frac{1}{Z}$$

and is therefore equal to the ratio of velocity to force:

$$Y = \frac{v}{F}$$

As we might expect, the unit of admittance is the inverse of the ohm, and is therefore called the **mho**. The more mhos, the greater the ease with which energy flows. The admittance values that we are concerned with in audiology are very small, and are thus expressed in **millimhos (mmhos)**.

Impedance involves the complex interaction of three familiar physical components: mass, stiffness, and friction. In **Fig. 1.18** mass is represented by the block, stiffness (or compliance) by the spring, and friction by the rough surface under the block. Let's briefly consider each of these components. Friction dissipates some of the energy being introduced into the system by converting it into heat. This component of impedance is called resistance (R). The effect of resistance occurs in-phase with the applied force (**Fig. 1.19**). Some amount of friction is always present. Opposition to the flow of energy due to mass is called **mass (positive) reactance (X)** and is related to inertia. The opposition due to the stiffness of a system is called **stiffness (negative) reactance (X_s)**, and is related to the restoring force that develops when an elastic element (e.g., a spring) is displaced.

Mass and stiffness act to oppose the applied force because these components are out-of-phase with it. They oppose the flow of energy by storing it in these out-of-phase components before effecting motion. First, consider the mass all by itself. At the same point in time (labeled 1) the applied force is maximal (in the upward direction) and the velocity of the block is zero (crossing the horizontal line in the positive direction). One quarter of a cycle later, at the time labeled 2, the applied force is zero and the velocity of the mass is now maximal (in the upward direction).

Fig. 1.18 The components of impedance are (1) mass reactance (X_m), represented by the block; (2) stiffness reactance (X_s), represented by the spring; and (3) resistance (R), represented by the rough surface under the block.

Hence, a sinusoidally applied force acting on a mass and the resulting velocity of the mass are a quarter-cycle (90°) out-of-phase. To appreciate this relationship, hold a weight and shake repetitively back and forth from right to left. You will feel that you must exert the most effort (maximal force) at the extreme right and left points of the swing, where the direction changes. Notice that the weight is momentarily still (i.e., its velocity is zero) at the extreme right and left points because this is where it changes direction. On the other hand, the weight will be moving the fastest (maximum velocity) as it passes the midpoint of the right-to-left swing, which is also where you will be using the least effort (zero force).

Now consider the spring all by itself at the same two times. At time 1, when the applied force is maximal (upward), the velocity of the spring is zero (crossing the horizontal line in the negative direction). One quarter-cycle later, at time 2, the applied force is zero, and the velocity of the spring is now maximal (downward). Hence, a sinusoidally applied force acting on a spring and the resulting velocity of the spring are a quarter-cycle (90°) out-of-phase. This occurs in the opposite direction of what we observed for the mass (whose motion is associated with inertia) because the motion of the spring is associated with restoring force. You can appreciate this relationship by alternately compressing and expanding a spring. You must push or pull the hardest (maximum applied force) at the moment when the spring is maximally expanded (or compressed), which is also when the spring is not moving (zero velocity) because it is about to change direction. Similarly, you will exert no effort (zero applied force) and the spring will be moving the fastest (maximum velocity) as it moves back through its "normal" position (where it is neither compressed nor expanded).

Notice that the mass and stiffness reactances are 180° out-of-phase with each other (**Fig. 1.19**). This means that the effects of mass reactance and stiffness reactance oppose each other. As a result, the **net reactance (X$_{net}$)** is the difference between them, so that

$$X_{net} = X_s - X_m$$

when stiffness reactance is larger, or

$$X_{net} = X_m - X_s$$

when mass reactance is larger. For example, if X$_s$ is 850 ohms and X$_m$ is 140 ohms, then X$_{net}$ will be 850 – 140 = 710 ohms of stiffness reactance. If X$_m$ is 1000

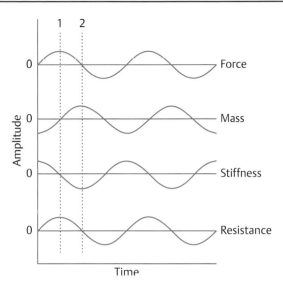

Fig. 1.19 Relationship between a sinusoidally applied force (top) and the velocities associated with mass, stiffness, and resistance. The dotted lines labeled 1 and 2 show two moments in time. Resistance is in-phase with the applied force (F). Mass and stiffness are 90° out-of-phase with force and 180° out-of-phase with each other.

ohms and X$_s$ is 885 ohms, then X$_{net}$ will be 1000 – 885 = 115 ohms of mass reactance.

The overall impedance is obtained by combining the resistance and the net reactance. This cannot be done by simple addition because the resistance and reactance components are out-of-phase. (Recall here the difference between scalars and vectors mentioned at the beginning of the chapter.) The relationships in **Fig. 1.20** show how impedance is derived from resistance and reactance. The size of the resistance component is plotted along the x-axis. Reactance is plotted on the y-axis, with mass (positive) reactance represented upward and stiffness (negative) reactance downward. The net reactance here is plotted downward because X$_s$ is greater than X$_m$, so that X$_{net}$ is negative. Notice that R and X$_{net}$ form two legs of a right triangle, and that Z is the hypotenuse. Hence, we find Z by the familiar Pythagorean theorem ($a^2 + b^2 = c^2$); which becomes $Z^2 = R^2 + X_{net}^2$. Removing the squares gives us the formula for calculating impedance from the resistance and reactance values:

$$Z = \sqrt{R^2 + X_{net}^2}$$

Resistance tends to be essentially the same at all frequencies. However, reactance depends on fre-

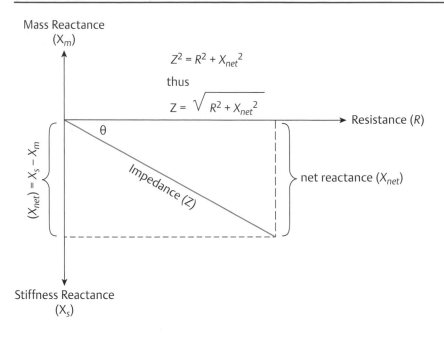

Mass Reactance
(X_m)

$$Z^2 = R^2 + X_{net}^2$$

thus

$$Z = \sqrt{R^2 + X_{net}^2}$$

Resistance (R)

θ

$(X_{net}) = X_s - X_m$

Impedance (Z)

net reactance (X_{net})

Stiffness Reactance
(X_s)

Fig. 1.20 Impedance (Z) is the complex interaction of resistance (R) and the net reactance (X_{net}, which is equal to $X_s - X_m$). Notice the impedance value is determined by the vector addition of the resistance and reactance. The angle (θ) between the horizontal leg of the triangle (resistance) and its hypotenuse (impedance) is called the phase angle.

quency (f) in the following way: (1) mass reactance is proportional to frequency,

$$X_m = 2\pi M$$

where M is mass; and (2) stiffness reactance is inversely proportional to frequency,

$$X_s = \frac{S}{2\pi f}$$

where S is stiffness. In other words, X_m gets larger as frequency goes up, and X_s gets larger as frequency goes down. Because of these frequency relationships, impedance also depends on frequency:

$$Z = \sqrt{R^2 = \left(\frac{S}{2\pi f} + 2\pi f M\right)^2}$$

In addition, there will be a frequency where X_m and X_s are equal, and thus cancel. This is the resonant frequency, where the only component that is opposing the flow of energy is resistance.

Admittance is the reciprocal of impedance,

$$Y = \frac{1}{Z}$$

and the components of admittance are the reciprocals of resistance and reactance: **conductance (G)** is the reciprocal of resistance,

$$G = \frac{1}{R}$$

stiffness (compliant) susceptance (B_s) is the reciprocal of stiffness reactance,

$$B_s = \frac{1}{X_s}$$

and **mass susceptance (B_m)** is the reciprocal of mass reactance

$$B_M = \frac{1}{X_m}$$

Stiffness susceptance is proportional to frequency (B_s increases as frequency goes up), and mass susceptance is inversely proportional to frequency (B_m decreases as frequency goes up). Net susceptance (B_{net}) is the difference between B_s and B_m. The formula for admittance is

$$Y = \sqrt{G^2 + B_{net}^2}$$

where B_{net} is ($B_s - B_m$) when B_s is bigger, and ($B_m - B_s$) when B_m is larger.

Up to this point we have discussed immittance in mechanical terms. **Acoustic immittance** is the term used for the analogous concepts when dealing with sound. The opposition to the flow of sound energy is called **acoustic impedance (Z_a)**, and its reciprocal is **acoustic admittance (Y_a)**. Thus,

$$Z_a = \frac{1}{Y_a}$$

and

$$Y_a = \frac{1}{Z_a}$$

When dealing with acoustic immittance, we use **sound pressure (p)** in place of force, and velocity is replaced with the velocity of sound flow, called **volume velocity (U)**. Thus, acoustic impedance is simply the ratio of sound pressure to volume velocity,

$$Z_a = \frac{P}{U}$$

and acoustic admittance is the ratio of volume velocity to sound pressure,

$$Y_a = \frac{U}{P}$$

The components of acoustic immittance are based on the acoustic analogies of friction, mass, and stiffness (compliance). Friction develops between air molecules and a mesh screen, which is thus used to model **acoustic resistance (R_a)**. **Mass (positive) acoustic reactance (+X_a)** is represented by a slug of air in an open tube. Here an applied sound pressure will displace the slug of air as a unit, so that its inertia comes into play. A column of air inside a tube open at one end and closed at the other end represents **compliant (negative) acoustic reactance (–X_a)** because sound pressure compresses the air column like a spring. The formulas and relationships for acoustic immittance are the same as those previously given, except that the analogous acoustic values are used. For example, acoustic impedance is equal to

$$Z_a = \sqrt{R_a^2 + X_a^2}$$

where X_a is the net difference between compliant acoustic reactance (–X_a) and mass acoustic reactance (+X_a). Similarly, the formula for acoustic admittance is

$$Y_a = \sqrt{G_a^2 + B_a^2}$$

where B_a is the net difference between compliant acoustic susceptance (+B_a) and mass acoustic susceptance (–B_a).

■ Expressing Values n Decibels

It is extremely cumbersome to express sound magnitudes in terms of their actual intensities or pressures for several reasons. To do so would involve working in units of watts/m² (or watts/cm²) and newtons/ml (or dynes/cm²). In addition, the range of sound magnitudes with which we are concerned in audiology

is enormous; the loudest sound that can be tolerated has a pressure that is roughly 10 million times larger than the softest sound that can be heard. Even if we wanted to work with such an immense range of cumbersome values on a linear scale, we would find that it is hard to deal with them in a way that has relevance to the way we hear. As a result, these absolute physical values are converted into a simpler and more convenient form called **decibels (dB)** to make them palatable and meaningful.

The decibel takes advantage of ratios and logarithms. Ratios are used so that physical magnitudes can be stated in relation to a reference value that has meaning to us. It makes sense to use the *softest sound that can be heard by normal people* as our **reference value**. This reference value has an *intensity* of

$$10^{-12} \text{ w}/\text{cm}^2$$

in MKS units, which corresponds to

$$10^{-16} \text{ w}/\text{cm}^2$$

in the cgs system. The same softest audible sound can also be quantified in terms of its *sound pressure.* This reference pressure is

$$210^{-5} \text{ N}/\text{m}^2$$

or

$$20 \ \mu\text{Pa}$$

in the MKS system.[1] In cgs units this reference pressure is

$$210^{-4} \text{ dynes}/\text{cm}^2$$

which the student will often find written as 0.0002 dynes/cm² in the older audiological literature.[2] The appropriate reference value (intensity or pressure, MKS or cgs) becomes the denominator of our ratio, and the intensity (or pressure) of the sound that is actually being measured or described becomes the numerator. As a result, instead of describing a sound that has an intensity of 10^{-10} w/m², we place this value into a ratio so we can express it in terms of how it

---

[1] One Pascal = 1 N/m². Thus, 10^{-6} N/m² = 1 micropascal (μPa), 10^{-5} N/m² = 10 μPa, and 2 × 10^{-5} N/m² = 20 μPa.
[2] Occasionally reported as 2 × 10^{-4} μbar or 0.0002 μbar, especially in the older literature.

compares to our reference value (which is 10^{-12} w/m^2). Hence, this ratio would be

$$\frac{10^{-10} \text{ w/m}^2}{10^{-12} \text{ w/m}^2}$$

This ratio reduces to simply 10^2.

Regardless of what this ratio turns out to be, it is replaced with its common logarithm because equal ratios correspond to different distances on a linear scale, but equal ratios correspond to equal distances on a logarithmic scale. In other words, the linear distance between two numbers with the same ratio relationship (e.g., 2 to 1) is small for small numbers and large for large numbers, but the logarithm of that ratio is always the same. For example, all of the following pairs involve 2/1 ratios. Even though the linear distance between the numbers in the pairs gets wider as the absolute sizes of the numbers get larger, the logarithm of all of the ratios stays the same (2/1 = 2, and log 2 is always 0.3) **(Table 1.4)**.

The general decibel formula is expressed in terms of *power* as follows:

$$PL = 10\log\frac{P}{P_o}$$

Here, PL stands for **power level** (in dB), P is the power of the sound being measured, and P_o is the reference power to which the former is being compared. The word *level* is added to distinguish the raw physical quantity (power) from the corresponding decibel value (which is a logarithmic ratio about the power). Similarly, intensity expressed in decibels is called **intensity level (IL)** and sound pressure expressed in decibels is called **sound pressure level (SPL)**.

Most sound measurements are expressed in terms of intensity or sound pressure, with the latter being the most common. The formula for decibels of **intensity level** is

$$IL = 10\log\frac{I}{I_o}$$

where IL is intensity level in dB, I is the intensity of the sound in question (in w/m^2), and I_o is the reference intensity (10^{-12} w/m^2). If the value of I is 10^{-10} w/m^2, then

$$IL = 10\log\frac{10^{-10} \text{ w/m}^2}{10^{-12} \text{ w/m}^2}$$

$$= 10\log\frac{10^{-10}}{10^{-12}} \text{ (notice that w/m}^2\text{cancels out}$$

$$= 10\log 10^{(-10)-(-12)}$$

$$= 10\log 10^2$$

$$= 10 \cdot 2$$

$$= 20 \text{ dB re:} 10^{-12} \text{ w/m}^2$$

Consequently, an absolute intensity of 10^{-10} w/m^2 has an intensity level of 20 dB re: 10^{-12} w/m^2, or 20 dB IL. The phrase "re: 10^{-12} w/m^2" is added because the decibel is a dimensionless quantity that has real meaning only when we know the reference value, that is, the denominator of the ratio.

The formula for decibels of **sound pressure level (dB SPL)** is obtained by replacing all of the intensity values with the corresponding values of *pressure squared* (because I ∝ p^2):

$$SPL = 10\log\frac{P^2}{P_o^2}$$

Table 1.4 All pairs of numbers that have the same ratio between them (e.g., 2:1) are separated by the same logarithmic distance even though their linear distances are different

Pairs of numbers with 2:1 ratios	Distances between the absolute numbers get wider	Logarithms of all 2:1 ratios are the same
2/1	1	0.3
8/4	4	0.3
20/10	10	0.3
100/50	50	0.3
200/100	100	0.3
2000/1000	1000	0.3

Here, p is the measured sound pressure (in N/m^2) and p_o is the reference sound pressure ($2 \times 10^{-5}\,N/m^2$, or 20 μPa). This form of the formula is cumbersome because of the squared values, which can be removed by applying the following steps:

$$SPL = 10\log\frac{p^2}{p_o^2}$$

$$SPL = 10\log\left(\frac{p}{p_o}\right)^2$$

$$SPL = 10 \cdot 2\log\left(\frac{p}{p_o}\right) \quad (\text{because } x^2 = 2\log x)$$

$$SPL - 20\log\left(\frac{p}{p_o}\right)$$

Therefore, the commonly used simplified formula for decibels of SPL is

$$SPL = 20\log\frac{p}{p_o}$$

where the multiplier is 20 instead of 10 as a result of removing the squares from the unsimplified version of the formula.

Let us go through the exercise of converting the absolute sound pressure of a sound into dB SPL. We will assume that the sound being measured has a pressure of $2 \times 10^{-4}\,N/m^2$. Recall that the reference pressure is $2 \times 10^{-5}\,N/m^2$. The steps are as follows:

$$SPL = 20\log\frac{2\ 10^{-4}\ N/m^2}{2\ 10^{-5}\ N/m^2}$$

$$= 20\log\frac{10^{-4}}{10^{-5}}(\text{notice that } N/m^2 \text{ cancels out})$$

$$= 20\log 10^{(-4)-(-5)}$$

$$= 20\log 10^1$$

$$= 201$$

$$= 20\ dB \quad re: 2 10^{-5}\ N/m \text{ (or } 20\ \mu Pa)$$

Hence, a sound pressure of $2 \times 10^{-4}\,N/m^2$ corresponds to a sound pressure level of 20 dB re: $2 \times 10^{-5}\,N/m^2$ (or 20 μPa), or 20 dB SPL.

What is the decibel value of the reference itself? In other words, what would happen if the intensity (or pressure) being measured is equal to the reference intensity (or pressure)? In terms of intensity, the answer is found by using the reference value ($10^{-12}\,w/m^2$) as both the numerator (I) and denominator (I_o) in the dB formula, so that

$$IL = 10\log\frac{10^{-12}\ w/m^2}{10^{-12}\ w/m^2}$$

$$= 10\log 1(\text{anything divided by itself equals 1})$$

$$= 1010$$

$$= 0\ dB\ re: 10^{-12}\ w/m^2$$

Consequently, the intensity *level* of the reference intensity is 0 dB IL. Similarly, 0 dB SPL means that the measured sound pressure corresponds to that of the reference sound:

$$SPL = 20\log\frac{10^{-5}\ w/m^2}{10^{-5}\ w/m^2}$$

$$= 20\log 1 \,(\text{anything divided by itself equals 1})$$

$$= 20\ 0$$

$$= 0\ dB \quad re: 2 10^{-5}\ N/m \text{ (or } 20\ \mu Pa)$$

Notice that 0 dB IL or 0 dB SPL means that the sound being measured is equal to the reference value; it does not mean "no sound." It follows that negative decibel values indicate that the magnitude of the sound is lower than the reference; for example, −10 dB means that the sound in question is 10 dB below the reference value.

◼ Sound Measurement

The magnitude of a sound is usually measured with a device called a **sound level meter (SLM)**. This device has a high-quality microphone that picks up the sound and converts it into an electrical signal that is analyzed by an electronic circuit, and then displays the magnitude of the sound on a meter in decibels of sound pressure level (dB SPL). An example of a SLM is shown in **Fig. 1.21**. Sound level meters are used to calibrate or establish the accuracy of audiometers and other instruments used to test hearing, as well as to measure noise levels for such varied purposes as determining whether a room is quiet enough for performing hearing tests or identifying potentially hazardous noise exposures. Sound level meters or equivalent circuits that perform the same function are also found as components of other devices, such as hearing aid test systems.

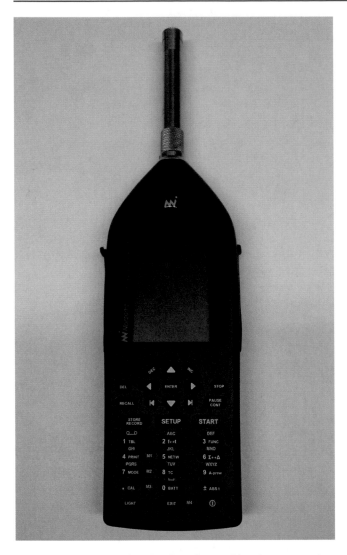

Fig. 1.21 An example of a digital sound level meter with a measuring microphone attached.

Fig. 1.22 An example of a piston phone acoustical calibrator (**a**) and barometer (**b**).

The characteristics of sound level meters are specified in ANSI standard S1.4 (2006). The accuracy of the measurements produced by a SLM is established using a compatible **acoustical calibrator**, which is a device that produces a known precise signal that is directed into the SLM microphone. **Fig. 1.22** shows an example of one type of acoustical calibrator, known as a **piston phone** because of the way it works. A barometer is shown to the right of the piston phone, which is needed because these measurements are affected by barometric pressure. For example, if the calibrator produces a signal that is exactly 114 dB SPL, then the SLM is expected to read this amount when it is connected to the calibrator (within certain tolerances allowed in the ANSI standard). If the meter reading deviates from the actual value of 114 dB

SPL, then its controls are adjusted to reset the meter to the right value, or it might be necessary to have the SLM repaired and recalibrated by the manufacturer or an instrumentation service company.

The microphone of a SLM picks up all sounds that are present at all frequencies within its operating range. At its **linear setting** the SLM measures the overall SPL for all of the sounds picked up by the microphone. In addition to the linear setting, SLMs also have weighting filters that change the emphasis given to certain parts of the spectrum, and may also have octave-band or third-octave-band filters, which measure only certain ranges of frequencies. We all know that turning up the bass control on a home stereo system makes the low pitches more pronounced, whereas turning the bass down makes the lows less noticeable. In other words, the bass control determines whether the low frequencies will be emphasized or de-emphasized. The treble control does the same thing for the high frequencies. The **weighting filters** or networks on a sound level meter do essentially the same thing, mainly by de-emphasizing the low frequencies. **Fig. 1.23** shows the three weighting networks found on the SLM. The y-axis is relative level in decibels, and may be thought of as showing how the weighting network changes the sound that originally entered the SLM through the microphone. A horizontal line at 0 dB refers to how the sound would be without the weighting network. In other words, 0 dB here means "unchanged," which corresponds to the linear setting of the SLM. The negative decibel values tell the amount by which the sound level is de-emphasized at each frequency.

The **A-weighting** network considerably de-emphasizes the low frequencies, as shown by its curve, which gets progressively more negative as frequency decreases below 1000 Hz. For example, the curve shows that the A-weighting network de-emphasizes sounds by ~ 4 dB at 500 Hz, 11 dB at 200 Hz, 19 dB at 100 Hz, and 30 dB at 50 Hz. This is analogous to turning the bass all the way down on a stereo system. The **B-weighting** network also de-emphasizes the lower frequencies, but not as much as the A-weighting. For example, the amount of reduction is only ~ 6 dB at 100 Hz. The **C-weighting** is barely different from a linear response. Sound level measurements made with these networks are expressed as decibels of A-, B-, or C-weighted sound pressure levels, or as **dBA**, **dBB**, and **dBC**, respectively. Measurements in dBA are commonly used when it is desirable to exclude the effects of the lower frequencies, and are especially useful in noise level measurements. Measurements in dBC are also commonly employed in noise level measurements. However, the B-scale is rarely used.

Sound level meters often have a set of built-in or attached **octave-band filters**, which is simply a group of filters that allows the SLM to "look at" a certain range of frequencies instead of all of them. In other words, the octave-band analyzer separates the overall frequency range into narrower ranges, which are each one octave wide, as illustrated in

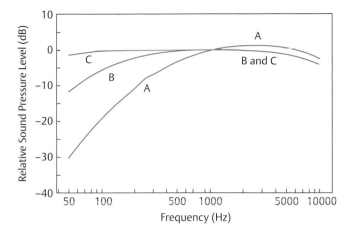

Fig. 1.23 Frequency response curves for the A-, B-, and C-weighting networks.

Fig. 1.24. For example, the range from 355 to 710 Hz is an octave-band because 710 = 2 × 355, and the bandwidth from 2800 to 5600 Hz is also an **octave-band** because 5600 = 2 × 2800. An **octave-band** is named according to its center frequency, although the center is defined as the geometric mean of the upper and lower cutoffs rather than the arithmetic midpoint between them. Hence, the 500 Hz octave-band goes from 355 to 710 Hz, and the 4000 Hz octave-band includes 2800 to 5600 Hz. The center frequencies and the upper and lower cutoff frequencies of the octave-bands typically used in acoustical measurements are listed in **Table 1.5**.

Measuring a noise on an octave-band by octave-band basis is called **octave-band analysis** and makes it possible to learn about the spectrum of a sound instead of just its overall level. An even finer level of analysis can be achieved by using **third-octave-band filters**, in which case each filter is one third of an octave wide. For example, the 500 Hz third-octave

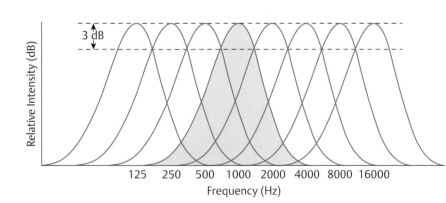

Fig. 1.24 A series of octave-bands representing those typically used in octave-band analysis. Notice the bands overlap at their 3 dB down points. The 1000 Hz octave-band is highlighted for clarity.

Table 1.5 Examples of octave-band center frequencies, and lower and upper cutoff frequencies

Center frequency (Hz)	Lower cutoff (Hz)	Upper cutoff (Hz)
31.5	22.4	45
63	45	90
125	90	180
250	180	355
500	355	710
1,000	710	1,400
2,000	1,400	2,800
4,000	2,800	5,600
8,000	5,600	11,200
16,000	11,200	92,400

Table 1.6 Combining decibels: Find the difference in decibels between the two sounds, and then add the corresponding decibel increment to the larger original decibel value

Difference in dB between original sounds	Increment in dB (add to larger original sound)
0	3.0
1	2.6
2	2.2
3	1.8
4	1.4
5	1.2
6	1.0
7	0.8
8	0.6
9	0.5
10	0.4
11	0.35
12	0.3
13	0.25
14	0.2
15	0.15
16	0.1

filter includes the frequencies between 450 and 560 Hz, and the 4000 Hz third-octave-band goes from 3550 to 4500 Hz. Octave-band and third-octave-band filters are useful when we want to concentrate on the sound level in a narrow frequency range without contamination from other frequencies. For example, it is usually better to measure the level of a 1000 Hz tone while using a filter centered around 1000 Hz than to do the same thing at the linear setting of the SLM because the filter excludes other frequencies; thus the results are not contaminated.

Even though we cannot get the spectrum of a noise from overall sound level measurements, we can combine **octave-band levels (OBLs)** or **⅓-OBLs** to arrive at the overall level of a sound. There are two ways to combine OBLs into overall SPL. The simpler approach involves adding the OBLs in successive pairs using the rules for adding decibels shown in **Table 1.6**. It is very easy to use this table. First, find the difference in decibels between the two sounds being combined. For example, if one sound is 80 dB and the other is 76 dB, then the difference between them is 4 dB. Then find the increment that corresponds to the difference. According to the table, the increment for a 4 dB difference is 1.4 dB. Now, just add this increment to the larger of the original two sounds. The larger value in our example is 80 dB, so we add the 1.4 dB increment to 80 dB (80 + 1.4 = 81.4). Hence, combining 80 and 76 dB results

in a total of 81.4 dB. To combine octave-bands into an overall level, simply arrange their OBLs from largest to smallest, and combine pairs successively using the increments in the table. A complete example is shown in Appendix A.

The more precise method for combining octave-band levels into an overall SPL is to use the following formula for logarithmic addition:

$$L = 10\log\sum_{i=1}^{n} 10^{L_i/10}$$

In this formula L is the overall (combined) level in dB SPL; n is the number of bands being combined; i is the ith band; and Li is the OBL of the ith band. An example showing how this formula is used may be found in Appendix A.

Table 1.7 Corrections (dBA weightings) to convert linear octave-band levels into a-weighted octave-band levels

Octave-band center frequency (Hz)	dBA weighting
31.5	−39.4
63	−26.2
125	−16.1
250	−8.6
500	−3.2
1000	0
2000	+1.2
4000	+1.1
8000	−1.1

The same methods can be used to combine octave-band levels into an A-weighted sound level (dBA), except that a correction factor is applied to each OBL. This correction factor is the amount by which the A-weighting de-emphasizes the level of the sounds within each octave-band. **Table 1.7** shows the corrections (dBA weightings) that can be used to convert linear octave-band levels into A-weighted octave-band levels. For example, dBA de-emphasizes the 125 Hz octave-band by 16.1 dB. Thus, if the 125 Hz OBL is 60 dB, we correct it to its dBA value by subtracting: 60 − 16.1 = 43.9 dB. A full example is shown in Appendix A. The formula for more precisely converting OBLs into dBA is as follows:

$$L_A = 10 \log \sum_{i=1}^{n} 10^{(Li+ki)/10}$$

The symbols here are the same as in the previous formula except L_A is now the overall (combined) level in dBA, and ki is the correction factor that must be applied to the OBL of the ith band to convert it into its equivalent value in dBA (which is the reason for the term Li + ki in the equation). Appendix A shows an example of how this formula is used.

■ Study Questions

1. Define and specify the units of measurement for the following terms: displacement, velocity, acceleration, force, work, and power.
2. Explain pressure and intensity, state the reference values for each of them, and explain why we have these reference values.
3. Explain what happens to the intensity of a sound with increasing distance from the sound source.
4. Define simple harmonic motion and explain how its characteristics are depicted by a sine wave.
5. Define the terms *cycle, period, frequency,* and *wavelength*, and explain how they are related to each other.
6. Define friction and explain why it causes damping.
7. Define complex periodic and aperiodic waves, and describe how their characteristics are shown on the waveform and spectrum.
8. What are resonant frequencies and how are they related to standing waves?
9. Define impedance and describe how it is related to mass and stiffness.
10. What are the formulas and reference values for intensity level and sound pressure level in decibels? Explain how the magnitude of a sound is expressed in decibels.

References

American National Standards Institute (ANSI). 2006. ANSI-S1.4–1983 (R2006). American National Standard Specification for Sound Level Meters. New York, NY: ANSI

Beranek LL. 1986. Acoustics. New York, NY: American Institute of Physics

Gelfand SA. 2010. Hearing: An Introduction to Psychological and Physiological Acoustics, 5th ed. Colchester, Essex, UK: Informa

Hewitt P. 1974. Conceptual Physics. Boston, MA: Little, Brown

Kinsler LE, Frey AR, Coppens AB, Sanders JB. 1982. Fundamentals of Acoustics, 3rd ed. New York, NY: Wiley

Peterson APG, Gross EE. 1972. Handbook of Noise Measurement, 7th ed. Concord, MA: General Radio

Sears FW, Zemansky MW, Young HD. 1982. University Physics, 6th ed. New York, NY: Addison Wesley

2 Anatomy and Physiology of the Auditory System

■ General Overview

Hearing and its disorders are intimately intertwined with the anatomy and physiology of the auditory system, which is composed of the ear and its associated neurological pathways. The auditory system is fascinating, but learning about it for the first time means that we must face many new terms, relationships, and concepts. For this reason it is best to begin with a general bird's-eye view of how the ear is set up and how a sound is converted from vibrations in the air to a signal that can be interpreted by the brain. A set of self-explanatory drawings illustrating commonly used anatomical orientations and directions is provided in **Fig. 2.1** for ready reference.

Fig. 2.2 shows how the structures of the hearing system are oriented within the head. The major parts of the ear are shown in **Fig. 2.3**. One cannot help but notice that the externally visible auricle, or pinna, and the ear canal (external auditory meatus) ending at the eardrum (tympanic membrane) make up only a small part of the overall auditory system. This system is divided into several main sections: The *outer ear* includes the auricle and ear canal. The air-filled cavity behind the eardrum is called the *middle ear*, also known as the tympanic cavity. Notice that the middle ear connects to the pharynx by the Eustachian tube. Medial to the middle ear is the *inner ear*. Three tiny bones (malleus, incus, and stapes), known as the ossicular chain, act as a bridge from the eardrum to the oval window, which is the entrance to the inner ear.

The inner ear contains the sensory organs of hearing and balance. Our main interest is with the structures and functions of the hearing mechanism. Structurally, the inner ear is composed of the vestibule, which lies on the medial side of the oval window; the snail-shaped cochlea anteriorly; and the three semicircular canals posteriorly. The entire system may be envisioned as a complex configuration of fluid-filled tunnels or ducts in the temporal bone, which is descriptively called the labyrinth. The labyrinth, which courses through the temporal bone, contains a continuous membranous duct within it, so that the overall system is arranged as a duct within a duct. The outer duct contains one kind of fluid (perilymph) and the inner duct contains another kind of fluid (endolymph). The part of the inner ear concerned with hearing is the cochlea. It contains the organ of Corti, which in turn has hair cells that are the actual sensory receptors for hearing. The balance (vestibular) system is composed of the semicircular canals and two structures contained within the vestibule, called the utricle and saccule.

The sensory receptor cells are in contact with nerve cells (neurons) that make up the eighth cranial (vestibuloacoustic) nerve, which connects the peripheral ear to the central nervous system. The auditory branch of the eighth nerve is often called the auditory or cochlear nerve, and the vestibular branches are frequently referred to as the vestibular nerve. The eighth nerve leaves the inner ear through an opening on the medial side of the temporal bone called the internal auditory meatus (canal), and then enters the brainstem. Here, the auditory portions of the nerve go to the cochlear nuclei and the vestibular parts of the nerve go to the vestibular nuclei.

The hearing process involves the following series of events. Sounds entering the ear set the tympanic membrane into vibration. These vibrations are conveyed by the ossicular chain to the oval window. Here, the vibratory motion of the ossicles is transmitted to the fluids of the cochlea, which in turn stimulate the sensory receptor (hair) cells of the organ of Corti. When the hair cells respond, they activate the neurons of the auditory nerve. The signal is now in the form of a neural code that can be processed by the nervous system.

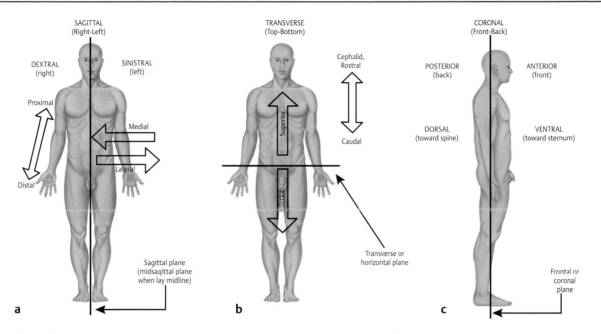

Fig. 2.1 **(a–c)** Commonly encountered anatomical planes, orientations, and directions.

The outer ear and middle ear are collectively called the **conductive system** because their most apparent function is to bring (conduct) the sound signal from the air to the inner ear. The cochlea and eighth cranial nerve compose the **sensorineural system**, so named because it involves the physiological response to the stimulus, activation of the associated nerve cells, and the encoding of the sensory response into a neural signal. The aspects of the central nervous system that deal with this neurally encoded message are generally called the **central auditory nervous system**.

■ Temporal Bone

To be meaningful, a study of the ear must begin with a study of the **temporal bone**. Most of the structures that make up the ear are contained within the temporal bone (**Fig. 2.2**). In fact, the walls of these structures and all of the bony aspects of the ear, except for the ossicles, are actually parts of the temporal bone itself. Recall from your anatomy class that the skeleton of the head is composed of 8 cranial bones and 14 facial bones. The right and left temporal bones compose the inferior lateral aspects of the cranium. Beginning posteriorly and moving clockwise, the temporal bone articulates with the occipital bone behind, the parietal bone behind and above, the sphenoid and zygomatic bones to the front, and the mandible anteriorly below. All of these connections, except for the articulation with the mandible, are firmly united, seam-like fibrous junctions called

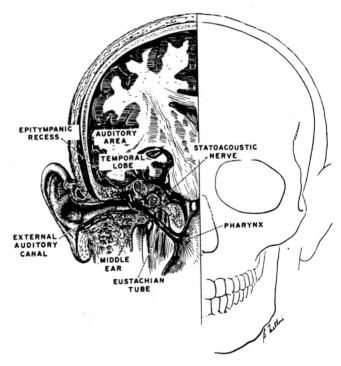

Fig. 2.2 The auditory system in relation to the brain and skull. (Courtesy of Abbott Laboratories.)

sutures. The articulation with the mandible is via the highly mobile **temporomandibular joint**.

Lateral and medial views of the temporal bone are shown in **Fig. 2.4**. The lateral surface of the bone faces the outside of the head and the medial surface faces the inside of the head. The temporal bone is composed of five sections, including the mastoid,

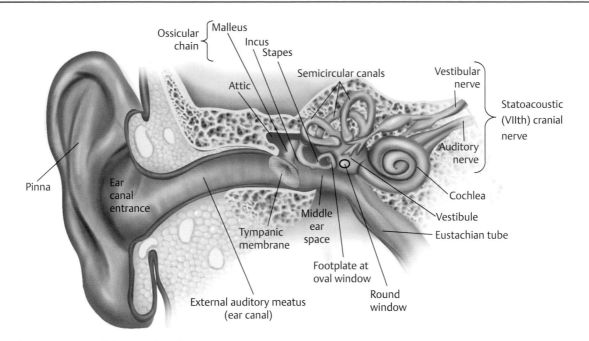

Fig. 2.3 The major parts of the peripheral ear.

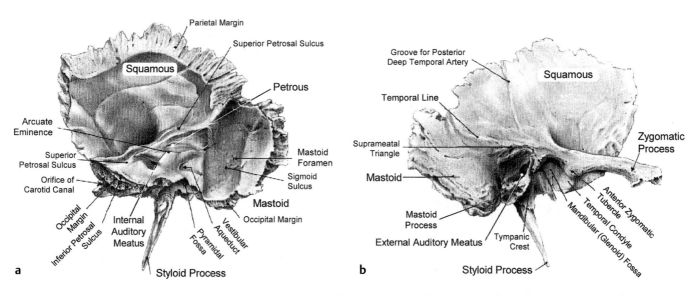

Fig. 2.4 **(a)** Lateral and **(b)** medial views of the right temporal bone. (Adapted from Proctor [1989], with permission.)

petrous, squamous, and tympanic parts, and the styloid process.

The **squamous part** is a very thin, fan-shaped portion on the lateral aspect of the bone. It articulates with the parietal bone posteriorly and superiorly, and with the sphenoid bone anteriorly. The prominent zygomatic process runs anteriorly to join with the zygomatic bone, forming the zygomatic arch. Just below the base of the zygomatic process is a depression called the **mandibular fossa**, which

accepts the condyle of the mandible to form the temporomandibular joint just anterior to the ear canal.

The **petrous part** is pyramid-shaped and medially oriented so that it forms part of the base of the cranium. This extremely hard bone contains the inner ear and the internal auditory meatus through which the eighth cranial nerve travels on its way to the brainstem, so that much of the discussion pertaining to the inner ear is also a discussion of this part of the temporal bone.

The **mastoid part** composes the posterior portion of the temporal bone. It extends posteriorly from the petrous part, below and behind the squamous part. The mastoid articulates with the occipital bone posteriorly and with the parietal bone superiorly. It has an inferiorly oriented, cone-shaped projection below the skull base called **mastoid process**. The mastoid contains an intricate system of interconnecting air cells that vary widely in size, shape, and number. These are connected with an anterosuperior cavity called the **tympanic antrum**, which is located just behind the middle ear cavity. An opening called the **aditus ad antrum** connects the antrum with the attic or upper part of the middle ear cavity. The roof of the antrum (and the middle ear) is composed of a thin bony plate called the **tegmen tympani**, which separates them from the part of the brain cavity known as the middle cranial fossa. Its medial wall separates it from the lateral semicircular canal of the inner ear. Notice that the middle ear, antrum, and air cells compose a continuous, air-filled system. Hence, it is not hard to imagine how an untreated middle ear infection can spread to the mastoid air cell system and beyond.

The tympanic part is inferior to the squamous and petrous parts and anterior to the mastoid. The tympanic part forms the inferior and anterior walls of the ear canal, as well as part of its posterior wall.

The **styloid process** is an anteroinferior pillar-like projection from the base of the temporal bone that varies widely in size. It does not contribute to the auditory structures but is of interest to us as the origin of several muscles involved in the speech mechanism.

these muscles are not vestigial in many lower animals that are able to orient their pinnae with respect to the location of a sound source.

The major landmarks of the pinna are highlighted in **Fig. 2.5**. Notice that the pinna is not symmetrical. For example, and most obviously, it has a flap-like extension that angles away from the skull in the backward direction, so that the pinna overlaps the side of the head posteriorly, superiorly, and inferiorly, but not anteriorly. It also has an intricate arrangement of ridges, bumps, and furrows. The entrance to the ear canal is at the bottom of a large, cup-shaped depression called the **concha**, and is partially covered by a posteriorly directed projection or ridge called the **tragus**. The ridged rim along most of the perimeter of the pinna is the **helix**. Starting at the very top of the pinna, the helix courses anteriorly and downward, making a hook-like turn in the posterior direction to form a shelf above the concha, which is the **crus of the helix**. Again, beginning at the top of the pinna, the helix courses downward along the posterior perimeter, reaching the **earlobe**, or **lobule**, at the bottom. The **scaphoid fossa** is the furrow just anterior to the helix as it courses down the posterior rim of the pinna. The ridge anterior to the scaphoid fossa is called the **antihelix**. The antihelix runs parallel with the helix and splits superiorly into the two **crura of the antihelix**. The splitting of the antihelix into two crura creates a triangle-shaped depression called the **triangular fossa**. If we follow the antihelix downward, it widens at the bottom to form the **antitragus**, an upward pointing mound that is located posteroinferior to the tragus and superior to the earlobe. The space or angle between the tragus and the antitragus is the **intertragic incisure**.

■ Outer and Middle Ear

The **outer ear** is composed of the pinna and the ear canal, ending at the eardrum. The **tympanic membrane** is generally considered to be part of the **middle ear** system, which includes the middle ear cavity and its contents, and "ends" where the ossicles transmit the signal to the inner ear fluids at the oval window.

Pinna

The externally visible aspect of the ear is an odd-shaped appendage called the **pinna** or **auricle**. The internal structure of the pinna is composed principally of elastic cartilage (except for the earlobe). It also contains some undifferentiated intrinsic muscle tissue, as well as several extrinsic muscles, although these are vestigial structures in humans. However,

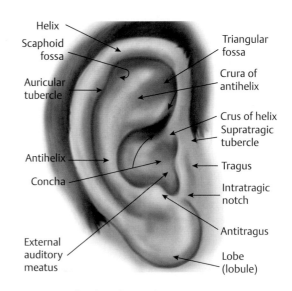

Fig. 2.5 Major landmarks on the pinna.

External Auditory Meatus

The ear canal is more formally called the **external auditory meatus (canal)**. On average, it is ~ 9 mm high by 6.5 mm wide, and is roughly 2.5 cm to 3.5 cm long. The ear canal is not quite a straight tube, but has two curves forming a slightly S-like pathway.

These curves usually make it difficult to get an unobstructed view of the eardrum, so that it is usually necessary to straighten the canal before looking inside with an otoscope. An otoscope is the familiar instrument used for examining the ear (**Fig. 2.6**). The ear canal is straightened by gently pulling up and back on the pinna, as illustrated in **Fig. 2.7**.

The external auditory meatus is lined with tight-fitting skin. However, the outer third of the canal is different from the inner two thirds in several ways. The underlying material is cartilage in the outer third and bone for the remainder of its length. The bony portion of the canal is derived from (1) the tympanic part of the temporal bone, which forms the floor and anterior wall, as well as the inferoposterior wall; (2) the squamous part, making up the roof and part of the posterior wall; and (3) the condyle of mandible, which contributes to the inferioanterior wall at the temporomandibular joint. The cartilaginous portion contains hairs as well as a plentiful distribution of **sebaceous (oil)** and **ceruminous (wax) glands**, although this is not the case for the bony portion of the canal. Sebaceous glands are also present in the concha. Their secretions serve lubricating and antimicrobial functions, and also help to keep the canal free of debris and even some foreign bodies and insects.

Tympanic Membrane

The external auditory meatus ends at the **tympanic membrane** or **eardrum,** which is tilted at an angle of ~ 55° to the canal. The tympanic membrane is firmly attached to the **tympanic sulcus**, a groove in the bony canal wall, by a ring of fibrocartilaginous connective tissue called the **tympanic annulus** (or **annular ligament**). The ring has a deficiency at the top due to a tiny interruption in the tympanic sulcus known as the **notch of Rivinus**. The eardrum is a smooth, translucent, and sometimes almost transparent membrane with an average thickness of only ~ 0.074 mm. It is slightly taller (~ 0.9 to 1.0 cm) than it is wide (~ 0.8 to 0.9 cm), and it is concave outward rather than flat. The peak of the cone-like inward displacement is called the **umbo**. Structurally, the eardrum is often described as having three layers, although more correctly there are four of them. The most lateral layer of the tympanic membrane is continuous with the skin of the ear canal, and the most medial layer is continuous with the mucous membrane of the middle ear. Sandwiched between them are two fibrous layers. One of them is composed of radial fibers reminiscent of the spokes of a wheel, and the other layer is made of essentially concentric circular fibers.

The tympanic membrane is connected to the malleus, which is the first of the three middle ear bones. Specifically, a long, lateral process of the malleus called the **manubrium** attaches almost vertically to the eardrum, with its tip at the umbo and continuing upward toward the position of 1 o'clock in the right

Fig. 2.6 Examples of otoscopes used for examining the ear, along with reusable and disposable specula. The speculum is the cone-shaped attachment that is inserted into the ear canal.

Fig. 2.7 The ear canal is straightened to facilitate otoscopic inspection by gently pulling up and back on the pinna.

ear and 11 o'clock in the left ear. This attachment of the manubrium of the malleus forms the **malleal prominence**. Ligamentous bands called the **anterior** and **posterior malleal folds** run from both sides of the malleal prominence to the notch of Rivinus, forming a triangular area between them on the eardrum. The largest part of the tympanic membrane lies *outside* or below the malleal folds, and is called the **pars tensa** ("tense part") because it contains all three layers described above. The superior area of the eardrum between the malleal folds *is missing* the fibrous layers, and is called the **pars flaccida** ("flaccid area") for this reason. It is also known as **Shrapnell's membrane**.

Fig. 2.8 shows some of the major landmarks that are identified when looking at the eardrum through an otoscope. In addition to the landmarks already mentioned, notice that the light from the otoscope is reflected back in a characteristic way, called the **cone of light** or **light reflex**. This reflection is seen as a bright area on the anteroinferior surface of the eardrum, radiating from the tip of the manubrium to the 5 o'clock position in the right ear and the 7 o'clock position in the left ear. It is often possible to identify one or more middle ear landmarks, especially when viewing relatively transparent eardrums.

Middle Ear

The cavity in the temporal bone behind the tympanic membrane is called the **middle ear**, **tympanum**, or **tympanic cavity**. The posterosuperior portion of the middle ear space is usually viewed as an "attic room" above the main tympanic cavity, and is called the **epitympanic recess** or the **attic**. This space accommodates the more massive portions of the two larger ossicles, the incus and the malleus. Using a certain amount of artistic license, **Fig. 2.9** depicts the middle

ear space as a box-shaped room. Keep in mind that the box is only an analogy used to describe *relative* directions and relationships. In addition, **Fig. 2.10** shows a more realistic drawing of the tympanic cavity and its contents looking backward toward its posterior wall. The tympanic membrane forms the lateral wall, and is shown folded downward to reveal the inside of the "room" in the figure. The middle ear really has irregularly shaped curved surfaces as in the other figures, *not* flat walls with right-angled corners. The floor of the tympanic cavity separates it from the **jugular bulb** below. The ceiling is the **tegmen tympani**, which is the thin bony plate that separates the tympanic cavity from the brain cavity above. Low down on the anterior wall (~ 3 mm up from the floor) is the opening of the **Eustachian tube** (sometimes called the **auditory tube**). The **internal carotid artery canal** is located on the other side of (i.e., anterior to) the anterior wall, just below the Eustachian tube. Just above the Eustachian tube is the **tensor tympani semicanal**, which contains the **tensor tympani muscle**. The tensor tympani semicanal and Eustachian tube are separated by a bony shelf or septum. There is a curved bony projection on the anterior/medial wall that points into the middle ear space, called the **cochleariform process**. The tendon of the tensor tympani muscle bends around the cochleariform process and proceeds in the lateral direction on its way to the malleus (**Fig. 2.10**).

The prominent bulge on the medial wall is the **promontory** of the basal turn of the cochlea. The **oval window** of the cochlea (with its attachment to the stapes) is located posterosuperior to the promontory, and the **round window** of the cochlea is posteroinferior to it. The **facial nerve canal prominence** is situated superior to the oval window.

The posterior wall separates the tympanic cavity from the mastoid. The **aditus ad antrum** is an opening located superiorly on the rear wall, and provides

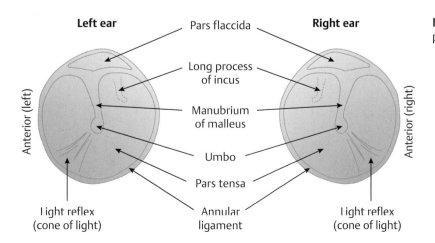

Fig. 2.8 Major otoscopic landmarks of the tympanic membrane.

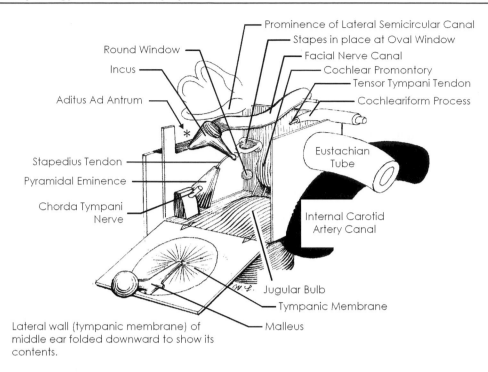

Prominence of Lateral Semicircular Canal
Round Window
Incus
Stapes in place at Oval Window
Facial Nerve Canal
Cochlear Promontory
Tensor Tympani Tendon
Aditus Ad Antrum
Cochleariform Process
Eustachian Tube
Stapedius Tendon
Pyramidal Eminence
Chorda Tympani Nerve
Internal Carotid Artery Canal
Jugular Bulb
Tympanic Membrane
Malleus
Lateral wall (tympanic membrane) of middle ear folded downward to show its contents.

Fig. 2.9 An artist's conceptualization of the middle ear cavity as a room, with the lateral wall (including the eardrum and attached malleus) folded down to reveal the inside. The stapes is shown in place in the oval window. (Adapted from Proctor [1989], with permission.)

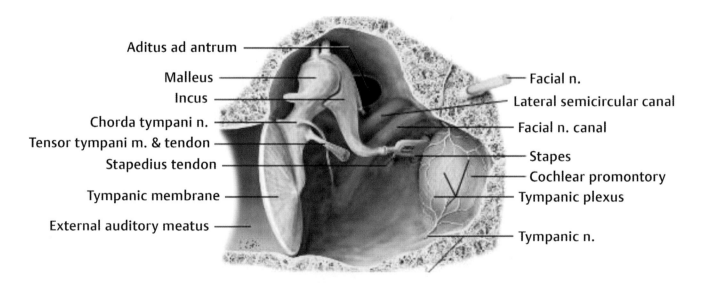

Aditus ad antrum
Malleus
Incus
Chorda tympani n.
Tensor tympani m. & tendon
Stapedius tendon
Tympanic membrane
External auditory meatus
Facial n.
Lateral semicircular canal
Facial n. canal
Stapes
Cochlear promontory
Tympanic plexus
Tympanic n.

Fig. 2.10 Artist's representation of the middle ear looking backward toward the posterior wall (m., muscle; n., nerve). (Adapted from Schuenke M, Schulte E, Schumacher U, Ross LM, Lamperti ED, Voll M. 2010. Head and Neuroanatomy [Thieme Atlas of Anatomy]. New York, NY: Thieme; Fig. 9.3b, p. 144, with permission.)

communication between the epitympanic recess of the middle ear cavity and the antrum of the mastoid air cell system. The **pyramidal eminence** or **pyramid** is a prominence on the posterior wall that contains the body of the **stapedius muscle**. The **stapedial tendon** exits from the apex of the pyramid and proceeds to the stapes. The **fossa incudis** is a recess on the posterior wall that accommodates the short process of the incus. The **chord tympani nerve** is a branch of the **facial (seventh cranial) nerve** that enters the middle ear from an opening laterally at the juncture of the posterior and lateral walls, runs just under the neck of the malleus, and leaves the middle ear cavity via the opening of the **anterior chordal canal (of Huguier)** that is anterior to the tympanic sulcus.

Ossicular Chain

Three tiny bones known as the ossicles or the **ossicular chain** transmit the sound-induced vibrations of the tympanic membrane to the cochlea via the oval window (**Fig. 2.11**). The ossicles are the smallest bones in the body, and include the **malleus, incus,** and **stapes**. Instead of being attached to other bones, the ossicular chain is suspended within the middle ear cavity by ligaments and tendons, as well as its attachments to the tympanic membrane and the oval window. The malleus ("hammer" or "mace") is ~ 8 to 9 mm long and weighs ~ 25 mg. Its **manubrium** (handle) is firmly embedded between the fibrous and mucous membrane layers of the eardrum, forming the lateral attachment of the ossicular chain. The neck of the malleus is a narrowing between its manubrium and head. Its lateral process produces a bulge on the eardrum that is often visible otoscopically. There is also an **anterior process** near the junction of the neck and manubrium. The head of the malleus connects with the body of the incus by a diarthrodial or double-saddle joint, the **incudomallear articulation**, such that these two bones move as a unit.

The incus, which is ~ 7 mm long and weighs roughly 30 mg, is commonly called the "anvil" but looks more like a tooth with two roots. The **short process** is posteriorly oriented and is accommodated by the fossa incudus on the back wall of the middle ear. The **long process** descends from the body of the incus, parallel with the manubrium of the malleus,

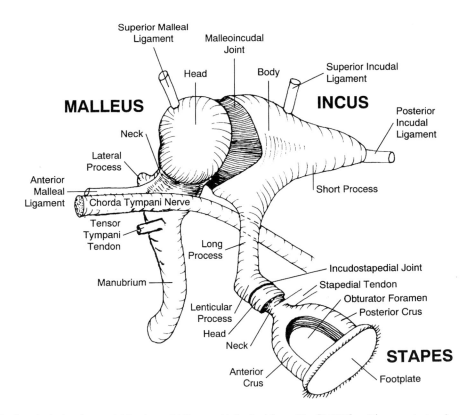

Fig. 2.11   The ossicular chain in place within the middle ear. (Adapted from Tos [1995], with permission.)

and then hooks medially to end at a rounded nodule called the **lenticular process**. In turn, the lenticular process articulates with the head of the stapes via a true ball-and-socket or enarthrodial joint called the **incudostapedial joint**.

The stapes bears a close resemblance to a "stirrup," which is its common name. Its head is connected via the neck to two strut-like processes called the **anterior** and **posterior crura**, which lead down to the oval shaped **footplate**. The opening between the crura and footplate is called the **obturator foramen**. The stapes weighs only 3 to 4 mg. It is ~ 3.5 mm long, and the footplate has an area of roughly 3.2 mm². The footplate is attached to the oval window by the **annular ligament**, forming the medial attachment of the ossicular chain.

In addition to its lateral attachment to the tympanic membrane and its medial attachment at the oval window via the annular ligament, the ossicular chain is also supported by several ligaments and the tendons of the two middle ear muscles. The **superior malleal ligament** runs from the roof (tegmen tympani) of the attic down to the head of the malleus. The **anterior malleal ligament** goes from the anterior tympanic wall to the anterior process of the malleus. The **lateral malleal ligament** extends from the bony margin of the notch of Rivinus to the neck of the malleus. **The posterior incudal ligament** (actually a fold of mucous membrane rather than a ligament) runs from the fossa incudus to the short process of the incus.

Middle Ear Muscles

The **tensor tympani muscle** is innervated by the **trigeminal (fifth cranial) nerve**. It is housed within the tensor tympani semicanal in the anterior middle ear wall superior to the Eustachian tube. This muscle is ~ 25 mm long and arises from the cartilage of the Eustachian tube, the walls of its semicanal, and the segment of sphenoid bone adjacent to the canal. The **tensor tympani tendon** bends around the cochleariform process and proceeds in the lateral direction to insert on the malleus at the top of the manubrium near the neck. Contraction of the tensor tympani pulls the malleus in the anteromedial direction, thereby stiffening the ossicular chain.

The **stapedius muscle** is the smallest skeletal muscle in the body, with an average length of only 6.3 mm. It is contained within the pyramidal eminence of the posterior wall of the tympanic cavity, and is innervated by the **facial (seventh cranial) nerve**. The **stapedius tendon** exists via the apex of the pyramidal eminence and runs anteriorly to insert on the posterior aspect of the neck of the sta-

pes. Contraction of the stapedius pulls the stapes posteriorly. Even though the middle ear muscles pull in more or less opposite directions, they both exert forces that are perpendicular to the normal motion of the ossicles, and their contraction has the effect of stiffening the ossicular chain, thereby reducing the amount of energy that is delivered to the inner ear.

The **acoustic reflex** refers to the reflexive middle ear muscle contraction that occurs in response to high levels of sound stimulation (Gelfand 1984, 2010). In humans this is at least principally a stapedius reflex, while the tensor tympani contracts as part of a startle reaction to very intense sounds, and also in response to certain kinds of nonacoustic stimulation such as an air jet directed at the eye. The acoustic reflex involves both muscles in some animals.

The fundamental aspects of the **acoustic (stapedius) reflex arc** are as follows (Borg 1973; Wiley & Block 1984). The sensory (afferent) pathway proceeds via the auditory nerve to the ventral cochlear nucleus, and then to the superior olivary complex on *both sides* of the brainstem (with the crossover to the opposite side by way of the trapezoid body). The motor (or efferent) pathway is followed bilaterally, and runs from the motor nuclei of the **facial (seventh cranial) nerve** on both sides, and then via the facial nerves to the stapedius muscles. The motor pathway for tensor tympani activation goes from the **trigeminal (fifth cranial) nerve** nuclei to the tensor tympani muscles via the trigeminal nerves. Because contraction of the stapedius and tensor tympani muscles stiffens the middle ear system, the transmission of low frequencies is reduced (Simmons 1959; Møller 1965; Rabinowitz 1976). This change has been observed as a decrease in hearing sensitivity or loudness for low-frequency sounds (Smith 1943; Reger 1960; Morgan & Dirks 1975), although these effects are not always found (Morgan, Dirks, & Kamm 1978).

The purpose of the acoustic reflex is not really known, although several theories have been proposed. The *protection theory* suggests the acoustic reflex protects the inner ear from potentially damaging sound levels. However, it is unlikely that this is its main purpose because the reflex has a delay (latency) that would make it an ineffective protection against sudden sounds, and the contraction adapts over time, limiting its protection against ongoing sounds. The *fixation theory* holds that the middle ear muscles maintain the appropriate positioning and rigidity of ossicles, and the *accommodation theory* states that the muscles modify the characteristics of the conductive system so that the absorption of sound energy is maximized. Simmons (1964) suggested the acoustic reflex improves the audibility of environmental sounds by attenuating internal sounds. This enhancement of signal-to-noise ratio would improve the survival rates for both the fox who is hunting for dinner and the rabbit who is trying to avoid being the main course. Similarly, Borg (1976) proposed that one of the purposes of the reflex is to improve the listener's dynamic range by attenuating low frequency sounds. Discussions of these and other reflex theories may be found in several sources (Jepsen 1963; Simmons 1964; Borg, Counter, & Rosler 1984).

Eustachian Tube

The **Eustachian (auditory) tube** provides for the aeration and drainage of the middle ear system, and makes it possible for air pressure to be the same on both sides of the eardrum. It runs from the anterior middle ear wall to the posterior wall of the nasopharynx behind the inferior nasal turbinate, as illustrated in **Fig. 2.12** and **Fig. 2.13**. In adults the Eustachian tube follows a 3.5 to 3.8 cm long course that is directed inferiorly, medially, and anteriorly, tilting downward at an angle of ~ 45°. However, it is important to be aware that the Eustachian tube is almost horizontal in infants and young children (see **Fig. 6.4** in Chapter 6). The first third of the tube beginning at the middle ear is surrounded by bone and the remainder is sur-

rounded by an incomplete ring of elastic cartilage. The meeting point of the **bony** and **cartilaginous portions** is called the **isthmus**. The lumen of the Eustachian tube is narrowest at the isthmus, where it is only 1 to 2 mm across compared with 3 to 6 mm in the remainder of the tube. A prominence on the pharyngeal wall, the **torus tubarius**, is formed by the cartilage of the Eustachian tube and other tissues (e.g., the salpingopalatine, salpingopharyngeous, and tensor palatini muscles).

The cartilaginous portion of the Eustachian tube is arranged as shown in **Fig. 2.14**. Notice that the cartilage hooks around the tube from above, forming the incomplete ring alluded to above. A portion of the tensor palatini muscle is attached to the hooked segment of the cartilage (**Fig. 2.13** and **Fig. 2.14**). At rest, the cartilage keeps the Eustachian tube closed (**Fig. 2.14a**). The lumen of the tube is opened when the cartilage is uncurled due to the pull exerted by the tensor palatini muscle (**Fig. 2.14b**). This occurs during swallowing, yawning, and other actions that cause the tensor palatini muscle to contract. Negative pressure develops in the middle ear (compared with the outside, atmospheric pressure) when this mechanism fails to open the Eustachian tube frequently and effectively. We have all experienced this phenomenon as fullness in the ears that is (hopefully) alleviated when the tube "pops open" due to a swallow, yawn, or some other maneuver. Swelling and/or blockage by mucus due to colds or allergy, and obstruction of the pharyngeal orifice by hypertrophic (enlarged) adenoids, are just a few of the causes of a nonpatent Eustachian tube. The resulting negative pressure within the closed-off middle ear space often precipitates the development of clinically significant middle ear disease.

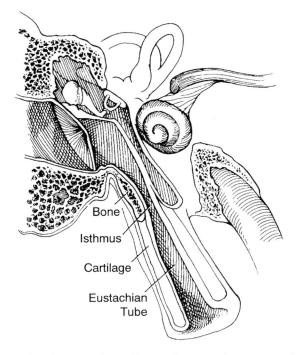

Fig. 2.12 The Eustachian tube in relation to the ear. Note that the bony portion of the tube meets the cartilaginous portion at the isthmus. (Adapted from Hughes [1985], with permission.)

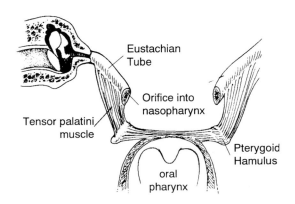

Fig. 2.13 Relationship of the Eustachian tube to the tensor palatini muscle, highlighting the parts of the muscle that arise from the tubal cartilage, hook around the pterygoid hamulus of the sphenoid bone, and insert into the palate. (Adapted from Hughes [1985], with permission.)

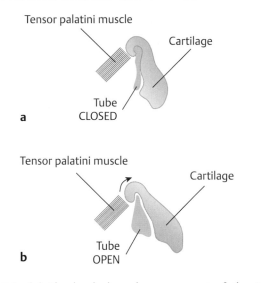

Fig. 2.14 **(a)** The hook-shaped arrangement of the Eustachian tube cartilage keeps the tube in the normally closed state. **(b)** The tube is opened when the cartilage hook is uncurled by action of the tensor palatini muscle.

■ Functioning of the Conductive Mechanism

Sound entering the outer ear is picked up by the tympanic membrane. The vibrations of the eardrum are transmitted to the ossicular chain, which vibrates essentially in the right-left plane. This vibration is represented as a rocking motion of the stapes footplate in the oval window, as shown in **Fig. 2.15**. The resulting inward and outward displacements of the oval window are thus transmitted to the cochlear fluid. However, instead of just serving as an inert passageway that allows sound to travel to the cochlea from the surrounding air, the conductive mechanism actually modifies sound in several ways that have a direct bearing on how and what we hear.

Head-Related Transfer Function

Sounds reaching the eardrum are affected by the acoustics of the external auditory meatus, which operates as a quarter-wavelength resonator because it is essentially a tube with one open end and one closed end (at the tympanic membrane). Sounds entering the ear will be enhanced if they are close to the resonant frequency range, resulting in a boost in the sound pressure level (SPL) reaching the eardrum, called the **ear canal resonance effect**. To deter-

mine this boost in level (or gain) at the eardrum, the sound presented from a loudspeaker is monitored by a microphone outside the patient's ear and also by a special kind of microphone that monitors the sound level inside the subject's ear canal, very close to the eardrum. The difference between these two measurements is the amount of gain provided by the ear canal resonance, shown as a function of frequency in **Fig. 2.16**. On this kind of graph, 0 dB means "unchanged," that is, that the SPL at the eardrum is the same as it is outside the person's ear. Positive values show the amounts of gain provided by the ear canal resonances (negative values mean that the level is lower at the eardrum than outside the ear). We see clearly that the resonance characteristics of the ear canal provide a sound level boost of as much as 15 to 20 dB in the frequency range from roughly 2000 to 5000 Hz. In addition, the middle ear has a resonant region between ~ 800 Hz and ~ 5000–6000 Hz (Zwislocki 1975). The resonant responses of the conductive system affect our hearing sensitivity for sounds at different frequencies, as discussed in Chapter 3.

The graph in **Fig. 2.16** is technically called the **head-related transfer function (HRTF)** because it shows how the sound reaching the eardrum is affected by the direction of the sound source relative to the head. In other words, the HRTF shows how the spectrum is changed by the acoustical path from the loudspeaker to the eardrum. Thus, it is sometimes

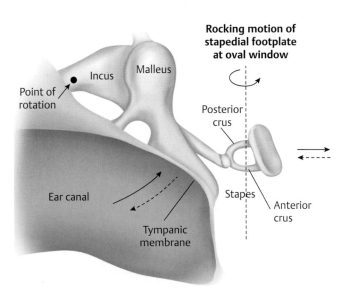

Fig. 2.15 The middle ear transmits the signal to the cochlea via a rocking motion of the stapedial footplate at the oval window. (After Bekesy [1941].)

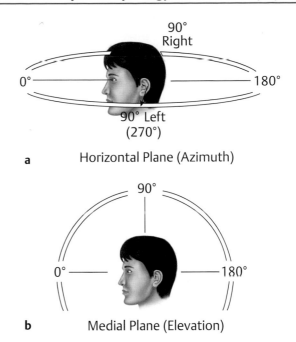

Fig. 2.16 Average head-related transfer functions (sound level at the eardrum compared with outside of the ear) for sounds presented from a loudspeaker directly in front of the subjects. (*Dotted line,* Wiener & Ross [1946]; *dashed line,* Shaw [1974]; *solid line.* Mehrgardt & Mellert [1977]) (From Mehrgardt & Mellert [1977], with permission of the *Journal of the Acoustical Society of America.*)

Fig. 2.17 Directions around the head. **(a)** The horizontal plane goes around the head horizontally from right to left, expressed in degrees of azimuth. **(b)** The medial (median) plane goes around the head vertically from front to back, expressed in degrees of elevation.

also called the **sound field to eardrum transfer function**. The HRTF actually reflects the accumulated effect of all factors that influence the sound on the way from the loudspeaker to the tympanic membrane, including acoustical shadows, reflections, and diffraction due to the head and body, as well as the ear canal resonance. This is why the figure caption specifies the direction of the loudspeaker. These acoustical effects depend on the direction of the sound and are important cues for directional hearing, or the ability to identify the location of a sound source and differences in locations between different sound sources.

Sound direction is described in terms of angles around the head (**Fig. 2.17**). The easiest way to describe the location of a sound source is to give its angle relative to the head (e.g., so many degrees to the right, so many degrees straight up from the front, etc.). The **horizontal plane** refers to horizontal directions around the head toward the right and toward the left. Horizontal directions are usually called angles of **azimuth.** For example:

0° azimuth is *straight ahead* (in front of your nose);

90° azimuth is directly *to the right* (in front of your right ear);

180° azimuth is *straight back* (directly behind your head); and

270° azimuth is directly *to the left* (in front of your left ear).

Thus, an azimuth of 45° means 45° to the right, and 315° azimuth is the same as 45° to the left. By

the way, it is perfectly fine to say "45° to the right" and "45° to the left." It is also acceptable (and often confusing) to use positive angles for one direction and negative values for the other, such as +60° azimuth for 60° to the right, and –60° azimuth for 60° to the left.

Azimuths of 0° and 180° are both dead center between the two ears. The same thing is true for **elevations** such as straight up above the center of the head, 45° upward from directly in front, 30° downward from directly in front, and 70° upward from straight back. These are examples of directions in the **medial (or median) plane**. The medial plane is the same as going around the head vertically in the *midsagittal anatomical plane,* so that all locations on the medial plane are equidistant from the two ears. In the medial plane, 0° is straight ahead, 90° is straight up, and 180° is straight back.

To appreciate how directional differences are represented acoustically at the ears, let us suppose that a loudspeaker is located at an azimuth of 45° to the right, as depicted in **Fig. 2.18a**. Even though the original sound is the same, it reaches the left ("far") ear differently than it does the right ("near") ear. The far ear is subjected to an acoustical shadow when the head obstructs the path of the sound (**Fig. 2.18b**).

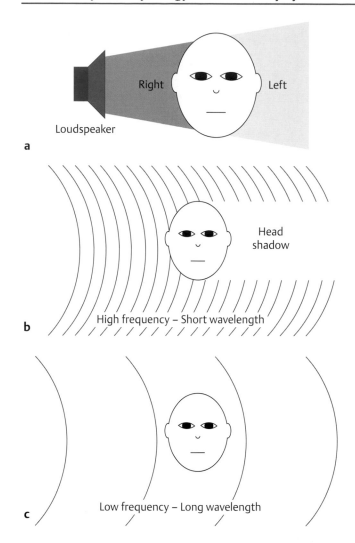

Fig. 2.18 **(a)** Sound coming from a loudspeaker off to the right side arrives differently at the two ears. **(b)** An acoustical shadow (the head shadow effect) occurs for high-frequency sounds because their wavelengths are small compared with the size of the head. **(c)** Because of their large wavelengths, low-frequency sounds are not subjected to a head shadow because they are able to bend around the head.

As a result, the sound reaches the far ear at a softer level than it reaches the near ear. This level disadvantage at the far ear is called the head shadow effect. The head shadow occurs for frequencies that can be obstructed by the head. This occurs for sounds with wavelengths that are short compared with the size of the head. Recall that wavelength gets shorter as frequency increases. Hence, the head shadow affects relatively higher frequencies, especially those over ~ 1500 Hz. This level difference between the ears is called an **inter-ear (interaural) intensity difference**.

The result of these differences at the eardrum can be seen by comparing the **head-related transfer functions** obtained when a loudspeaker is positioned at different locations around the head. **Fig. 2.19** illustrates the **azimuth effect** by showing how the head-related transfer functions are different for the right ear when a loudspeaker is at an azimuth of 45° to the right compared with when is 45° to the left (i.e., 45° versus 315°). The sound level at the right eardrum is greater when the sound comes from 45° to the right ("near ear") compared with when it comes from 45° to the left ("far ear"). Notice that the shape of the curve also changes depending on the azimuth. This graph shows the results at two representative azimuths. Curves obtained from many azimuths all around the head would reveal a continuum of these kinds of differences (Shaw 1974).

Low frequencies have wavelengths that are long relative to the size of the head, so that diffraction can occur. In other words, they are able to bend around the head to the far ear with little if any loss of level (**Fig. 2.18c**). However, the sound will arrive at the near ear earlier than at the far ear, constituting an **inter-ear (interaural) time difference**. Interaural intensity and time differences provide the principal cues needed for directional hearing.

Pinna Effect

What does the pinna do for us? It has long been known that any amplification provided by the pinna is essentially negligible in spite of its funnel-like appearance, and that its main contribution to hearing is in the realm of sound source localization (Bekesy & Rosenblith 1958). (To appreciate the importance of the pinna in directional hearing, one has only to watch a cat orient its pinnae toward a sound source.) The pinna provides sound localization cues because its asymmetrical and irregular shape, ridges, and depressions modify the spectrum of a sound in a way that depends on the direction of the source (Blauert 1983). The simplest example is that sounds coming from the rear are obstructed by the pinna so that some of the high-frequency components of their spectra are attenuated compared with the same sounds arriving from the front. These kinds of pinna-related spectral differences are particularly important when inter-ear sound differences are negligible or absent. This is the case for localizations in the medial plane and/or when trying to localize sounds with just one ear.

The Middle Ear Transformer

The sound signal that reaches the ear in the form of air vibrations must be transmitted to the cochlea, which is a fluid-filled system. The impedance of the

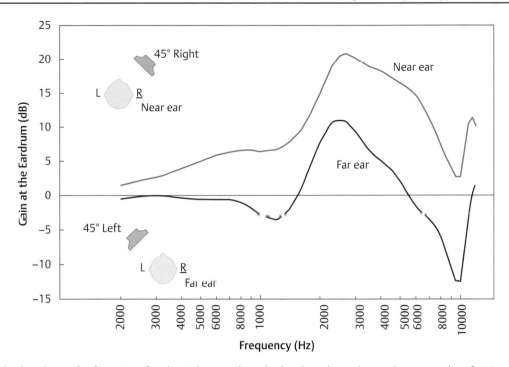

Fig. 2.19 Head-related transfer functions for the right ear when the loudspeaker is located at azimuths of 45° to the right ("near ear" situation) versus 45° to the left ("far ear" situation). Based on the data of Shaw (1974) and Shaw & Vaillancourt (1985).

cochlear fluids is much greater than the impedance of the air. As a result, most of the sound energy would be reflected back if airborne sound were to impinge directly on the cochlear fluids, and only ~ 0.1% of it would actually be transmitted. This situation is analogous to the reflection of airborne sound energy off the water's surface at the beach, which is why you cannot hear your friends talking when your head is under the water. The middle ear system overcomes this impedance mismatch by acting as a mechanical *transformer* that boosts the original signal so that energy can be efficiently transmitted to the cochlea.

The transformer function of the middle ear is accomplished by the combination of three mechanisms: (1) the area ratio advantage of the eardrum to the oval window, (2) the curved membrane buckling effect of the tympanic membrane, and (3) the lever action of the ossicular chain. The largest contribution comes from the **area advantage**. Here, the force that is exerted over the larger area of the tympanic membrane is transmitted to the smaller area of the oval window, just as the force applied over the head of a thumbtack is concentrated onto the tiny area of its point (**Fig. 2.20**). Pressure is force divided by area (p = F/A), so that concentrating the same force from a larger area of the eardrum down to a smaller area of the oval window results in a proportional boost in the pressure at the oval window.

The **curved membrane buckling** mechanism is illustrated in **Fig. 2.21**. The eardrum curves from its rim at both ends to its attachment to the manubrium toward the middle. As a result, eardrum vibration involves greater displacement for the curved membranes and less displacement for the manubrium, which might be envisioned as a buckling effect. A boost in force accompanies the smaller displacement of the manubrium because the product of force and displacement must be the same on both sides of a lever (F1 × D1 = F2 × D2). The third and smallest contributor to the middle ear transformer mechanism is the **lever action of the ossicular chain**. **Fig. 2.22** shows how the malleus constitutes the longer leg of this lever and the incus is the shorter leg, as well as the axis of rotation.

How much of a boost does this transformer mechanism provide? To answer this question we can plug some representative values into the relationships just discussed. The area of the eardrum is roughly 85 mm²; however, only about two thirds of this area vibrates effectively (Bekesy, 1960), so that the effective area of the eardrum is something like 56.7 mm². The area of the oval window is roughly 3.2 mm². Hence, the area ratio is 56.7 to 3.2, or 17.7 to 1. The ossicular lever ratio is ~ 1.3 to 1. So far, the total advantage is 17.7 × 1.3 = 23 to 1. In terms of pressure the decibel value of this ratio would be

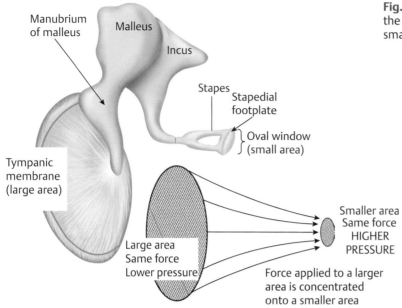

Manubrium of malleus

Malleus

Incus

Stapes

Stapedial footplate

Oval window (small area)

Tympanic membrane (large area)

Large area
Same force
Lower pressure

Smaller area
Same force
HIGHER
PRESSURE

Force applied to a larger area is concentrated onto a smaller area

Fig. 2.20 The area advantage involves concentrating the force applied over the tympanic membrane to the smaller area of the oval window.

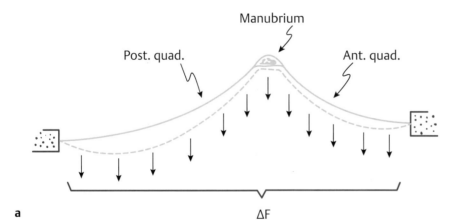

Manubrium

Post. quad.

Ant. quad.

ΔF

a

Fig. 2.21 **(a)** The curved membrane buckling principle involves a boost in force at the manubrium because it moves with less displacement than the curved eardrum membrane. **(b)** Variations in the amount of displacement are shown by concentric contours in this photograph and corresponding drawing of the vibration pattern of the cat's eardrum at 600 Hz. The two areas of concentric contours on both sides of the manubrium show that the eardrum's vibration pattern agrees with the curved membrane principle. (From Tonndorf & Khanna [1970], with permission of the *Annals of Otology, Rhinology, and Laryngology*.)

AXIS OF ROTATION

INCUS

MALLEUS

600Hz 11dB

b

30°

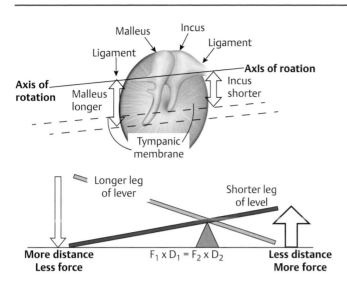

Fig. 2.22 Axis of rotation and relative lengths of the longer (malleus) and shorter (incus) legs of the ossicular lever. (Based in part on Bekesy [1941].)

20 × log (23/1) = 27 dB. However, if we add the curved membrane buckling advantage of 2 to 1, the ratio becomes 23 × 2 = 46 to 1. In decibels of pressure, the total advantage now becomes 20 × log (46/1) = 33 dB. This is only an approximation; the actual size of the pressure advantage varies considerably with frequency (Nedzelnitsky 1980).

■ Inner Ear

The Cochlea

Recall the inner ear is set up like a duct inside of a duct. The outer duct is called the **osseous** or **bony labyrinth** because its walls are made of the surrounding bone. The inside duct is made of membranous materials and is thus called the **membranous labyrinth.** The osseous and membranous labyrinths are represented in **Fig. 2.23**.

It is useful to "build" a simple model of this apparently complicated system, as in **Fig. 2.24a**. This model will represent the auditory part of the labyrinth, the cochlea. The outer, bony duct is represented by a steel pipe that is closed at the back end. The inner, membranous duct is represented by a pliable rubber hose (or a long balloon) with a closed-off end that is inserted almost all the way into the pipe. The left and right sides of the pliable hose are glued to the inner right and left sides of the pipe, forming three cham-

bers. The middle chamber is completely enclosed by the rubber hose. The upper chamber is above the rubber hose and the lower chamber is below the rubber hose. We now pour water that contains blue food coloring into the rubber hose. Hence, the middle chamber contains blue water. Then we pour water that contains red food coloring into one of the outer chambers, and we find that the red water fills both of the outer chambers. This occurs because the rubber hose does not extend all the way to the far end of the pipe, so that the two outer chambers are jointed at that end. We then close off the open ends of the ducts with transparent plastic so that the water does not leak out. We now have a model of a duct inside of a duct. It has two outer chambers filled with red water that are separated by an inner chamber filled with blue water. In addition, the outer chambers are continuous at the back end of the pipe.

Notice the similarities between our pipe model in **Fig. 2.23a** and an artist's representation of a cochlea (**Fig. 2.24b**) that has been "uncurled" from its snail shell configuration. Here the upper duct is called the scala vestibuli and the lower duct is called the scala tympani. They are separated by a middle duct, called the scala media. A liquid called **endolymphatic fluid** or **endolymph** fills the scala media, whereas the two outer ducts are filled with a different liquid called **perilymphatic fluid** or **perilymph**. The two outer ducts meet at the far end of the tube at an opening called the **helicotrema**. The stapes at the oval window is at the base of scala vestibuli, and the round window is at the basal end of the scala tympani. The scala media is separated from the scala vestibuli above it by Reissner's membrane, and from the scala tympani below it by the **basilar membrane**. Notice that the basilar membrane is narrowest at the base and becomes progressively wider toward the apex.

Perilymph is similar to most extracellular fluids in the sense that it contains a large concentration of sodium. On the other hand, endolymph is virtually unique among extracellular fluids because it contains a high concentration of potassium. The same fluids are contained in the balance portion of the inner ear, as discussed below. The membranous labyrinths of the hearing and balance systems are connected by a tiny duct called the **ductus reuniens**, forming one continuous endolymph-filled system. Another conduit, called the **endolymphatic duct**, leads from the membranous labyrinth in the vestibule to the **endolymphatic** sac partly located in a niche in the petrous part of the temporal bone and between the layers of dura in the posterior cranial fossa. In addition, the **cochlear aqueduct** leads from an opening in the scala tympani to the subarachnoid space.

The cochlear duct is ~ 35 mm long and is coiled in the form of a cone-shaped spiral staircase. The

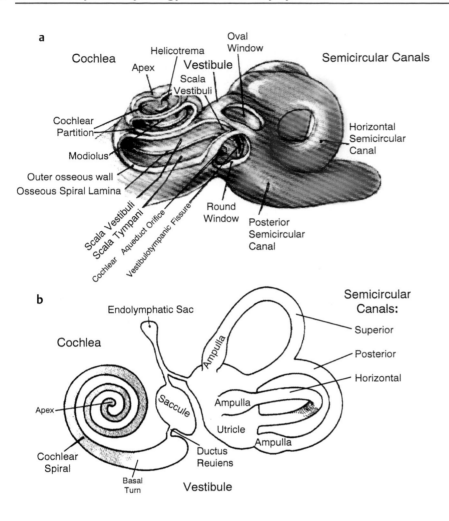

Fig. 2.23 The major landmarks of the osseous and membranous labyrinths. (Adapted from Proctor [1989], with permission.)

resulting arrangement looks like a 5 mm high snail shell that is 9 mm wide at its base and tapers toward the apex (**Fig. 2.23**). The superstructure of the spiral duct is a bony shelf called the **osseous spiral lamina** that makes ~2¾ turns around a central core called the **modiolus**, as shown in **Fig. 2.25**. **Fig. 2.25a** also shows that the medial side of the membranous duct (scala media) is attached to the lateral lip of the bony shelf, and follows it from base to apex. (Inside the cochlea, "medial" means toward the center core of the spiral, and "lateral" means toward the outer perimeter of the spiral, or away from the center core.) **Fig. 2.25b** shows how the cochlea would appear if cut down the center and opened to reveal the inside arrangement. Here we see several cross-sectional views of the cochlear duct going around the modiolus. The osseous spiral lamina forms a shelf that divides each section of the duct into an upper and lower part. The section of each duct above the shelf is the scala vestibuli and the section below the shelf is the scala tympani. The membranous duct that is attached to the lip of the shelf in **Fig. 2.25a**

is not shown in **Fig. 2.25b**; however, it would continue across the duct to form the middle chamber, the scala media. The osseous spiral lamina is actually composed of two plates separated by a space that serves as a passageway for nerve fibers. In addition, the core of the modiolus itself is hollow and leads to the **internal auditory meatus** (**Fig. 2.25b**), providing a conduit for the auditory nerve and blood supply to the cochlea.

Fig. 2.26 is a cross section of one part of the cochlear duct, showing the scala media between the scala vestibuli above and the scala tympani below, as well as auditory nerve cells coursing through the osseous spiral lamina toward the modiolus. A close-up view emphasizing the structures inside the scala media is shown in **Fig. 2.27**. Both of these figures are oriented so that the modiolus is toward the left (medial) and the outer wall of the cochlea is toward the right (lateral). The outer wall of the cochlear duct is covered with a band of fibrous connective tissue called the **spiral ligament**. The top of the osseous spiral lamina is covered by a thickened band of peri-

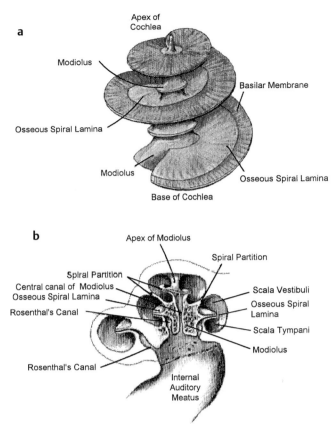

Fig. 2.24 **(a)** A model made of a rubber hose glued within a steel pipe to represent an uncurled cochlea. **(b)** Conceptual drawing of an uncoiled cochlea.

Fig. 2.25 **(a)** The superstructure of the cochlea is a bony shelf called the osseous spiral lamina that spirals around a central core called the modiolus. **(b)** Cross section through the cochlea showing the cochlear duct coiling around the modiolus. The center of the modiolus is hollow and leads to the internal auditory meatus. (Adapted from Proctor [1989], with permission.)

osteum called the **limbus**. The **basilar membrane** is a fibrous membrane that runs horizontally from the osseous spiral lamina to the spiral ligament. Reissner's membrane is a thin membrane that goes from the top of the medial aspect of the limbus to the spiral ligament at an upward angle of ~ 45°. The endolymph-filled scala media is contained within these borders, with the perilymph-filled scalae vestibuli and tympani above and below, respectively.

The rounded space formed by the concave lateral side of the limbus is called the **internal spiral sulcus**. The **organ of Corti** is the sensory organ for hearing, and sits on the basilar membrane lateral to the internal spiral sulcus. The **tectorial membrane** arises from the upper lip of the limbus and forms the overlying membrane of the organ of Corti. The tectorial membrane is mainly composed of collagen fibers that give it considerable tensile strength and make it quite compliant (Zwislocki, Chamberlain, & Slepecky 1988). The lateral margin of the tectorial membrane attaches via a net of fibers to the lateral supporting

cells of the organ of Corti. Attached to the spiral ligament is a rich network of capillaries called the **stria vascularis** that maintain the chemical environment of the scala media.

The organ of Corti is a complex arrangement of sensory hair cells along with various accessory cells and structures. The conspicuous upside-down "Y" seen roughly in the center of the organ of Corti composes the **pillars** or **rods of Corti**. These pillar cells enclose a triangular space called the **tunnel of Corti**. The thin lines running across the tunnel are auditory nerve fibers (discussed later). Medial to the tunnel of Corti is a single row of **inner hair cells (IHCs)** and lateral to it are three rows of **outer hair cells (OHCs)**. These cells are called hair cells because they are topped by tufts of microscopic hairs called stereocilia. The stereocilia extend upward from the **cuticular plate**, which is a thickening on the top of the hair cell. Only one inner hair cell and three outer hair cells are shown in **Fig. 2.27** because this drawing cuts across the cochlear tube, whereas these rows of cells

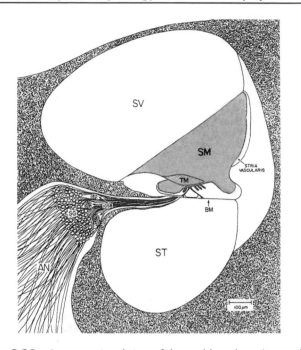

Fig. 2.26 Cross-sectional view of the cochlear duct. (SV, scala vestibuli; SM, scala media; ST, scala tympani; TM, tectorial membrane; BM, basilar membrane; IGSB, intraganglionic spiral bundle, principally composed of efferents; SG, spiral ganglion; AN, auditory nerve.) (From Kiang et al [1986], with permission of *Hearing Research*.)

(along with all of the organ of Corti) course up the length of the duct. A variety of supporting cells are also identified in the figure, although it is not necessary to address them individually in an introductory discussion. Auditory nerve cells or fibers from the hair cells enter the osseous spiral lamina through openings called the **habenula perforata**.

An impervious layer called the **reticular lamina** is formed by the tops of the hair cells, as well as by the upper ends of the tunnel cells and other supporting cells. The reticular lamina isolates the underlying structures of the organ of Corti from the rest of the scala media above them. Moreover, the fluid in the spaces below the reticular lamina is similar to the perilymph of the scala tympani[1] which provides the sodium-rich environment that is needed for the functioning of the hair cells and unmyelinated nerve fibers in the organ of Corti. In addition, endolymph must be kept out because it is toxic to the hair cells.

---

[1] It was previously thought to be a separate fluid known as cortilymph.

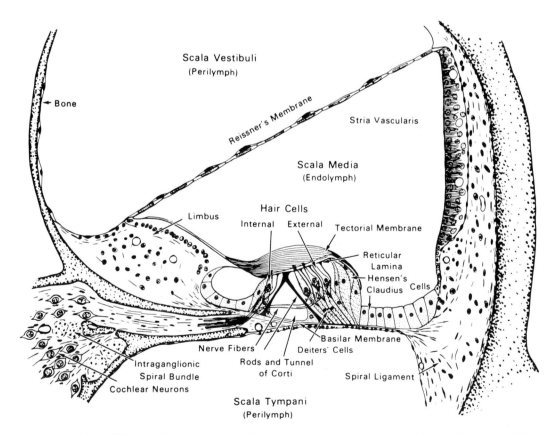

Fig. 2.27 Cross-sectional view of the cochlear duct emphasizing the organ of Corti in the scala media. (Adapted from Davis [1962], with permission of the *Journal of the Acoustical Society of America*.)

Fig. 2.28 shows the upper surface of the reticular lamina. Here we can easily see the three rows of outer hair cells topped by a W- or V-shaped cluster of stereocilia. The tops of the inner hair cells are identified by the row of stereocilia bunches located toward the right side of the figure. The stereocilia on top of the IHCs have a very wide U shape even though they seem to form a straight line at first glance. The tectorial membrane overlays the reticular lamina. The stereocilia of the OHCs are firmly attached to the undersurface of the tectorial membrane. On the other hand, it appears that the stereocilia of the IHCs are not attached to the tectorial membrane.

Electrical voltage differences called **resting potentials** exist between different parts of the cochlea. The perilymph is usually considered to be the reference point, so that its voltage is 0 millivolts (mV). Compared with the perilymph, the endolymph has polarity of about +100 mV, and is called the **endocochlear potential** (Peak, Sohmer, & Weiss 1969). The electrical potential inside the hair cells is called the **intracellular potential**, and is about –40 mV in the IHCs and –70 mV in the OHCs (Dallos 1986).

Hair Cells

There are ~ 3500 inner hair cells and 12,000 outer hair cells in each ear. Schematic representations of the two kinds of cochlear hair cells are shown in **Fig. 2.29**. The IHCs are flask-shaped, whereas the OHCs are tube-like. Both types have rows of different-size stereocilia protruding from the cuticular plates at their top ends. There is also a noncuticular area containing another kind of cilium called the **basal body** or **rudimentary kinocilium** just beyond the tallest row of stereocilia. In spite of the similarities between inner and outer hair cells, one cannot help but notice their many differences. We have already seen that the inner and outer hair cells differ substantially in number, occupy different locations in the organ of Corti, and relate differently to the tectorial membrane. We shall see that they have different neural connections as well. Notice in the drawings that the distribution of cellular structures is also different for the two types of cells. The inner hair cells have concentrations of Golgi apparatus, mitochondria, and other organelles associated with the extensive metabolic activity needed to support the sensory reception process. The outer hair cells contain **contractile proteins** and several structural characteristics that are usually associated with muscle cells. In fact, the OHCs are able to shorten and lengthen (both pull and push) in response to neural signals and chemical agents. Their **motility** is important for the normal

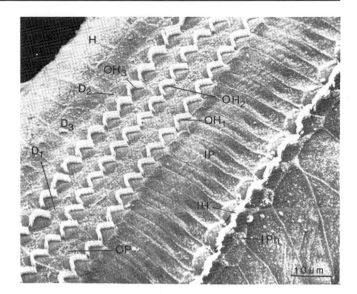

Fig. 2.28 The upper surface of the reticular lamina. Notice the stereocilia extending upward from the single row of inner hair cells (IH) and the three rows of outer hair cells (OH1, OH2, OH3). The cilia are white in the figure. This picture is oriented so that the medial side of the duct (modiolus) is toward the right and the lateral or outer side (spiral ligament) is toward the left. (D1–D3, Deiters' cells; OP and IP, outer and inner pillar cells; IPh, inner phalangeal cells; H, Hensen's cells.) (From Lim [1986a], with permission of *Hearing Research*.)

operation of the cochlea. The interested student will readily find several more detailed explanations of this and related issues elsewhere (Lippe 1986; Dallos 1988; Pickles 1988; Brownell 1990; Gelfand 2010).

The hair cells are activated when their stereocilia are bent toward the basal body. The basal body is at

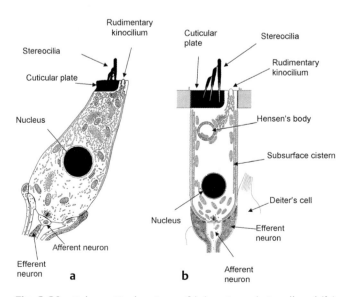

Fig. 2.29 Schematic drawings of **(a)** an inner hair cell and **(b)** an outer hair cell. (From Lim [1986b], with permission.)

the base of the W- or V-shaped arrangement of the stereocilia, which is oriented toward the spiral ligament on the outer wall of the cochlear duct, that is, away from the modiolus (**Fig. 2.28**). Thus, *hair cells respond when their stereocilia are caused to bend toward the lateral wall of the duct, or away from the modiolus.* The reason why the hair cell responds when the stereocilia bend in a particular direction requires a closer look at the stereocilia themselves. **Fig. 2.30** shows a close-up of a representative bunch of stereocilia. Notice that there are various kinds of tiny filaments or **cross-links** between the stereocilia.

Fig. 2.31 highlights the kind of filament that goes *upward* from the top of a shorter cilium to the side of a taller one. These filaments are known as a **tip-links**, as well as upward-pointing and tip-to-side cross-links. The mechanism of hair cell activation is based on this relationship (Pickles, Comis, & Osborne 1984; Hudspeth 1985; Pickles & Corey 1992), and is illustrated in **Fig. 2.32**. Bending of the stereocilia in the direction just described pulls or stretches the upward-pointing cross-link, as in the figure panel labeled "Excitation." Pulling the filament opens a **pore** (analogous to a trapdoor) on the top of the shorter cilium, which permits ions to flow through it, thereby activating the cell. Bending of the stereocilia in the opposite direction compresses the filaments so that the pore is closed, as shown in the figure panel labeled "Inhibition." This appears to be the mechanism by which mechanical-to-electrochemical transduction occurs in the hair cells. The result-ing response of the hair cell is then transmitted to the adjoining auditory neurons.

Innervation of the Cochlea

The cochlear hair cells are connected to the auditory nervous system by their synapses with auditory nerve fibers within the organ of Corti. These nerve fibers go through the habenula perforata leading to their cell bodies to form the **spiral ganglia** located in **Rosenthal's canal** of the modiolus, and then proceed into the internal auditory meatus (**Fig. 2.25b, Fig. 2.26,** and **Fig. 2.27**). The neural fibers twist like the fibers of a rope to form the auditory nerve. In general, neurons originating from the apex of the cochlea are arranged toward the core of the nerve trunk and those from the base of the cochlea spi-

Fig. 2.31 Upward-pointing (tip-to-side) cross-links going from the top of a shorter cilium upward to the side of a taller one are shown by arrows and the close-up in the insert. A row-to-row cross-link is also shown (*white arrowhead*). These filaments are usually called tip-links. (From Pickles, Comis, & Osborne [1984], with permission of *Hearing Research*.)

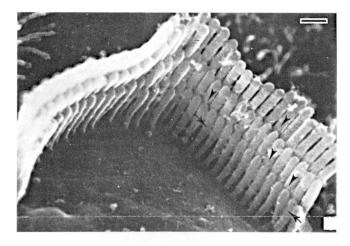

Fig. 2.30 Cross-linking filaments between stereocilia. *Arrows* show side-to-side cross-links between adjacent stereocilia. *Arrowheads* show upward-pointing or tip-to-side cross-links that go from the top of a shorter cilium upward to the side of another cilium in the next taller row. (From Furness & Hackney [1986], with permission of *Hearing Research*.)

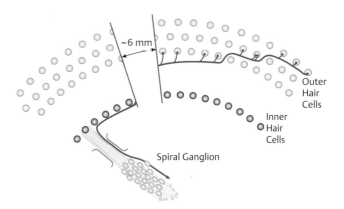

Fig. 2.32 Bending of the stereocilia in one direction leads to excitation by stretching upward-pointing cross-links, thereby opening a pore that permits ions to flow. Bending in the opposite direction causes inhibition because the pore closes. (From Pickles, Comis, & Osborne [1984], with permission of *Hearing Research.*)

Fig. 2.33 The distribution of auditory neurons to the inner and outer hair cells. (From Spoendlin H. 1978. The afferent innervation of the cochlea. In: Naunton RF, Fernandez C, eds. *Electrical Activity of the Auditory Nervous System.* New York, NY: Academic Press.)

ral are closer to the outside. The innervation of the cochlea involves both afferent and efferent neurons. The **afferent** nerve supply is made up of *ascending* sensory neurons that send signals from the cochlea to the nervous system. The **efferent** nerve supply includes a much smaller population of *descending* neurons that send signals from the nervous system to the cochlea.

Afferent Innervation

The afferent auditory nerve supply is unequally distributed between the inner and outer hair cells and involves two different kinds of neurons (Spoendlin 1969, 1975, 1978; Kiang, Rho, Northrop, Liberman, & Ryugo 1982; Liberman 1982a). These relationships are shown in **Fig. 2.33** and **Fig. 2.34**. Approximately 95% of the afferent auditory neurons supply the inner hair cells and the remaining 5% go to the outer hair cells. Each IHC exclusively receives ~ 20 nerve fibers that come to it directly in the radial direction from the habenula perforata. The wiring diagram is much different for the much smaller number of afferent fibers that supply the OHCs. These neurons bypass the IHCs, cross under the tunnel of Corti **(Fig. 2.27)**, turn and travel ~ 0.6 mm along the spiral toward the base of the cochlea, and then send collateral fibers to ~ 10 *different* OHCs. In addition, each OHC receives collateral fibers from several different neurons. Because of the paths that they follow, the neurons that go to the IHCs are called **inner radial fibers** and the ones that go to the OHCs are called **outer spiral fibers**. All of these fibers are unmyelinated while they are inside the organ of Corti.

After exiting the organ of Corti, the inner radial fibers from the IHCs continue in the modiolus as **type I auditory neurons**. These fibers are large-diameter, myelinated, bipolar sensory neurons. A bipolar neuron has a cell body located somewhere along the axon as opposed to being at one end. Outer spiral fibers from the OHCs continue as **type II auditory neurons**, which are unmyelinated, small in diameter, and pseudo-monopolar rather than bipolar. Type I and type II auditory neurons are illustrated just below the spiral ganglion in **Fig. 2.34**. Most if not all of what we know about the functioning of auditory nerve fibers is derived from the type I neurons. In summary: (1) the IHCs are innervated by inner radial fibers that continue outside the organ of Corti as type I auditory neurons; and (2) the OHCs are innervated by outer spiral fibers that continue outside the organ of Corti as type II auditory neurons.

Efferent Innervation

The cochlea receives efferent signals from the nervous system via the **olivocochlear bundle (Rasmussen's bundle)**, which is a series of descending pathways that go from the superior olivary complex to the cochlea (Guinan 2006). Approximately 1600 efferent neurons from the olivocochlear bundle enter the temporal bone along with the vestibular branch of the eighth nerve, and then split off to enter the cochlea, where they are then distributed to the hair cells. The endings of the efferent neurons have vesicles containing the chemical neurotransmitter acetylcholine, and they communicate differently with the inner and outer hair cells.

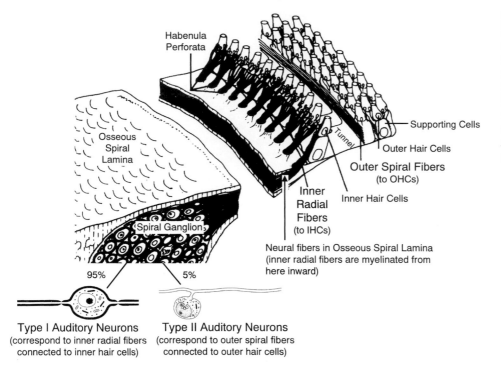

Fig. 2.34 Associations between inner hair cells, inner radial fibers, and type I auditory neurons in the spiral ganglion; and outer hair cells, outer spiral fibers, and type II auditory neurons. (Based on Spoendlin H. The afferent innervation of the cochlea. In: Naunton RF, Fernandez C, eds. *Electrical Activity of the Auditory Nervous System.* ©1978 by Academic Press.)

The distribution of efferent fibers is the opposite of that for the afferents, that is, most of them go to the outer hair cells. The attachments of the efferent neurons are also different for the two groups of hair cells. Efferent neurons synapse *directly* with OHCs. As a result, efferent neurons act on OHCs before they synapse with their afferent neurons (presynaptically). However, this is not the case for the inner hair cells. Here, the efferent fiber synapses with the *afferent neurons that are associated with the inner hair cells,* so that their effect is postsynaptic. In other words, the efferent neuron acts directly on an outer hair cell, but for inner hair cells the efferent fiber acts on the afferent neuron downstream of its synapse with the hair cell.

■ Vestibular Organs and Innervation

The sensory receptor organs of the vestibular system share the bony and membranous labyrinths with the cochlea (**Fig. 2.23**). The balance end organs are located posterior to the cochlea and include the **utricle** and **saccule**, which are within the vestibule, as well as the **semicircular canals**.

Each ear contains three semicircular canals that respond to angular acceleration, that is, circular

motions such as turning one's head. These canals are at right angles to each other so that they can respond to angular motion in any direction. Each canal has an **ampulla**, which is a widening anteriorly where it joins the vestibule as shown in **Fig. 2.35**. The ampulla contains a receptor organ called the crista. The base of the crista contains the **vestibular hair cells** and their supporting cells. These hair cells are very similar to cochlear hair cells, except that they have a large **kinocilium** instead of a basal body. The top portion of the crista is the **cupula**, a mound-shaped gelatinous mass that blocks the flow of endolymph in the canal, much like a swinging door. The stereocilia of the hair cells extend into the cupula. The vestibular hair cell synapses with vestibular neurons below it, which are part of the eighth cranial nerve.

The operation of the semicircular canals is quite straightforward. First, consider a simple experiment with a bowl of water that illustrates the concept. If you quickly revolve the bowl clockwise, you will notice the motion of the water lags behind the motion of the bowl. This occurs because of the inertia of the water (due to its mass), as well as the ability of the water to move within the bowl. In relative terms, the lagging behind of the water when the bowl moves clockwise is the same as if the bowl had stood still and the water moved counterclockwise. In this experiment the bowl represents the head and the water represents the endolymph within a

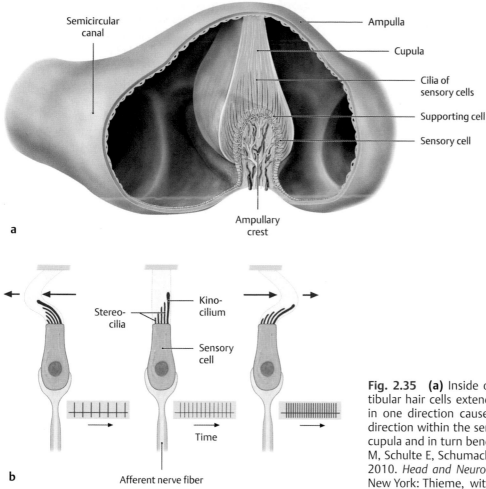

Semicircular canal

Ampulla

Cupula

Cilia of sensory cells

Supporting cell

Sensory cell

Ampullary crest

a

Stereo-cilia

Kino-cilium

Sensory cell

Time

b

Afferent nerve fiber

Fig. 2.35 **(a)** Inside of the ampulla, the cilia of the vestibular hair cells extend into the cupula. **(b)** Head turning in one direction causes endolymph flow in the opposite direction within the semicircular canals, which deflects the cupula and in turn bends the hair cell cilia. (From Schuenke M, Schulte E, Schumacher U, Ross LM, Lamperti ED, Voll M. 2010. *Head and Neuroanatomy* [*Thieme Atlas of Anatomy*]. New York: Thieme, with permission.)

semicircular canal. Similarly, the endolymph in the semicircular canals will lag behind when the head turns, which is the same as the motion of the endolymph in the opposite direction. For example, turning the head to the right causes a relative motion of the endolymph to the left in the horizontal (lateral) semicircular canals.

Recall that the cupula crosses the ampulla of the canal like a swinging door. Thus, the flow of the endolymph in the semicircular canals will deflect the cupula. Because the hair cell cilia extend into the cupula, deflection of the cupula also bends the cilia, thereby stimulating the hair cells, which in turn transmits their response to the underlying neurons. As **Fig. 2.35** shows, the response of the hair cells is excitatory (the neurons fire faster) when the stereocilia bend toward the kinocilium, and inhibitory (the neurons fire slower) when they bend away from it. As illustrated in the left panel of the figure, the hair cells are oriented in the horizontal (lateral) canal so that the endolymph flow deflecting the cupula

toward the utricle (utriculopedal flow) is excitatory, whereas endolymph flow away from the ampulla (utriculofugal flow) is inhibitory. The right panel in the figure shows that the opposite arrangement exists in the two vertical semicircular canals.

The utricle and saccule respond to gravity and linear acceleration, which means motion in a straight line (such as front–back, right–left, or up–down). The sensory receptor organs of the utricle and saccule are called the **maculae**. Each macule contains vestibular hair cells that synapse with the eighth nerve neurons. Their cilia project up into a gelatinous material called the **otolith membrane**, on top of which are found calcium carbonate crystals called **otoliths**. For this reason, the utricle and saccule are also called the **otolith organs**. The hair cells are stimulated when the otolith bears down on the otolith membrane, thereby deflecting the cilia. This can be caused by gravity or by linear acceleration, in which case the inertia of the otoliths causes them to lag behind the movement of the head. The otolith organs can respond to gravity or linear acceleration in any direction because of their orientation inside the vestibule and the way in which the hair cells are arranged along each macule. The saccule is approximately vertical and the utricle is roughly horizontal. In addition, hair cells are organized with opposite orientations on each side of a curved "line" (the **striola**) along each macule. Consequently, motion in any direction will cause some hair cells to be stimulated (i.e., their stereocilia will bend toward the kinocilium).

■ Functioning of the Sensorineural Mechanism

Stimulation is transmitted to the cochlear fluids by the in-and-out motions of the stapedial footplate at the oval window at the base of the cochlea. The oval window leads into the upper chamber (scala vestibuli). Hence, a given inward motion will cause the fluids to be displaced downward, pushing downward on the basilar membrane, and a given outward motion will displace the fluids and basilar membrane upward. The trick is to translate this vibratory stimulation into the bending of the hair cell stereocilia in the right direction, which we already know is necessary to activate the sensory process. In addition, the mechanism for accomplishing this activity must account for our ability to hear different pitches.

Traditional Theories

Historically, two kinds of classical theories have attempted to explain how basilar membrane vibrations are converted into neural signals that distinguish between different frequencies. In the **resonance place theory**, Helmholtz (1895) proposed that the basilar membrane was constructed of segments that resonated in response to different frequencies, and that these segments were arranged according to location (place) along the length of the basilar membrane. To achieve this tuning, the segments at different locations would have to be under different degrees of tension. (We all know that changing the tension on a guitar string changes its pitch, and that musicians adjust this tension to tune the instrument.) According to resonance theory, a sound entering the cochlea causes the vibration of the segments that are tuned to (resonate at) the frequencies that it contains. Because these resonators are laid out according to place, the locations of the vibrating segments signal which frequencies are present. In contrast, **temporal** (or **frequency**) **theories** of hearing, like Rutherford's (1886) "telephone theory," claimed that the entire cochlea

responds as a whole to all frequencies instead of being activated on a place-by-place basis. Here, all aspects of the stimulus waveform would be transmitted to the auditory nerve (like a telephone receiver connected to the telephone wire), and then the frequency analysis is accomplished at higher levels in the auditory system.

The resonance theory had several significant problems, two of which will be mentioned. Sharply tuned resonators damp very slowly, so they would have to continue vibrating long after the stimulus is gone. This after-ringing would be like a never-ending echo that does not exist, and would preclude useful hearing if it did. In addition, this theory cannot explain why we hear a pitch corresponding to 100 Hz when we are presented with a stream of clicks at a rate of 100 per second, or when we are presented with several harmonics of 100 Hz (e.g., 1200, 1300, and 1400 Hz). After all, how can the 100 Hz segment of the basilar membrane respond when a 100 Hz signal is not physically present?

Temporal theory had its own problems. For example, damage to a certain part of the cochlea results in a hearing loss for certain frequencies but not for others (e.g., basal damage causes high-frequency hearing loss). Yet temporal theory says that location and frequency are unrelated. In addition, the auditory nerve must be able to carry all the information in the sound wave. Neurons code information in the form of individual all-or-none neural discharges (described later in this chapter). There is an *absolute refractory period* of ~ 1 millisecond between discharges during which they cannot fire, no matter how powerful the stimulus might be. It would be no problem for a neuron to fire 410 times per second for a 410 Hz signal, or 873 times per second for an 873 Hz signal, but the 1 millisecond refractory period limits the maximum firing rate to roughly 1000 times per second. Hence, temporal theory could not explain how we hear the frequencies well above ~ 1000 Hz.

The resonance model of place theory and the old temporal theories that denied place coding in the cochlea were both wrong. Place coding is very much real, but it operates according to the **traveling wave** model (Bekesy 1960), discussed later. Temporal coding also exists. Even though neurons cannot respond to all of the individual cycles, it has been shown they can follow the periodicity of a sound for frequencies as high as ~ 5000 Hz on a probability basis, even though they actually fire in response to relatively few individual cycles (e.g., Kiang 1965). In other words, even though a particular neuron may not discharge very often, when it does fire it will do so in synchrony with a certain phase of the stimulus. The synchronous nature of neural discharges with respect to a certain phase of the signal is called **phase locking**.

The **volley principle** (Wever 1949) proposed that several neurons operating *as a group* could fire in response to each cycle of a high-frequency sound, even though none of them can do so individually. This is possible if one neuron fires in response to one cycle, and another neuron fires in response to the next cycle (while the first nerve cell is still in its refractory period), etc. The **place-volley theory** (Wever & Lawrence 1954) involves the combined operation of both place and temporal mechanisms. Low frequencies are handled by temporal coding, high frequencies by place, and an interaction of the two mechanisms occurs for the wide range of frequencies between the two extremes.

Traveling Wave Theory

Bekesy's (1960[2]) **traveling wave theory** describes how frequency is coded by place in the cochlea. Contrary to resonance theory, Bekesy found that the basilar membrane is not under any tension, but that its elasticity is essentially uniform. Because the basilar membrane gets wider going toward the top, the apex, the result is a *gradation of stiffness* along its length, going from *stiffest at the base* (near the stapes) to *least stiff at the apex* (near the helicotrema). As a result of this stiffness gradient, sounds transmitted to the cochlea develop a special kind of wave pattern on the basilar membrane that always travels

from the base up toward the apex, called the **traveling wave**.

The characteristic traveling wave pattern is shown in **Fig. 2.36**. In this diagram, the x-axis represents the distance in millimeters up the basilar membrane from the stapes. In the figure the base of the cochlea would be toward the left and the apex of the cochlea would be toward the right. The y-axis represents the relative amount of basilar membrane displacement. The outer dashed lines represent the *envelope* of the traveling wave displacement pattern along the basilar membrane. It shows that the traveling wave involves a displacement pattern that (1) gradually increases in amplitude as it moves up the basilar membrane, (2) reaches a peak at a certain location, and (3) decays in amplitude rather quickly just beyond the peak. The four solid lines inside the envelope represent the *instantaneous displacements* of the basilar membrane at four phases of the wave cycle. In other words, the instantaneous displacement of the basilar membrane changes from moment to moment, proceeding from **a** to **b** to **c** to **d**, and so on. If these four instantaneous displacement curves were expanded into a complete set, then they would fill the shape of the traveling wave envelope. Imagine a movie in which each successive frame contains one of the instantaneous displacements, arranged in order. The resulting movie image would be a wave that travels up the cochlea (from left to right in the figure) with the overall shape of the traveling wave envelope indicated by the dashed lines.

The location (place) of the traveling wave peak along the basilar membrane depends on the frequency of the sound. In other words, the traveling wave is the mechanism that translates signal frequency into place of stimulation along the basilar membrane. High frequencies are represented toward

---

[2] Bekesy's work on the traveling wave is largely reproduced in his book *Experiments in Hearing* (1960). For simplicity, the book is cited here as a general reference for this body of work; however, the figures cite the original sources.

Fig. 2.36 Characteristics of the traveling wave. This particular traveling wave was generated by a 200 Hz stimulus, and peaked at a distance of ~ 29 mm from the base of the cochlea. (Based on Bekesy [1953].)

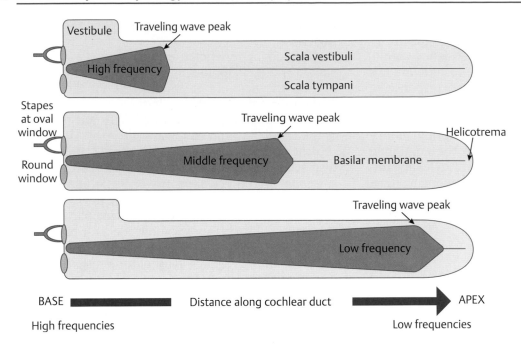

Fig. 2.37 The traveling wave is the place coding mechanism of the cochlea. The artist's conceptualization shows that the traveling wave peak occurs toward the base of the cochlea for high frequencies and toward the apex for low frequencies.

the base of the cochlea, and successively lower frequencies are represented closer and closer to the apex, as illustrated in **Fig. 2.37**. The traveling wave brings the stimulus to the appropriate location for a given frequency, which involves motion *along* the length of cochlear duct. However, the stereocilia must be bent away from the modiolus in order for the hair cells to respond. In other words, the traveling wave moves *along* the cochlear duct (in the longitudinal direction) but the stereocilia must be bent *across* the duct (in the *radial* direction). This would be a problem if the basilar membrane was free on both sides so that its displacement would generate forces only in the *longitudinal* direction, as in **Fig. 2.38a**, but this is not the case. The basilar membrane is actually attached along both sides, at the osseous spiral lamina medially and at the spiral ligament laterally. As a result, the traveling wave will also cause a *radial* force to be applied *across* the duct near the traveling wave peak, as in **Fig. 2.38b**. (This type of effect can be approximated by jiggling the free end of a bed sheet when its sides are tucked under the sides of the mattress.)

This radial force near the traveling wave peak causes the stereocilia to bend away from the modiolus, thereby activating the hair cells by the following mechanism (Davis 1958). The medial attachment of the basilar membrane is at the tip of the osseous spiral lamina. Hence, up or down motions will cause the basilar membrane to pivot around this point. The hair cells and reticular lamina also follow this motion. On the other hand, the tectorial membrane

is attached at the lip of the limbus, so that it has a different pivot point than the reticular lamina. As a result of these different pivot points, upward and downward deflections will cause the reticular lamina and the tectorial membrane to move relative to one another. Moreover, the increasing curvature of the cochlear spiral has an enhancing effect because it concentrates vibrations toward the outer wall of the duct, especially for lower frequencies (Manoussaki, Dimitriadis, & Chadwick 2006). The stereocilia extend between these two differently hinged mem-

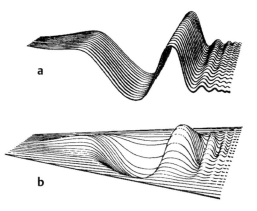

Fig. 2.38 **(a)** Imagined basilar membrane vibration pattern if it were not fixed along its sides. **(b)** Actual basilar membrane vibration pattern, with forces in the radial direction in the vicinity of the traveling wave peak. (From Tonndorf [1960], with permission of the *Journal of the Acoustical Society of America*.)

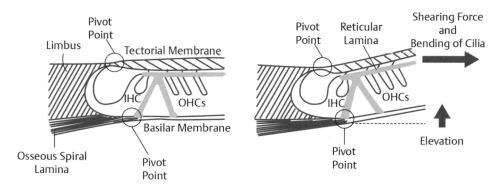

Fig. 2.39 Relative motion between the basilar and tectorial membranes places a shearing force on the stereocilia so they are bent away from the modiolus when the cochlear duct is displaced upward. OHCs, outer hair cells; IHC, inner hair cell. (Based on Davis [1958].)

branes, and are therefore subjected to a **shearing** action or shearing force when displacement of the duct causes these two membranes to move relative to each other. This shearing action bends the cilia away from the modiolus when the cochlear duct is displaced upward, as illustrated in **Fig. 2.39**. The OHC cilia are sheared because they are attached to the tectorial membrane, and the IHC cilia are sheared because of the drag imposed on them by the surrounding fluid when the membranes are displaced (Dallos, Billone, Durrant, Wang, & Raynor 1972). The result is activation of the hair cells leading to the excitation of their associated auditory neurons. [Shearing can sometimes occur with downward deflections because the flexibility of the tectorial membrane allows it to bend over the internal sulcus (e.g., Steel 1983).]

The electrochemical activity involved in the hair cell response activity produces electrical signals called **receptor potentials**, which can be monitored with electrodes. One of these receptor potentials is an AC (alternating current) signal that faithfully represents the stimulus waveform, called the **cochlear microphonic**. The other receptor potential is the **summating potential**, which appears as a deviation or shift in the DC (direct current) baseline.

The Cochlear Amplifier

Recall that the outer hair cells are directly connected to the tectorial membrane, receive neural signals from the olivocochlear bundle, and have the capability of motility. These characteristics constitute an active, micromechanical system that sensitizes and fine-tunes the responsiveness of the cochlea, known as the **cochlear amplifier** (Davis 1983). In other words, the cochlear amplifier enhances the signal received by the inner hair cells so they can be activated by faint sound levels and respond faithfully to

narrow frequency ranges. This mechanism accounts for the sensitivity needed to hear soft sounds and the ability to hear fine frequency distinctions. **Fig. 2.40** shows an example of the sharply tuned response (tuning curve) of a normal cochlea that is seen only in live animals with healthy cochleas (Russell & Sellick 1977; Khanna & Leonard 1982; Sellick, Patuzzi, & Johnstone 1982). In particular, the sharp peak is dependent on the integrity of the outer hair

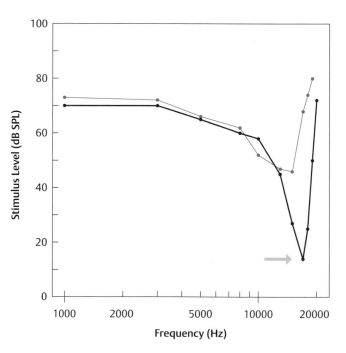

Fig. 2.40 The sharply peaked curve reveals the very narrow, mechanical tuning of the basilar membrane in a completely healthy cochlea (*arrow*). The sharp peak is lost when the integrity of the cochlea is compromised, or postmortem, as shown by the other curve. (Idealized curves based on findings by Sellick et al [1982].)

cells (e.g., Kiang, Liberman, Sewell, & Guinan 1986). Notice that the sharp peak is missing for the other curve in the figure, representing a situation where these conditions have not been met. The stria vascularis appears to be the source of metabolic energy for the cochlear amplifier. These active processes also appear to be responsible for the ability of the cochlea to *produce* sounds called **otoacoustic emissions** that can be picked up by sensitive microphones in the ear canal (Chapter 11).

Auditory Nerve Responses

Neurons produce *all-or-none electrical discharges* called **action potentials** which are recorded as **spikes**, as illustrated in **Fig. 2.41**. The number of spikes per second is called the **firing** or **discharge rate**. Auditory neurons have a certain ongoing firing rate even when they are not being stimulated, called the **spontaneous firing rate (Fig. 2.41a)**. Stimulation causes the firing rate to increase (**Fig. 2.41b**), and raising the stimulus level causes the neuron to fire even faster (**Fig. 2.41c**), at least within certain limits. The faintest sound level that induces a response from a neuron is called its **threshold**.[3]

Fig. 2.42 shows that an auditory neuron has a **dynamic range** over which its firing rate increases with stimulus level, after which the firing rate **saturates** or stops growing as the stimulus level increases further. Auditory neurons vary in threshold over a

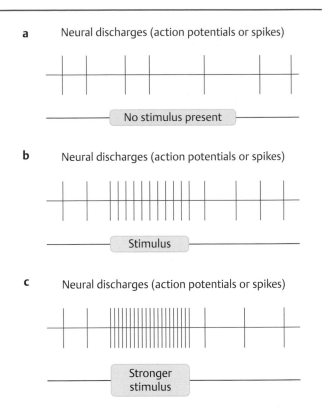

a Neural discharges (action potentials or spikes)

No stimulus present

b Neural discharges (action potentials or spikes)

Stimulus

c Neural discharges (action potentials or spikes)

Stronger stimulus

Fig. 2.41 Idealized firing rates of an auditory neuron **(a)** in the absence of stimulation (spontaneous rate), **(b)** with a relative weaker stimulus, and **(c)** with a relatively stronger stimulus.

[3] Auditory neurons often respond with a reduction in firing rate from the spontaneous rate at bare threshold levels, above which increasing stimulus levels result in an increasing firing rate.

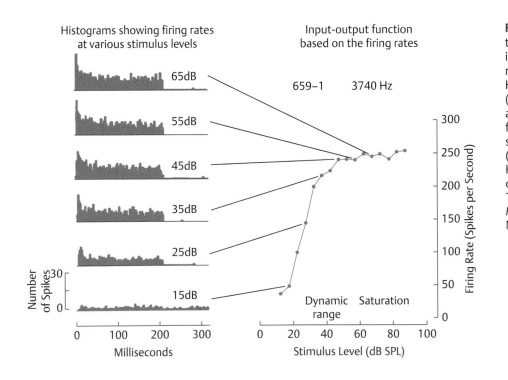

Fig. 2.42 The firing rate of an auditory neuron increases as the stimulus intensity increases within its dynamic range, and eventually plateaus. Left: Histograms showing firing rates. (Notice that the discharge pattern has an initial peak followed by an ongoing firing rate that continues during the stimulus.) Right: Input-out function. (Adapted from Salvi, Henderson, & Hamernik [1983]. Physiological bases of sensorineural hearing loss. In: Tobias JV, Schubert ED, eds. *Hearing Research and Theory,* Vol. 2. New York, NY: Academic Press.)

range of ~ 60 dB or more, and their dynamic ranges are ~ 25 dB wide for some groups of auditory neurons and ~ 40 dB or more for others (e.g., Sachs & Abbas 1974; Liberman 1988). These gradations of thresholds and dynamic ranges contribute to the ability of the auditory nerve to represent a wide range of sound intensities.

Auditory neurons represent frequency information by both place and temporal coding. The place coding mechanism is represented by the tuning curves in **Fig. 2.43** (Kiang 1965). Each tuning curve shows the range of frequencies to which a given nerve fiber responds at different levels of stimulation. A given curve was obtained here by finding the threshold for a particular neuron for many different frequencies. Let us concentrate on the curve highlighted by the arrow because it shows a complete set of thresholds over a wide range of frequencies. The narrow part of the curve shows that the neuron responds to a very limited range of frequencies at relatively soft levels (downward on the y-axis). The peak of the curve shows the lowest threshold of the neuron, and the frequency where this occurs is its **characteristic frequency (CF)**. The CF is 5000 Hz for the highlighted curve. The orderly arrangement of CFs reflects the places along the length of the cochlea where the neurons are connected (e.g., Liberman 1982b). The neuron responds to a slightly wider range of frequencies around its CF as the stimulus level is raised (upward on the y-axis). If the stimulus is raised high enough, then the neuron will respond to a wide range of frequencies extending well below its characteristic frequency. This phenomenon appears as the "tail" on the low-frequency side of the curve. However, the neuron is not responsive to much higher frequencies even when they are presented at very intense stimulus levels.

Another way to look at how auditory neurons respond to stimuli is illustrated by the graphs in **Fig. 2.44**. They show responses from four neurons that have characteristic frequencies of 540, 1170, 2610, and 2760 Hz. They were tested by presenting a click and then measuring how many times each neuron fires as a function of time since the onset of the click. Such a time delay is called a **latency**. This is done many times, and the number of spikes is then tallied for each latency. On each graph, latency is shown along the x-axis, and the number of spikes is shown vertically, as indicated in the insert. These graphs are called **post-stimulus time (PST) histograms** because tallies are shown on a histogram, and the histograms are arranged according to the time since ("post") the stimulus. The peaks show that the neurons tended to fire at certain latencies but not at other times. The latencies to the first peak get shorter as the characteristic frequency gets higher.

Fig. 2.43 Tuning curves of auditory neurons with a variety of characteristic frequencies. The y-axis shows signal intensity as decibels below some maximum value (0 dB indicates the most intense sound used, and –100 dB is 100 dB below that most intense sound). The *arrow* refers to material in the text. (Reproduced from *Discharge Patterns of Single Fibers in the Cat's Auditory Nerve* by NYS Kiang, with permission of The MIT Press, Cambridge, MA, © 1965, p. 87.)

Fig. 2.44 Selected post-stimulus time (PST) histograms showing the number of spikes (vertically) at different latencies since the onset of the click (horizontally). The PST histograms are shown for four nerve fibers with characteristic frequencies of 540,1170, 2610, and 2760 Hz. (Adapted from *Discharge Patterns of Single Fibers in the Cat's Auditory Nerve* by NYS Kiang, with permission of The MIT Press, Cambridge, MA, © 1965, p. 28.)

This occurs because it takes less time for the traveling wave to reach high-frequency locations near the base of the cochlea and more time for it to reach low-frequency places near the apex. The latencies between the successive peaks in each graph are equal to the period of each neuron's characteristic frequency (or 1/CF). The peaks alternate with times when there is little, if any, neural firing, which reveals temporal coding for individual cycles of the tone; spikes are timed to the upward deflections of the basilar membrane, and spaces (inhibition) occur when it is deflected downward. [For neurons with higher CFs (not shown), the later peaks clump together because the time between them (1/CF) gets very short; they eventually disappear when the neuron cannot fire fast enough due to its refractory period.]

Temporal coding for tones is revealed by the **period histogram**, which is a graph that shows the timing of neural firings during the presentation of a pure tone. The four period histograms in **Fig. 2.45** show the firing patterns produced by the same neuron during the presentation of pure tones at 412, 600, 900, and 1000 Hz. In each graph, the number of spikes is shown on the y-axis, and time during a tone is shown along the x-axis. Each x-axis is labeled with dots that are spaced at intervals equal to the period of the pure tone (2427 ms for 412 Hz, 1667 ms for 600 Hz, 1111 ms for 900 Hz, and 1000 ms or 1 millisecond for 1000 Hz). In each case, notice that the neural firing peaks line up with the periods of the tones (the dots), revealing a temporal representation of the signal frequency in the neuron's firing pattern.

Neural representations of the signal can also be viewed by measuring the overall response of the auditory nerve as a whole. In this case, we present a click or some other brief sound that can cause a very large number of neurons to fire at more or less the same time (synchronously). The result is the auditory nerve's **compound** or whole-nerve **action potential (AP)**. An idealized example is shown in **Fig. 2.46a**. This kind of waveform is really the average of many individual responses, and is obtained with techniques regularly used in clinical practice (discussed in Chapter 11). The compound AP has a major negative peak called **N1** that is usually followed by a second peak (**N2**), and often by a third peak as well (**N3**, not shown). It is quantified in terms of the amplitude and latency of the N1 peak. These parameters are shown as a function of stimulus level on an **amplitude-latency function** such as the one shown in **Fig. 2.46b**. Notice that the amplitude of N1 increases and its latency decreases as the level of the click stimulus increases. In other words, raising the intensity of the stimulus causes the AP to become bigger and occur sooner.

Fig. 2.45 Selected period histograms showing that neural firing during a pure tone is timed to the period of the tone. Dots along each x-axis correspond to the multiples of the period of the tone. (Adapted from Rose, Brugge, Anderson, & Hind [1967], with permission of the *Journal of Neurophysiology*.)

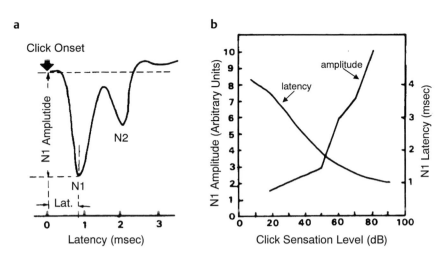

Fig. 2.46 **(a)** Idealized auditory nerve compound action potential. **(b)** Typical amplitude-latency function of the compound action potential based on findings by Yoshie (1968). (From Gelfand [2010], by courtesy of Informa, Inc.)

■ The Central Auditory Pathways

In this section we will track the major aspects of the ascending central auditory nervous system, as well as briefly overview the olivocochlear pathways and the central connections of the vestibular system.

Afferent Auditory Pathways

The major pathways of the **central auditory nervous system** from the cochlea to the auditory cortex are depicted in **Fig. 2.47**. Notice that the auditory pathway is quite *redundant*. Information originating from each ear is carried by pathways on both sides of the brain. The neural connections have what might be called a "series-parallel" wiring diagram. This is simpler than it sounds. A series circuit is like a string of cheap Christmas lights and a parallel circuit is like a string of expensive Christmas lights. The cheap string of lights has a single set of wires that go from bulb to bulb to bulb. We all know what happens if even one of the bulbs breaks: it interrupts the flow of electricity down the line so that all the lights go out. This does not happen with an expensive string of lights because the electricity goes to each bulb without passing through the preceding ones. Hence, if 3 bulbs blow in a string of 12, the remaining 9 bulbs will still light up. The term "series-parallel" is used because *the two arrangements exist together* in the central auditory pathways. For example, points A and C are connected by many neural fibers ("wires"); some of them go from A to B to C, and others bypass B on their way from A to C. As a result of the redundant pathways, a given lesion (analogous to a cut wire or

a blown bulb) that occurs *within* the *central* auditory pathway rarely causes a loss of hearing *sensitivity* because the signal is usually also represented along an alternative route. However, this does *not* mean that a central lesion does not cause auditory impairments. On the contrary, significant disturbances are caused by central lesions because they affect the processing of auditory information that allows you to determine sound locations, differentiate among sounds and background noises, and interpret speech.

What are the major pathways of the ascending auditory system? The auditory nerve exits the temporal bone through the internal auditory meatus and enters the brainstem at a location called the **cerebellopontine angle**, which is a term that describes the relationship of the pons and cerebellum in this area. The auditory nerve fibers, constituting the **first-order neurons** of the auditory pathway, terminate at either the **ventral cochlear nucleus** or the **dorsal cochlear nucleus**, where they synapse with the next level of nerve cells, called **second-order neurons.** Some second-order neurons go to the **superior olivary complex** on the same (ipsilateral) side of the brainstem, but a majority will decussate (cross to the opposite side) via the **trapezoid body** and proceed along the contralateral pathway. The fibers that cross over will either synapse with the opposite superior olivary complex or ascend in the contralateral **lateral lemniscus.** As a result, each superior olivary complex receives information from both ears, so that **bilateral representation** exists as low as this low level in the auditory nervous system.

Third-order neurons arise from the superior olivary complex and rise via the lateral lemniscus. Fibers also originate from the nuclei of the lateral lemniscus. Notice here that the pathway rising out of the lateral lemniscus contains neurons that originated from several different levels. Neurons ascending from this point may synapse at the **inferior colliculus** or may bypass the inferior colliculus on their way to the next level. Neurons originating from the inferior colliculus and those that bypass it ascend via the **brachium of the inferior colliculus** to terminate at the medial geniculate body of the **thalamus**. This is the last subcortical way station in the auditory pathway, and all ascending neurons that reach the medial geniculate body will synapse here. Neurons from the medial geniculate then ascend along a pathway called the **auditory radiations (auditory geniculocortical** or **thalamocortical radiations)** to the **auditory cortex** located in the transverse **temporal (Heschl's) gyrus**.

Recall that crossovers between the two sides of the brain occur beginning with second-order neurons from the cochlear nuclei, so that **bilateral** representation exists as low as the superior olivary complex. **Commissural tracts** also connect auditory nuclei on the two sides at the levels of the lateral lemniscus (via the **commissure of Probst**), the inferior colliculus (via the **commissure of the inferior colliculus**), and the auditory cortex (via the **corpus callosum**). However, communication does not occur between the medial geniculate bodies on the two sides.

Functioning of the Central Auditory System

The central auditory pathways include a variety of different kinds of neurons, and we find many different kinds of firing patterns as well. Several examples are shown in **Fig. 2.48**, where the *on-response* that is typical of auditory nerve fibers is identified as *primary-like*. The other examples are descriptively named according to their appearance as *choppers, build-up* units, *onset* units, and *pausers*. These are not the only types of firing patterns found in the central auditory system. For example, there are also fibers that respond to stimulus offset, and others have discharge patterns that decay exponentially over time. Neurons in the auditory cortex generally do not respond more than a few times to ongoing stimuli, but are more receptive to novel stimuli. For example, they might respond only at the beginning and end of a stimulus; only to sounds that rise, fall, or modulate in frequency; only to sounds coming from a certain direction; or only to moving sound sources.

The responses of central auditory neurons depend on the origin of the signal, as well as on the nature of the signal. Recall that information from both ears is represented in the pathways on both sides of the head as low as the superior olivary complex, and that there are commissural pathways between the two

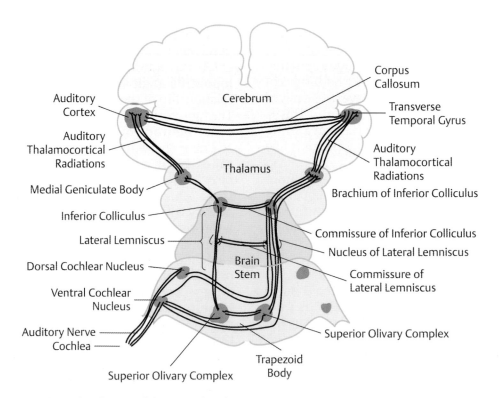

Fig. 2.47   The major nuclei and pathways of the central auditory nervous system.

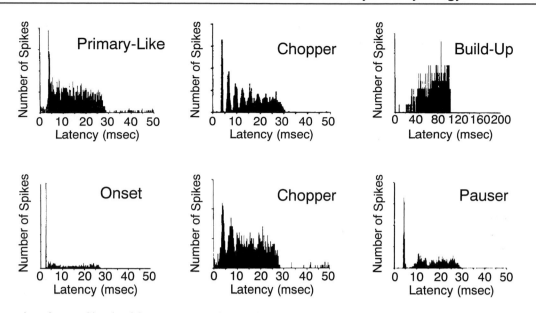

Fig. 2.48 Examples of several kinds of firing patterns observed in central auditory neurons (obtained from neurons in the cochlea nucleus). (Adapted from Rhode [1985], with permission of the *Journal of the Acoustical Society of America*.)

sides at all levels through the cortex, except for the medial geniculates. Nerve cells that receive inputs originating from the two sides are excited and/or inhibited in a manner that depends on the interaction of the two inputs. **Fig. 2.49** shows how cells in the superior olivary complexes on each side of the head receive signals from the cochlear nuclei on both sides of the head. In this diagram, ipsilateral (same side) signals are inhibitory and contralateral (opposite side) signals are excitatory; however, just about all excitatory/inhibitory combinations actually exist. This kind of arrangement allows the cells in various nuclei at all levels, including the cortex, to respond to the inter-ear time and intensity differences discussed earlier, and underlies much of our directional hearing ability and other binaural perceptions.

The systematic organization of frequency by location is called **tonotopic organization**, and is seen at every level of the auditory system from the cochlea up to and including the cortex. Tonotopic relationships are determined by measuring the characteristic frequencies of many individual cells for each nucleus, and have been reported for the auditory nerve (e.g., Liberman 1982b; Keithley & Schreiber 1987), cochlear nuclei (e.g., Rose, Galambos, & Hughes 1959), superior olivary complex (e.g., Tsuchitani & Boudreau 1966), lateral lemniscus (e.g., Aitkin, Anderson, & Brugge 1970), inferior colliculus (e.g., Rose, Greenwood, Goldberg, & Hind 1963), medial geniculate bodies (e.g., Aitkin & Webster 1971), and the cortex (e.g., Woolsey 1960; Talavage et al 20004).

For example, **Fig. 2.50** shows the frequency map for the S-shaped lateral superior olive of the cat, and **Fig. 2.51** is a classical composite summary picture showing the layout of frequencies by place for various areas of the animal cortex. More contemporary work has reviewed six arrangements from low to high frequencies in the human auditory cortex (Talavage et al 2004).

Efferent Auditory Pathways

The efferent neurons that communicate with the organ of Corti are derived from the superior olivary complexes on both sides of the brainstem, constituting the **olivocochlear bundle (OCB)**, also known as Rasmussen's bundle (Rasmussen 1946; Warr 1978). The major aspects of the OCB are depicted in **Fig. 2.52**, where we readily see that there are two systems rather than one. The **uncrossed olivocochlear bundle (UOCB)** is the olivocochlear pathway derived from the same side of the head as the cochlea in question. Most of its fibers are from the area of the **lateral superior olive (LSO)** and terminate at the afferent fibers of the *inner* hair cells, and some of its fibers are from the vicinity of the **medial superior olive (MSO)** and go to the *outer* hair cells. The opposite arrangement exists for the **crossed olivocochlear** bundle (COCB), whose neurons originate on the opposite side of the brainstem and cross along the floor of the fourth ventricle to the side of the

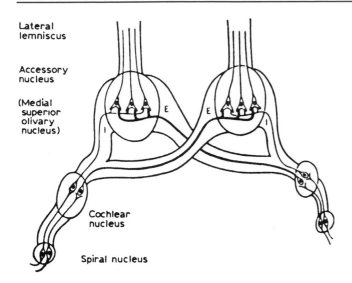

Fig. 2.49 Schematic diagram of binaural (ipsilateral and contralateral) inputs to cells in the superior olivary complex. E, excitatory; I, inhibitory. (From van Bergeijk [1962], with permission of the *Journal of the Acoustical Society of America*.)

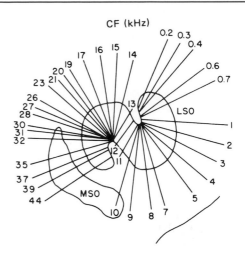

Fig. 2.50 Tonotopic organization in the S-shaped lateral superior olive (cat). (Adapted from Tsuchitani & Boudreau [1966], with permission of the *Journal of Neurophysiology*.)

cochlea in question. Here, most of the fibers are from the MSO and go to the *outer* hair cells, while a much smaller number come from the LSO and terminate at the *inner* hair cells. In other words, the uncrossed olivocochlear bundle extends mainly from the LSO to the afferent neurons of the IHCs, and the crossed olivocochlear bundle extends mainly from the MSO to the OHCs.

The olivocochlear bundle is by no means the only descending neural pathway in the auditory system. We have already seen that efferent signals influence the transmission system of the middle ear by innervating the stapedius and tensor tympani muscles. In addition, higher centers exert influences over lower

ones at many levels of the auditory system, with some efferents going to the ear and others going to lower centers within the nervous system itself (e.g., Harrison & Howe 1974; Winer, Diamond, & Raczkowksy 1977). For example, some of these efferent connections descend to lower levels from the cortex, lateral lemniscus, and inferior colliculus, and are received by various central auditory centers such as the medial geniculates and the inferior colliculi.

■ Central Vestibular Pathways

The vestibular neurons join to compose the *vestibular branch* of the eighth (vestibuloacoustic) nerve, with the **vestibular (Scarpa's) ganglia** in the inter-

a	Low frequencies (apex of cochlea)
b	High frequencies (apex of cochlea)
AI	Auditory area AI
AII	Auditory area AII
AIII	Auditory area AIII
INS	Insula
SF	Suprasylvian fringe
EP	Posterior ectosylvian gyrus

Fig. 2.51 Composite diagram of the tonotopic organization of the cerebral cortex. (Adapted from Woolsey [1960], in *Neural Mechanisms of the Auditory and Vestibular System*, GL Rasmussen and WF Windel, eds., by courtesy of CC Thomas, Publisher.)

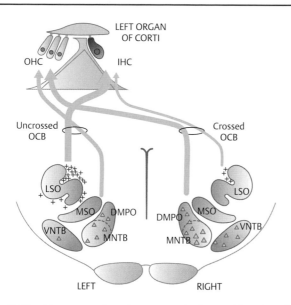

Fig. 2.52 The crossed and uncrossed olivocochlear bundles. Thicker arrows show that most of the fibers from the crossed olivocochlear bundle (OCB) go from the medial superior olive (MSO) to outer hair cells, and most of the fibers from the uncrossed OCB go from the lateral superior olive (LSO) to inner hair cells. (MNTB, medial nucleus of the trapezoid body; VNTB, ventral nucleus of the trapezoid body; DMPO, dorsal perolivary nucleus; OHC, outer hair cell; IHC, inner hair cell.) (Adapted from Warr WB. The olivocochlear bundle: its origins and terminations in the cat. In: Naunton RF, Fernandez C, eds. *Electrical Activity of the Auditory Nervous System.* ©1978 by Academic Press; pp. 43–65.)

Hearing By Bone-Conduction

Hearing usually involves receiving a sound in the form of vibrating air particles. This "regular route" is called air-conduction. It is also possible to hear by **bone-conduction**, which means that the sound is transmitted via vibrations of the bones of the skull. Bone-conduction can be initiated by air conducted sounds that are intense enough to set the bones of the skull into vibration, or by directly activating the bones of the skull with a vibrator made for this purpose. In clinical audiology, air-conduction signals are presented from earphones or loudspeakers, and bone-conduction stimuli are presented from a bone-conduction vibrator.

Air-conduction and bone-conduction result in the same cochlear activity, that is, the initiation of traveling waves and displacements of the hair cell cilia. **Fig. 2.53** shows how the skull vibrates when stimulated at different frequencies with a bone-conduction vibrator at the forehead (Bekesy 1932). At 200 Hz the whole skull vibrates as a unit in the same (forward–backward) direction as the applied vibrations. It continues to vibrate in the forward–backward direction at 800 Hz, but the pattern changes so that the front and back of the skull vibrate out-of-phase with each other. By 1600 Hz the skull begins to vibrate in four

nal auditory meatus. After entering the brainstem at the cerebellopontine angle, the vestibular nerve goes to the **vestibular nuclei** on the same side, and also sends a branch directly to the cerebellum. There are actually four (the superior, inferior, lateral, and medial) vestibular nuclei on each side. The details of the central vestibular pathways are beyond the scope of an introductory text, but the beginning student should be aware of the breadth of these connections, if only to appreciate the multiplicity of factors that contribute to our ability to maintain balance and body orientation in space. The vestibular nuclei communicate with the nuclei of the nerves that control eye movements while the head is turning, most notably with the **third (oculomotor)** and **sixth (abducens) cranial nerves.** These connections compose the **medial longitudinal fasciculus,** which coordinates eye motion with vestibular activity. The vestibular nuclei also communicate with the vestibulospinal tracts, which influence skeletal muscle tone and antigravity muscle reflexes, as well as the cerebellum, cerebral cortex, and the vestibular nuclei on the other side of the brain.

Fig. 2.53 Skull vibration patterns initiated by bone-conduction stimulation applied to the forehead at **(a)** 200 Hz, **(b)** 800 Hz, and **(c)** 1600 Hz. (Based on Bekesy [1932].)

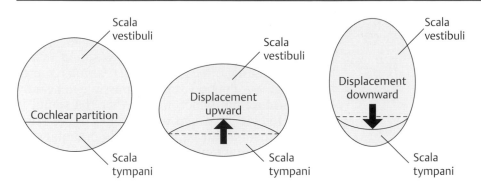

Fig. 2.54 Basilar membrane displacements due to distortional bone-conduction. (Based on Tonndorf [1962].)

segments, involving right–left as well as front-back displacements.

Skull vibrations activate the cochlea by three mechanisms, including inner ear, middle ear, and even outer ear components (Tonndorf et al 1966). All three components are similarly important above ~ 1000 Hz, but the middle and outer ear mechanisms take on a dominant role in the lower frequencies (Tonndorf et al 1966). The *inner ear component* of bone-conduction primarily involves a **distortional** mechanism, as illustrated conceptually in **Fig. 2.54**. Vibrations of the temporal bone cause the cochlear capsule (the circle) to be distorted in a manner that is synchronized with the stimulus (represented by the flattened and elongated ovals). Because the scala vestibuli has a larger volume than the scala tympani, the distortions of the fluid-filled capsule result in compensatory upward and downward displacement of the basilar membrane (represented by the lines within the circle and ovals). The distortional mechanism is supplemented and modified by a **compressional** mechanism (Bekesy 1932). Here, temporal bone vibrations alternately compress and expand the cochlear capsule. When compressed, the cochlear fluids push outward at the oval and round windows. The greatest amount of bulging occurs at the *round* window because it is much more compliant than the oval window. As a result the fluid is displaced downward from the scala vestibuli toward the scala tympani and the round window, displacing the basilar membrane as well **(Fig. 2.55a)**. This displacement is enhanced because the total surface area of the scala vestibuli and the vestibule is larger than that of the scala tympani **(Fig. 2.55b)**.

The *middle ear component* of bone-conduction is illustrated in **Fig. 2.56**. The ossicles are represented by pendulums because they are essentially suspended within the middle ear, where they can move relative to the rest of the head. Notice that the pendulums (the ossicles) vibrate in the left–right direction. A bone-conduction vibrator at the mastoid

process causes the skull to vibrate in the left-right direction, which will also induce left–right motions of the ossicles **(Fig. 2.56a)**. However, the inertia of the suspended ossicular chain will cause its motion to lag behind the motion of the head, which means that the ossicles will be moving relative to the head. This relative movement effects a rocking motion of the stapedial footplate in the oval window, thereby transmitting the signal to the cochlear fluids. The middle ear contribution is called **ossicular-lag or inertial** bone-conduction for this reason. In contrast, a bone vibrator at the forehead would shake the head in the front–back direction. This vibration is at right angles to the motion of the ossicular chain, so that ossicular motion would not be initiated at low frequencies where the head moves only in the same plane as the vibrator **(Fig. 2.56b)**.

The *outer ear component* of bone-conduction is due to **acoustical radiations**, and is sometimes called **osseotympanic** bone-conduction. The vibra-

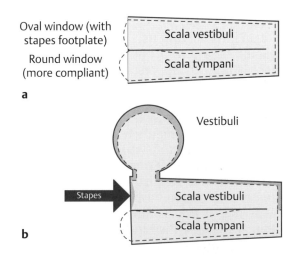

Fig. 2.55 (a,b) Principles of compressional bone-conduction. (Based on Bekesy [1932].)

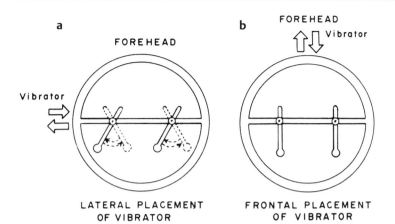

Fig. 2.56 Inertial or ossicular-lag bone-conduction occurs when a vibrator at the mastoid process shakes the skull in the same direction as ossicular chain motion **(a)**, but not when a vibrator at the forehead shakes the skull perpendicular to it **(b)**. (Based on Barany [1938]. From Gelfand [2010], by courtesy of Informa.)

tions of the cartilaginous canal wall are radiated into the ear canal itself, and are then picked up by the tympanic membrane and transmitted to the cochlea via the air-conduction route. You can easily appreciate the outer ear component of bone-conduction by clicking your teeth together, first without touching your ears and then while firmly (but gently) closing off your ear canals with the palms of your hands. The sound will be noticeably louder under the second, occluded, condition because it enhances the effect of the outer ear bone-conduction mechanism by preventing low frequencies from being lost.

This **occlusion effect** has several clinical ramifications that will become apparent in forthcoming chapters.

■ Study Questions

1. Describe the major anatomical components of the outer, middle, and inner ear.
2. Explain why the sound produced by a loudspeaker somewhere in a room is different when it reaches the eardrum.
3. Explain why it is necessary for the middle ear system to amplify the sound reaching the tympanic membrane, and how this is done.
4. How does the vibration entering the cochlea result in activation of the hair cells?
5. What is the traveling wave and how does it relate to our ability to hear different frequencies?
6. Describe the similarities and differences between the inner and outer hair cells in terms of their structures, attachments, and functions.
7. How are different sound levels represented in the behavior of auditory neurons?

8. How are different frequencies represented in the behavior of auditory neurons?
9. How do the outer, middle, and inner ear contribute to hearing by bone-conduction?
10. Describe the major neural pathways from the ears to the auditory cortex.

References

Aitkin LM, Anderson DJ, Brugge JF. Tonotopic organization and discharge characteristics of single neurons in nuclei of the lateral lemniscus of the cat. J Neurophysiol 1970;33(3):421–440

Aitkin LM, Webster WR. Tonotopic organization in the medial geniculate body of the cat. Brain Res 1971; 26(2):402–405

Barany E. A contribution to the physiology of bone conduction. Acta Otolaryngol Suppl 1938;26:1–223

Bekesy G. Zur Theorie des Horens bei der Schallaufnahme durch Knochenleitung. Ann Phys 1932;13:111–136

Bekesy G. Uber die Messung der Schwingungsamplitude der Gehorknochelchen mittels einer kapazitiven Sonde. Akust Zeits 1941;6:1–16

Bekesy G. Description of some mechanical properties of the organ of Corti. J Acoust Soc Am 1953;25:770–785

Bekesy G. 1960. Experiments in Hearing. New York, NY: McGraw-Hill.

Bekesy G, Rosenblith WA. 1958. The mechanical properties of the ear. In: Stevens SS, ed. Handbook of Experimental Psychology. New York, NY: Wiley; 1075–1115

Blauert J. 1983. Spatial Hearing: The Psychophysics of Human Sound Localization. Cambridge, MA: MIT Press

Borg E. On the neuronal organization of the acoustic middle ear reflex. A physiological and anatomical study. Brain Res 1973;49(1):101–123

Borg E. 1976. Dynamic characteristics of the intraaural middle reflex. In: Feldman AS, Wilber LA, eds. Acoustic Impedance and Admittance-The Measurement of Middle Ear Function. Baltimore, MD: Williams & Wilkins; 236–299

Borg E, Counter A, Rosler G. 1984. Theories of middle ear muscle function. In: Silman S, ed. The Acoustic Reflex: Basic Principles and Clinical Applications. Orlando, FL: Academic Press; 63–99

Brownell WE. Outer hair cell electromotility and otoacoustic emissions. Ear Hear 1990;11(2):82–92

Dallos P. Neurobiology of cochlear inner and outer hair cells: intracellular recordings. Hear Res 1986;22: 185–198

Dallos P. Cochlear neurobiology: revolutionary developments. ASHA 1988;30(6-7):50–56

Dallos P, Billone MC, Durrant JD, Wang C, Raynor S. Cochlear inner and outer hair cells: functional differences. Science 1972;177(4046):356–358

Davis H. Transmission and transduction in the cochlea. Laryngoscope 1958;68(3):359–382

Davis H. Advances in the neurophysiology and neuroanatomy of the cochlea. J Acoust Soc Am 1962;34:1377–1385

Davis H. An active process in cochlear mechanics. Hear Res 1983;9(1):79–90

Furness DN, Hackney CM. High-resolution scanning-electron microscopy of stereocilia using the osmium-thiocarbohydrazide coating technique. Hear Res 1986;21(3):243–249

Gelfand SA. 1984. The contralateral acoustic reflex threshold. In: Silman S, ed. The Acoustic Reflex: Basic Principles and Clinical Applications. Orlando, FL: Academic Press; 137–186

Gelfand SA. 2010. Hearing: An Introduction to Psychological and Physiological Acoustics, 5th ed. Colchester, Essex, UK: Informa

Guinan JJ Jr. Olivocochlear efferents: anatomy, physiology, function, and the measurement of efferent effects in humans. Ear Hear 2006;27(6):589–607 [Erratum in Ear Hear 28, 129 (2007)]

Harrison JM, Howe ME. 1974. Anatomy of the descending auditory system (mammalian). In: Keidel WD, Neff WD, eds. Handbook of Sensory Physiology, Vol. 511. Berlin, Germany: Springer; 363–388

Helmholtz H. 1895. Die Lehre von der Tonempfindugen (trans. by A. Ellis, On the Sensation of Tones)

Hudspeth AJ. The cellular basis of hearing: the biophysics of hair cells. Science 1985;230(4727):745–752

Hughes GB, Ed. 1985. Textbook of Clinical Otology. New York, NY: Thieme-Stratton

Jepsen O. 1963. The middle ear muscle reflexes in man. In: Jerger J, ed. Modern Developments in Audiology. New York, NY: Academic Press; 194–239

Keithley EM, Schreiber RC. Frequency map of the spiral ganglion in the cat. J Acoust Soc Am 1987;81(4): 1036–1042

Khanna SM, Leonard DGB. Basilar membrane tuning in the cat cochlea. Science 1982;215(4530):305–306

Kiang NYS. 1965. Discharge Patterns of Single Fibers in the Cat's Auditory Nerve. Cambridge, MA: MIT Press

Kiang NYS, Liberman MC, Sewell WF, Guinan JJ. Single unit clues to cochlear mechanisms. Hear Res 1986;22: 171–182

Kiang NYS, Rho JM, Northrop CC, Liberman MC, Ryugo DK. Hair-cell innervation by spiral ganglion cells in adult cats. Science 1982;217(4555):175–177

Liberman MC. Single-neuron labeling in the cat auditory nerve. Science 1982a;216(4551):1239–1241

Liberman MC. The cochlear frequency map for the cat: labeling auditory-nerve fibers of known characteristic frequency. J Acoust Soc Am 1982b;72(5):1441–1449

Liberman MC. Physiology of cochlear efferent and afferent neurons: direct comparisons in the same animal. Hear Res 1988;34(2):179–191

Lim DJ. Functional structure of the organ of Corti: a review. Hear Res 1986a;22:117–146

Lim DJ. Effects of noise and ototoxic drugs at the cellular level in the cochlea: a review. Am J Otolaryngol 1986b;7(2):73–99

Lippe WR. Recent developments in cochlear physiology. Ear Hear 1986;7(4):233–239

Manoussaki D, Dimitriadis EK, Chadwick RS. Cochlea's graded curvature effect on low frequency waves. Phys Rev Lett 2006;96(8):088701

Mehrgardt S, Mellert V. Transformation characteristics of the external human ear. J Acoust Soc Am 1977; 61(6):1567–1576

Møller AR. An experimental study of the acoustic impedance of the middle ear and its transmission properties. Acta Otolaryngol 1965;60:129–149

Morgan DE, Dirks DD. Influence of middle-ear muscle contraction on pure-tone suprathreshold loudness judgments. J Acoust Soc Am 1975;57(2):411–420

Morgan DE, Dirks DD, Kamm C. The influence of middle-ear muscle contraction on auditory threshold for selected pure tones. J Acoust Soc Am 1978;63(6): 1896–1903

Nedzelnitsky V. Sound pressures in the basal turn of the cat cochlea. J Acoust Soc Am 1980;68(6):1676–1689

Peak WT, Sohmer HS, Weiss TF. Microelectrode recordings of intracochlear potentials. MIT Res Lab Elect Quart Rep 1969;94:293–304

Pickles JO. 1988. An Introduction to the Physiology of Hearing, 2nd ed. London, UK: Academic Press

Pickles JO, Comis SD, Osborne MP. Cross-links between stereocilia in the guinea pig organ of Corti, and their possible relation to sensory transduction. Hear Res 1984;15(2):103–112

Pickles JO, Corey DP. Mechanoelectrical transduction by hair cells. Trends Neurosci 1992;15(7):254–259

Proctor B. 1989. Surgical Anatomy of the Ear and Temporal Bone. New York, NY: Thieme

Rabinowitz WM. 1976. Acoustic-reflex effects on the input impedance and transfer characteristics of the human middle-ear. Unpublished. Ph.D. dissertation. Cambridge, MA: MIT

Rasmussen GL. The olivary peduncle and other fiber projections of the superior olivary complex. J Comp Neurol 1946;84:141–219

Reger SN. Effect of middle ear muscle action on certain psycho-physical measurements. Ann Otol Rhinol Laryngol 1960;69:1179–1198

Rhode WS. The use of intracellular techniques in the study of the cochlear nucleus. J Acoust Soc Am 1985; 78(1 Pt 2):320–327

Rose JE, Brugge JF, Anderson DJ, Hind JE. Phase-locked response to low-frequency tones in single auditory nerve fibers of the squirrel monkey. J Neurophysiol 1967;30(4):769–793

Rose JE, Galambos R, Hughes JR. Microelectrode studies of the cochlear nuclei of the cat. Bull Johns Hopkins Hosp 1959;104(5):211–251

Rose JE, Greenwood DD, Goldberg JM, Hind JE. Some discharge characteristics of single neurons in the inferior colliculus of the cat: 1. Tonotopic organization, relation of spike-counts to tone intensity, and firing patterns of single elements. J Neurophysiol 1963;26:294–320

Russell IJ, Sellick PM. Tuning properties of cochlear hair cells. Nature 1977;267(5614):858–860

Rutherford W. A new theory of hearing. J Anat Physiol 1886;21(1):166–168

Sachs MB, Abbas PJ. Rate versus level functions for auditory-nerve fibers in cats: tone-burst stimuli. J Acoust Soc Am 1974;56(6):1835–1847

Salvi R, Henderson D, Hamernik R. 1983. Physiological bases of sensorineural hearing loss. In: Tobias JD, Schubert ED, eds. Hearing Research and Theory, Vol. 2. New York, NY: Academic Press; 173–231

Schuenke M, Schulte E, Schumacher U, Ross LM, Lamperti ED, Voll M. 2010. Head and Neuroanatomy (THIEME Atlas of Anatomy). New York, NY: Thieme

Sellick PM, Patuzzi R, Johnstone BM. Measurement of basilar membrane motion in the guinea pig using the Mössbauer technique. J Acoust Soc Am 1982;72(1):131–141

Shaw EAG. Transformation of sound pressure level from the free field to the eardrum in the horizontal plane. J Acoust Soc Am 1974;56(6):1848–1861

Shaw EAG, Vaillancourt MM. Transformation of sound-pressure level from the free field to the eardrum presented in numerical form. J Acoust Soc Am 1985; 78(3):1120–1123

Simmons FB. Middle ear muscle activity at moderate sound levels. Ann Otol Rhinol Laryngol 1959;68:1126–1143

Simmons FB. Perceptual theories of middle ear muscle function. Ann Otol Rhinol Laryngol 1964;73:724–739

Smith HD. Audiometric effects of voluntary contraction of the tensor tympani muscles. Arch Otolaryngol 1943; 38:369–372

Spoendlin H. Innervation patterns in the organ of Corti of the cat. Acta Otolaryngol 1969;67(2):239–254

Spoendlin H. 1978. The afferent innervation of the cochlea. In: Naunton RF, Fernandez C, eds. Electrical Activity of the Auditory Nervous System. London, UK: Academic Press; 21–41

Spoendlin H. Neuroanatomical basis of cochlear coding mechanisms. Audiology 1975;14(5–6):383–407

Steel KP. The tectorial membrane of mammals. Hear Res 1983;9(3):327–359

Talavage TM, Sereno MI, Melcher JR, Ledden PJ, Rosen BR, Dale AM. Tonotopic organization in human auditory cortex revealed by progressions of frequency sensitivity. J Neurophysiol 2004;91(3):1282–1286

Tonndorf J. Shearing motion in scala media of cochlear models. Proj Rep USAF Sch Aviat Med 1960;32:238–244

Tonndorf J. Compressional bone conduction in cochlear models. J Acoust Soc Am 1962;34:1127–1132

Tonndorf J, et al. Bone conduction: studies in experimental animals; a collection of seven papers. Acta Otolaryngol Suppl 1966;213:1–132

Tonndorf J, Khanna SM. The role of the tympanic membrane in middle ear transmission. Ann Otol Rhinol Laryngol 1970;79(4):743–753

Tos M. 1995. Manual of Middle Ear Surgery: Vol. 2, Mastoid Surgery and Reconstructive Procedures. Stuttgart, Germany: Thieme

Tsuchitani C, Boudreau JC. Single unit analysis of cat superior olive S segment with tonal stimuli. J Neurophysiol 1966;29(4):684–697

van Bergeijk WA. Variation on a theme of Bekesy: a model of binaural interaction. J Acoust Soc Am 1962; 34:1431–1437

Warr WB. 1978. The olivocochlear bundle: Its origins and terminations in the cat. In: Naunton RF, Fernandez C, eds. Electrical Activity of the Auditory Nervous System. London, UK: Academic Press; 43–65

Wever EG. 1949. Theory of Hearing. New York, NY: Dover

Wever EG, Lawrence M. 1954. Physiological Acoustics. Princeton, NJ: Princeton University Press

Wiener FM, Ross DA. The pressure distribution in the auditory canal in a progressive sound field. J Acoust Soc Am 1946;18:401–408

Wiley TL, Block MG. 1984. Acoustic and nonacoustic reflex patterns in audiologic diagnosis. In: Silman S, ed. The Acoustic Reflex: Basic Principles and Clinical Applications. New York, NY: Academic Press; 387–411

Winer JA, Diamond IT, Raczkowski D. Subdivisions of the auditory cortex of the cat: the retrograde transport of horseradish peroxidase to the medial geniculate body and posterior thalamic nuclei. J Comp Neurol 1977;176(3):387–417

Woolsey CN. 1960. Organization of cortical auditory system: a review and a synthesis. In: Rasmussen GL, Windel WF, eds. Neural Mechanisms of the Auditory and Vestibular System. Springfield, IL: Charles C Thomas; 165–180

Yoshie N. Auditory nerve action potential responses to clicks in man. Laryngoscope 1968;78(2):198–215

Zwislocki J. 1975. The role of the external and middle ear in the sound transmission. In: Tower DB, Eagles EL, eds. The Nervous System: Vol. 3, Human Communication and Its Disorders. New York, NY: Raven Press; 45–55

Zwislocki JJ, Chamberlain SC, Slepecky NB. Tectorial membrane. I: Static mechanical properties in vivo. Hear Res 1988;33(3):207–222

Measurement Principles and the Nature of Hearing

Physical attributes such as a person's height, body temperature, or blood sugar can be measured directly. This is not so for sensory and perceptual capabilities such as hearing. To find out about what a person can hear and how these sounds are perceived we must, in effect, ask her. In other words, hearing assessment relies for the most part on *presenting a stimulus and measuring the response* to that stimulus. Raising one's hand when a sound is heard, repeating a test word, judging which of two sounds is louder than the other, and even the electrical activity of the nervous system ("brain waves," so to speak) elicited by a sound are all responses. The trick is to contrive the stimulus-response situation in a way that is (1) **valid**, which means that we are really testing what we think is being tested, and (2) **reliable**, which means that the same results will be obtained if the test is repeated.

We must also be aware of the nature of the measurement being made and its limitations. For example, there is a major difference between whether a person can hear a sound presented at one particular intensity, as opposed to what is the smallest intensity that she needs to just barely hear the presence of that sound. The first test classifies a person according to whether she falls into the group of people who can hear that sound or the group who cannot hear it; the second test classifies her hearing along a continuum. Finally, we need to know that how a person responds is affected by more than whether she did or did not hear the stimulus sound. Responses are often affected by confounding influences that are built into the testing approach (e.g., how the last response affects the next one) and the criteria employed by the person taking the test (e.g., how sure she must be before saying "yes").

■ Scales and Measurements

Scales of Measurement

Most tests and other measures of hearing can be viewed in terms of the classic nominal, ordinal, interval, and ratio scales of measurement described by Stevens (1975). In a **nominal scale**, subjects or observations are simply categorized into different groups, but there is *no* order or hierarchy among the groups. Some examples include grouping people according to gender (male/female) or eye color (brown/blue/hazel), or classifying paintings by subject type (landscape/portrait/still life). On the other hand, if there is also some hierarchy or order among the observations or categories, then we have an **ordinal scale**. For example, we might ask subjects to specify their relative preferences for different kinds of paintings, or to organize the paintings according to relative price. Here, there is an orderly progression from group to group, but the spacing between groups is different. For example, several paintings might be rank ordered according to their prices, which are $10, $25, $100, $150, and $175. Because we know the relative order of the observations, the information on ordinal scales can be described in terms of medians and percentiles.

An ordinal scale becomes an **interval scale** when the spacing between categories or observations is equal, such as the hours on a clock or degrees of temperature in Fahrenheit or Celsius. Notice that the spacing is the same between any successive two points on the scale: There is 1 hour from 6 am to 7 am and there is also 1 hour from 10 pm to 11 pm; and there is one degree from 30°C to 31°C and also from 99°C to 100°C. An interval scale allows us to use most kinds of calculations so information can now be described in terms of means (averages) and standard deviations. However, ratios may not be used because there is no true zero point. **Ratio scales** have all the characteristics of interval scales plus a true zero point (an inherent origin). Length and temperature on the Kelvin scale (where 0 is absolute zero) are typical examples of ratio scales, as are loudness in *sones* and pitch in *mels,* described later in this chapter. All mathematical calculations can be used with ratio scale information, including the use of ratios, geometric means, and decibels.

Classical Measurement Methods

The classical techniques that have been used to measure hearing and other senses are the methods of limits, adjustment, and constants (or constant stimuli). Other testing methods are also available, such as the direct scaling approaches (discussed below) as well as the clinical techniques (discussed later). Sophisticated *adaptive testing methods* (see, e.g., Gelfand, 1998) are usually employed in research applications, but they have clinical uses as well. We will describe each of the methods of limits, adjustment, and constants in the context of a test to find the subject's **threshold** of hearing for a pure tone signal, which is simply the lowest intensity level at which the subject is able to hear. However, these methods can also be used for other kinds of measurements,

such as determining the smallest perceptible difference in intensity or frequency between two sounds.

The **method of limits** is illustrated in **Fig. 3.1.** The subject is presented with one tone at a time, and he responds by indicating whether the stimulus was heard ("yes" or +) or not heard ("no" or –) after each presentation. The tester controls the level of the stimulus and changes it in fixed steps (e.g., 2 dB at a time) in one direction (ascending or descending) until the responses change from "yes" (+) to "no" (–), or from "no" (–) to "yes" (+). Each set of presentations is called a run. Eight runs are shown in the figure. Descending runs begin above the subject's expected threshold, and the stimulus level is lowered until the tone first becomes inaudible. Ascending runs start below the subject's threshold, and the level is raised until the tone is first heard. Notice that the crossover point varies from run to run, so the best estimate of the threshold is the average of several runs. Testing biases are minimized by averaging across an equal number of ascending and descending runs with different starting levels, as illustrated in the figure.

In the **method of adjustment**, the stimulus level changes continuously rather than in fixed steps, and is controlled by the subject herself. To find her threshold, the subject increases (or decreases) an unmarked level control until the tone first becomes audible (or inaudible). *Bracketing,* or increasing and decreasing the level alternately until a change point is reached, is a commonly employed modification of the methods of adjustment and limits.

Stimulus (dB)	Run:	1	2	3	4	5	6	7	8
34		+						+	
32		+						+	
30		+		+				+	
28		+		+				+	
26		+		+		+		+	
24		+		+		+		+	
22		+		+		+		+	
20		+		+	+	+		+	
18		+	+	+	–	+		+	
16		+	–	–	–	+	+	–	+
14		+	–		–	–	–		–
12		–	–		–		–		–
10			–		–		–		–
8			–		–		–		–
6			–				–		–
4			–						–
Threshold (dB) per run:		13	17	17	19	15	15	17	15
Mean Threshold: 16 dB									

Fig. 3.1 Eight "runs" being used to find the threshold of hearing with the method of limits. (From Gelfand [1998], p. 247, by courtesy of Marcel Dekker, Inc.)

The methods of limits and adjustment are sequential techniques because one presentation level depends on the response to the previous one. In contrast, the **method of constant stimuli (constants)** uses an equal number of stimuli at each of several predetermined levels, which are presented to the subject in random order. The "yes" (+) and "no" (–) responses are tallied for each of the levels used. The threshold is then obtained by calculating the level that corresponds to 50% from these tallies. **Fig. 3.2** shows an example in which the percentage of "yes" (+) responses is calculated on the basis of 50 random tone presentations at 11 levels from 0 dB to 10 dB sound pressure level (SPL). The tallies are converted into percentages, which are then plotted on a graph known as a **psychometric function**. The 50% point on the psychometric function is usually considered to be the threshold, which corresponds to 7.5 dB in this example. The method of constants is very accurate, but it can be inefficient because many presentations are "wasted" at levels well above and well below the threshold (**Fig. 3.2**).

Direct Scaling

In direct scaling the subject directly establishes the correspondence between physical sounds and how they are perceived. The major approaches are partition scales and ratio or magnitude scales. The loudness (sone) and pitch (mel) scales discussed later in this chapter were developed using the magnitude and ratio scaling methods. With **partition scales** the subject is presented with a range of intensities or frequencies, and is asked to divide (partition) this range into equally spaced categories on the basis of how she perceives them.

Ratio scales are developed by ratio estimation or production. In **ratio estimation** the subject is presented with pairs of tones and describes (estimates) how they are related in the form of a ratio. For example, compared with the first one, the second tone might be twice as loud, half as loud, four times louder, etc.; or its pitch might be half as high, one-quarter as high, twice as high, etc. The opposite approach is **ratio production**. Here, the subject is asked to adjust (produce) the intensity of a tone until it sounds twice or half as loud as another tone, or to change the frequency of a tone so that its pitch is one-quarter, half, or twice that of another tone.

Magnitude scales are similar to ratio scales, except they use numbers (magnitudes) instead of ratios or fractions. In **magnitude estimation** the subject is presented with stimuli along a continuum (e.g., intensity) and is asked to assign numbers to each of them in a way that reflects the magnitude of the perception (e.g., loudness). The results show the relationship between physical stimuli and their perception, as in **Fig. 3.3**. There are two major variations of the magnitude estimation method. In one approach the subject is presented with a "standard" tone called a **modulus** and is told that it has a magni-

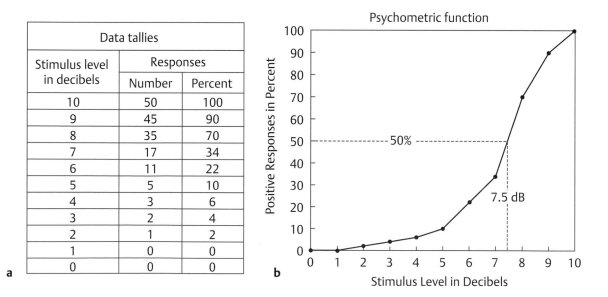

Data tallies		
Stimulus level in decibels	Responses	
	Number	Percent
10	50	100
9	45	90
8	35	70
7	17	34
6	11	22
5	5	10
4	3	6
3	2	4
2	1	2
1	0	0
0	0	0

a

b

Fig. 3.2 Illustration of the method of constant stimuli. The **(a)** data tallies are used to plot a **(b)** psychometric function, on which the 50% point constitutes the threshold.

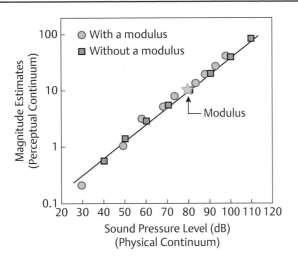

Fig. 3.3 Magnitude estimates showing the perceptual values of a range of intensities. Notice that similar results are obtained with and without a modulus. (Based on data by Stevens [1956].)

tude of, say, "10." She then hears other tones at other intensities and is asked to describe (estimate) their magnitudes with numbers that are proportional to the modulus. A tone that is twice as loud as the modulus is rated 20; 40 means four times louder; and 2 means one-fifth as loud. The alternative approach is to omit the modulus. In this case the subject is asked to provide a rating for each sound using numbers that represent how they are perceived. Similar results are obtained with and without the modulus, as illustrated in the figure. The opposite of magnitude estimation is **magnitude production**. Here the subject is presented with numbers and must adjust the intensity (or frequency) to produce a tone with the corresponding loudness (or pitch).

Magnitude scales have been developed for a large number of sensations, and it is even possible to make **cross-modality matches**, that is, to express a perception from one sensory modality in terms of a different sense. Cross-modality matching can be useful audiologically by facilitating the ability to assess a patient's perception of loudness in terms of perceived line length (Hellman & Meiselman 1988; Hellman 1999).

■ The Nature of Normal Hearing

Audiology is concerned with the normal and abnormal aspects of hearing, its place in the communicative process, and the clinical evaluation and management of patients with auditory impairments.

The area of science that deals with the perception of physical stimuli is called psychophysics. Hence, in addition to being an aspect of audiology, the science that deals with perception of sound is also known as **psychoacoustics**.

The Range of Hearing

Minimal Audible Levels

It is useful to conceive of a range of hearing that includes sounds that are audible and tolerable. The lower curves in **Fig. 3.4** show the faintest audible sounds or **thresholds** of normal people in decibels of sound pressure level (dB SPL) as a function of frequency. The striking feature of these curves is they are not flat. Instead, the SPL needed for a sound to be barely audible depends on its frequency to a major extent. Hearing thresholds are reasonably sensitive between ~ 100 and 10,000 Hz, and become poorer (i.e., more intensity is needed to reach threshold) as frequency increases and decreases above and below this range. In addition, hearing is most sensitive (i.e., the least amount of intensity is needed to reach threshold) in the 2000 to 5000 Hz range. The resonant responses of the conductive system are largely responsible for the lower thresholds in this most sensitive frequency range (see Chapter 2).

The sound levels needed to achieve minimum audibility also depend on how they are obtained. Notice that the curve labeled "MAF" is ~ 6 to 10 dB lower (i.e., better or more sensitive) than the curves labeled "MAP." **Minimal audible pressure (MAP)** is based on monaural (one ear) thresholds that are obtained with earphones. First, the subject's threshold is obtained with an appropriate method. Then the sound pressure that corresponds to that threshold is measured as it actually exists under the earphone in the subject's ear canal. A commonly used alternative approach is to measure the sound in a 6-cc *coupler*, which is a special measurement cavity standardized for this purpose. We shall see that the latter method is used to calibrate audiological instruments. In contrast, **minimal audible field (MAF)** values are based on the binaural (two ear) thresholds of subjects listening to sounds presented from a loudspeaker in an echo-free (*anechoic*) room. After determining the threshold, the subject leaves the room and is replaced by a microphone that measures the sound as it exists in the same location previously occupied by the subject's head.

The discrepancy between the MAF and MAP thresholds has been known as the "missing 6 dB," and was a problematic issue for quite some time. However, it appears that the MAF-MAP difference is

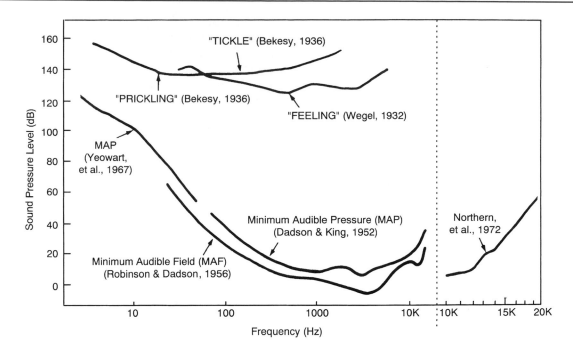

Fig. 3.4 Minimal audible levels (MAP and MAF curves) and maximum tolerable levels in decibels of sound pressure level (dB SPL) as a function of frequency from selected studies cited in the figure. The frequency scale is expanded above 10,000 Hz for clarity. (Adapted from Gelfand [1998], p. 283, by courtesy of Marcel Dekker, Inc.)

more apparent than real because it is accounted for by a combination of factors, including binaural versus monaural hearing, physiologic noise that masks stimuli presented under earphones, real ear versus coupler measurements, and other technical factors (Killion 1978).

Upper Limits of Hearing

The upper levels of usable hearing depend on how they are defined. The threshold of *uncomfortable loudness* occurs at ~ 100 dB SPL (Hood & Poole 1970; Morgan, Wilson, & Dirks 1974), although higher values of ~ 111 to 115 dB SPL have been reported by Sherlock and Formby (2005). However, the threshold is much higher for sensations such as feeling, tickle, and pain. These unpleasant and potentially intolerable sensations are generally *tactile* rather than auditory in nature, and occur roughly between 120 and 140+ dB SPL, depending on the nature of the sensation. Several examples are shown in **Fig. 3.4**. In contrast to the threshold sensitivity curves, the upper limits of hearing are relatively flat across the frequency range for both uncomfortable loudness and tactile sensations.

Temporal Summation

The threshold for a sound is not affected by its duration unless it becomes *shorter* than approximately one third of a second. When a sound is shorter than ~ 300 milliseconds, then its threshold increases when its duration decreases, and vice versa (**Fig. 3.5a**). In general, a ten-times increase in duration can be offset by a 10 dB decrease in intensity, and a 10-times (or decade) decrease in duration can be offset by a 10 dB increase in intensity. This phenomenon is called **temporal summation** or **temporal integration**. An example of this *time-intensity trade* is as follows: Suppose a person's threshold is 18 dB for a tone that is 250 milliseconds long. If we reduce the duration of the tone by 10 times, to only 25 milliseconds, then the person's threshold will increase by 10 dB to 28 dB. Similarly, if the threshold of a tone lasting 25 milliseconds is 28 dB, then increasing its duration by 10 times, to 250 milliseconds, will cause the threshold to improve by 10 dB to 18 dB. The same relationship also applies to the loudness of a sound; for example, a 40 dB tone lasting 25 milliseconds will sound as loud as a 50 dB tone if increase its duration by 10 times, to 250 milliseconds.

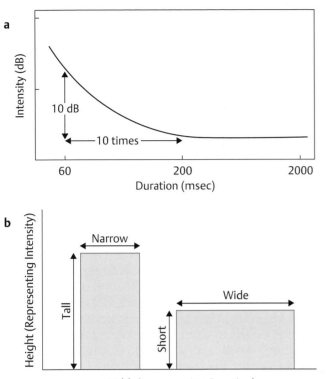

Fig. 3.5 (a) Temporal summation involves a trade-off in which a 10-times change in duration can be offset by a complementary 10 dB intensity change. (b) The area of each rectangle represents the amount of energy that is present, and is the same regardless of whether it is (1) high and narrow (more intense and shorter in duration) or (2) short and wide (less intense and longer in duration).

Temporal summation reflects the ear's ability to integrate energy within a time frame of roughly one third of a second. The principle is illustrated in **Fig. 3.5b**, where the area of each rectangle represents the amount of energy present. Notice that the area (energy) is the same regardless of whether the rectangle is (1) high and narrow (representing more intense and shorter in duration) or (2) short and wide (representing less intense and longer in duration). Students with photographic experience will recognize that this phenomenon is similar to the trade-off between lens opening and shutter speed.

Differential Sensitivity

The smallest perceptible difference between two sounds is called a **difference limen (DL)** or the **just noticeable difference (jnd)**. For example, the smallest intensity difference that can be distinguished between two sounds is the DL for intensity. Because *delta* (Δ) is the symbol for "change," the intensity DL is often called ΔI. If ΔI is the intensity difference needed to tell two sounds apart, then one of those sounds has an intensity of I and the other one has an intensity of I + ΔI (**Fig. 3.6**). Analogous terms apply to just noticeable differences for other aspects of sounds. For example, the difference limen for frequency, **D**f, is the smallest discernible difference between the frequencies of two sounds, f and f + **D**f.

The values of ΔI and **D**f are *absolute* difference limens because they specify the actual physical difference needed to tell two sounds apart. However,

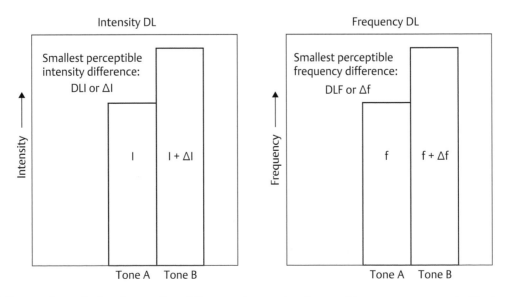

Fig. 3.6 The difference limen (DL) is the smallest difference that can be discerned between two sounds. The intensity DL, or ΔI, is the smallest noticeable intensity difference between two sounds, I and I + ΔI. The frequency DL, or Δf, is the smallest perceptible frequency difference between two sounds, f and f + Δf.

common experience tells us that the physical size of a DL is not the same under all conditions. For example, we all know that the additional illumination provided by a tiny night-light is very noticeable in the dark of night but is totally indiscernible during the day. In other words, the size of ΔI depends on the size of I. For this reason, we are especially interested in the *relative* difference limen that considers both the DL as well as the starting value. The relative DL is equal to ΔI/I and is called the **Weber fraction**. The notion that the Weber fraction (ΔI/I) is a constant value (k) is called **Weber's law**. In numerical terms, Weber's law says that ΔI/I = k.

These principles become clear when we consider a classic, albeit hypothetical, experiment described by Hirsh (1952) aimed at answering the question: "If we already have a certain number of candles, how many more candles must be added in order for us to notice a difference in brightness?" The "results" are given in **Table 3.1**. The first column gives the original numbers of candles (I), which might be 10, 100, 1000, 10,000, or even 100,000. The additional candles needed to tell a difference (the DL or ΔI) in each case are in the second column, and the new totals (I + ΔI) are in the third column. The fourth column, labeled "Weber fraction," shows the raw ratios of ΔI/I in each case, and the last column, labeled "Weber's law," shows the results of simplifying each of these fractions. The results are obvious: the more candles you start with (I), the more candles you must add (ΔI) to tell a difference, but the relative size of the increase (ΔI/I) is always the same (ΔI/I = k = 0.1).

Difference Limens for Intensity and Frequency

Although the relative difference limen for intensity follows Weber's law for white noise (e.g., Houtsma, Durlach, & Braida 1980), the value of ΔI/I improves

to some extent with increasing sensation level for pure tones (e.g., Jesteadt, Wier, & Green 1977). **Sensation level (SL)** is simply the number of decibels above threshold, so that 0 dB SL means "at threshold" and 40 dB SL means 40 dB above threshold. For example, Jesteadt et al (1977) found the values of ΔI/I are roughly 0.4 near threshold, 0.3 at 40 dB SL, 0.2 at 60 dB SL, and somewhat smaller at high intensities. Hence, there appears to be a "near miss to Weber's law" for the intensity difference limen in the sense that ΔI/I is not quite constant. The size of ΔI/I appears to be reasonably constant in the middle frequencies, but it is not clear whether this holds true for all audible frequencies.

The difference limen for frequency becomes larger (wider) as frequency increases and also as sensation level decreases (Wier, Jesteadt, & Green 1977). At the readily audible and comfortable level of 40 dB SL, the size of **D**f is ~ 1 Hz at 200 Hz and 400 Hz, and 2 Hz at 1000 Hz, 3 Hz at 2000 Hz, 16 Hz at 4000 Hz, and 68 Hz at 8000 Hz. In terms of the Weber fraction, **D**f/f is smallest (~ 0.002) between 600 Hz and 2000 Hz, and gets larger for the frequencies below and above this range. All of these values become larger (poorer) as the intensity decreases toward threshold.

Temporal Discriminations

The closest analogy in the time domain to the intensity and frequency DLs just discussed would be the difference limen for signal duration. Here the subject must determine which one of two signals lasted for a longer period of time. The difference limen for duration (Dt) becomes larger (longer) as the overall duration of the signal (t) increases, and the Weber fraction, Dt/t, is not constant (Abel 1972; Dooley & Moore 1988). However, this is by no means the only kind of time-related discrimination in hearing.

Table 3.1 Illustration of the Weber fraction (ΔI/I) and Weber's law (ΔI/I = k) with make-believe data showing how many candles must be added to several originally present candles (I) to produce a difference limen (ΔI) for brightness

Original candles, I	Additional candles, ΔI	New total, I + ΔI	Weber fraction, ΔI/I	Weber's law, ΔI/I = k
10	1	11	1/10	0.1
100	10	110	10/100	0.1
1,000	100	1,100	100/1,000	0.1
10,000	1,000	11,000	1,000/10,000	0.1
100,000	10,000	110,000	10,000/100,000	0.1

The shortest perceptible time interval or **temporal resolution** is typically on the order of 2 to 3 milliseconds in young, normal individuals, and can be measured by gap detection as well as other approaches (e.g., Fitzgibbons & Wightman 1982; Buus & Florentine 1985; Green 1985; Fitzgibbons & Gordon-Salant 1987). The stimulus used for **gap detection testing** is usually a pair of noises that are presented in rapid succession, separated by a very short break or gap. The duration of this gap is varied according to an appropriate method of measurement, and the subject's task is to determine whether a gap can or cannot be heard. The shortest discernible gap is the **gap detection threshold**. These principles are illustrated in **Fig. 3.7**. The same results are obtained if the subject is asked whether she heard one continuous sound or two of them in succession. However, an interval of ~ 20 milliseconds is needed if the subject must indicate which of two distinguishable signals came first, or the **perceived order** (Hirsh 1959).

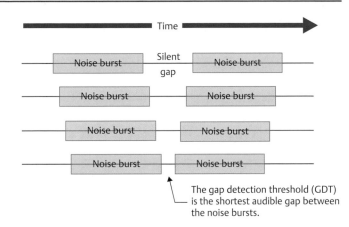

Fig. 3.7 Gap detection testing involves listening for a brief gap between two sounds (noise bursts) presented in rapid succession. The gap detection threshold (GDT) is simply the shortest gap that can be heard.

Loudness and Pitch

Loudness and pitch refer to how we *perceive* the *physical attributes* of intensity and frequency, respectively. It may seem odd to make this distinction since everyone knows sounds with greater intensities are louder than sounds with smaller intensities, and higher frequencies have higher pitches. These generalities are true. However, we will see that there is far from a one-for-one relationship between the perceptual world of loudness and pitch and the physical world of intensity and frequency.

Loudness Level

We have already seen that sounds of different frequencies are not equally audible (**Fig. 3.4**). In other words, different SPLs are needed to reach threshold at different frequencies; for example, 10 dB SPL may be audible at one frequency but not at another frequency. The same thing applies to loudness: even though tone A and tone B have the same intensity, one of them is likely to be louder than the other. In other words, loudness depends on frequency. We may now ask how much intensity is needed at each of two different frequencies for one tone to be perceived just as loud as the other tone. For example, how many decibels would it take for a 100 Hz tone to sound *equally loud* as a 1000 Hz tone at 40 dB SPL? To answer this question we may present a 1000 Hz tone at 40 dB alternately with various levels of a 100 Hz tone, and ask the subject whether each 100 Hz tone is louder, softer, or equally loud as the 1000 Hz

reference tone. Alternatively, we might have the subject adjust the level of a 100 Hz tone until it sounds just as loud as a reference tone of 1000 Hz at 40 dB. The same procedure would then be repeated with other frequencies until we have developed a list of the SPLs at many different frequencies that all sound equally loud as the 40 dB, 1000 Hz tone. It makes sense that if all of these sounds are equally loud as the 1000 Hz, 40 dB reference tone, then they are also equal in loudness to each other. We could then plot these equally loud SPLs as a function of frequency, and draw a smooth line through them.

The results look like the curve labeled "40 Phons" in **Fig. 3.8**. Notice this curve corresponds to an SPL of 40 dB *at* 1000 Hz, but that the SPLs are quite different at the other frequencies. For example, this curve tells us that all of the following tones *sound equally loud* even though their SPLs are different:

78 dB at 50 Hz
54 dB at 200 Hz
43 dB at 500 Hz
40 dB at 1000 Hz (*the reference*)
39 dB at 2000 Hz
40 dB at 5000 Hz

Because all of these sounds are equally loud we say they have the same **loudness level**. The loudness level curve is called a **loudness level contour**, **equal loudness contour**, or **Fletcher-Munson curve**. The number 40 does not mean 40 dB. Instead, it refers to the loudness level of the sounds along the curve, that is, all of the SPLs at different frequencies that are perceived to be equally loud as a 1000 Hz reference

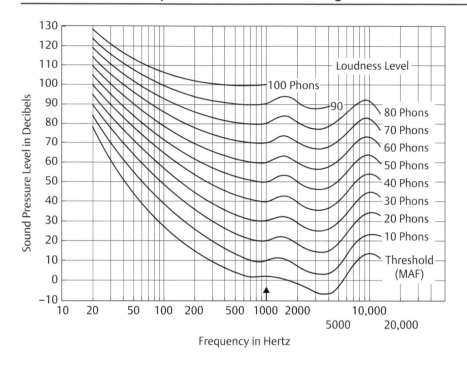

Fig. 3.8 Equal loudness-level or phon curves (based on values from ISO-226, 2003) and binaural free-field auditory threshold curve (based on values from ANSI S3.6-2010 and ISO 389-7, 2005). Notice how the number of phons corresponds to the number of decibels at 1000 Hz.

frequency at 40 dB SPL. To avoid confusing loudness and intensity, the loudness level of this curve is said to be "40 phons" (as distinguished from decibels). The **phon** is the *unit of loudness level*. By convention, the number of phons corresponds to the number of decibels *at* 1000 Hz. As a result, an equal-loudness contour is also called a **phon curve**. Hence, we have been discussing the *40 phon curve*. The other phon curves in **Fig. 3.8** were obtained in the same manner used to generate the 40 phon curve, except that the loudness balances were made to different levels of the 1000 Hz reference tone (e.g., 1000 Hz at 20 dB for the 20 phon line, 80 dB for the 80 phon line, etc.).

The equal-loudness contours flatten as intensity increases, particularly for the lower frequencies. This is analogous to what we saw when we compared the effect of frequency on auditory thresholds versus maximum listening levels. As a result, the distance in decibels between a softer phon curve and a much louder phon curve is narrower for the low frequencies than for higher frequencies. For example, 10 phons corresponds to ~ 30 dB at 100 Hz and 10 dB at 1000 Hz, whereas 100 phons corresponds to ~103 dB at 100 Hz and 100 dB at 1000 Hz. As a result, the spread between 10 phons and 100 phons is 90 dB wide at 1000 Hz but only 73 dB wide at 100 Hz. In other words, a 73 dB increase at 100 Hz sounds like a 90 dB increase at 1000 Hz.

These curves are not just some esoteric effect confined to the laboratory. It is an experience familiar to anyone who has ever changed the volume con-

trol on a stereo system: A musical selection that has a natural sound when it is being played softly will become "boomy" when the volume is increased, and a natural-sounding loud selection begins to sound "tinny" when the volume is decreased. This is one of the reasons why there are *bass* (low pitch) and *treble* (high pitch) controls on stereo systems. We turn down the bass after raising the volume to counteract the disproportionate loudness boost in the low frequencies, which results when the intensity is increased. Similarly, we turn up the bass after lowering the volume to counteract the disproportionate drop in low-frequency loudness, which occurs when the intensity is decreased.

Loudness

Phon curves show equally loud relationships among different sounds but they do not show how loudness is related to intensity. This would require a scale of loudness as a function of intensity of the type described in the earlier discussion of magnitude and ratio scales (e.g., as in **Fig. 3.3**). The loudness-intensity relationship based on methods of this type is called the **sone scale** (Stevens, 1975; ANSI S3.4-2007), and is illustrated in idealized form in **Fig. 3.9**. The *unit of loudness* is called the **sone**. By convention, the reference intensity for the sone scale is a 1000 Hz tone at 40 dB, and its loudness is 1 sone. The sone scale expresses loudness as ratios. Hence, the tone that is

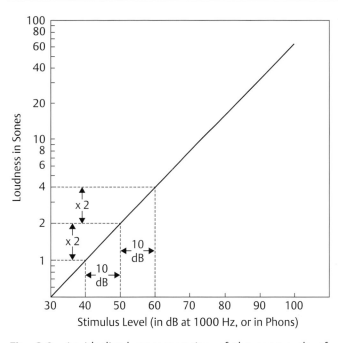

Fig. 3.9 An idealized representation of the sone scale of loudness. Notice that a doubling or halving of loudness in sones corresponds to a 10 dB (or 10 phon) increase or decrease in level (*dotted lines*). (More precisely, the function actually curves downward below ~ 40 phons (ANSI-S3.4–2007.).

The exponent *e* describes the slope of the line that relates loudness to intensity (it will suffice to say *k* is a constant). This relationship is **Stevens' power law** (1975), which more generally states that the magnitude of a perception is equal to a power (exponent) of the magnitude of the stimulus. The slope of the loudness function is ~ 0.6, so that L = $10^{0.6}$. A slope (exponent) of 1.0 means that the perception has a one-to-one relationship to the size of the stimulus. The slope of 0.6 means that loudness increases at a slower rate than intensity increases. Other perceptions such as brightness also have exponents that are less than 1.0. On the other hand, exponents greater than 1.0 are encountered for percepts that increase faster than the physical stimulus level; electric shock is a noteworthy example.

The Critical Band

Loudness is related to the bandwidth of the sound. Suppose we have a sound made up of two frequencies that are just 10 Hz apart (e.g., 995 Hz and 1005 Hz). We then slowly move these two tones farther apart in frequency so that the separation between them increases. We will find that the loudness of this sound stays the same until the separation reaches a certain critical width. Beyond this, making the separation between the two frequencies any wider will cause the sound to become louder even though the intensity is still the same; the wider the separation, the louder the sound becomes. The same phenomenon occurs using a band of noise that starts out narrow and gets wider and wider: the loudness stays the same until a certain bandwidth is reached, but it becomes louder as the bandwidth widens beyond that point, as illustrated in **Fig. 3.10**. This bandwidth, where perceptual changes occur, is called the **critical band** (Scharf 1970) and is one of several indicators of the frequency-selective nature of the ear. The critical bandwidth becomes broader as the center frequency gets higher above ~ 1000 Hz, as shown in **Fig. 3.11**. However, the student should avoid the trap of thinking of a fixed series of individual bands that are arranged one next to the other. Instead, critical bands may be conceived of as overlapping on a smooth continuum, so that there would be a critical bandwidth no matter what the center frequency might be.

twice as loud as 40 dB (1 sone) would be 2 sones; the tone that is four times as loud is 4 sones; the tone that is half as loud would be 0.5 sone; etc. Notice the distinction between *loudness in sones* and *loudness level in phons*. At other frequencies than 1000 Hz the level of the sound would be expressed in phons (which are uniformly equivalent to decibels only at 1000 Hz). Comparing dotted lines in the figure reveals that a level increase of about 10 dB (or 10 phons) results in a doubling of loudness (e.g., 1 to 2 sones, 2 to 4 sones, etc.), and a 10 dB decrease results in a halving of loudness (e.g., 2 to 1 sone; 1 to 0.5 sone).

The sone scale is shown as a straight line[1] in the figure, and both axes of the graph are logarithmic. The logarithmic scale is clearly indicated on the y-axis, and is implicit for the x-axis because decibels are logarithmic values. A straight line on a log-log graph indicates an exponential or power relationship. Consequently, we can say that loudness (L) is a *power function* of intensity (I), or

$$L = kI^e$$

Pitch

Even though we can detect sound frequencies as low as ~ 2 Hz, the lowest frequency that is associated with "tonality" or a perceptible pitch is ~ 20 Hz. There is also a minimum duration necessary before a sound

---

[1] In actuality, the sone curve arches downward below ~ 40 phons (ANSI-S3.4, 2007).

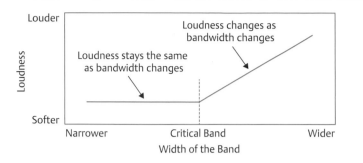

Fig. 3.10 Loudness increases when the bandwidth of a sound becomes wider than the critical band.

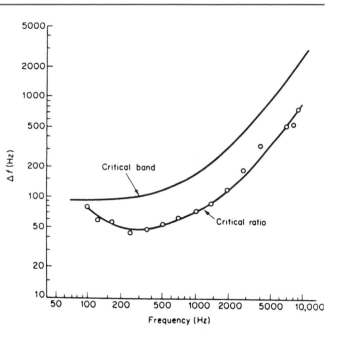

Fig. 3.11 Width of the critical band (Df [Hz]) and the masking critical ratio as a function of center frequency. (Adapted from Zwicker, Flottorp, & Stevens [1957], with permission of the *Journal of the Acoustical Society of America.*)

takes on a tonal quality, which is ~ 10 milliseconds for frequencies above 1000 Hz. Lower-frequency sounds must be on long enough for us to hear several cycles (periods) in order for tonality to be perceived (e.g., 15 milliseconds at 500 Hz and 60 milliseconds at 50 Hz).

Just as the sone scale relates intensity and loudness, the relationship between pitch and frequency is depicted by the **mel scale**, in which the *unit of pitch* is the **mel** (Stevens 1975). The reference point for the mel scale is a 1000 Hz tone at 40 phons, which has a pitch of 1000 mels. Following what we know about the nature of ratio scales, 2000 mels is twice as high as (twice the pitch of) 1000 mels, 500 mels is half as high, etc. An idealized example of the mel scale is shown in **Fig. 3.12**.

Notice that the relation between frequency and pitch is somewhat S-shaped rather than linear, and that the frequency range of 16,000 Hz is "compressed" into a pitch range of only ~ 3300 mels. (This point is highlighted by the dashed lines labeled 16,000 Hz and 3300 mels extending to the upper right end of the curve.) Let's see what this means. A doubling of pitch from 1000 mels to 2000 mels corresponds to a tripling of frequency from 1000 Hz to roughly 3000 Hz, as illustrated by the guidelines and shaded region in the figure. In other words, doubling the frequency from 1000 Hz to 2000 Hz results in *less than* a doubling of the pitch. We would expect that doubling the pitch again from 2000 mels should bring us to 4000 mels. However, this does not happen. Instead, the maximum pitch that is attainable within the entire audible frequency range is less than ~ 3500 mels.

There is disagreement between the musical pitch scale and the psychoacoustic pitch scale in mels, even though neither of them is wrong. For example, the range from 100 to 200 Hz and the range from 1000 to 2000 Hz are both musical octaves. An **octave**

is a 2-to-1 ratio. However, these two doublings of frequency (on the x-axis) do not correspond to equal distances in mels (on the y-axis). You can see this for yourself by drawing vertical pencil lines from 100, 200, and 2000 Hz on the x-axis up to the curve, and then extending them horizontally to the y-axis, just like the dotted lines already printed at 1000 Hz and ~ 3000 Hz. The distance in mels on the y-axis between the 100 and 200 Hz lines will be smaller than the distance between the 1000 and 2000 Hz lines.

Pitch of Complex Tones

The pitch of complex tones depends to a large extent upon the perception of the harmonics in the sound as opposed to the place of maximal displacement along the cochlear spiral. This phenomenon is demonstrated most dramatically by the perception of the **missing fundamental** or **residue pitch** (Seebeck 1841; Schouten 1940). In this case, a subject is presented with a complex periodic sound composed of only the *high* frequency harmonics of some fundamental but *without any energy present at the fundamental frequency itself.* For example, the sound might be composed of components at only 1800 Hz, 2000 Hz, 2200 Hz, and 2400 Hz. These are all harmonics

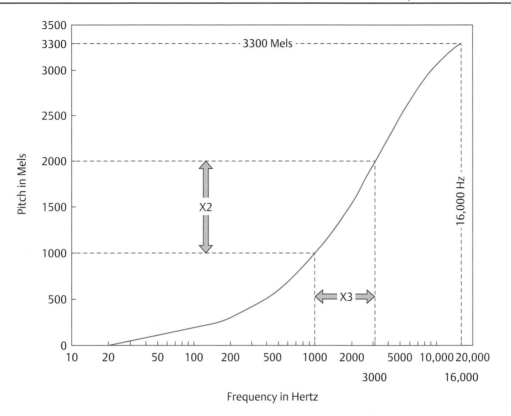

Fig. 3.12   The mel scale of pitch is shown here by an idealized curve based on data tabulations by Beranek (1988). It shows the relationship between pitch in mels and frequency in hertz.

of 200 Hz, but the spectrum of the sound does not contain 200 Hz. In this case, the subject perceives the pitch associated with 200 Hz (the missing fundamental) even though the absence of any energy at 200 Hz makes it impossible for that location on the basilar membrane to be activated. The hypothetical spectrum of this sound is shown in **Fig. 3.13**, where the location of the perceived but absent 200 Hz component (the missing fundamental or residue pitch) is represented by the shaded bar. The perception of the missing fundamental appears to depend upon pattern recognition of some aspect of the harmonics within the auditory nervous system.

A related phenomenon is the perception of **periodicity** or **repetition pitch**, which is the perception of a pitch when a sound is pulsed on and off. For example, if a subject listens to a high-frequency tone that is interrupted every 10 milliseconds (which is the period of a 100 Hz tone), then she will perceive a pitch corresponding to 100 Hz (Thurlow & Small 1955). Perceptions of this type are not surprising because the auditory system is equipped with mechanisms for coding frequency information on the basis of temporal factors as well as place.

■ Audible Distortions

It is possible to hear frequencies that are not actually present in the stimulus. These responses are called **distortion products** and are produced by **nonlinear distortions** in the cochlea. A distortion product is any signal that is present at the output of a system (in this case, what we hear) that was not present at the input to the system (the sound entering the ear). To understand the concept of a nonlinear response and distortion products, consider what happens when you hold a flexible ruler at one end and shake it. The motion of the free end of the ruler (the output) will include several frequencies above and beyond the rate at which you are shaking it (the input), which is understandable because the flexibility of the ruler causes it to bounce and wobble when shaken. These extra frequencies in the motion of the free end are distortion products.

The simplest distortion products occur when tones are presented at high levels, resulting in the generation of **aural harmonics** that are heard by the subject. For example, an original or "primary" tone presented at 500 Hz may cause the ear to generate

Fig. 3.13 A missing fundamental or residue pitch of 200 Hz is perceived (represented by the shaded bar) when we are presented with a complex tone composed of just the harmonics of 200 Hz.

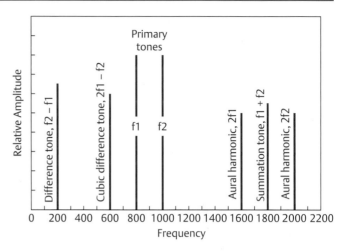

Fig. 3.14 Examples of distortion products produced by 800 Hz and 1000 Hz tones.

signals at multiples (harmonics) of 500 Hz, so that the person will hear 500 Hz plus 1000 Hz, 1500 Hz, etc. **Fig. 3.14** shows two examples of aural harmonics. The primary tone at 800 Hz (f1) produced the aural harmonic at 1600 Hz (2 × f1). Similarly, the primary tone at 1000 Hz (f2) generated the aural harmonic at 2000 Hz (2 × f2).

If two primary tones that are *close together* in frequency (e.g., f1 = 1000 Hz and f2 = 1005 Hz) are presented simultaneously, then their representations in the cochlea will be cyclically in-phase and out-of-phase, so that the combination alternates between reinforcement and cancellation. The result is a tone that waxes and wanes, or modulates, at a rate equal to the difference between the two tones, as illustrated in **Fig. 3.15**. For example, primary tones of 1000 Hz and 1005 Hz will be heard as a 1000 Hz tone that modulates or beats at a rate of five times per second (because 1005 – 1000 = 5 Hz).

Two primary tones (f1 and f2) that are relatively far apart in frequency will be heard as two separate tones; however, they may interact to produce audible **combination tones**. Several examples of combination tones are shown in **Fig. 3.14**, where the primary tones are 800 Hz (f1) and 1000 Hz (f2). A **difference tone** is often heard when the primary tones are presented at relatively high sensation levels. As its name implies, this distortion product occurs at the frequency equal to the difference between the two primaries (f2 – f1), which is 1000 – 800 = 200 Hz in this example. It is sometimes possible to hear a **summation tone** at the frequency equal to the sum of the two primaries (f1 + f2). which is 1800 Hz in the figure. Another distortion product is the **cubic difference tone** that occurs at the frequency corresponding to 2f1 – f2. For primaries of 800 Hz and

1000 Hz, the cubic difference tone occurs at 2(800) – 1000 = 600 Hz, as shown in the figure. The cubic difference tone is audible even when the primary tones are relatively soft, and is of particular interest in audiology because of its applications in otoacoustic emissions assessment (Chapter 11).

Masking

We are all familiar with some variation of the expression "I didn't hear you because the water was running." This is masking. More formally, **masking** is the interference with the ability to hear one sound (the **signal**) because of the presence of a second sound (the **masker**). In other words, an otherwise audible signal is rendered inaudible by the presence of the masker. The typical masking procedure involves a few simple steps:

1. Find the threshold for a signal, such as a tone.
2. Add a masker, such as a noise.
3. Find the threshold of the tone again, this time in the presence of the masking noise.

The second threshold obtained in the presence of the masker will be higher, revealing that the noise has masked the tone. In fact, comparing the second threshold to the first one tells us how much of an effect the noise had on the audibility of the tone.

Suppose the threshold of a signal is 8 dB when it is presented alone, or "in quiet," as represented by the **unmasked threshold** in **Fig. 3.16**. Retesting the signal's threshold in the presence of a masking noise results in a **masked threshold** of 22 dB. In other words, the level of the tone had to be increased by 14 dB to be heard over the noise. The amount by

Fig. 3.15 The interaction of two similar tones, **(a)** f1 = 1000 Hz and **(b)** f2 = 1005 Hz, results in the perception of **(c)** audible beats at a rate of f2 – f1 = 5 times per second.

Fig. 3.16 Numerical example showing how the threshold of a tone is 8 dB in quiet and 22 dB in the presence of a masking noise, revealing the noise has caused 14 dB of masking.

which the masked threshold is elevated or "shifted" is called a **threshold shift**. Hence, the masking noise caused a 14 dB threshold shift from 8 dB to 22 dB. The size of the threshold shift shows the *amount of masking* caused by the noise. In other words, there was 14 dB of masking because the noise caused the threshold of the tone to shift by 14 dB.

The frequency and intensity of a masker determines which signals it will mask and how much masking it will produce. To see the effects of the masker's frequency, it must be either a narrow band of noise or a pure tone. For example, a 1000 Hz masker could be either a 1000 Hz *tone* or a *narrow*

band of noise that is centered around 1000 Hz. Similar masking patterns are obtained either way (Wegel & Lane 1924; Egan & Hake 1950; Ehmer 1959a,b).

Fig. 3.17 shows the masking effects produced by various intensities of four different masker frequencies: 250 Hz, 500 Hz, 1000 Hz, and 2000 Hz. The masker frequency is indicated at the top of each frame, and the number next to each curve shows the level of the masker (in dB SPL) that produced it. These are called **masking patterns**. The frequencies of the *test signals* are shown along the abscissa, and the *amount of masking* (threshold shift) produced by a masker is shown on the ordinate. In other words, the

Fig. 3.17 Masking patterns showing the amount of masking (threshold shift) as a function of signal frequency produced by 250 Hz, 500 Hz, 1000 Hz, and 2000 Hz maskers. The numbers near each individual curve correspond to the levels of the masker. (Adapted from Ehmer [1959a], with permission of the *Journal of the Acoustical Society of America*.)

decibel values on the y-axis show how much the signal threshold was shifted by the masker: if the height of a curve is 25 dB at 1000 Hz, this means that the masker caused 25 dB of masking at 1000 Hz. In other words, the 1000 Hz threshold was raised 25 dB above its unmasked threshold due to the noise. Similarly, if the curve is at 0 dB at 500 Hz, this means that the 500 Hz threshold in the presence of the noise is the same as it was with no noise at all (i.e., there was no masking at this frequency).

These masking patterns tell us a lot about the nature of masking. First, the amount of masking increases (the curves get higher) as the masker level increases. Second, more masking is produced at frequencies close to the frequency of the masker than at more distant frequencies. For example, the curve for a 500 Hz masker has a peak at 500 Hz, indicating that it produces more masking at 500 Hz than it does above and below this frequency; and the 1000 Hz masker produces the most masking at 1000 Hz. Third, the masking pattern produced by a low-level masker (e.g., 20 dB) tends to be narrow and essentially symmetrical around the masker frequency. As the intensity of the masker increases, the range of frequencies that it masks becomes wider and extends asymmetrically upward in frequency. For example, an intense 1000 Hz masker is able to mask frequencies higher than 1000 Hz but it has very little effect at frequencies below 1000 Hz. In addition, comparing one frame to the other in the figure reveals that masking patterns are quite wide for low-frequency maskers and become progressively narrower for higher-frequency maskers. The notion that masking extends to frequencies that are higher than the masker, but not below it, is called **upward spread of masking**.

These masking patterns can be understood in terms of the excitation patterns of the signal and masker along the basilar membrane, as represented schematically in **Fig. 3.18**. Recall that the traveling wave envelope rises gradually on the basal (high-frequency) side of its peak and then falls rapidly on the apical (low-frequency) side. In addition, the excitation pattern becomes larger as the intensity of a sound increases. As a result, the broad trailing part of the excitation pattern produced by a lower-frequency masker is able to encompass the excitation pattern of a higher-frequency signal (**Fig. 3.18a**). However, the leading side of the excitation pattern produced by a higher-frequency masker is not able to envelop the excitation pattern of a lower-frequency signal (**Fig. 3.18b**).

Fig. 3.19 shows the masking of tones by white noise (Hawkins & Stevens 1950). Here, the lowest curve represents the unmasked thresholds of pure tones as a function of frequency, and the other curves

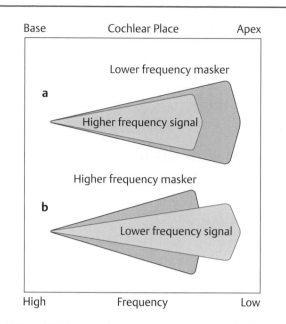

Fig. 3.18 **(a)** The cochlear excitation pattern of a lower-frequency masker is able to envelop that of a higher-frequency signal, but **(b)** the excitation pattern of a higher-frequency masker does not encompass that of a lower-frequency signal.

show the masked thresholds produced by various levels of the noise, indicated by the numbers above each curve. Notice that increasing the masking noise level by 10 dB also causes the masked threshold to increase by 10 dB. In other words, the amount of masking is a linear function of masker level, as illustrated in **Fig. 3.20**.

The noise levels in **Fig. 3.19** are expressed in **spectrum level**, which is the *level per cycle* of the noise. For the benefit of the mathematically oriented student, spectrum level (dB_{SL}) is obtained by applying the formula

$$dB_{SL} = dB_o - 10\log BW$$

where dB_o is the overall power of the noise and BW is its bandwidth. For example, if a noise that is 10,000 Hz wide has an overall power level of 95 dB, then its spectrum level is 55 dB, because:

$$dB_{SL} = dB_o - 10\log BW$$

$$= 95 - 10\log 10,000$$

$$= 95 - 10\left(4\right) = 95 - 40 = 55$$

Fig. 3.19 Masked thresholds in dB SPL of pure tones as a function of frequency for various levels of a white noise masker. The lowest curve shows unmasked thresholds. The amount of masking produced by a given noise level at a particular frequency can be found by subtracting the corresponding unmasked threshold (from the lowest curve) from the masked threshold. The masker levels near each curve are expressed in decibels of spectrum level. (Adapted from Hawkins & Stevens [1950], with permission of the *Journal of the Acoustical Society of America*.)

Fig. 3.20 The amount of masking produced by a masker increases linearly with increases in masker level. Notice that a 10 dB increase in the level of the masker (x-axis) causes a 10 dB increase in the amount of masking for the signal (y-axis). (Adapted from Hawkins & Stevens [1950], with permission of the *Journal of the Acoustical Society of America*.)

Notice that the bandwidth is converted into its decibel equivalent (10 log BW), which is then subtracted from the power level (the equivalent of dividing the power by the bandwidth) to arrive at the level per cycle or spectrum level.

Critical Band for Masking or Critical Ratio

Is all of the white noise actually needed to mask a particular tone, or is a particular frequency masked by only a certain range or bandwidth within the noise that is around it? Fletcher (1940) found that the masked threshold for a tone increases as the bandwidth of the masking noise around it gets wider. However, once a certain bandwidth is reached, then any farther widening of the noise does not cause any more masking. Hence, only a certain **critical band** within the white noise is actually helping to mask the tone at the center of that band, whereas the parts of the noise above and below this range do not help to mask the tone (**Fig. 3.21**).

At the masked threshold, the power of the signal (S) is equal to the power of the noise (N) inside the critical band (CB), or S = CB × N (Fletcher, 1940). Consequently, the *critical band for masking* is actually a **critical ratio** because CB = SNR, or $dB_S - dB_N$

when expressed in decibels. For example, the 1000 Hz threshold is 58 dB when the masking noise is 40 dB, so that the critical ratio is 58 − 40 = 18 dB, which corresponds to 63.1 Hz when it is converted back to frequency (Hawkins & Stevens 1950). In other words, when white noise is used to mask a 1000 Hz tone, the only part of the noise that actually does the masking is a 63 Hz wide band of the noise around 1000 Hz. The masking critical ratio is shown as a function of frequency in **Fig. 3.11**, along with the critical band that was discussed earlier. In general, the critical band tends to be ~ 2.5 times wider than the critical ratio for masking (Scharf 1970).

Psychoacoustic Tuning Curves

We have already seen that a masking pattern shows the *threshold shifts* at many different signal frequencies that are produced by a certain *fixed masker* (e.g., a 1000 Hz narrow band of noise at, say, 40 dB). We can also address masking in terms of finding what *masker levels* at different frequencies are needed to just mask a certain *fixed signal* (e.g., Christovich 1957; Small 1959; Zwicker & Schorn 1978). **Fig. 3.22** illustrates this concept and an example of typical results. The filled circle in the graph represents the

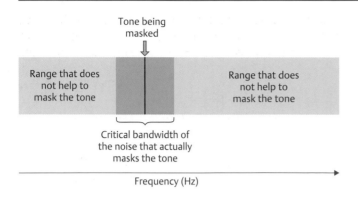

Fig. 3.21 The critical band for masking is the limited bandwidth within a noise that actually contributes to masking a tone whose frequency is at the center of that band.

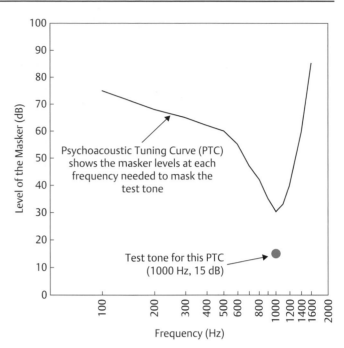

Fig. 3.22 An example of a psychoacoustic tuning curve (PTC). This PTC shows the masker levels at each frequency needed to keep a 15 dB, 1000 Hz tone just masked. The frequency and level of the tone are represented by the filled circle for illustrative purposes. (Based on material by Zwicker & Schorn [1978].)

frequency and intensity of a fixed test signal, which happens to be a 1000 Hz pure tone at 15 dB. Maskers at many different frequencies are used to mask this fixed signal, and the resulting masker levels are then graphed as a function of frequency, shown by the curve in the figure. This kind of masking diagram is called a **psychoacoustic tuning curve (PTC)** because of its resemblance to auditory nerve fiber tuning curves; however, it is *not* the "perceptual replica" of a neuron's response area. Instead, the PTC takes on this shape because the closer the frequency of the masker gets to the frequency of the test tone, the lower its level has to be to mask that tone. As a result, the PTC provides a good representation of the ear's frequency selectivity.

Central and Temporal Masking

Until now, we have been considering masking in terms of two sounds that are in the same ear at the same time, or **simultaneous monaural masking**. However, masking effects can also occur when one or both of these conditions are not met. **Central masking** refers to the masking of a sound in one ear due to a masker in the *other* ear, and is the result of interactions in the lower portions of the central auditory nervous system (e.g., Zwislocki, Buining, & Glantz 1968; Zwislocki 1973). Overall, central masking occurs principally in the higher frequencies, and the threshold shifts that it produces are much smaller than what occurs by monaural masking.

Temporal masking occurs when the signal and masker are not presented at the same time (e.g., Pickett 1959; Elliott 1962a,b; Wilson & Carhart 1971). Here, a very brief signal (often a click) is presented either before or after a brief masker, as illustrated

in **Fig. 3.23**. In **forward masking** the masker comes before the signal so that the masking effect operates forward in time. **Backward masking** occurs when the signal comes before the masker, so that the masking operates backward in time. Forward masking effects occur for intervals of up to roughly 100 milliseconds between the masker and the signal, whereas backward masking is effective for intervals up to ~ 50 milliseconds between the signal and masker. Temporal masking effects involve interactions between the representations of the signal and masker in the auditory nervous system, but there may be some overlapping of the excitation patterns within the cochlea when the intervals between the signal and masker are very brief.

Binaural Hearing

Binaural hearing is the general term used to describe the nature and effects of listening with two ears instead of just one. Every aspect of binaural hearing is fascinating, beginning with a phenomenon that is so fundamental to our perception of sound we actually fail to realize its existence. Specifically, we perceive *one world* through *two ears* (Cherry 1961). This

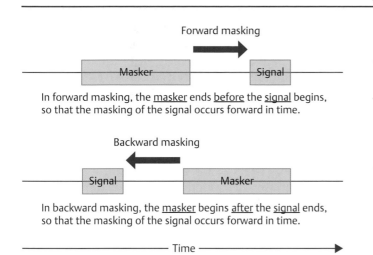

Forward masking

In forward masking, the <u>masker</u> ends <u>before</u> the <u>signal</u> begins, so that the masking of the signal occurs forward in time.

Backward masking

In backward masking, the <u>masker</u> begins <u>after</u> the <u>signal</u> ends, so that the masking of the signal occurs forward in time.

Time ⟶

Fig. 3.23 Temporal masking occurs when the masker and the signal do not overlap in time.

phenomenon is called **binaural fusion**. In formal terms, it means that the separate signals received by the two ears are perceived as a *single, fused auditory image*. Recall that similar sounds are rarely identical at the two ears. Instead, there are inter-ear differences in intensity, time, and spectrum. Binaural fusion occurs as long as there is some similarity between these two signals, particularly for the frequencies below ~ 1500 Hz. Under typical listening conditions the fused image is perceived as coming from a location outside of the head (extracranially); however, it is heard inside the head (intracranially) when the signals are presented through earphones. It is easy to experience extra- versus intracranial locations using a home stereo system by listening to a CD recording first from loudspeakers and then through earphones.

Earlier in this chapter, we learned that beats are heard when two tones of slightly different frequencies are presented to the same ear. **Binaural beats** can be heard when one of the tones is presented to the right ear and the other tone is presented to the left ear as long as the tones are relatively low in frequency (optimally between ~ 300 and 600 Hz). Unlike monaural beats, which are due to interactions in the cochlea, binaural beats result from interactions between the neural representations of the tones from the two ears within the central nervous system.

Binaural Sensitivity and Loudness

The threshold of hearing is ~ 3 dB lower (better) when listening with two ears compared with just one (e.g., Shaw, Newman, & Hirsh 1947). This advantage is called **binaural summation**. In addition to

more sensitive absolute thresholds binaurally than monaurally, binaural hearing results in more acute differential sensitivity, that is, smaller difference limens, for intensity and frequency. For example, Jesteadt and Wier (1977) found that difference limens are larger (poorer) monaurally than binaurally by a factor of 1.65 to 1 for intensity and 1.44 to 1 for frequency.

Binaural summation also occurs for loudness, so that a given sound level is perceived to be roughly 1.2 to 1.5 times as loud binaurally compared with its monaural loudness (see, e.g., Moore & Glasberg 2007; Sivonen & Ellermeier 2011).

Masking Level Differences

The binaural **masking level difference** occurs for abstract sounds such as tones as well as for speech (Hirsh 1948; Licklider 1948; Durlach 1972). It is easily understood in terms of the following example. A 500 Hz tone is presented to one ear at a level well above threshold. A masking noise is then also presented to that ear and its level is adjusted until it just masks the tone. This is the typical situation in monaural masking and is illustrated in **Fig. 3.24a**. Let's use the letter **S** to represent the signal (the tone), **N** to stand for the noise, and **m** to mean monaural. Using this shorthand, monaural masking is written as S_mN_m. The same masking outcome occurs if the tone is presented binaurally and the noise is also presented binaurally (**Fig. 3.24b**). Using **o** to mean "the same in both ears," the second situation would be called S_oN_o because the signal is the same in both ears (S_o), and is being just masked by a noise that is the same in both ears (N_o).

Let us see what happens when we start with the S_oN_o situation and simply *invert the phase of the signal in just one ear* (so that it is positive in the right ear whenever it is negative in the left ear, and vice versa). This situation is called $S_\pi N_o$, where π means "*antiphasic* (or 180° out-of-phase) at the two ears," and is illustrated in **Fig. 3.24c**. Strangely, the tone becomes audible again with $S_\pi N_o$, even though the noise and signal levels are the same as they were for S_oN_o. In other words, just changing the phase of the signal between the ears from S_oN_o to $S_\pi N_o$ causes the tone to become *unmasked*. This unmasking effect will also occur if the noise is made antiphasic while keeping the tone the same at the two ears, written as S_oN_π. This *release from masking* relies upon binaural interactions as low as the superior olivary complex. Now that the tone has become audible, the noise must be raised even further to mask the tone again. The number of decibels that the noise must be raised to mask

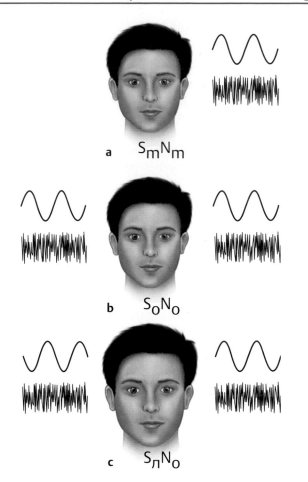

a S_mN_m

b S_oN_o

c $S_\pi N_o$

Fig. 3.24 Masking level differences (MLDs) for the **(a)** S_mN_m, **(b)** S_oN_o, and **(c)** $S_\pi N_o$ conditions.

the tone again is called the **masking level difference (MLD)**. In other words, the MLD is the difference between (1) the noise level needed to mask the signal for $S_\pi N_o$ (or S_oN_π) and (2) the noise level needed to mask the signal for S_oN_o. In normal individuals this difference is ~ 13 to 15 dB for frequencies below ~ 500 Hz. The MLD provides us with a way to look at some of the binaural processes that make it possible for us to hear and communicate effectively in spite of noise and reverberant conditions.

Directional Hearing: Localization and Lateralization

The notions of directional hearing, inter-ear (interaural) differences, and spectral cues were introduced in Chapter 2. In addition, it has already been mentioned that the binaurally fused image is **lateralized** intracranially when listening through earphones and **localized extracranially** when listening in a sound field. The most fundamental explanation for how

binaural hearing provides for directionality is known as the **duplex theory**. According to the duplex theory, the main cues for determining the direction of a sound source are **interaural intensity differences (IIDs)** and **interaural time differences (ITDs)**, with IIDs taking on the principal role for the high frequencies and ITDs predominating for the low frequencies. In other words, sound sources can be localized because slightly different signals reach the two ears, and the characteristics of these interaural differences depend on the direction of the sound source relative to the head. There are no interaural differences when the sound source is directly in front of or behind the listener, or elsewhere in the median plane, because these locations are equally distant from the two ears. As a result, median plane localizations depend upon the **spectral variations** that result from the effects of the pinna, head, and torso. It is no wonder that front-back confusions occur more often than other kinds of localization errors.

The Minimal Audible Angle

In addition to sound localization, we must also be able to distinguish between two sound sources. Just as we express locations in degrees around the head, the separation between two sound sources is also given in degrees. The smallest perceptible separation between two sound sources is called the **minimal audible angle (MAA)** and might be thought of as a difference limen for localization. We can distinguish between sound sources that are only 1° to 2° apart if they are directly in front of the head, but the MAA gets larger (poorer) as the two sounds move off to the side (Mills 1972). In fact, there is an ambiguous zone called the "cone of confusion" on each side of the head where a pair of sound source directions cannot be distinguished because both of them are facing the same ear. Along with front-back confusions, this cone of confusion highlights the importance of head movements for effective localization. The MAA is acute in front of the head because small changes in location here cause noticeable changes in inter-ear differences. This is not the case on the side of the head, where interaural differences are already very large (favoring the near ear), so the two sound sources must be far apart (a large MAA) before there will be any distinguishable change in inter-ear differences.

An advanced note is in order here: There are actually two kinds of minimal audible angles, depending on whether the two sounds are *presented one after the other* (sequentially) or *at the same time* (concurrently). They both involve distinguishing locations, but the *concurrent* MAA also involves identifying the two sound sources. For this reason the concurrent MAA is also affected by spectral differences between the two sounds (Perrott 1984).

The Precedence Effect

Sounds are reflected back when they hit a surface, creating echoes. In rooms and other enclosures, there will be multiple echoes that cause the sound in the room to linger after the original or direct sound, called **reverberation**. As a result, we are often presented with multiple signals coming from different directions. Yet we are usually aware of just the original or direct sound, and we rarely have any difficulty telling the direction of its source. The perception of the direct sound and its correct direction is due to a principle known as the **precedence effect**, **first wavefront law**, or **Haas effect**. The precedence effect is illustrated most simply as follows: Suppose a click is presented to both ears through earphones, but the click arrives at the right ear a few milliseconds prior to arriving at the left ear. Instead of hearing two separate clicks, the listener will hear a single fused image that appears to be coming from the leading right ear (Wallach, Newman, & Rosenzweig 1949). Similarly, if a sound is presented from one of two separated loudspeakers followed by an "echo" coming from the other loudspeaker, then the listener will hear only one sound coming from the leading speaker (Haas 1951). In other words, the direction of the first-arriving signal determines the perceived direction of the sound. This effect occurs for delays up to ~ 40 milliseconds. Two separate signals are perceived by the time the delay reaches 50 milliseconds, in which case a distinct echo is heard.

■ Study Questions

1. Describe the characteristics of the nominal, ordinal, interval, and ratio scales of measurement, and give examples for each.

2. Explain how hearing thresholds are determined using the methods of limits, adjustment, and constant stimuli.

3. Describe how auditory thresholds are influenced by (a) stimulus frequency and (b) stimulus duration.

4. Define the difference limen, and distinguish between ΔI and the Weber fraction.

5. Explain the distinction between sound level and frequency versus loudness and pitch.

6. Explain the sone scale and how it is an example of Stevens' power law.

7. Describe how equal loudness levels are depicted by phon curves.

8. Define audible distortions and describe two examples of them.

9. What is masking and how is it affected by the level and frequency of the masker?

10. Define binaural hearing and give three examples of how we benefit from it.

References

Abel SM. Duration discrimination of noise and tone bursts. J Acoust Soc Am 1972;51(4):1219–1223

American National Standards Institute (ANSI). 2010. American National Standard Specifications for Audiometers. ANSI S3.6-2010. New York, NY: ANSI

American National Standards Institute (ANSI). 2007. American National Standard Procedure for the Computation of Loudness of Steady Sounds. ANSI S3.4-2007 (R2012). New York, NY: ANSI

Beranek LL. 1988. Acoustical Measurements, rev. ed. New York, NY: Acoustical Society of America

Buus S, Florentine M. 1985. Gap detection in normal and impaired listeners: the effect of level and frequency. In: Michelsen A, ed. Time Resolution in Auditory Systems. New York, NY: Springer; 159–179

Caussé R, Chavasse P. Difference entre L'ecout binauriculaire et monauriculaire pour la perception des intensites supraliminaires. Comp R Soc Biol 1942;139:405

Cherry EC. 1961. Two ears—but one world. In: Rosenblith WA, ed. Sensory Communication. Cambridge, MA: MIT Press; 99–117

Christovich LA. Frequency characteristics of masking effect. Biophysics (Oxf) 1957;2:743–755

Dirks DD, Malmquist C. Shifts in auditory thresholds produced by pulsed and continuous contralateral masking. J Acoust Soc Am 1965;37:631–637

Dooley GJ, Moore BCJ. Duration discrimination of steady and gliding tones: a new method for estimating sensitivity to rate of change. J Acoust Soc Am 1988; 84(4):1332–1337

Durlach NI. 1972. Binaural signal detection: equalization and cancellation theory. In: Tobias JV, ed. Foundations of Modern Auditory Theory, Vol. 2. New York, NY: Academic Press; 369–462

Egan JP, Hake HW. On the masking pattern of a simple auditory stimulus. J Acoust Soc Am 1950;22:622–630

Ehmer RH. Masking patterns of tones. J Acoust Soc Am 1959a;31:1115–1120

Ehmer RH. Masking by tones vs. noise bands. J Acoust Soc Am 1959b;31:1253–1256

Elliott LL. Backward masking: monotic and dichotic conditions. J Acoust Soc Am 1962a;34:1108–1115

Elliott LL. Backward and forward masking of probe tones of different frequencies, J Acoust Soc Am 1962b;34:1116–1117

Fitzgibbons PJ, Gordon-Salant S. Temporal gap resolution in listeners with high-frequency sensorineural hearing loss. J Acoust Soc Am 1987;81(1):133–137

Fitzgibbons PJ, Wightman FL. Gap detection in normal and hearing-impaired listeners. J Acoust Soc Am 1982;72(3):761–765

Fletcher H. Auditory patterns. Rev Mod Phys 1940;12:47–65

Fletcher H, Munson MA. Loudness: its definition, measurement and calculation. J Acoust Soc Am 1933;5:82–108

Gelfand SA. 1998. Hearing: An Introduction to Psychological and Physiological Acoustics, 3rd ed. New York, NY: Marcel Dekker

Green DM. 1985. Temporal factors in psychoacoustics. In: Michelsen A, ed. Time Resolution in Auditory Systems. New York, NY: Springer; 122–140

Haas H. Ober den Einfachechos auf die Horsamkeit von Sprache. Acoustica 1951;1:49–58 [1972. On the influence of a single echo on the intelligibility of speech. J Audio Eng Soc 20, 146–159.]

Hawkins JE, Stevens SS. The masking of pure tones and of speech by white noise. J Acoust Soc Am 1950;22:6–13

Hellman RP. Cross-modality matching: a tool for measuring loudness in sensorineural impairment. Ear Hear 1999;20(3):193–213

Hellman RP, Meiselman CH. Prediction of individual loudness exponents from cross-modality matching. J Speech Hear Res 1988;31(4):605–615

Hirsh IJ. The influence of interaural phase on interaural summation and inhibition. J Acoust Soc Am 1948;20:536–544

Hirsh IJ. 1952. The Measurement of Hearing. New York, NY: McGraw-Hill

Hirsh IJ. Auditory perception of perceived order. J Acoust Soc Am 1959;31:759–767

Hood JD, Poole JP. Investigations upon the upper physiological limit of normal hearing. Int Audiol 1970;9:250–255

Houtsma AJM, Durlach NI, Braida LD. Intensity perception XI. Experimental results on the relation of intensity resolution to loudness matching. J Acoust Soc Am 1980;68(3):807–813

International Organization for Standardization (ISO). 2003. Acoustics—Normal Equal-Loudness-Level Contours. ISO-226. Geneva, Switzerland: ISO

International Organization for Standardization (ISO). 2005. Acoustics—Reference Zero for Calibration of Audiometric Equipment—Part 7: Reference Threshold of Hearing under Free-Field and Diffuse-Field Listening Conditions. ISO 389-7. Geneva, Switzerland: ISO

Jesteadt W, Wier CC, Green DM. Intensity discrimination as a function of frequency and sensation level. J Acoust Soc Am 1977a;61(1):169–177

Jesteadt W, Wier C. Comparison of monaural and binaural discrimination of intensity and frequency. J Acoust Soc Am 1977;61(6):1599–1603

Killion MC. Revised estimate of minimum audible pressure: where is the "missing 6 dB"? J Acoust Soc Am 1978;63(5):1501–1508

Licklider JCR. The influence of interaural phase relations upon the masking of speech by white noise. J Acoust Soc Am 1948;20:150–159

Marks LE. Binaural summation of the loudness of pure tones. J Acoust Soc Am 1978;64(1):107–113

Mills AW. 1972. Auditory localization. In: Tobias JV, ed. Foundations of Modern Auditory Theory, Vol. 2. New York, NY: Academic Press; 301–348

Moore BC, Glasberg BR. Modeling binaural loudness. J Acoust Soc Am 2007;121:1604–1612

Morgan DW, Wilson RH, Dirks DD. Loudness discomfort level under earphone and in the free field: the effect of calibration. J Acoust Soc Am 1974;56:577–581

Perrott DR. Concurrent minimum audible angle: a re-examination of the concept of auditory spatial acuity. J Acoust Soc Am 1984;75(4):1201–1206

Pickett JM. Backward masking. J Acoust Soc Am 1959; 31:1613–1715

Scharf B. 1970. Critical bands. In: Tobias JV, ed. Foundations of Modern Auditory Theory, Vol. 1. New York, NY: Academic Press; 157–202

Schouten JF. The residue, a new concept in subjective sound analysis. Proc Kon Ned Akad 1940;43:356–365

Seebeck A. Beohchtungen über einige Bedingungen der Entstehung von Tonen. Ann Phys Chem 1841;53:417–436

Shaw WA, Newman EB, Hirsh IJ. The difference between monaural and binaural thresholds. J Exp Psychol 1947;37(3):229–242

Sherlock LP, Formby C. Estimates of loudness, loudness discomfort, and the auditory dynamic range: normative estimates, comparison of procedures, and test-retest reliability. J Am Acad Audiol 2005;16(2):85–100

Sivonen VP, Ellermeier W. Binaural loudness. In: Florentine M, Popper AN, Fay RR, eds. Loudness. New York, NY: Springer; 2011:169–197

Small AM. Pure tone masking. J Acoust Soc Am 1959; 31:1619–1625

Stevens SS. The direct estimation of sensory magnitudes – loudness. Am J Psychol 1956;69(1):1–25

Stevens SS. 1975. Psychophysics. New York, NY: Wiley.

Thurlow WR, Small AM. Pitch perception of certain periodic auditory stimuli. J Acoust Soc Am 1955;27:132–137

Wallach H, Newman EB, Rosenzweig MR. The precedence effect in sound localization. Am J Psychol 1949; 62(3):315–336

Wegel RL, Lane CE. The auditory masking of pure tone by another and its probable relation to the dynamics of the inner ear. Physiol Rev 1924;23:266–285

Wier CC, Jesteadt W, Green DM. Frequency discrimination as a function of frequency and sensation level. J Acoust Soc Am 1977;61(1):178–184

Wilson RH, Carhart R. Forward and backward masking: interactions and additivity. J Acoust Soc Am 1971;49(4):1254–1263

Zwicker E, Flottorp G, Stevens SS. Critical band width in loudness summation. J Acoust Soc Am 1957;29:548–557

Zwicker E, Schorn K. Psychoacoustical tuning curves in audiology. Audiology 1978;17(2):120–140

Zwislocki J. 1973. In search of physiological correlates of psychoacoustic characteristics. In: Møller AJ, ed. Basic Mechanisms in Hearing. New York, NY: Academic Press; 787–808

Zwislocki JJ, Buining E, Glantz J. Frequency distribution of central masking. J Acoust Soc Am 1968;43(6): 1267–1271

4 The Audiometer and Test Environment

◼ The Audiometer

The principal tool used in the process of evaluating a patient's auditory functioning is the **audiometer**. Fundamentally, the audiometer is nothing more than an electronic device that produces and delivers sounds to the patient. What makes the audiometer unique is that these sounds are very specific: we know precisely what is being presented to the patient, and we can be confident that these sounds will be consistent from audiometer to audiometer. A basic audiometer should make it possible to perform the most fundamental audiological tests, which involve determining how much intensity is needed for a patient to hear pure tones at different frequencies. The **pure tone audiometer** must be able to produce pure tones at certain frequencies, precisely control the levels of these tones, and deliver them to the patient in the manner intended by the audiologist. A typical pure tone audiometer is shown in **Fig. 4.1**.

The components of an audiometer are shown in **Fig. 4.2**. The **power switch** controls the electrical supply to the instrument, and there is often a power indicator lamp to show whether it is on or off. Test tones are presented to the patient by turning them on and off with a button called the **interrupter**. The **frequency control** is used to select among the various test frequencies. Most audiometers include the frequencies 125, 250, 500, 750, 1000, 1500, 2000, 3000, 4000, 6000, and 8000 Hz. The pure tones themselves are produced by a circuit within the audiometer called a pure tone oscillator. There is a **stimulus** or **tone mode switch** that allows the test tone to be presented either continuously on or pulsed on and off at a regular rate. Another mode produces a warble tone, which means that the frequency varies periodically (e.g., 1000 Hz ± 5%) rather than staying steady over time. This feature is not commonly found in basic audiometers. The intensity of the test signal is controlled by the **attenuator** or **Hearing Level control**. (*Frequency dial, attenuator* or *HL dial,* and *dial readings* are convenient terms that continue to be used even though many digital instruments have replaced dials with other kinds of controls.) Unlike common volume controls, attenuators are **calibrated**, which means that the markings on the attenuator refer to *specific physical values and increments.* Setting the attenuator to "45 dB HL" will cause the sound coming out of the earphone to have a sound pressure level (SPL) that actually corresponds to 45 dB HL; and changing the attenuator setting by 5 dB means the sound pressure level will really change by 5 dB. Most audiometers have attenuators that are calibrated in 5 dB steps, and more sophisticated models also provide for testing in 1 dB, 2 dB, or some other step size. The range of intensities that can be tested usually goes from as low as –10 dB HL up to 115 dB HL for air-conduction and ~ 70 dB for bone-conduction. The

Fig. 4.1 An example of a basic pure tone audiometer. (Courtesy of Grason-Stadler, Inc.)

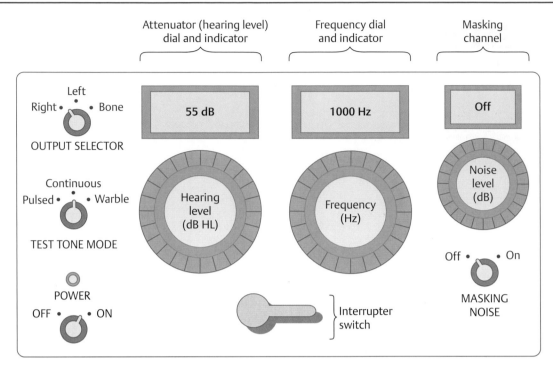

Fig. 4.2 Components of audiometers.

testable range varies for each type of signal and is indicated on the audiometer.

Finally, an **output selector** is used to direct the signal to the right or left earphone, or to the **bone-conduction vibrator**. **Fig. 4.3** shows examples of typical audiometric earphones and a bone-conduction vibrator. The standard audiometric headset includes a headband that holds two earphones, each of which is surrounded by a rubber cushion. They are often called supra-aural earphones because the earphone/cushion combination is worn over the ear. This is in contrast to the less frequently used circumaural earphones, which have cushions that fit around the ears. **Insert earphones** have a pliable earpiece that is inserted into the external auditory canal, and are also used for various clinical purposes, as discussed in Chapters 5 and 9. A **bone-conduction vibrator** is usually held against the mastoid by a spring-like headband.

The audiometer described so far would be considered a single-channel instrument because it can produce only one signal. However, many pure tone audiometers have a second channel that can produce a **masking noise**. The second channel has its own interrupter switch and attenuator. The noise signal is produced by a circuit inside the audiometer called a noise generator. It is premature to discuss masking at this point, except to say that we might need to put a masking noise into the left ear to prevent it from hearing the test tones that are being presented to the right ear.

Fig. 4.3 Examples of **(a)** standard supra-aural audiometric earphones, **(b)** a bone-conduction vibrator, and **(c)** insert receivers.

Clinical audiometers such as the one depicted in **Fig. 4.4** include all of the features of pure tone audiometers, plus a wide array of features that enable them to perform sophisticated tests with tones and many other kinds of signals. These instruments also

Fig. 4.4 Example of a state-of-the-art clinical audiometer that is able to perform a wide variety of clinical tests. (Courtesy of Grason-Stadler, Inc.)

include microphones; inputs for tape and CD players that are used to present recorded tests; patient response microphones; an intercom system; a patient response signal; computer interface; etc. Some instruments provide for testing in the 8000 to 16,000 Hz range, and are identified as **extended high-frequency audiometers**. In addition, the output selector of a clinical audiometer provides a wide choice of **output transducers**, such as (1) the right or left earphone, (2) the right or left insert receiver, (3) the bone-conduction vibrator, (4) loudspeakers, and (5) any *combination* of these. How many and which ones of these and other functions are provided varies by manufacturer and model. In fact, the term *clinical audiometer* is really professional jargon for an instrument that is sufficiently versatile and accurate to meet the extensive clinical needs of an audiologist. Technically, audiometers are actually specified in terms of type based on standards for the functions they provide and the accuracy of these capabilities (ANSI S3.6-2010).

■ Hearing Level

Recall from Chapter 3 that our actual hearing sensitivity in decibels of sound pressure level (dB SPL re: 2×10^{-5} N/m^2 or 20 μPa) is not the same at every frequency. For example, the average normal person needs 26.5 dB SPL just to barely hear a 250 Hz tone, but only 7.5 dB SPL to just hear a 1000 Hz tone. **Table 4.1** shows what the normal threshold SPLs are when using typical audiometric earphones. We consider these values to be **normal reference values**—more technically, **reference equivalent threshold sound pressure levels (RETSPLs)**—because they are the physical intensities needed by normal people to reach the threshold of hearing. In fact, when we say a person has a "hearing loss," we really mean that she requires higher SPLs than these values to just hear a sound; the more her thresholds deviate from these reference values, the worse is her hearing loss.

It is inconvenient to have different reference values at every frequency, particularly when they are "odd" numbers like 47.5, 13.5, 7.5, and 11. Life would be more pleasant if we could use the same number to represent the normal value at every frequency, especially if that reference could have a convenient value like zero. How can we make that happen?

Even though the reference values in **Table 4.1** have different sound pressure levels, they are all just barely audible—and therefore equally audible. In other words, these different physical intensities are the *same* with respect to *hearing*. Hence, we can say that each of these different *sound pressure levels* has the same *hearing level*.

Table 4.1 Reference values (reference equivalent threshold sound pressure levels [RETSPLs]) for standard supra-aural audiometric earphones expressed as the sound pressure levels (dB SPL in a 6-cc coupler, type NBS-9A) corresponding to 0 dB hearing level (HL)[a]

Frequency (Hz)										
125	250	500	750	1000	1500	2000	3000	4000	6000	8000
TDH-49 and -50 earphones										
47.5	26.5	13.5	8.5	7.5	7.5	11.0	9.5	10.5	13.5	13.0
TDH-39 earphones										
45.0	25.5	11.5	8.0	7.0	6.5	9.0	10.0	9.5	15.5	13.0

[a]Adapted from ANSI S3.6-2010.

What is the **hearing level** of each of these threshold sounds? Because each of the SPLs in **Table 4.1** is the softest sound that can be heard, it makes sense to say that they constitute the reference values for hearing. We already know that a reference has a decibel value of zero. In other words, each of these threshold SPL values corresponds to a *hearing level (HL) of 0 dB,* or simply *0 dB HL.* Now we can say it takes 26.5 dB SPL to reach 0 dB HL at 250 Hz, 7.5 dB SPL to reach 0 dB HL at 1000 Hz, and 10.5 dB SPL to reach 0 dB HL at 4000 Hz.

The circles in **Fig. 4.5** show these normal threshold reference values as a function of frequency in terms of both SPL (**Fig. 4.5a**) and hearing level (**Fig. 4.5b**). Notice that the SPL graph is read upward whereas the HL graph is read downward. The curved line in **Fig. 4.5a** demonstrates that these thresholds have different physical values in dB SPL, but they fall along a straight line at 0 dB HL in **Fig. 4.5b** because they have the same hearing levels. We might say that hearing level considers each reference SPL value to be 0 dB HL. For illustrative purposes, the threshold curve of a person with a hearing loss at high frequencies is shown by the triangles in the figure. The hearing loss (triangles) is seen as a deviation from the normal values (the circles). Notice how much easier it is to think of "normal" as a straight line.

Let us now put the idea of hearing level together with the audiometer. The attenuator dial on the audiometer reads in decibels of hearing level (dB HL), and all of the reference values shown in **Table 4.1** are built into the audiometer's circuitry. When the tester sets the attenuator dial to any value in dB HL, the audiometer automatically adds the reference value needed to produce the corresponding physical intensity. For example, when the frequency is set to 1000 Hz (where the reference value is 7.5 dB SPL), an attenuator setting of 0 dB HL causes the audiometer to produce a tone of

$$0 + 7.5 = 7.5 \text{ dB SPL}$$

and an attenuator setting of 55 dB HL results in

$$55 + 7.5 + 62.5 \text{ dB SPL}$$

If the frequency is set to 500 Hz (where the reference value is 13.5 dB SPL), then 0 dB HL yields

$$0 + 13.5 = 13.5 \text{ dB SPL}$$

and 65 dB HL would result in a tone of

$$65 + 13.5 = 78.5 \text{ dB SPL}$$

For most purposes, the SPLs are transparent to us and we deal only in terms of the hearing level values in dB HL.

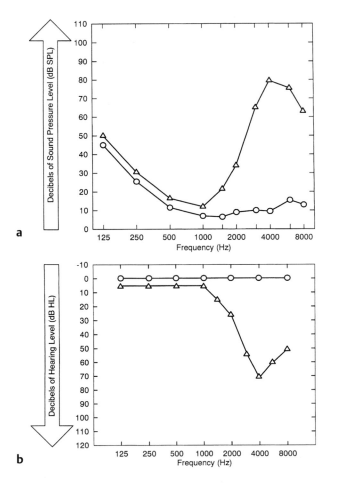

a

b

Fig. 4.5 Normal hearing thresholds (circles) as a function of frequency appear **(a)** as a curved line representing different physical values in dB SPL and **(b)** as a straight line representing the same hearing values in dB HL. The triangles show the thresholds of a person who has a hearing loss in the higher frequencies in **(a)** dB SPL and **(b)** dB HL. Notice how intensity increases upward in frame **(a)** and downward in frame **(b)**. (Adapted from Gelfand [1981], with permission.)

■ Audiometer Calibration

We need to know what sound is actually being presented to the patient. For example, when the frequency dial says "1000 Hz" and the attenuator says "40 dB HL," the audiometer should actually be producing a 1000 Hz tone at 40 dB HL. For this reason, there are **national** and **international standards** that specify the physical characteristics of the sounds that are produced by an audiometer. These standards also specify the tolerances for these characteristics, which means how far the actual sounds are allowed to deviate from the standard values. Most of these requirements are contained in the *American National Standard Specifications for Audiometers* (ANSI S3.6 2010). **Calibration** is the process of making sure that an instrument is really doing what it is supposed to be doing. In this case, it is the process of making sure the audiometer is in compliance with the applicable standards. When an audiometer is calibrated to the ANSI S3.6-2010 standard, it is said to be calibrated to **ANSI/ISO Hearing Level**, and we say that the values are expressed in *decibels of ANSI/ISO Hearing Level,* or *dB re: ANSI-2010* (or similar terminology). The term *ANSI/ISO* reflects the corresponding international standards, ISO 389-1–5,7 (1994a–c, 1998, 2005, 2006), as well as the ANSI standard.

Air-Conduction Calibration

An audiometer is calibrated with a **sound level meter** to ensure that the correct SPLs are being presented to the patient. More sophisticated calibration measurements employ other instruments as well. For example, a **frequency counter** is used to determine whether the test frequencies are within acceptable limits. Other instruments such as **oscilloscopes** and **distortion analyzers** are used to determine the timing characteristics of the test signal and the types and amounts of distortions that might be present. An audiometer calibration system incorporating many of these components is illustrated in **Fig. 4.6**.

Air-conduction calibration involves measuring the sounds produced by the earphones, and is done separately for each earphone. As shown in **Fig. 4.6**, the earphone is placed on an **NBS-9A coupler**, which is a metal cavity having a volume of 6 cc. This coupler is used because it roughly approximates the acoustical characteristics of the ear, and is often called a **6-cc coupler** or an **artificial ear**. A high-quality microphone is located at the bottom of the coupler. The microphone is connected to the audiometer calibrator or sound level meter, which measures the actual sound pressure level being produced by the earphone. Notice that the microphone measures the sound coming from the audiometer earphone is a very specific way, as it exists within the 6-cc coupler. The accuracy of the sound level meter itself is often confirmed using a **sound level calibrator**, which is a device that produces a precisely controlled signal (**Fig. 4.7**).

Fig. 4.6 Air-conduction calibration using an audiometer calibration system. Notice that the audiometer's earphone is mounted on an artificial ear (6-*cc* coupler). (Courtesy of Quest Technologies, Inc.)

Fig. 4.7 Example of a sound level calibrator used to confirm the accuracy of the sound level meter. The sound level meter's microphone is inserted into the depression at the end of the calibrator, which is then set to produce one or more precisely known test signals. (Courtesy of Quest Technologies, Inc.)

Table 4.1 shows the reference values specified by the ANSI S3.6-2010 standard for TDH-39, TDH-49, and TDH-50 supra-aural earphones (Telephonics). We will use the values for TDH-49 and TDH-50 earphones for the purpose of illustration because these are the values most commonly used. However, reference values will be provided for other types of receivers as well.

The reference values for Etymotic ER-3A and Aero EARtone 3A insert receivers are shown in **Table 4.2**. The reference values for insert earphones are obtained using special types of **2-cc couplers** or **occluded ear simulators** instead of the 6-cc NBS-9A coupler described for use with standard audiometric earphones. Special measurement couplers are used because insert receivers are placed *into* the ear canal instead of being worn over the ear, and are used for many hearing aid measurements.

Extended high-frequency audiometry involves testing patients in the frequency range from 8000 through 16,000 Hz, and requires the use of special *insert* receivers or *circumaural* earphones. The insert receivers look like the ones we saw in **Fig. 4.3**, and an example of circumaural earphones is shown in **Fig. 4.8**. Normal reference values (RETSPL) for extended high-frequency audiometry are provided for Etymotic ER-2 insert receivers and Sennheiser HDA200 circumaural earphones in **Table 4.3**. The outputs of the insert receivers are tested with an occluded ear simulator. Because of their shape, a *flat plate adapter* is used to couple circumaural earphones to the artificial ear.

It is very simple to perform a *sound level calibration check* once we know the reference SPLs and the equipment has been set up as shown in **Fig. 4.6**. The

Fig. 4.8 Circumaural earphones used for extended high-frequency audiometry. (Photography courtesy of Sennheiser electronic GmbH & Co. KG.)

following procedure is used at each test frequency and for both earphones:

1. Select the frequency.
2. Set the attenuator to a convenient level, such as 70 dB HL. (We use a high level so that the intensity of the tone will be well above any noise levels in the room.)
3. Turn on the tone.
4. Read the meter on the audiometer calibrator (or sound level meter) to measure the actual sound pressure level that is produced by the earphone.

Table 4.2 Reference values (RETSPLs) for etymotic ER-3A and EARtone 3A insert receivers expressed as the sound pressure levels (in two kinds of measurement couplers used for this purpose) corresponding to 0 dB hearing level (HL)[a]

Frequency (Hz)										
125	**250**	**500**	**750**	**1000**	**1500**	**2000**	**3000**	**4000**	**6000**	**8000**
dB SPL in HA-2 coupler										
26.0	14.0	5.5	2.0	0.0	2.0	3.0	3.5	5.5	2.0	0.0
dB SPL in HA-1 coupler										
26.5	14.5	6.0	2.0	0.0	0.0	2.5	2.5	0.0	−2.5	−3.5
dB SPL in occluded ear simulator										
28.0	17.5	9.5	6.0	5.5	9.5	11.5	13.0	15.0	16.0	15.5

[a]Adapted from ANSI S3.6-2010, which also provides details about how the insert receiver is attached to the measurement device in each case.

Table 4.3 Reference values (RETSPLs) for extended high-frequency audiometry at 8000 to 16,000 Hz for insert and circumaural earphones expressed as the sound pressure levels (dB re: 20 µPa) corresponding to 0 dB hearing level (HL)[a]

Frequency (Hz)						
8000	**9000**	**10,000**	**11,200**	**12,500**	**14,000**	**16,000**
Etymotic EA-2 insert receivers (dB SPL in occluded ear simulator)						
19.0	16.0	20.0	30.5	37.0	43.5	53.0
Sennheiser HDA 200 circumaural earphones (dB SPL in flat plate coupler)						
17.5	19.0	22.0	23.0	27.5	35.0	56.0

[a]Adapted from ANSI S3.6-2010, which also provides details about how the insert receiver is attached to the measurement device in each case.

5. Compare the actual sound pressure level to what it is supposed to be.
6. Record any difference.

A calibration worksheet such as the one shown in **Table 4.4** facilitates the procedure and also serves as a permanent record of the calibration and its results. Let us examine one of the measurements on this worksheet. The level of the 500 Hz tone should be 83.5 dB SPL, which is equal to the dial setting of 70 dB plus the 13.5 dB reference value (which is built into 0 dB HL). The calibrator meter showed that its level was actually only 81.3 dB for the right earphone. Thus, the 500 Hz tone produced by this audiometer and earphone was 2.2 dB less than it should have been. The ANSI S3.6-2010 standard requires that all sound pressure levels (and force levels for bone-conduction) should be within ± 3 dB of their expected values up to 5000 Hz, and ± 5 dB at and above 6000 Hz. Thus, our 2.2 dB difference is within the acceptable range of tolerances. The worksheet in **Table 4.4** reveals that SPLs are within ± 3 dB of the expected values for all of the other frequencies as well.

An audiometer is considered to be out of calibration if it deviates from the reference values in the standard by an amount that exceeds the allowable tolerances. There are three ways to handle this situation: (1) Its internal settings can be adjusted so that the audiometer's output is brought into calibration. (2) The instrument might have to be repaired. (3) A "correction chart" can be posted, which shows how to adjust test results before recording them.

It is also necessary for the attenuator (hearing level) dial to be calibrated for **linearity**. A linearity check is done by changing the attenuator setting throughout its entire range to make sure that every 5 dB dial change actually results in a 5 dB change in SPL at the earphone. The standard requires the linearity of an audiometer's attenuator to be accurate within ± 1 dB per 5 dB step.[1]

A frequency calibration is required to ensure each test frequency is within a certain percentage of the nominal value. The tolerance limits for frequency accuracy are between ± 1% and ± 2%, depending on the audiometer's type, according to ANSI S3.6.-2010. Specifically, the frequency must be accurate within ± 1% for type 1, type 2, and extended high-frequency audiometers, and ± 2% for type 3 and type 4 instruments. For example, if the dial is set to 1000 Hz, then the frequency must actually be between 990 and 1010 Hz for type 1 and type 2 audiometers, and between 980 and 1020 Hz for types 3 and 4. Sweep frequency audiometers (in which the frequency increases continuously from low to high over a certain period of time) must be accurate within ± 5% of the frequency indicated on the audiogram, so that the actual frequency must be between 950 and 1050 Hz when the audiogram reads 1000 Hz.

Other calibrations are also required, although these are usually done by a service technician because

---

[1] Although 5 dB is the typical step size, many audiometers provide for testing at smaller increments as well. Thus, to be very specific, the standard dictates that the tolerance for hearing level increments up to 5 dB must be accurate to within 1 dB or three tenths of the interval, whichever is smaller.

Table 4.4 *Example of a pure tone air-conduction calibration worksheet*

	Frequency (Hz)										
	125	250	500	750	1000	1500	2000	3000	4000	6000	8000
Right ear Reference SPLs for 0 dB HL	47.5	26.5	13.5	8.5	7.5	7.5	11.0	9.5	10.5	13.5	13.0
Attenuator dial setting (dB HL)	70	70	70	70	70	70	70	70	70	70	70
Expected SPL at 70 dB HL dial setting	117.5	96.5	83.5	78.5	77.5	77.5	81.0	79.5	80.5	83.5	83.0
Actual SPL measured	117.0	96.5	81.3	78.0	77.5	78.2	82.0	79.0	81.5	83.0	83.0
Calibration error	–0.5	0	–2.2	–0.5	0	0.7	1.0	–0.5	1.0	–0.5	0
Left ear Reference SPLs for 0 dB HL	47.5	26.5	13.5	8.5	7.5	7.5	11.0	9.5	10.5	13.5	13.0
Attenuator dial setting (dB HL)	70	70	70	70	70	70	70	70	70	70	70
Expected SPL at 70 dB HL dial setting	117.5	96.5	83.5	78.5	77.5	77.5	81.0	79.5	80.5	83.5	83.0
Actual SPL measured	116.0	97.0	84.0	78.5	78.0	79.0	83.0	78.8	81.0	84.0	83.7
Calibration error	–1.5	0.5	0.5	0	0.5	1.5	2.0	–0.7	0.5	0.5	0.7

Abbreviations: HL, hearing level; SPL, sound pressure level.

they require either a complete audiometric calibration system or a variety of special instruments. Some of these measurements involve determining the amount of harmonic distortion, rise and fall times, switching parameters, etc.

In addition to periodic electroacoustic calibrations such as the ones just described, it is desirable for **biological calibrations** to be done as frequently as possible. This is done by checking the thresholds of someone whose hearing levels are already known. Biological calibrations should also include a general listening check, which is done to make sure that the instrument is working well overall, and to make sure that there is no static, extraneous noises, broken wires, or other apparent problems. For example, a broken earphone wire or contact is often discovered by listening to the test tone while wiggling the wires between the hands. It is far better to find out that the left earphone is intermittently dead during a five-minute listening check in the morning than to figure out you have a problem in the middle of a clinical evaluation.

Bone-Conduction Calibration

The bone-conduction system can be calibrated using an **artificial mastoid** or **mechanical coupler**, as shown in **Fig. 4.9**. This type of measurement is usually done by a service technician because most clinical facilities do not own their own artificial mastoids. The basic concept is analogous to what is done with the earphone and artificial ear, but involves reference values in terms of the force needed to achieve 0 dB HL for bone-conduction. **Table 4.5** shows the reference values used for bone-conduction calibration according to the ANSI S3.6-2010 standard. These values are called **reference equivalent threshold force levels (RETFLs)** because they show the force (in dB re: 1 mN) needed to achieve 0 dB HL with bone-conduction stimulation.

A useful method for biological bone-conduction calibration is based on the premise that air-conduction and bone-conduction thresholds are the same in patients who have sensorineural hearing losses (Chapter 5). The technique requires that the

Fig. 4.9 **(a)** An artificial mastoid used for the calibration of bone-conduction signals. **(b)** Close-up view of a bone-conduction vibrator being tested on the artificial mastoid. The output of the artificial mastoid is connected to a sound level meter. In effect, the artificial mastoid transduces the vibrations of the bone-conduction vibrator into an electrical signal that can be read on the sound level meter. (Photographs courtesy of Brüel & Kjaer.)

air-conduction system be properly calibrated, and requires access to patients who are known to have reliable sensorineural hearing losses. The biological calibration procedure is done at each frequency where bone-conduction testing is done (usually up to 4000 Hz), as follows: (1) Obtain and record the air-conduction threshold. (2) Obtain the bone-conduction threshold and record the number of decibels indicated on the attenuator dial. (3) Find the difference between the air-conduction hearing level and the bone-conduction dial reading. This is the amount by which the bone-conduction dial reading must be corrected to indicate the correct bone-conduction threshold. For example, if the air-conduction threshold is 40 dB and the dial reading of the bone-conduction threshold is 50 dB, then the difference is –10 dB. In other words, 10 dB needs to be subtracted from the bone-conduction dial reading in order for it to be correct (for this frequency and subject). (4) Correction values are obtained for several patients with sensorineural losses (using steps 1 to 3) to arrive at average corrections for each frequency, which are then posted on a correction chart. The more subjects used to establish the averages, the more confidence you can have in the correction factors.

The following example will show why the biological bone-conduction calibration method cannot validly be done with normal subjects. Suppose a subject responds at –10 dB HL for air-conduction and bone-conduction, which are the softest levels produced by the audiometer. It *seems* that both thresholds are –10 dB HL, but the reality might be that the patient could have heard one or both signals at an even lower level. This is a big problem if we are interested in knowing the difference between the two dial readings at threshold, which is the basis of the biological bone conduction calibration.

Table 4.5 Reference values for audiometric bone-conduction vibrators, expressed as reference equivalent threshold force levels (RETFLs) in dB Re: 1 mN, when measured on an artificial mastoid (mechanical coupler)[a]

Frequency (Hz)							
250	500	750	1000	1500	2000	3000	4000
At mastoid							
67.0	58.0	48.5	42.5	36.5	31.0	30.0	35.5
At forehead							
79.0	72.0	61.5	51.0	47.5	42.5	42.0	43.5

[a]Adapted from ANSI S3.6-2010.

Calibrating the Speech Signal

Many audiological procedures use various kinds of speech stimuli. These are either recordings that are directed into the audiometer, or may involve "live voice," which means that the audiologist herself speaks into a microphone. Both types of signals involve using the audiometer's **VU** or **monitoring meter**, which is similar to the level monitoring meter found on almost every stereo system and tape recorder. In effect, the VU meter tells whether the level of the incoming signal is appropriate. For the system to be calibrated, the input signal must achieve 0 dB VU. If the VU meter reads –3 dB, then the signal will be 3 dB less than the attenuator dial reading, and +2 dB means the signal will be 2 dB greater than what the dial says. If the meter is "pinned" to the end on the plus side, then you have no idea of how high the signal is, and you can also assume it is being distorted. In the live voice situation, the audiologist talks into the microphone while monitoring her speech on the VU meter, and adjusts an input level dial so that her average speech peaks fall at 0 dB on the VU meter. Hence, presenting speech in this way is called **monitored live-voice (MLV)** testing. Recorded speech tests usually have a 1000 Hz **calibration tone** on the recording. The level of the calibration tone corresponds to the average level of the speech peaks. The input level dial on the audiometer is adjusted so that this calibration tone is at 0 dB VU.

The reference level (RETSPL) for speech signals is 12.5 dB higher than the reference level (RETSPL) for a 1000 Hz pure tone. This relationship between the reference levels of the 1000 Hz tone and the speech signal is used because it results in agreement between the pure tone thresholds and speech reception thresholds (Chapters 5, 8, and 14) in normal-hearing listeners (Jerger, Carhart, Tillman, & Peterson 1959). **Table 4.6** shows these reference levels for various kinds of audiometric transducers and testing conditions. For example, the 1000 Hz RETSPL is 7.5 dB SPL for TDH-49 and -50 earphones, so that the reference level for speech is 20 dB SPL. For practical purposes, this reference actually refers to the level of the calibration tone on the speech test recording. It means that when the 1000 Hz calibration tone is adjusted to zero on the VU meter, it will then have a magnitude of 20 dB SPL at the earphone when the attenuator dial is set to 0 dB HL.

The calibration procedure uses the recorded calibration tone the same way we calibrated the pure tone system, except that the selectors are set to "speech" and the reference level is now 20 dB SPL (for a TDH-49 earphone): The attenuator is set to 70 dB HL and we turn on the speech recording to play the calibration tone. We expect the calibration tone be measured as 70 + 20 = 90 dB SPL in the artificial ear.

Table 4.6 Reference values for speech stimuli corresponding to 0 dB hearing level (HL) for various audiometric transducers[a]

Transducer	Reference level in dB[b]
Supra-aural earphones	
TDH-49 and TDH-50	20.0
TDH-39	19.5
Insert receivers	
HA1 or HA2 coupler	12.5
Occluded ear simulator	18.0
Circumaural earphones	
Sennheiser HDA200 Flat plate coupler	19.0
Bone vibrators	
Mastoid	55.0
Forehead	63.5
Sound field	
0° azimuth	14.5
45° azimuth	12.5
90° azimuth	11.0

[a]Adapted from ANSI S3.6-2010.
[b]RESPLs for earphones and loudspeakers; RETFLs for bone vibrators.

Sound Field Calibration

Sound field testing means that the test sounds are delivered into the test room by loudspeakers instead of through earphones or a bone-conduction vibrator. The signal from the loudspeaker is transmitted through the air and picked up by the microphone of the sound level meter, which is placed where the patient's head would normally be located.

Recall from Chapters 2 and 3 that hearing in a sound field is affected by the head-related transfer function as well as by whether the individual is listening monaurally or binaurally. For these reasons, the ANSI S3.6-2010 standard provides different reference levels (RETSPLs) for sound field testing for monaural and binaural listening when the loudspeaker is located directly in front of the patient (0° azimuth), as well as for monaural listening with loudspeakers at azimuths of 45° and 90° (i.e., to the side). These values are shown for commonly tested frequencies[2] in **Fig. 4.10** and for speech in **Table 4.6**. As with earphone calibration, a relatively high attenuator dial setting (e.g., 70 dB HL) is used so that the sound level measurements can be made well above any room noise.

The Test Environment and Ambient Noise

We know from experience that you must talk louder to be heard in a noisy room than in a quiet room. This occurs because of **masking**, whereby one sound interferes with the ability to hear other sounds. Consequently, we must be sure audiological testing is done in a room quiet enough so that the softest test sounds used will not be masked by any noise in the room. In practical terms, this means that the ambient noise level in the test room must be low enough to allow us to measure thresholds down to 0 dB HL at each audiometric test frequency by both air-conduction and bone-conduction, and in a sound field.

Audiological Testing Rooms

To meet the need for an appropriately quiet environment, audiological testing is performed in specially constructed, sound-isolated rooms. These testing suites can be purchased from several manufacturers or can be locally constructed. Although we will describe only the commercial booths, the same goals must be addressed when testing rooms are constructed locally.

Commercial audiometric booths come as either single rooms, like the one shown in **Fig. 4.11**, or two-room suites, as in **Fig. 4.12**. A patient's-eye view of the inside of a typical booth is shown in **Fig. 4.13**. When single-room booths are used, the patient stays in the booth and the tester and equipment are located on the outside. Two-room suites include a patient room and

---

[2] Because of acoustical considerations, sound field testing uses frequency-modulated tones or narrow-band noises centered around these audiometric frequencies instead of pure tones.

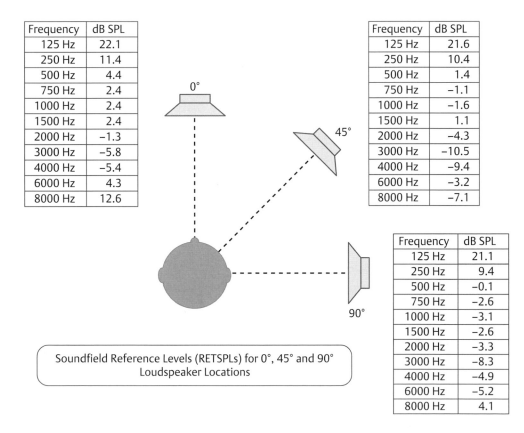

Frequency	dB SPL
125 Hz	22.1
250 Hz	11.4
500 Hz	4.4
750 Hz	2.4
1000 Hz	2.4
1500 Hz	2.4
2000 Hz	−1.3
3000 Hz	−5.8
4000 Hz	−5.4
6000 Hz	4.3
8000 Hz	12.6

Frequency	dB SPL
125 Hz	21.6
250 Hz	10.4
500 Hz	1.4
750 Hz	−1.1
1000 Hz	−1.6
1500 Hz	1.1
2000 Hz	−4.3
3000 Hz	−10.5
4000 Hz	−9.4
6000 Hz	−3.2
8000 Hz	−7.1

Frequency	dB SPL
125 Hz	21.1
250 Hz	9.4
500 Hz	−0.1
750 Hz	−2.6
1000 Hz	−3.1
1500 Hz	−2.6
2000 Hz	−3.3
3000 Hz	−8.3
4000 Hz	−4.9
6000 Hz	−5.2
8000 Hz	4.1

Soundfield Reference Levels (RETSPLs) for 0°, 45° and 90° Loudspeaker Locations

Fig. 4.10 Reference levels [reference equivalent threshold sound pressure levels (RETSPLs)] for sound field testing at commonly tested audiometric frequencies for binaural listening when the loudspeakers are located at 0°, 45°, and 90° azimuth. (Based on ANSI S3.6-2010.)

Fig. 4.11 Example of a single-room audiological testing chamber. (Photograph courtesy of Industrial Acoustics Corporation, Inc.)

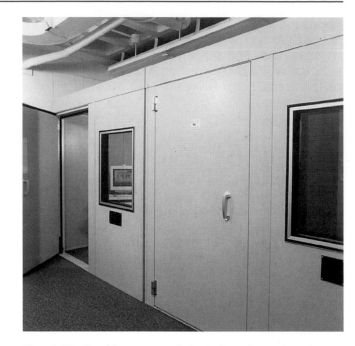

Fig. 4.12 Double-room audiological testing suites. Instrumentation can be seen through the control room window. (Photograph courtesy of Industrial Acoustics Company, Inc.)

a control room. The noise levels permitted in audiometric booths, which are outlined in the next section, actually apply to the patient room. However, the control room should be as quiet as possible, especially if any live-voice speech testing is done. Room size is a critical issue because money and space are always limited. The patient room should be as large as possible, especially for sound field testing and/or pediatric evaluations. The tester's room must be large enough to comfortably accommodate the equipment, the tes-

ter, and an observer. In addition, space planning must account for at least the *outside* dimensions of the test suite, room for the doors to swing open, and wheelchair access. Stretcher access should also be taken into account, depending on the setting, and the space needed for wheelchairs and/or stretchers must consider whether turns must be made to enter and exit.

The walls, ceilings, floors, and doors are usually constructed of 4 inch thick panels composed of metal sheets filled with sound-attenuating material. To minimize

Fig. 4.13 The inside of a typical audiological testing booth from the patient's perspective.

reverberation within the room the metal surfaces facing into the sound-treated chamber are covered with holes, giving the appearance of pegboard (except for the floor, which is typically carpeted). Single-walled booths are one panel thick. Double-walled booths are made of two layers of panels, usually with dead air space between them, and provide more sound isolation than single-walled rooms. The type of room construction is dictated by the amount of sound attenuation that is needed in light of the noise levels at the location in question.

Several other measures are taken to ensure that the acoustical isolation provided by the chamber is not compromised: the doors should close with tight seals; the windows between the patient and tester rooms are made of multiple panes of glass with dead air spaces between them; and prewired jack panels are used so that holes do not have to be made to pass wires between the rooms. The test booth often "floats" on vibration isolators to minimize the transmission of vibrations through the structures of the building into the test booth. Air enters and leaves the booths via a sound-muffled ventilation system. It might be noted that vibration isolation and muffled ventilation systems are often problem areas with noncommercial booths that are constructed locally. It is preferable to use incandescent lights because they do not produce any noise; however, fluorescent lighting can be used if care is taken to mount their noisy ballasts or starters outside the booth.

---

[3] The characteristics of bandwidths are specified in the ANSI S1.11 (2009) standard.

Maximum Permissible Ambient Noise Levels

How quiet must it be in an audiological testing room? The ambient noise in the audiometric booth is measured with a sound level meter. We could measure this noise in overall SPL or in dB-A (see Chapter 1), but values such as these do not tell us how the room noise will affect *each* of the audiometric frequencies. It is more useful to determine how much noise exists in the vicinity of each audiometric testing frequency. (Recall from Chapter 3 that a given tone is masked most by noise that is close to it in frequency, and that lower-frequency sounds can often mask higher-frequency sounds.) To do this we must first specify a range of frequencies (a bandwidth) to be considered around each frequency. This is done in terms of **octave-bands** and **third-octave-bands**.[3] An octave-band is a range of frequencies that is an octave wide and a third-octave-band is a frequency range that is one third of an octave wide. These bandwidths are shown in **Table 4.7**. For example, the 500 Hz octave-band includes the range of frequencies between 354 and 707 Hz. Here, we say 500 Hz is the center frequency, and that 354 and 707 Hz are the lower and upper cutoff frequencies, respectively. The range of frequencies between the lower and upper cutoffs is called the **bandwidth**. Similarly, the 500 Hz third-octave-band has a bandwidth of 116 Hz between cutoff frequencies of 445 and 561 Hz. These bandwidths are used when specifying the maximum allowable room noise levels for each audiometric frequency.

Table 4.7   Octave-bands and third-octave-bands for the audiometric test frequencies[a]

Center frequency	Octave-bands			Third-octave-bands		
	Lower limit	Upper limit	Bandwidth	Lower limit	Upper limit	Bandwidth
125	88	176	88	111	140	29
250	177	354	177	223	281	58
500	354	707	354	445	561	116
1000	707	1414	707	891	1122	232
1500	1061	2121	1061	1336	1684	347
2000	1414	2828	1414	1782	2245	463
3000	2121	4243	2121	2673	3367	695
4000	2828	5657	2828	3564	4490	926
6000	4243	8485	4243	5345	6735	1389
8000	5657	11,314	5657	7127	8980	1853

[a]All numbers are in hertz (calculations subject to rounding errors).

To determine whether a given room is sufficiently quiet for audiological testing, the ambient noise levels in the room are measured with a sound level meter that has a set of octave-band or third-octave-band filters. The sound pressure level within an octave-band is called an **octave-band level (OBL)**, and the sound pressure level within a third-octave-band is called a **third-octave-band level (third-OBL)**. These ambient room noise levels are then compared with the **maximum permissible ambient noise levels** specified by the ANSI S3.1-1999 (R2008) standard. The maximum allowable room noise levels that apply when testing the frequencies between 250 and 8000 Hz are shown in **Table 4.8** and **Table 4.9**. **Table 4.8** shows the octave-band levels of the noise at center frequencies of 125 Hz to 8000 Hz, and **Table 4.9** shows the respective third-octave-band levels. These two tables are used in the same way; the choice between them depends only on whether the room noise was measured using a sound level meter with octave or third-octave filters. We will assume the use of a sound level meter with octave filters and refer only to **Table 4.8**; but the same principles apply to third-octave-band levels and **Table 4.9**.

The octave-band levels in **Table 4.8** are the maximum ambient room noise levels that will still allow a normal-hearing patient to hear a tone presented as low as 0 dB HL.[4] Two sets of maximum octave-band levels are given for each frequency, one with "ears covered" and one with "ears uncovered." The higher maximum room noise levels for "ears covered" apply only when the patient is wearing earphones, so that both ears are covered. The lower (stricter) maximum room noise levels apply whenever the ears are not covered with earphones, which occurs during bone-conduction and sound field testing. Higher noise levels are allowed in the room when earphones are being worn because they act as earmuffs that reduce the amount of room noise reaching the eardrum. For example, the maximum room noise at 1000 Hz has an OBL of 13 dB with the ears uncovered and 26 dB with the ears covered by supra-aural earphones. The allowable room noise is 13 dB higher with the ears covered because the earphone and cushion are expected to reduce (attenuate) the noise entering the ear by 13 dB. The noise level actually getting into the ear is 13 dB in either case. Separate sets of maximum permissible noise levels are given for supra-aural earphones and insert receivers because they provide different amounts of sound isolation.

---

[4] Actually, these permissible noise levels are expected to cause no more than a 2 dB change in threshold at 0 dB HL, which is too small to be of any clinical significance.

Table 4.8 Maximum octave-band levels (OBLs) (in dB) allowed when testing in the 250–8000 Hz range[a,b] with ears covered and with ears uncovered (based on ANSI S3.1-1999 [R2008]); the ears uncovered values must be used if bone-conduction or sound field tests are done

Octave-band center frequency	Ears covered		Ears not covered
	Supra-aural earphones	Insert receivers	
125 Hz	39	67	35
250 Hz	25	53	21
500 Hz	21	50	16
1000 Hz	26	47	13
2000 Hz	34	49	14
4000 Hz	37	50	11
8000 Hz	37	56	14

[a]If 125 Hz is also tested, then the maximum allowable OBL at 125 Hz is lowered to 29 dB for ears uncovered, 35 dB for supra-aural earphones, and 59 dB for insert receivers.
[b]If the *lowest* test frequency is 500 Hz, then the maximum allowable OBLs are raised to 44 dB at 125 Hz and 30 dB at 250 Hz for ears uncovered, 49 dB at 125 Hz and 35 dB at 250 Hz for supra-aural earphones, and 78 dB at 125 Hz and 64 dB at 250 Hz for insert receivers.

Table 4.9   Maximum third-octave-band levels (in dB) allowed when testing in the 250–8000 Hz range[a,b] with ears covered and with ears uncovered (based on ANSI S3.1-1999 [R2008]); the ears uncovered values must be used if bone-conduction or sound field tests are done

| Third-octave-band center frequency | Ears covered | | Ears not covered |
	Supra-aural earphones	Insert receivers	
125 Hz	34	62	30
250 Hz	20	48	16
500 Hz	16	45	11
800 Hz	19	44	10
1000 Hz	21	42	8
1600 Hz	25	43	9
2000 Hz	29	44	9
3150 Hz	33	46	8
4000 Hz	32	45	6
6300 Hz	32	48	8
8000 Hz	32	51	9

[a]If 125 Hz is also tested, then the maximum allowable third-OBL at 125 Hz is lowered to 24 dB for ears uncovered, 30 dB for supra-aural earphones, and 54 dB for insert receivers.
[b]If the *lowest* test frequency is 500 Hz, then the maximum allowable third-OBLs are raised to 39 dB at 125 Hz and 25 dB at 250 Hz for ears uncovered, 44 dB at 125 Hz and 30 dB at 250 Hz for supra-aural earphones, and 73 dB at 125 Hz and 59 dB at 250 Hz for insert receivers.

The "ears uncovered" ambient noise standards should be met by all rooms where bone- conduction and/or sound field testing is done. The less stringent "ears covered" standards are appropriate only when testing is limited to air-conduction measurements, such as screening programs and certain industrial testing settings. Perusal of the footnotes in **Table 4.8** and **Table 4.9** reveals that higher noise levels become acceptable at low frequencies when the range of frequencies being tested changes from (a) 125 to 8000 Hz to (b) 250 to 8000 Hz to (c) 500 to 8000 Hz. Using the maximum noise levels for the 250 to 8000 Hz range is no problem (and is usually desirable) because (1) most clinical testing is limited to this 250 to 8000 Hz range, and (2) patients who need to be tested at 125 Hz usually have hearing losses that are so severe that ambient noise is not an issue for them anyway. However, even though limiting the testable range to ≥ 500 Hz is appropriate for screening and some industrial hearing conservation programs, it is not desirable for clinical purposes.

The maximum permissible ambient noise levels in **Table 4.8** and **Table 4.9** must be met to obtain thresholds as low as 0 dB HL. The presence of higher noise levels will limit the kind of testing that can be done in the room. For example, if the actual noise in the test room exceeds the appropriate maximum allowable levels by 15 dB, then the lowest measurable threshold in that room will be 15 dB HL. If the noise levels are 30 dB higher than the permissible maximum, then the lowest measurable threshold will be 30 dB HL. In addition, meeting the "ears covered" noise requirements but not meeting the "ears uncovered" standards can distort the comparison between air-conduction and bone-conduction thresholds, which is a fundamental diagnostic consideration in clinical audiology (see Chapter 5). Hence, ambient room noise is not just a technicality but is a primary limiting factor in clinical testing.

Unfortunately, compliance with room noise standards appears to be astonishingly poor. Frank and Williams (1993) studied the noise levels of 136 test rooms in a variety of different types of audiological facilities. Only 14% of the rooms met the standards for "ears uncovered" for either 125 to 8000 Hz or 250 to 8000 Hz ranges, and only 37% of the rooms met the standards for testing at 500 to 8000 Hz. Compliance with room noise requirements for "ears covered" was better but still quite disappointing, at 50% for testing either 125 to 8000 Hz or 250 to 8000 Hz, and 82% for testing 500 to 8000 Hz.

It is often necessary to do hearing screening tests in "quiet" rooms in schools or other buildings rather than in sound-isolated environments of the type we have been assuming thus far. Here the goal is to separate those who are *probably* normal from those who should be referred for complete evaluations. The general screening approach is to determine whether the patient can hear several pure tones at a fixed level, such as 25 dB HL, on a pass/fail basis. The screening level that is chosen not only must be adequate to separate probably normal from possibly impaired hearing, but it must also be appropriate for the room in which the testing is being done. For example, if the screening level is to be 25 dB HL, then the ambient room noise can be *no more than 25 dB* above those values in **Table 4.8** and **Table 4.9** (which apply to testing at 0 dB HL). In other words, the ambient noise levels in the room are as much of a limiting factor for screening tests as they are for clinical testing. These points apply equally to hearing screenings that are being done in therapy rooms as part of speech-language pathology or other evaluations.

■ Study Questions

1. Describe the functions of the following audiometer controls: (a) attenuator (hearing level control), (b) frequency control, (c) interrupter switch, (d) output selector.
2. Describe and contrast between supra-aural earphones, insert receivers, and the bone-conduction vibrator.
3. Explain the difference between decibels of hearing level (dB HL) and decibels of sound pressure level (dB SPL).
4. Why do we calibrate audiometers, and what is the difference between electroacoustic and biological calibrations?
5. What instruments are used for the calibration of audiometric earphones, and what are the major steps in the process?
6. What are the similarities of and differences between bone-conduction calibration and air-conduction calibration.

7. Describe how the calibration of speech signals is different from the calibration of pure tone signals.
8. How does sound field calibration differ from earphone calibration?
9. Why do we have standards for maximum allowable noise levels in audiological testing rooms, and what are the implications of using a room that fails to meet these standards?
10. Describe the major characteristics and considerations involved in the design and selection of audiological testing rooms.

References

American National Standards Institute (ANSI). 2008. Maximum Permissible Ambient Noise Levels for Audiometric Test Rooms. ANSI S3.1-1999 (R2008). New York, NY: ANSI

American National Standards Institute (ANSI). 2009. American National Standard Specification for Octave-Band and Fractional-Band Analog and Digital Filters. ANSI S1.11-2004 (R2009). New York, NY: ANSI

American National Standards Institute (ANSI). 2010. American National Standard Specifications for Audiometers. ANSI S3.6-2010. New York, NY: ANSI

Frank T, Williams DL. Ambient noise levels in audiometric test rooms used for clinical audiometry. Ear Hear 1993;14(6):414–422

Gelfand SA. 1981. Hearing: An Introduction to Psychological and Physiological Acoustics. New York, NY: Marcel Dekker

International Organization for Standardization (ISO). 1994a. Acoustics—Reference Zero for Calibration of Audiometric Equipment—Part 2: Reference Equivalent Threshold Sound Pressure Levels for Pure Tone and Insert Earphones. ISO 389-2. Geneva, Switzerland: ISO

International Organization for Standardization (ISO). 1994b. Acoustics—Reference Zero for Calibration of Audiometric Equipment–Part 3: Reference Equivalent Threshold Force Levels for Pure Tones and Bone Vibrators. ISO 389-3. Geneva, Switzerland: ISO

International Organization for Standardization (ISO). 1994c. Acoustics—Reference Zero for Calibration of Audiometric Equipment—Part 4: Reference Levels for Narrow-Band Masking Noise. ISO 389-4. Geneva, Switzerland: ISO

International Organization for Standardization (ISO). 1998. Acoustics—Reference Zero for Calibration of Audiometric Equipment—Part 1: Reference Equivalent Threshold Sound Pressure Levels for Pure Tone and Supraaural Earphones. ISO 389-1. Geneva, Switzerland: ISO

International Organization for Standardization (ISO). 2005. Acoustics—Reference Zero for Calibration of Audiometric Equipment—Part 7: Reference Threshold of Hearing under Free-Field and Diffuse-Field Listening Conditions. ISO 389-7. Geneva, Switzerland: ISO

International Organization for Standardization (ISO). 2006. Acoustics—Reference Zero for Calibration of Audiometric Equipment—Part 5: Reference Equivalent Threshold Sound Pressure Levels for Pure Tones in the Frequency Range 8 kHz to 16 kHz. ISO 389-5. Geneva, Switzerland: ISO

Jerger JF, Carhart R, Tillman TW, Peterson JL. Some relations between normal hearing for pure tones and for speech. J Speech Hear Res 1959;2(2):126–140

5 Pure Tone Audiometry

■ Hearing Threshold

We often conclude that someone has a hearing loss because we have to talk at a louder than normal level for that person to hear us. Even though we cannot directly experience the degree of that person's hearing loss, we can appreciate its magnitude in terms of how loud we must speak to be heard. This is certainly *not* the only manifestation of a hearing impairment, but it does highlight an important point: We can quantify the degree of a patient's hearing loss in terms of the magnitude of the stimulus needed for him to respond to it. The smallest intensity of a sound that a person needs to detect its presence is called his **threshold** for that sound. For clinical purposes, we define the threshold as the lowest intensity at which the patient responds to the sound at least 50% of the time.

The sounds used to test a person's hearing must be clearly specified so that his thresholds are both accurate and repeatable. The test sounds used to determine the degree of hearing loss are usually pure tones of different frequencies. Recall from Chapter 4 that the normal threshold value at each frequency is said to be 0 dB **Hearing Level (HL)**. Also recall the actual physical magnitude (in decibels of sound pressure level, dB SPL) needed to produce 0 dB HL is specified in the American National Standard Specifications for Audiometers (ANSI S3.6-2010), which corresponds to several international (ISO) standards (see Chapter 4). Hearing thresholds are thus given in **decibels of hearing level** or **dB HL**, which is more completely expressed as "dB HL re: ANSI-2010," "dB HL re: ANSI/ISO," or "dB HL re: ANSI-1969" (because the original version was published in 1969).

In the most general terms, a person has "normal hearing" if his thresholds are close to the norm and a "hearing loss" if the tones must be presented at higher intensities for them to be heard. In other words, the amount of the hearing loss is expressed in terms of how many decibels above 0 dB HL are needed to reach the person's threshold. For example, when we say a patient has a hearing loss of 55 dB HL, we mean his ear problem has caused his threshold to be elevated to the extent that it is 55 dB higher than 0 dB HL.

Test signals can be presented by **air-conduction** or **bone-conduction**, or in **sound field**. Thresholds are obtained by both air and bone-conduction because a comparison between the two sets of results enables us to distinguish between different kinds of hearing losses, as will be explained later. Sound field testing involves presenting signals from loudspeakers, and is discussed later in this chapter.

■ Air-Conduction Testing

Air-conduction testing usually involves presenting the test signals from standard audiometric (supra-aural) earphones, as shown in **Fig. 5.1**. Insert earphones can also be used for air-conduction testing. Recall from Chapter 4 that insert earphones go into the ear canals instead of being worn over the ears. They are useful when facing several problem situations, but the convenience of standard earphones makes them the method of choice under routine conditions.

Earrings and most eyeglasses (except contact lenses) must be removed for both comfort and proper fitting of the earphones. It is also necessary to remove any other objects (e.g., headbands or other hair adornments) that could interfere with the placement of the headset (or the bone vibrator that will be used later). Hearing aids should be removed, turned off, and put away during the test. Chewing gum and candy must be disposed of. The audiologist should check to see whether putting pressure on the

Fig. 5.1 Arrangement of the earphones for air-conduction-tion testing.

Fig. 5.2 Arrangement of the bone-conduction vibrator at the mastoid process for bone-conduction testing.

external ear seems to cause the ear canal to close. This is important because the pressure exerted by the earphones might similarly cause collapse of the ear canals, and give the false impression of a conductive hearing loss. We will return to the issue of ear canal collapse later in this chapter. Finally, the clinician gently places the headset on the patient, being careful that the earphone receivers are located over the entrances to the ear canals. It is not desirable to allow the patient to apply the headset because the fit may not be optimal. If the patient is allowed to do this, then the clinician must check the fit and make any necessary adjustments.

■ Bone-Conduction Testing

Bone-conduction is tested by applying a vibratory stimulus to the skull, which is transmitted to the cochlea and heard as sound. To do this, a **bone-conduction vibrator** is placed on the mastoid process or forehead, and is held in place by a spring headband. Even though mastoid versus forehead placement of the bone vibrator is an arguable issue (see below), mastoid placement is recommended here and is the more commonly used method. **Fig. 5.2** illustrates the proper placement of a bone-conduction vibrator for the mastoid process.

The bone-conduction vibrator itself is encased in a small plastic shell as shown in **Fig. 4.3c** of Chapter 4. The part that comes in contact with the skin is a disk with a flat surface having an area of 1.75

cm^2. Most American audiometers use the Radioear B-71 bone-conduction vibrator, which is the one in the figure. Radioear's model B-72 is also available but is less commonly used. The B-71 and B-72 vibrators have replaced the older B-70 model, which does not have a disk-shaped contact area.

Before putting the bone vibrator on the patient, one must identify any structural aberrations or other problems that would affect the proper placement. Common problems are hair under the vibrator, oily skin, and oddly shaped or narrow mastoids that make it hard to place the vibrator without it slipping. Pathologies and surgically modified structures are less common but equally important. Earrings, glasses, hearing aids, etc., as well as gum and candy, should already have been removed prior to air-conduction testing. The vibrator is gently placed on the mastoid process on one side, and the other end of the spring band is placed gently on the opposite side of the head (usually just anterior to the opposite ear). The vibrator should be placed so that the surface of its disk sits flatly on the skin of the mastoid process without touching the pinna. The vibrator should be held to the head with a force corresponding to a least 400 g to achieve adequate reliability (Dirks 1964) and 5.4 newtons to meet ANSI S3.6-2010 standards.

Placement variations on the mastoid can result in threshold differences. For this reason, many audiologists have the patient listen to a readily audible 500 Hz bone-conduction tone while they shift the vibrator around on the mastoid. The vibrator is then kept in the location where the tone sounds loudest. To minimize the chances that the vibrator will shift once it has been placed, it is wise to instruct the patient to keep her head still and not to talk during bone-conduction testing. The patient should also be instructed to tell you if the vibrator moves in any way. It is also a good idea to provide a strain relief so that an unintentional tug on the wire will not dislodge the vibrator. This can be done with a small clip or by looping the wire under the patient's collar.

Occlusion Effect

We have been assuming that the ears are not covered by the earphones while bone-conduction is being tested. This is the typical method, and the results obtained this way are called **unoccluded** bone-conduction thresholds. In contrast, **occluded** bone-conduction thresholds are obtained when one or both ears are covered with the earphones. A stronger signal reaches the cochlea when bone-conduction signals are presented with the ears occluded compared with unoccluded. This boost is called the **occlusion effect.** As a result, occluded bone-conduction thresholds are lower (better) than unoccluded ones, and a given bone-conduction signal will sound louder with the ears covered compared with when the ears are open. An occlusion effect occurs when the cartilaginous section of the ear canal is occluded, but not when the bony portion is blocked. It is also absent when there is a disorder of the conductive system. The occlusion effect can be used clinically to help determine whether a conductive impairment is present in the form of the Bing test (described later in this chapter), as well as to help determine how much noise is needed for masking during bone-conduction testing (Chapter 9). The occlusion effect is discussed further in Chapters 2 and 9.

The magnitude of the occlusion effect is found by simply comparing the bone-conduction thresholds obtained when the ears are occluded and unoccluded. **Fig. 5.3** shows the mean occlusion effects obtained at various frequencies by various studies. The figure shows that the occlusion effect occurs for frequencies up to ~ 1000 Hz, and that it is largest at lower frequencies. The size of the occlusion effect also varies considerably among individuals. This variability is reflected by the differences among the means shown in the figure.

Mastoid versus Forehead Bone-Conduction

There is a long-standing controversy about whether the best vibrator placement is at the forehead or at the mastoid, and it has not been definitively resolved.

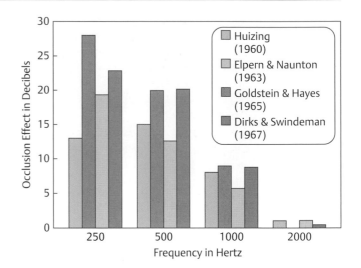

Fig. 5.3 Mean occlusion effects at different frequencies from various studies.

Forehead placement has several advantages in terms of higher test-retest reliability and lower intersubject variability; however, the sizes of these benefits are probably too small to be of serious clinical significance (Studebaker 1962; Dirks 1964).

A practical forehead advantage has to do with the fact that mastoid vibrators can shift rather easily, and on rare occasions even pop off. In contrast, forehead placement is very stable, provided the vibrator is held in place with a holder that encircles the head.

Another advantage of forehead placement has to do with the middle ear component of bone-conduction provided by the inertial lag of the ossicular chain (Chapter 2). Recall that this component involves a relative movement of the ossicles in the right–left direction with respect to the head. At low frequencies, the side-to-side motion of the middle ear bones is activated by the right–left vibrations produced by a mastoid bone vibrator, but not by the front–back vibration caused by a forehead bone vibrator. Thus, the middle ear component makes a bigger contribution to the normal bone-conduction threshold (which we call 0 dB HL) with mastoid placement than with forehead placement. By interfering with the ossicular lag mechanism, some conductive disorders can elevate bone-conduction thresholds to the extent that they depend on the middle ear component. Hence, conductive pathologies have a bigger effect on bone-conduction thresholds with mastoid placement than at the forehead (Link & Zwislocki 1951; Studebaker 1962; Dirks & Malmquist 1969). This is undesirable because we like to think of bone-conduction thresholds as testing the cochlea directly.

In spite of various forehead placement advantages, mastoid placement enjoys a practical advantage that is of overwhelming clinical relevance. The strength of the vibration that is needed to reach threshold is smaller when the vibrator is on the mastoid than when it is on the forehead. This was shown in **Table 4.5** of Chapter 4, where the reference force levels were smaller for the mastoid than for the forehead. Because it takes less vibratory energy to reach threshold at the mastoid, the maximum hearing level produced by a bone vibrator will also be greater at the mastoid than on the forehead. For example, the highest testable bone-conduction threshold at some frequency might be 70 dB HL at the mastoid but only 55 dB HL at the forehead. Hence, a wider range of bone-conduction thresholds can be tested with mastoid placement. For this reason, we often say bone-conduction has a wider **dynamic range** at the mastoid than on the forehead.

A second advantage of mastoid placement has to do with the concept that there is no interaural attenuation (IA) for bone-conduction, so that the signal reaches both cochleae equally. This is really a half-truth. There is no IA for bone-conduction at the *forehead,* but the fact is that IA for *mastoid* bone-conduction is often as much as 15 dB at 2000 Hz and 4000 Hz (see Chapter 9). For example, suppose a patient has 4000 Hz air-conduction thresholds that are 50 dB HL in the right ear and 65 dB HL for the left. The *forehead* bone-conduction threshold will be 50 dB HL, reflecting the better sensitivity of the right cochlea, but there is still the possibility of a 15 dB air-bone-gap in the left ear. We shall see in Chapter 9 that this situation requires retesting with masking. On the other hand, it is quite possible that the bone-conduction thresholds will be 50 dB HL at the *right mastoid* and 65 dB HL at the *left mastoid.* Hence, the existence of IA for mastoid bone-conduction is an advantage for mastoid placement because it can avert the need for unnecessary masking under some conditions.

Some audiologists routinely test forehead bone-conduction while the patient is also wearing the air-conduction headset. This technique is called "forehead-occluded bone-conduction." One argument for this arrangement is that the dynamic range problem that comes with placing the vibrator at the forehead can be overcome by a boost in the bone-conduction signal that results from covering the ears with the earphones, due to the occlusion effect. However, the occlusion effect is simply too variable for this argument to be plausible. This approach does facilitate some aspects of testing because the patient is set up for all tests from the start, but it tends to be quite uncomfortable after a while.

■ Pretesting Issues and Considerations

Talk Before You Test

You want to establish a working rapport with the patient, but this is certainly not the only reason to talk to him before testing. A case history should be taken at this point. If a case history form was completed in advance, then this is the time to review it with the patient for clarification of pertinent details. Always ask if there have been any changes since the last time he was seen. This is also the time when the clinician observes the patient to develop a clinical picture of his auditory status, communicative strategies, and related behaviors. For example, does the patient favor one ear, watch the talker's face and lips, lean toward the talker, ask for repetition, respond as though a question was misheard, have aberrant speech or voice characteristics, or look to his wife for clarification? These are only a few of the questions that go through the clinician's mind during the pretest interview. The information gathered during the interview will be combined with the formal test results to reach a clinical audiologic impression, and will be important in planning the patient's aural rehabilitation. In addition, the impressions gathered here will be useful when giving the patient test instructions, and in making other decisions about test administration.

Look Before You Touch

The clinician should assess whether there are any apparent structural abnormalities and asymmetries of the head in general and the ears in particular, and perform an otoscopic inspection prior to testing. For example, is there evidence of active ear disease, eardrum perforations, atresia, exostoses, external ear abnormalities, or impacted cerumen (see Chapter 6)? Besides leading to appropriate referrals, this information may affect how testing is done and/or interpreted. Test procedures will have to be modified if there is a collapsing ear canal or a mastoid process that cannot properly support a bone-conduction vibrator.

Orientation of the Patient

The patient should be seated in a reasonably comfortable chair. Armrests are very desirable because they make almost every kind of response method (e.g., hand or finger raising) easier for the patient.

Chairs that swivel or lean back should be avoided because the movements are noisy and distracting, and can pose a safety problem for some patients.

Whether the patient should be seated facing toward or away from the tester has always been a controversial question. Many audiologists prefer to have the patient seated with her back to the clinician so that she will not receive inadvertent clues about when test signals are being presented. The unintended cues might come from seeing (1) the tester's behavior (e.g., changes in facial expression or head position while presenting a tone) or (2) the reflections of indicator lamps on the audiometer that light up when the interrupter button is pressed.

The other point of view is that the patient should face the clinician for several reasons. (1) Subtle patient behaviors that can affect the test outcome can be observed. For example, the clinician can notice eye movements or the beginnings of incomplete finger motions when the tone is presented 5 dB lower than the level where the patient actually decides to raise her hand. This often means that the patient is being too strict about when to respond, and therefore she should be reinstructed. (2) Many patients need encouragement and/or retraining during the test. Reinforcing correct response behaviors and retraining the patient is more effective and more pleasant when you can see one another. (3) Most speech audiometric tests (Chapter 8) involve verbal responses spoken by the patient. This means that the accuracy of the audiologist's own hearing can affect the test results. Hence, being able to see the patient's lips and face makes it more likely that the results are due to the patient's hearing ability and not due to errors made by the clinician. But what about inadvertent cues? The answer to this question is that indicator lights are easily covered (as is one's mouth if live-voice speech audiometry is being done), and that controlling one's own behavior is a valuable skill for clinicians to develop. Moreover, the ability to control the apparent cues provided by one's facial expressions can be a valuable clinical skill when dealing with patients who have functional hearing losses. Functional, or nonorganic, hearing impairments are discussed in Chapter 14.

As a compromise, the patient may be seated so that she faces the clinician at an angle between full face and profile. This permits the clinician to see the patient, but it limits the patient to a peripheral view of the clinician.

Patient Responses

The patient can indicate that she heard a tone by pushing a response button that causes a response lamp to light up on the audiometer, raising her hand

or finger, or verbally (e.g., saying "yes" when a tone is heard). The response is expected to have two components: an *on response* (e.g., finger is raised) when the tone begins, and an *off response* (e.g., finger is lowered) when the tone stops. Because test tones are presented in ascending levels starting from below the patient's threshold, there is often a brief hesitation or *latency* when the patient responds to the first (faintest) tone. However, there is usually no delay in responding to subsequent, higher-level tones. Silent responses like hand (or finger) raising and pushing a button are preferable for two reasons: (1) They are clear-cut actions that give the tester an unambiguous indication of when the patient heard the tone. (2) They do not interfere with the ability to hear the test tones because they are silent. Of course, modified and special modes of responding are often needed for young children and for difficult-to-test patients of various kinds.

Although the ASHA (2005) guidelines do permit verbal responses (e.g., saying "yes"), it is recommended that they should generally be avoided, if possible. The obvious reason for avoiding verbal responses is that test tones will be masked by the patient's own voice if she happens to respond while a tone is being presented. A second reason is that some patients do not limit themselves to saying "yes" when a tone is heard. Some patients occasionally say "no" when a tone has not been heard for a while. Others add comments like "I'm not sure" or "I think I hear it," thus increasing the chances that the patient will be talking while the tone is being presented. Comments such as these also force the tester to decide whether the tone was heard instead of keeping this decision with the patient.

Some clinicians have the patient indicate the ear in which the tone was heard, others consider this approach to be undesirable, and still others ask the patient to indicate laterality on an ad hoc basis. The simplest approach for routine cases is probably to avoid the issue of laterality when instructing the patient, and to give her the option of indicating sidedness if she asks. Having the patient indicate the sidedness of the tone in an appropriate manner is often useful in special cases and with children.

Test Instructions

The patient must know exactly what to do during the test. For this reason, test instructions should be explicit and clear. However, they also must be appropriate to the patient, which means that the same set of instructions cannot be given to every patient. Always remember that patients are calmer and more cooperative when they understand what is going on, what to expect, and what they have to do. With these points in mind, the following is a typical set of instructions for pure tone, air-conduction testing:

The idea of this test is to find out the softest sounds you can hear. You're going to hear tones from these earphones. There will be many tones, one at a time. Some of the tones will be loud, but most of them will be very faint, and many of them will be too soft to hear. Your job is to raise your hand every time you hear a tone, no matter how faint it is, and to put your hand down whenever you don't hear any tones. We will test one ear and then the other one. Remember, raise your hand every time you hear a tone, no matter how faint it is. Do you have any questions?

■ Determining the Pure Tone Threshold

Several techniques to obtain pure tone thresholds are accepted by the audiological community, such as the Carhart-Jerger (1959) modification of the Hughson-Westlake (1944) approach, and the ANSI (2004) and ASHA (2005) testing methods. That these respected methods are not identical highlights the point that there is no one method that is the singularly "right" way to test pure tone thresholds. However, these methods agree on the most important issues, and their similarities reveal a consensus of general approach within the audiological community.

The clinical threshold for a tone is generally defined as the lowest hearing level at which it can be heard for at least 50% of the presentations on ascending runs. In addition to this, the Carhart-Jerger (1959) method requires at least three responses at this level, whereas the ANSI (2004) and ASHA (2005) approaches require at least two, therefore taking less time. The two- and three-response rules appear to yield essentially the same results (Harris 1979; Tyler & Wood 1980). The typical test signal is a continuous pure tone lasting 1 to 2 seconds. However, pulsed tones and warble tones may also be used (ASHA 2005), and provide similar results with an easier listening task for many patients, especially those with tinnitus (Hochberg & Waltzman 1972; Mineau & Schlauch 1997; Burk & Wiley 2004; Franklin, Johnson, Smith-Olinde, & Nicholson 2009).

Familiarization and Ballpark Threshold Estimate

Testing begins by *familiarizing* the patient with a 1000 Hz test tone and making a ballpark guesstimate of approximately where the threshold might be. The

traditional Carhart-Jerger (1959) method did this by first presenting a test tone lasting 1 to 2 seconds at ~ 30 dB HL if the patient seems to be normal, or at 70 dB HL if he appears to have a hearing impairment. If the patient does not respond to the first tone, then its level would be raised in 15 dB steps until the tone is heard.

Contemporary guidelines (ANSI 2004; ASHA 2005) recommend using either of two methods. One technique involves first presenting a test tone lasting 1 to 2 seconds at 30 dB HL, which is followed by 50 dB HL if the 30 dB HL tone was inaudible. If the patient still does not hear the 50 dB HL tone, then its level is raised in 10 dB steps until the patient responds. The alternative approach is to begin presenting the tone at the lowest attenuator setting, and then gradually increase its level until the patient responds.

Threshold Search

After a ballpark estimate is obtained, the threshold search procedure is then begun, which uses the following strategy:

1. Each test tone is presented for 1 to 2 seconds.
2. We want the threshold to be *approached from below*, so testing starts at a level that is known to be below the patient's threshold. This can usually be done by simply setting the tone to 10 dB below where the patient responded during familiarization, and then present it to him.
3. The level of the tone is then raised in *5 dB* steps until the patient responds.
4. The tone is now decreased by *10 dB* (or 15 dB) and presented again, in which case it should again be inaudible. This is done so that the threshold can again be approached from below. [Sometimes a patient will respond at this lower level. When that happens the tone is decreased another *10 dB* (or 15 dB) and presented, and so on, until it is inaudible.]
5. The level of the tone is then raised in *5 dB* steps until the patient responds.

Steps 3 and 4 are repeated until the clinical threshold criterion is achieved. In other words, the clinician *lowers* the level of the next tone by 10 dB after every "yes" response, and *raises* the level of the next tone by 5 dB after every "no" response. The tone presentations should be reasonably irregular in their timing rather than following any rhythmic pattern.

In summary, the pure tone testing procedure can be thought of as having two parts. First, we raise or lower the intensity of the tone in fairly large steps to quickly find the ballpark location of the threshold. Once we know the general location of the threshold, we switch to a more formal threshold determination strategy in which the threshold is approached from below in 5 dB steps. This involves two tactics, which are illustrated in **Fig. 5.4**: (1) Whenever the patient does not hear the tone (–), we *increase* the level of the next tone by 5 dB ("up 5" after a "no"). (2) Whenever the patient hears the tone (+), we *decrease* the level of the next tone by 10 dB ("down 10" after a "yes"). It is no wonder this is known as the **up-5 down-10** technique.

A Step-by-Step Example

The threshold search procedure itself is easily understood by going through a typical example. The example shows how to do the procedure and also reveals why it works. We will illustrate only one "threshold search." However, the student should remember that a separate threshold is needed for every test frequency for both ears, and for both air and bone-conduction. The threshold search procedure is therefore performed many times for each patient. The example is portrayed in **Fig. 5.5**. The numbers along the abscissa represent each of the individual presentations of the test tone, or trials. The ordinate shows the hearing levels of the tones presented to the patient. It is assumed that all of the necessary preliminary procedures have been done, and that we are ready to begin the actual testing process.

We begin by presenting the tone at 30 dB HL. The patient does not respond, implying that 30 dB was not heard. This situation is indicated by the – for trial 1 at 30 dB HL. Since the 30 dB HL starting level is not audible, we increase the level of the tone to 50 dB HL

for the next trial. This time the patient does respond, indicated by the + for trial 2 at 50 dB HL. We can now estimate that the threshold is between 30 and 50 dB HL. If the patient did not hear the 50 dB HL tone, we would have raised the level in 10 dB steps until he did. On the other hand, if the patient heard the tone at the initial level of 30 dB HL, we would have lowered it in 10 dB steps until he could no longer hear the tone. In either case, the idea is to rapidly find the approximate range of the threshold, so that we do not waste any effort.

Because the tone was heard at 50 dB HL in trial 2, the tone is lowered by 10 dB and is next presented at 40 dB HL in trial 3 *("down 10" after a "yes")*. The patient hears the tone (+) at 40 dB in trial 3, so we drop its level by 10 dB and present it at 30 dB HL in trial 4.

The patient responds to the tone (+) at 30 dB HL in trial 4, so we again reduce its level by 10 dB and present the tone at 20 dB HL in trial 5. The patient does not hear the 20 dB HL tone (–). The rule now tells us to raise the level by 5 dB to 25 dB HL for trial 6 *("up 5" after a "no")*.

The tone is not heard at 25 dB HL in trial 6 (–). Hence, it is presented 5 dB higher in trial 7. The patient does not hear the 30 dB HL tone in trial 7. Thus, the "up 5" rule calls for trial 8 to be presented at 35 dB HL, which is heard (+) by the patient. Notice how trials 5 through 8 constitute an "ascending run" that ends in a "yes" (+) response for trial 8. In other words, we have approached the response from below.

The + response at 35 dB HL in trial 8 means that the tone must be presented 10 dB lower, at 25 dB HL,

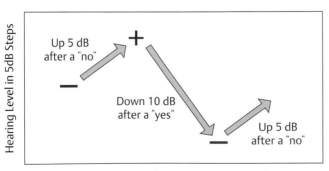

Fig. 5.4 Conceptual illustration of the "up-5 down-10" technique typically used in pure tone audiometry.

Fig. 5.5 Hypothetical threshold search for a patient whose threshold is 35 dB HL. A + indicates the patient heard the presentation, and a – shows that the patient did not hear the tone. Notice that the hearing level of a trial is raised by 5 dB following a – (the "up 5" rule) and is lowered by l0 dB following a + (the "down 10" rule), which causes the tester to search for responses in a series of ascending runs.

in trial 9 *("down 10" after a "yes")*. The patient does not hear the tone at 25 dB HL in trial 9 (–), or at 30 dB HL in trial 10 (–), but he does hear the tone at 35 dB HL in trial 11 (+). Thus, we have again approached a response from below in 5 dB steps, completing a second ascending run (trials 9–11)) ending in a + outcome at 35 dB HL. This completes the threshold search for this tone using a criterion of two responses out of four theoretical presentations, and establishes the threshold to be 35 dB HL. In other words, 35 dB HL is the patient's threshold because it is the lowest level at which he responded to the tone at least 50% of the (theoretically four) presentations, with at least two responses at that level.

We would still need one more ascending run if we wanted to use a three-response criterion. This exercise is shown in trials 12 through 14. Because 35 dB HL was heard in trial 11, the "down 10" rule now calls for us to present trial 12 at 25 dB HL, where we find no response (–). Trial 13 is thus presented at 30 dB HL according to the "up 5" rule. Because the tone is still not heard (–) at 30 dB HL, it is raised again by 5 dB, to be presented at 35 dB HL in trial 14. The patient hears the 35 dB HL tone in trial 14 (+), completing a third ascending run.

In other words, 35 dB HL is the lowest level at which the patient responded to at least 50% of (theoretically six) presentations, with at least three responses at that level.

Test Frequencies and Testing Order

Clinical pure tone thresholds are routinely tested in the frequency range from 250 to 8000 Hz. The threshold at 125 Hz is also obtained when there is an appreciable hearing loss in the low frequencies. High-frequency audiometry, which involves testing at frequencies above 8000 Hz, is sometimes done for special purposes, such as when monitoring patients who are at risk for ototoxicity.

Pure tone thresholds are routinely tested separately for each ear, followed by bone-conduction testing. For air-conduction, the right ear is tested before the left ear unless there is reason to believe that one ear is better than the other. In the latter case, the apparently better ear is tested before the poorer one. Of course, special circumstances often call for flexibility in one's testing approach. Typical examples include evaluating young children, difficult-to-test patients, or those with poor reliability.

Air-conduction traditionally has been tested for the octave frequencies from 250 to 8000 Hz. In this case, pure tone thresholds are obtained in the following order for each ear:

1000, 2000, 4000, 8000, retest at 1000, 500, 250 Hz

The 1000 Hz retest is done as a reliability check and is expected to be within ±5 dB of the first 1000 Hz threshold in that ear, and the lower (better) of the two is considered the threshold. The semioctaves (750, 1500, 3000, and 6000 Hz) are tested whenever there is a difference of ≥ 20 dB between two adjacent octave frequencies (e.g., 3000 Hz is tested if the thresholds at 2000 and 4000 Hz differ by 20 dB or more).

In contrast, the current ASHA (2005) guidelines include 3000 and 6000 Hz among the regularly tested frequencies. Here, the test order for each ear is

1000, 2000, 3000, 4000, 6000, 8000, retest at 1000, 500, 250 Hz

In this case, 750 Hz is tested if the 500 and 1000 Hz thresholds differ by ≥ 20 dB, and 1500 Hz is tested if the 1000 and 2000 Hz thresholds are ≥ 20 dB apart.

So, which group of frequencies should one routinely use? In principle, the author is inclined to side with the ASHA (2005) guidelines, but it makes sense to weigh the value of the added information gained by an extra pure tone threshold against the cost of obtaining it. Patient fatigue and clinician time must be considered because other tests will follow, and pure tone thresholds often have to be repeated with masking. The ANSI (2004) method includes the commonsense recommendation to include semioctaves depending on the intended purpose of the test. Thus, it seems prudent to include 3000 and 6000 Hz when conditions make this feasible, and certainly when they are needed for the intended purpose of the test. For example, we will see in a later chapter that 3000 Hz is often needed for medico-legal purposes. However, it is essential to test semioctaves when one finds a ≥ 20 dB spread between adjacent octave frequencies.

Bone-conduction is usually tested from 250 to 4000 Hz, traditionally in the following order:

1000, 2000, 4000, 1000, 500, 250 Hz

However, the ASHA (2005) guidelines add 3000 Hz, in which case the test order becomes:

1000, 2000, 3000, 4000, retest at 1000, 500, 250 Hz

Many audiologists do not perform the 1000 Hz reliability check or test semioctaves by bone-conduction unless there is reason to do so. However, a 3000 Hz bone-conduction threshold is quite desirable if that frequency was tested by air-conduction.

■ False Responses

A **false-positive** response means that the patient responds when he should not have responded. In contrast, a **false-negative** response means that he fails to respond when he should have responded. False-negative responses can occur for several reasons. Equipment problems or tester errors can prevent a signal from reaching the patient, or cause it to be presented in a manner that was not intended. Some patients are confused by tinnitus if their ear noises are similar to the test tones. The patient may not have fully understood the instructions or learned the proper mode of response. For example, some elderly patients have extremely strict criteria for when they will consider the tone present (i.e., they want to be very sure the tone is there) before they will respond. As we shall see in Chapter 14, there are also patients who do not respond because they are trying to make their hearing appear to be worse than it really is for conscious or unconscious reasons. False-negative responses can also occur for technical reasons, such as collapsed ear canals and standing waves, which are discussed later.

False-positive responses make thresholds difficult to obtain and unreliable from test to test. Some false positives are caused by tactile stimulation and/or acoustical radiations (discussed later). Others are the result of confusion between test tones and tinnitus. Many false-positive responses are behavioral and are often due to misunderstood or improperly learned instructions, or to very lax response criteria. Behaviorally based false positives can often be reduced by refamiliarizing the patient with the test tones and reinstructing him about exactly when and how to respond.

The tester can inadvertently encourage false positives by presenting tones rhythmically. Remembering that most of the tones are hardly audible to begin with, learning the tester's rhythm makes the patient expect tones at certain times, thus biasing him to respond at those times.

A difficult situation can develop if a patient's *false* response coincidentally occurs at just the "right" moment after a *real* tone presentation. Because the false response had every appearance of being a real one, the tester might even confirm its correctness for the patient. This problem can interact with rhythmic tone presentations. Not only does presenting the tones in a rhythmic pattern cause the patient to expect tones at certain intervals, but a rhythmic pat-

tern also makes it more likely that the false responses will occur at the "right" times.

■ Avoiding Equipment Problems and Tester Errors

Several strategies can minimize equipment problems and tester errors. Daily equipment checks are the first line of defense. Errors due to incorrect equipment settings can be minimized by establishing a set of "start-up" positions that are always the same (e.g., frequency at 1000 Hz, HL dial at 0 dB, input selector to "tone," output selector to right earphone, etc.). By always resetting the audiometer to these initial setup positions after each patient, the clinician can avoid errors caused by a control inadvertently set at the wrong position. An added benefit of resetting the audiometer is never having a control in the wrong position. Simply returning everything to the start-up position and then setting up the test from a "clean slate" is a lot easier and more effective than looking for the error. The ultimate version of this strategy is possible with digital audiometers that automatically return to their default positions when they are turned on. One should not be too eager to use the reset button or to turn the power off and (after waiting) on again. However, this can be the only solution when a digital audiometer "locks up" because of programming bugs or design flaws.

■ Recording Pure Tone Thresholds on the Audiogram

The Audiogram Form

The patient's thresholds at each frequency are recorded on an **audiogram**, which is usually shown as a graph. Many audiologists record the information for both ears on the same audiogram form, whereas others use a separate graph for each ear. The audiogram form and symbols recommended by ASHA (1990) are shown in **Fig. 5.6**. Frequency is shown on the abscissa, going from 125 Hz on the left to 8000 Hz on the right, and it is customary to label the frequency axis along the top. Notice that octaves are equally spaced. In other words, the distance covered by any doubling of frequency (e.g., 125 to 250 Hz, 1000 to 2000 Hz, 1500 to 3000 Hz, and 4000 to 8000 Hz) is always the same. This means that the frequency scale on an audiogram is logarithmic. Hearing level is shown in dB HL (ANSI/ISO or ANSI S3.6-2010) along the y-axis, with intensity increasing from −10 dB HL

Fig. 5.6 The audiogram form and symbols keys recommended by ASHA (1990).

at the top to the maximum level (120 dB HL in the figure) at the bottom.

An audiogram form can be of any convenient size but its *relative dimensions* are critical. Specifically, the distance covered by one octave must be equal to the distance covered by 20 dB. We could also say that it is made up of squares that are 1 octave wide by 20 dB high. The relative dimensions are important so that the configuration of a patient's audiogram will always have the same perspective. If the relative dimensions were not uniform, then the shape of the same hearing loss might have a steeply sloping appearance on one form and a shallow slope on another form.

Masking Noise Levels

The table below the audiogram in **Fig. 5.6** is used to record the amount of masking noise that has been used, if any. Masking is covered in Chapter 9. Here, "AC" means masking that is used during air-conduction testing, and "BC" means masking that is used during bone-conduction testing. Notice that this table refers to the ear that receives the masking noise (the "nontest ear") as opposed to the ear being tested.

Audiogram Symbols

All audiogram forms should always include a key that explicitly describes the symbols used to plot information on the audiogram. **Fig. 5.6** shows the symbols recommended by ASHA (1990). Do not be frustrated by the fact that many of the symbols refer to concepts that are unfamiliar at this point. It would be redundant to expand upon the symbol descriptions given in the key, except to highlight some key concepts and the most commonly used symbols. **"Unmasked"** means thresholds that were obtained in the way already described in this chapter, and **"masked"** means that the threshold was obtained with noise in the opposite ear. For air-conduction, the unmasked symbols are a circle for the right ear and an X for the left ear, and the masked symbols are respectively a triangle and a square.

The bone-conduction symbols refer to where the bone vibrator is located, which can be on the right or left mastoid or on the forehead. The right unmasked and masked mastoid bone-conduction symbols are < and [, and the equivalent left symbols are a > and], respectively. The student will soon learn that bone-conduction signals are picked up by the better cochlea no matter where the vibrator is placed. Hence, the unmasked "right" and "left" mastoid bone-conduction symbols (< and >) really refer to the position of the vibrator and not necessarily which ear heard the signal. In recognition of this point, some audiologists prefer to use the "unspecified" bone-conduction symbol unless masking has been used. Unlike air-conduction symbols, which are drawn on the grid line for the test frequency, the bone-conduction symbols are drawn near the frequency grid line. This is done to make the audiogram more readable.

The sound field threshold is represented by an **S** and is described on the key as "unspecified" because either or both of the two ears could have heard the signal (discussed later in this chapter).

If there is no response to a signal at the maximum level provided by the audiometer, then a downward-pointing arrow is added to the symbol. No-response symbols should be located on the audiogram at the highest testable level. For example, if there is no response to a bone-conduction tone at a maximum testable level of 70 dB HL, then the no-response symbol would be placed at 70 dB HL.

To make it easier to distinguish left ear and right ear symbols on the same audiogram, it has been traditional to plot right symbols in red and left symbols in blue or black. However, this convention is probably overemphasized because the red/blue distinction is lost whenever information must be shared: standard photocopying, faxes, carbon paper, and NCR paper produce single-color copies; printed material comes in black-and-white; and certain blues and reds do not photocopy well. Hence, although the use of red and blue is very convenient and desirable, it is no longer strictly required.

Numerical Audiograms

Instead of plotting symbols on a graph, many audiologists prefer to record the results numerically in tabular form. The disadvantages of numerical audiograms are largely related to the issue of whether one can visualize the audiometric pattern from the numbers. However, numerical audiograms have practical advantages when it comes to rapidly recording results and making calculations about masking (Chapter 9). Tabular arrangements of audiometric records are valuable when comparing audiograms over time, in which case the serial audiograms are recorded on separate lines of a table, one under the other. They also lend themselves to computerized record keeping. "No responses" should be indicated on numerical audiograms along with the maximum testable level. For example, a noresponse to a maximum bone-conduction signal of 70 dB HL could be written as "NR70," "70NR," "70+," or "70↓." However, just writing "NR" is ambiguous because one does not know what the highest level was, and the practice of writing the next-higher level (75 in this case) is very misleading.

Some audiologists (including the author) prefer to use the numerical format during the course of the evaluation and then plot the *final* threshold values onto a graphic audiogram. This approach takes advantage of the ease with which numbers can be written and used for calculations, and also results in a very neat graph that represents the "bottom line," rather than being cluttered by numerous extra symbols.

■ Automatic Audiometry

Computerized Audiometry

Pure tone audiometry does not always have to be done manually. It can also be done automatically with **microprocessor** or **computerized audiometers.** These instruments are programmed to test the patient (who responds by pressing a button) according to the same strategies that are used in manual audiometry, and can also be programmed for masking. Microprocessor audiometers can be useful for such large-scale testing applications as screening and industrial hearing conservation programs, provided the population being tested is able and willing to follow the test instructions. However, they are poorly suited for clinical use where patient variability and tester flexibility are the rule rather than the exception.

Another form of automatic audiometry involves the self-recording or tracking method, and is discussed in the next section.

Bekesy (Self-Tracking) Audiometry

Bekesy (1947) described an easy way in which a person is able to record her own thresholds by pressing and releasing a response button. The audiometer has a motor that continuously changes the attenuator setting at a fixed rate, so the hearing level is always changing (usually at 2.5 dB/second). The patient's response button controls the direction in which the attenuator moves. Specifically, the level increases as long as the button is not being pressed, and decreases as long as the button is being held down. The patient listens for the test tone, presses the button when the tone is audible, and releases it when the tone cannot be heard. Thus, pressing and releasing the button causes the intensity of the tone to rise and fall. The motor also controls a recorder, and the recorder pen moves up and down on a special audiogram form as the tone level rises and falls.

Fig. 5.7 shows how self-recording audiometry works. The y-axis shows the level of the tone in dB HL, with intensity increasing downward just as it does on a regular audiogram. The x-axis shows the progression of time while the threshold is being tracked. The dashed horizontal line represents the patient's threshold. The zigzag shows the pattern tracked by the recorder pen, which represents the level of the tone on the paper. In this example, the test tone is initiated at a low level ("start" on the graph). The patient does not press the button because the tone is inaudible. Hence, the level increases steadily until the patient realizes that she can now hear the tone, and responds at point **a**. This causes the motor to reverse direction, so that the intensity starts decreasing, and the pen moves upward on the audiogram (arrow 1). The tone then falls below her threshold, and the patient releases the button in response to the tone's inaudibility at point **b**. Releasing the button causes the motor to reverse direction again, so that the intensity starts rising, represented by the line drawn downward on the audiogram (arrow 2). The patient responds to the reappearance of the tone at point **c**, at which point she presses the button, and the process continues as described until the test is discontinued. This process causes the intensity of the tone to rise and fall around the patient's threshold, and the midpoint of the resulting zigzag pattern is

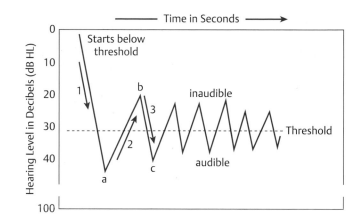

Fig. 5.7 Bekesy (self-tracking) audiometry.

taken as her threshold. [The attentive student will have noticed that the reversal points overshoot the dashed line representing threshold. This reflects (1) how far above (or below) the "threshold" value the intensity must be before the patient decides that it is present (or absent); and (2) her reaction time, which is how long it then takes her to press the button.]

In the example, we have been assuming that the frequency of the test tone stays the same during the procedure just described, so that the Bekesy audiogram is for one frequency. This type of testing is called **fixed-frequency** (or discrete-frequency) Bekesy audiometry. In **sweep-frequency** Bekesy audiometry, the frequency changes slowly over time, so that the patient's thresholds are tracked across the audiometric frequency range. Bekesy audiometry is covered in further detail in Chapter 10.

■ Comparing Air and Bone-Conduction Thresholds

Remember that the outer and middle ears collectively make up the conductive mechanism, and the cochlea and auditory nerve compose the sensorineural mechanism (Chapter 2). Comparing the air-conduction thresholds to the bone-conduction thresholds allows us to figure out whether a hearing loss is coming from a problem located in the conductive mechanism or in the sensorineural mechanism, or from a combination of the two. **Fig. 5.8** represents the whole peripheral hearing mechanism. It is divided into two halves, representing the conductive mechanism (outer and middle ear) and the sensorineural mechanism (cochlea and auditory nerve). The

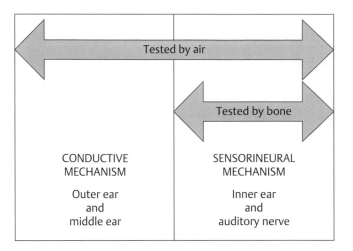

Fig. 5.8 Air-conductiontion tests the entire system. Bone-conductiontion is said to "bypass" the conductive mechanism, so it tests only the inner ear (and auditory nerve).

Table 5.1 Air and bone-conductiontion thresholds and air-bone-gaps, and the parts of a hearing loss represented by each

	Audiometric measure	Represents
	Air-conduction threshold	Whole hearing loss
Minus	Bone-conduction threshold	Sensorineural part of the hearing loss
Equals	Air-bone-gap	Conductive part of the hearing loss

entire ear is tested by air-conduction because the signal from an earphone must be processed through the outer, middle, and inner ear and the auditory nerve. This notion is represented by the arrow labeled "tested by air" in the figure. All of these parts must be working properly for the air-conduction threshold to be normal, and a problem in any one (or more) of these locations would cause a hearing loss by air-conduction. Hence, the air-conduction threshold shows the total amount of hearing loss that is present. However, it cannot distinguish between a problem coming from one part of the ear versus the other. In contrast, the bone-conduction signal "bypasses" the outer and middle ear and directly stimulates the cochlea.[1] Hence, bone-conduction is considered to test just the sensorineural mechanism. This idea is represented by the arrow labeled "tested by bone" in the figure.

We can deduce the location of a problem from the following principles: (1) air-conduction tests the whole ear, and (2) bone-conduction tests the sensorineural part of the ear. Thus, a difference between the air and bone-conduction thresholds implies that

there is a problem with the conductive system. The difference between the air-conduction threshold (AC) and the bone-conduction threshold (BC) at the same frequency is called an **air-bone-gap (ABG)**; that is, **AC – BC = ABG**. **Table 5.1** summarizes the relationship between the air and bone-conduction thresholds and the air-bone-gap, as well as the implications of each of these three audiometric measures.

Fig. 5.9a represents an ear in which the thresholds are 55 dB HL by air-conduction and 55 dB HL by bone-conduction. It is assumed that the air and bone-conduction thresholds are both obtained at the same frequency. The bone-conduction threshold tells us that 55 dB HL of the loss is coming from the sensorineural part of the ear, and the air-conduction threshold indicates that the whole loss is 55 dB HL. Consequently, the sensorineural part of the loss (55 dB HL) accounts for the total amount of the loss (55 dB HL). The air-bone-gap here is 55 – 55 = 0 dB. From

[1] It is useful to think in these terms even though it is not an altogether pristine concept. Bone-conductiontion also involves outer and middle ear components, and bone-conductiontion thresholds can be affected by conductive pathologies. This is why quotes are used when we say that the conductive mechanism is "bypassed." However, that bone-conductiontion thresholds principally represent hearing sensitivity at the cochlea is fundamentally correct and of great practical significance

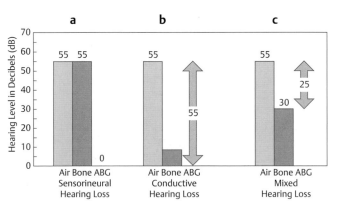

Fig. 5.9 Air-conductiontion (*Air*) and bone-conductiontion (*Bone*) thresholds in cases of **(a)** sensorineural hearing loss, **(b)** conductive hearing loss, and **(c)** mixed hearing loss. The difference between the air and bone-conductiontion thresholds is called the air-bone-gap (*ABG*) and represents the part of the loss coming from the conductive mechanism.

this information we can easily figure out that the whole loss is coming from the sensorineural mechanism, and also that the conductive mechanism must be okay. This kind of impairment is called a **sensorineural hearing loss.** It is indicated by air and bone-conduction thresholds that are equal, or at least very close to one another. Sensorineural losses can be caused by a disorder of the cochlea or auditory nerve, or both. The combination term *sensorineural* is used to highlight the fact that we cannot distinguish between cochlear (sensory) and eighth nerve (neural) disorders from the audiogram.

Fig. 5.9b shows another case in which the air conduction threshold is 55 dB HL. In this case, however, the bone-conduction threshold is normal at 0 dB HL. This means that none of the hearing loss is coming from the sensorineural mechanism, which leaves the conductive mechanism as the only possible culprit. The size of the air-bone-gap in this case is 55 – 0 = 55 dB. Therefore, this 55 dB HL hearing loss is coming from the conductive mechanism, that is, the outer and/or middle ear. This kind of hearing loss is called a **conductive hearing loss.** It is revealed by a hearing loss by air-conduction but essentially no hearing loss by bone-conduction.

It is also possible to have a hearing loss that is partly due to a sensorineural problem and partly to a conductive problem, called a **mixed hearing loss.** The mixed loss concept is shown in **Fig. 5.9c**. The 55 dB HL air-conduction threshold is the total amount of hearing loss coming from all sources, and the bone-conduction threshold of 30 dB HL represents the part of the loss that is due to problems in the sensorineural mechanism. If 30 dB of the 55 dB HL loss is coming from the sensorineural problem, then the remaining amount of 55 – 30 = 25 dB (which is the air-bone-gap) must be due to problems in the conductive system. In other words, the sensorineural part of a mixed loss is shown by the bone-conduction threshold, and its conductive component is represented by the air-bone-gap.

In principle, the air-bone-gap should be 0 dB unless there is a problem with the conductive mechanism. But this is not always the case, which is why it is suggested from the outset that the air-bone-gap should be at least 10 dB wide before it is considered significant. Let us see why this is so. One reason has to do with test-retest reliability. A given clinical threshold measurement is generally considered to be reliable within ± 5 dB. Applying ± 5 dB of variability to both the air and bone-conduction measurements at the same frequency means that the spread between them (the air-bone-gap) can be as wide as 10 dB. Another reason has to do with the statistical relationship between air and bone-conduction thresholds: it is the mean air-conduction threshold that equals the

mean bone-conduction threshold. In other words, air and bone-conduction thresholds are equal in normal ears *on average*, so that the normal air-bone-gap is 0 dB *on average*. Consequently, there must also be normal ears with at least some amount of air-bone-gap, and even ears in which bone-conduction is poorer than air-conduction. This statistical distribution is such that most air and bone-conduction thresholds are within ± 10 dB of each other (Studebaker 1967; Frank, Klobuka, & Sotir 1983). These points also explain why it is possible and perfectly acceptable for a bone-conduction threshold to be a bit poorer than the air-conduction thresholds at the same frequency (a so-called reverse air-bone-gap or *bone-air gap*), even if everything is done correctly. Most certainly, a clinician should not "adjust" a bone-conduction threshold that is too high down to where it "should be." In addition, one should be wary of the fact that bone-conduction may be worse than air-conduction because of an error. This often occurs if the bone vibrator slips or if it was improperly placed when it was applied.

■ Basic Audiogram Interpretation

A typical normal audiogram is shown in **Fig. 5.10**. All of the air-conduction thresholds are in the vicinity of 0 dB HL for both ears. In addition, the air-and bone-conduction thresholds are very close to one another at each frequency, so that there are no significant air-bone-gaps. Why do we bother testing bone-conduction in a case such as this one, where the hearing is clearly normal? The reason for testing bone-conduction, even when the air-conduction thresholds are normal, is because 0 dB HL is the *average* threshold for normal people, so that thresholds lower than 0 dB HL are expected to be found in many people, especially in children (Eagles, Wishik, & Doerfler 1967). A middle ear problem in a person who normally has –15 dB HL thresholds can cause these thresholds to shift up to 0 or 5 dB HL. Here, the hearing sensitivity is within the normal range but there is also a conductive disorder. In cases such as this, testing bone-conduction would show a 15 to 20 dB air-bone-gap, thus revealing the problem. However, omitting bone-conduction testing would cause such a conductive impairment to be missed.

A **pure tone average (PTA)** is usually calculated for each ear. The PTA, which is simply the mean of the air-conduction thresholds at 500, 1000, and 2000 Hz, is an attempt to summarize the degree of hearing loss. **Table 5.2** shows the various categories of degrees of hearing loss. It indicates that pure tone averages up to 15 dB HL are considered to be within

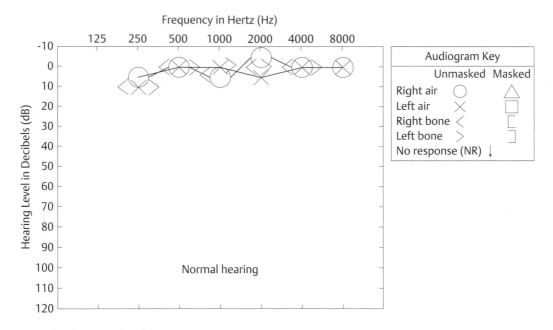

Fig. 5.10   An example of a normal audiogram.

the normal limits. The patient in **Fig. 5.10** has pure tone averages of 0 dB HL for the right ear and 2 dB for the left ear, which are well within this normal range.

The pure tone average was originally based on the 500, 1000, and 2000 Hz thresholds because it often agrees with hearing ability for speech (Fletcher 1929). The PTA is usually compared with a measure of hearing for speech called the **speech recognition (reception) threshold (SRT)**,[2] and significant differences between the PTA and SRT are of clinical significance (Chapters 8 and 14).

For this reason, 500, 1000, and 2000 Hz have come to be known as the "*speech frequencies.*" However, this is a misnomer because adequate speech recognition actually depends on a much wider range of frequencies. Moreover, this three-frequency pure tone average often fails to agree with the SRT, especially when the shape of the pure tone audiogram slopes sharply. A **two-frequency pure tone average** based on the best two of these three frequencies (usually 500 and 1000 Hz) is often used instead of the three-frequency PTA under these circumstances (Fletcher 1950). It is sometimes necessary to compare the SRT to the single frequency with the best threshold

Table 5.2   Typically used categories to describe the degree of hearing loss based on the pure tone average

Pure tone average in dB HL	Degree of hearing loss
< 15	Normal hearing
16–25	Slight hearing loss
26–40	Mild hearing loss
41–55	Moderate hearing loss
56–70	Moderately severe hearing loss
71–90	Severe hearing loss
≥ 90	Profound hearing loss

(often 500 Hz, and sometimes 250 Hz) to achieve agreement between the pure tone and speech results (Gelfand & Silman 1985, 1993).

The air-conduction thresholds in **Fig. 5.11** reveal that this patient has a hearing loss in both ears. A loss in both ears is said to be **bilateral.** The left ear was tested at 1500 Hz because there was a spread of [3]20 dB between the thresholds at 1000 and 2000 Hz. The three-frequency pure tone averages are 52 dB HL in the right ear and 50 dB HL in the left ear, so that the degree of hearing loss would be considered moderate according to **Table 5.2.** Because this audiogram has quite a slope, we would also calculate two-frequency PTAs based on 500 and 1000 Hz. These are 45 dB HL

---

[2] The SRT is the lowest level (in dB HL) at which a patient can correctly repeat spondee words 50% of the time. Spondee words have two syllables with equal emphasis on *both* syllables (e.g., *baseball* or *greyhound*). See Chapter 8

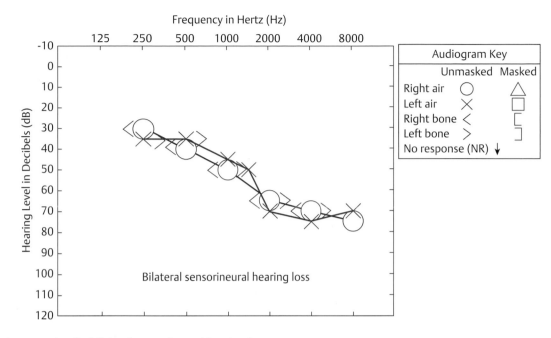

Fig. 5.11 An example of a bilateral sensorineural hearing loss.

for the right ear and 40 dB for the left. The type of loss in this example is sensorineural because the air and bone-conduction thresholds are essentially the same at each frequency, that is, there are no significant air-bone-gaps. This implies that the underlying disorders are located in the cochleae and/or eighth nerve. Finally, the configuration (shape) of the audiogram slopes downward with increasing frequency. It is easily understood why the interpretation of this audiogram would read as follows: "Moderate sloping sensorineural hearing loss, bilaterally."

Fig. 5.12 is an example of a bilateral conductive hearing loss. It is the audiogram of a child who has middle-ear infections in both ears. The air-conduction thresholds are between 25 and 45 dB HL, but all of the bone-conduction thresholds are in the vicinity of 0 dB HL. According to the criteria shown in **Table 5.2**, the losses would be considered to be in the mild range because the pure tone averages are 30 dB HL for the right ear and 38 dB for the left ear. **Table 5.3** shows how to calculate each of the air-bone-gaps in this figure. Overall, we can see that the air-bone-gaps account for virtually the entire hearing losses of both ears. In broad terms, the configurations of these losses could be described as flat; however, notice that there is a slight tent-like shape for the right ear.

The patient whose audiogram is shown in **Fig. 5.13** has a **unilateral** conductive hearing loss because it involves just one ear. The normal left ear has a pure

tone average of 2 dB. The impaired right ear has a mild hearing loss with a fairly flat configuration and a pure tone average of 32 dB HL. The hearing loss in the right ear is conductive because the bone-conduction thresholds approximate 0 dB HL in both ears. Let us calculate a couple of the air-bone-gaps for illustrative purposes. The air-bone-gap is 30 dB at 500 Hz because the air and bone-conduction thresholds at this frequency are 35 dB HL and 5 dB HL, respectively. Similarly, the air-bone-gap at 4000 Hz is 25 – 0 = 25 dB.

Fig. 5.14 shows the audiogram of a patient with normal hearing in his right ear and a sensorineural hearing loss in his left ear. The hearing loss is sensorineural because the air and bone-conduction thresholds are essentially the same. The patient's thresholds were tested at 1500 Hz for the left ear because of the large drop-off between 1000 and 2000 Hz. Notice, however, that there was no response at the maximum testable bone-conduction levels of 70 dB HL for both 2000 and 4000 Hz. This is not a problem at 2000 Hz, where the air-conduction threshold is only 75 dB HL, but we really *do not know for sure* whether or not there is an air-bone-gap at 4000 Hz, where the air-conduction threshold is 90 dB HL. For the purpose of discussion, we accept the fact that other findings have confirmed that this loss is completely sensorineural.

The normal right ear shown in **Fig. 5.14** has a pure tone average is 0 dB HL. The impaired left ear has a

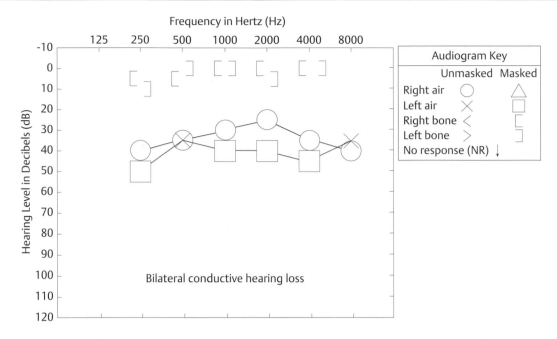

Fig. 5.12 An example of a bilateral conductive hearing loss. Each of the air-bone-gaps is enumerated in **Table 5.3**. (Notice that both unmasked and masked symbols are used in this figure and subsequent ones.)

three-frequency pure tone average of 38 dB HL and a two-frequency PTA of 20 dB HL. Even if one of these averages agrees with the speech reception threshold, both of them clearly understate the amount of hearing loss in the higher frequencies. This shows how misleading it can be to describe a hearing loss solely on the basis of the pure tone average. It is for this reason that the configuration of the hearing loss must

not be overlooked. Hence, one might interpret this audiogram as indicating "a unilateral severe high-frequency hearing loss in the left ear, with normal hearing sensitivity in the right ear." The "severe" designation here is borrowed from the degrees of loss shown in **Table 5.2**. This is technically a misuse of the term because the degrees of loss shown in the table really apply only to the pure tone average, and are

Table 5.3 How to calculate each of the air-bone-gaps in the audiogram shown in **Fig. 5.12**

Frequency	Ear	AC threshold (dB HL)	minus	BC threshold (dB HL)	equals	Air-bone-gap (dB)
250 Hz	Right	40	–	5	=	35
	Left	45	–	10	=	35
500 Hz	Right	35	–	5	=	30
	Left	35	–	0	=	35
1000 Hz	Right	30	–	0	=	30
	Left	40	–	0	=	40
2000 Hz	Right	25	–	0	=	25
	Left	40	–	5	=	35
4000 Hz	Right	35	–	0	=	35
	Left	45	–	0	=	45

Abbreviations: AC, air-conduction; BC, bone-conduction

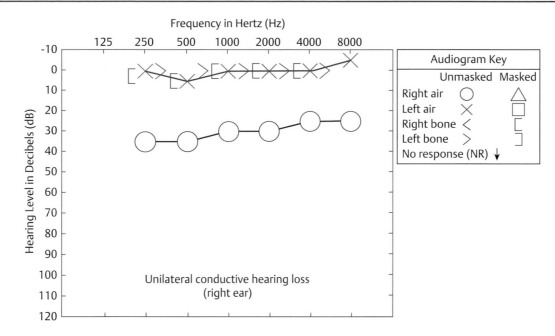

Fig. 5.13   An example of a unilateral conductive hearing loss in the right ear (with normal hearing in the left ear).

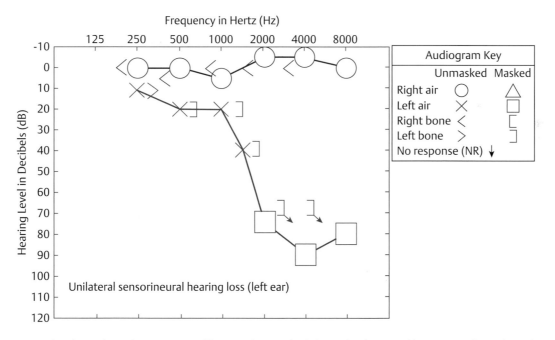

Fig. 5.14   An example of a unilateral sensorineural hearing loss in the left ear (with normal hearing in the right ear).

intended to imply how much the hearing loss affects overall sensitivity for speech. Yet it has become common practice to describe parts of the audiogram in these terms as well. (The author has never been quite comfortable with this usage, but finally has come to terms with the fact that it is here to stay.)

The audiogram in **Fig. 5.15** shows a bilateral **asymmetrical** sensorineural hearing loss because there is a hearing loss in both ears, but the thresholds are worse in one ear than in the other. In this example, the right ear has a two-frequency pure tone average of 48 dB HL and a three-frequency PTA

Fig. 5.15   An example of an asymmetrical sensorineural hearing loss that is worse in the right ear.

of 55 dB HL, and is noticeably worse than the left ear, which has two- and three-frequency PTAs of 28 and 32 dB HL, respectively. The criteria for classifying asymmetries as clinically significant are discussed in Chapter 10.

A **mixed hearing loss** occurs when both sensorineural and conductive impairments coexist in the same ear. In this case, the bone-conduction thresholds show the sensorineural portion of the loss, and the conductive component is represented by the air-bone-gap. The overall extent of the hearing loss is shown by the air-conduction thresholds. **Fig. 5.16** shows an example of a bilateral mixed hearing loss in which the pure tone averages are 67 dB HL in the right ear and 75 dB HL in the left ear. The bone-conduction thresholds show that the sensorineural components are similar for the two ears, sloping from ~ 10 to 15 dB HL at 250 Hz down to 55 to 60 dB HL at 4000 Hz. The air-bone-gaps are also similar for the two ears and also from one frequency to the other in this audiogram. However, it must be stressed that this is *not* always the case.

■ Sensation Level

Recall that *sound pressure level* expresses a sound's magnitude in decibels compared with a physical reference (which is 2×10^{-5} N/m^2). In contrast, *hear-*

ing level indicates the magnitude of a sound compared with the average threshold of that sound for the population of normal people. Hence, 0 dB HL will correspond to a different number of dB SPL at each frequency, as shown in **Table 4.1** of Chapter 4. For example, 0 dB HL corresponds to 13.5 dB HL at 500 Hz. Similarly, 0 dB HL corresponds to 7.5 dB at 1000 Hz, and 0 dB HL at 4000 Hz will have a sound pressure level of 10.5 dB. However, we often want to know the intensity of a sound above an *individual* person's threshold. This is called **sensation level (SL)**. For example, 25 dB SL means that the sound in question is 25 dB above the patient's threshold.

Consider a patient whose l000 Hz threshold is 30 dB HL, which means that she can just perceive the tone when it is 30 dB above 0 dB HL. In other words, 30 dB HL is *at her threshold*. Hence, 30 dB HL *for her* corresponds to a *sensation level* of 0 dB. This is so because one's own threshold is the reference value for sensation level, and a reference value has a level of 0 dB. Consequently, a threshold corresponds to 0 dB SL. Now, suppose we present this patient with a l000 Hz tone at 65 dB HL. This tone is 35 dB *above her threshold;* therefore, its *sensation level* is 35 dB SL.

As an exercise, let us determine the sensation levels for various tones using the audiograms just described. A 500 Hz tone at 70 dB HL would have sensation levels of (a) 70 dB SL in each ear for **Fig. 5.10**, (b) 30 dB SL for the right ear and 35 dB SL for the left ear in **Fig. 5.11**, and (c) 15 dB SL for both ears in **Fig. 5.16**. Now consider

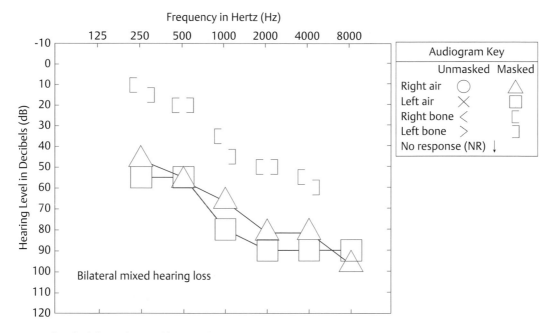

Fig. 5.16 An example of a bilateral mixed hearing loss.

several tones with different frequencies, all of which are presented at 90 dB HL. For the left ear in **Fig. 5.14**, 90 dB HL would correspond to 70 dB SL at 500 Hz, 50 dB SL at 1500 Hz, 15 dB SL at 2000 Hz, and 0 dB SL at 4000 Hz. Using the right ear in **Fig. 5.16**, the sensation levels of these 90 dB HL tones would be 45 dB SL at 250 Hz, 25 dB SL at l000 Hz, and l0 dB SL at 2000 Hz.

■ Factors That Affect Pure Tone Results

Many factors can affect the validity and reliability of the audiogram. The implications of calibration, regular instrumentation checks, and an appropriate test environment were covered in Chapter 4. We have also covered such issues as patient seating, instructions, false responses, etc. In this section we will address several very real phenomena that nonetheless produce incorrect outcomes on the audiogram. We will also briefly look at a couple of audiometric configurations that sometimes reveal possible errors. These points are introduced after covering basic audiometric interpretation because they require some basic understanding of audiograms and hearing losses. However, it will be apparent that these issues need to be in your mind while you are testing the patient.

Standing Waves

The distance between the eardrum and the diaphragm of the earphone can be very close to the wavelength of an 8000 Hz tone (which is ~ 4.25 cm or 1.68 inches). If they just match, then a standing wave can develop in the ear canal. Under these conditions the tone and its reflections within the ear canal will be 180° out-of-phase, which will *cancel* the tone. This will cause the patient's 8000 Hz threshold to be higher than its real value. A standing wave artifact is generally suspected if the 8000 Hz threshold is appreciably below the threshold at 4000 Hz. It is confirmed if altering the fit or orientation of the earphone causes the 8000 Hz threshold to get better, in which case the improved threshold is more likely to be the correct one. Using insert receivers can be helpful in these cases. These points should be kept in mind with respect to 6000 Hz as well, because standing wave problems are occasionally found at this frequency.

Tactile Responses

Patients with very severe hearing losses who cannot hear the sounds being presented might still respond if they *feel* the vibrations produced by the bone vibrator or earphones (Nober 1970). These **tactile**

responses are most likely to occur at low frequencies (especially 125 and 250 Hz), where the skin is more sensitive to vibratory stimulation.

Tactile responses cause two kinds of problems. First, they can give the false impression that the patient's thresholds are better than they actually are, or that the patient has hearing where there is none. For example, the tactile threshold at 250 Hz might be 75 dB HL when the actual threshold would have been 90 dB HL or even no-response. Second, a false bone-conduction threshold due to a tactile response can create an artificial air-bone-gap, so that a sensorineural hearing loss would appear to be mixed. For example, suppose a patient has an 85 dB HL sensorineural loss. A tactile response to bone-conduction at 45 dB HL would give the false impression that this is an 85 dB HL mixed loss that includes a 40 dB air-bone-gap.

Dealing with tactile responses often involves simply asking the patient if the stimulus was heard or felt. However, this is not always possible with young children, especially those with very severe hearing losses who have had little or no experience with sound.

Acoustical Radiations

The bone-conduction vibrator can cause a sound to be radiated into the air. The radiations then enter the ear canal, and may be heard via the air-conduction route. These acoustical radiations are sometimes heard at presentation levels that are below (better than) the patient's true bone-conduction threshold. This causes a false air-bone-gap above 2000 Hz, which is usually most prominent at 4000 Hz (Bell, Goodsell, & Thornton 1980; Shipton, John, & Robinson 1980; Frank & Crandell 1986). The artificial high-frequency air-bone-gap can make a sensorineural loss appear to be mixed. For example, hearing the acoustical radiations produced by a 55 dB HL bone-conduction tone can cause a 75 dB HL sensorineural loss to appear to include a 20 dB air-bone-gap.

The problem of acoustical radiations is easily alleviated by inserting earplugs into the ears during bone-conduction testing, but this is certainly not needed on a routine basis. Frank and Crandell (1986) suggested that bone-conduction should be retested with earplugs when there is an air-bone-gap of > 10 dB above 2000 Hz and no other evidence of conductive impairments.

Collapsed Ear Canals

It is possible for the pressure from the earphones to cause the cartilaginous portion of the ear canal to collapse during air-conduction testing (Ventry,

Chaiklin, & Boyle 1961). Collapse of the ear canal obstructs the flow of sound while the earphone pressure is being applied, and results in (1) an apparent high-frequency conductive hearing loss and (2) poor test-retest reliability. An example is shown in **Fig. 5.17**. The size of the air-bone-gap artifact can range from 10 to 50 dB HL (Coles 1967). The problem is more common in elderly patients than in other groups because tissue elasticity often becomes reduced with age, but the incidence rate is unclear because of variability among samples. For example, Marshall, Martinez, and Schlaman (1983) found collapsed ear canals in none of their elderly subjects, whereas Randolph and Schow (1983) reported a 36% incidence rate.

One must be alert to the possibility of a collapsed ear canal when there is an air-bone-gap that is greater in the higher frequencies, because this artifact can lead to misdiagnosis. The traditional ways to confirm and overcome this artifact involve (1) inserting a tube into the ear canal to hold it open, or (2) removing the earphone from the headset and holding it loosely at the ear to do away with the pressure. Two other methods are now preferred. One is to retest with insert earphones, which by their very nature hold the canals open. The other method is to retest the air-conduction thresholds while the patient is holding his jaw open (Reiter & Silman 1993). Before doing this, the patient should be asked whether he has any problems that would contraindicate the jaw opening technique (e.g., temporomandibular joint disorders). This technique alleviates the collapsed ear canal effect because the mandible contributes to the wall of the external auditory meatus, so that the movements involved in jaw opening can distort and therefore open the collapsed canal. Reiter and Silman (1993) found that similar thresholds are obtained with insert earphones and the open jaw method. They suggested that patients with air-bone-gaps can be screened for ear canal collapse by retesting them with the jaw open at 4000 Hz, which is where the artifact is usually largest. A collapsed ear canal is suspected if the air-conduction threshold improves by ≥ 15 dB with the jaw open.

Configurations That Should Be Confirmed

Several audiometric configurations can indicate the presence of a possible error. Hearing losses that are unilateral or identical for the two ears are audiometric configurations that should be confirmed because they could also be due to artifacts, errors, and/or false responses.

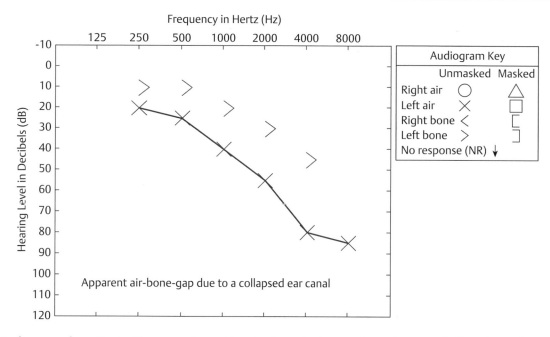

Fig. 5.17 Audiogram of a patient with a sensorineural hearing loss who has a collapsed ear canal effect. Notice how the ear canal collapse makes the loss appear to be mixed, and how the size of the apparent air-bone-gap gets larger as frequency gets higher. Only one ear is represented for clarity.

Unilateral hearing losses can be caused by equipment problems affecting one earphone, especially when there is no response at all for one ear. The most likely culprits are damaged earphone wires or jacks that have been dislodged from their sockets. A typical tester error that can cause a false unilateral loss is setting the output selector to the wrong transducer. Under these conditions, the clinician should (1) listen to the sounds produced by both earphones, and (2) retest the patient with the earphones reversed (i.e., right phone on left ear, left phone on right ear). It is often wise to do a Stenger test to rule out a functional component when faced with a unilateral loss (Chapter 14).

Identical thresholds in both ears usually means a symmetrical hearing loss, but it sometimes indicates that the clinician tested the same ear twice. It is wise to double-check if there is any question that this error may have occurred.

■ Supplemental Pure Tone Tests

Occlusion Effect and Audiometric Bing Test

Recall that the occlusion effect (1) causes a low-frequency bone-conduction threshold to be lower (better) than it would be with the ear uncovered,

and (2) occurs when the conductive mechanism is normal but not when there is a conductive disorder. The Bing test was originally a tuning fork technique used to determine whether the occlusion effect is present (see below). The audiometric Bing test uses a bone-conduction vibrator in place of a tuning fork. Because the audiometric Bing test also reveals the *size* of the occlusion effect, it is used to help determine how much noise is required when bone-conduction is tested with masking (Chapter 9), and this is the major use of the test.

The **audiometric Bing test** is administered as follows. Bone-conduction thresholds are obtained in the regular way, with the ears uncovered. The low-frequency (< 1000 Hz) thresholds are then retested while the test ear is occluded by one of the earphones. The other earphone is located on the opposite side of the head (usually between the opposite ear and eye, or high on the opposite cheek) but *not* covering the other ear. The audiometric Bing test is positive if the occluded thresholds are significantly better (lower) than the unoccluded thresholds. A positive result means that the occlusion effect is present, and suggests that a conductive disorder is not present. This would occur when the ear is normal or when the hearing loss is sensorineural. The size of the occlusion effect is simply the difference between the occluded and unoccluded thresholds at any given frequency. The test is negative if the occluded and unoccluded thresholds are essentially the same, indicating that the occlusion effect is absent. This result suggests that there is a problem with the conductive mechanism and implies that the hearing loss is either conductive or mixed.

Sensorineural Acuity Level (SAL) Test

The **Sensorineural Acuity Level (SAL) test** (Jerger & Tillman 1960) is an indirect technique for estimating bone-conduction thresholds that can be useful when standard bone-conduction testing methods produce equivocal results. The SAL test is discussed further in Chapter 9 because it involves a masking technique.

Tuning Fork Tests

Tuning forks were used to test hearing long before the development of the audiometer. A set of tuning forks used for this purpose is shown in **Fig. 5.18**. Four of the more well known of these tests are the Schwabach, Weber, Bing, and Rinne tests. Even though the Schwabach test is rarely if ever used anymore, it is still worthy of some discussion because it uses interesting principles and highlights the limitations of methods that compare the patient to the tester. The Weber, Bing, and Rinne tests are still used, and can also be done audiometrically. **Table 5.4** summarizes the outcomes and clinical implications associated with these three tests.

Schwabach Test

The Schwabach test is a technique for estimating a patient's hearing sensitivity by bone-conduction. The test has two principal characteristics: (1) it makes

Fig. 5.18 A complete set of tuning forks used for hearing assessment.

use of the fact that the tone produced by a tuning fork becomes softer with time after it has been struck due to damping, and (2) the patient's hearing is expressed in relative terms compared with the examiner's hearing ability. This comparison is done by timing how long the tuning fork is heard by the patient and how long it is heard by the examiner. The basic procedure involves placing the base of the vibrating fork on the patient's mastoid process until the tone fades away. The clinician then moves the fork to his own mastoid and times how long he can hear it. Compared with how long the examiner can hear the tone, it is expected that the patient will hear the tone (1) for a shorter period of time if she has a sensorineural loss; (2) for a longer period of time (or perhaps the same length of time) if she has a conductive loss; and (3) for

Table 5.4 Outcomes and diagnostic implications of the most commonly used tuning fork tests

Test	Outcome	Diagnostic implications
Weber	Sound lateralized to midline or both ears equally	Normal (or sensorineural loss)
	Better ear	Sensorineural loss
	Poorer ear	Conductive loss
Bing	Positive (occluded louder)	Normal or sensorineural loss
	Negative (no difference)	Conductive loss
Rinne	Positive (air > bone)	Normal or sensorineural loss
	Negative (bone > air)	Conductive loss

the same amount of time if she has normal hearing. Schwabach outcomes are problematic when dealing with mixed losses. The Schwabach test provides a relative estimate of hearing at best, and its validity is completely dependent on the tenuous assumption that the examiner really has normal hearing. It is not surprising this test is rarely if ever used.

Weber Test

The Weber test is used to help determine whether a unilateral hearing loss is sensorineural or conductive. It is a **lateralization** test because the patient is asked to indicate the direction from which a sound appears to be coming. Before starting this test, the patient should be advised that it *is* possible for the tone to be heard from the good side *or* the poorer side, or any other location for that matter. The procedure involves putting the base of the vibrating tuning fork somewhere on the midline of the skull, most commonly on the center of the forehead or the top of the head. The audiometric Weber test uses the bone-conduction vibrator instead of tuning forks. The patient is asked to indicate *where* the tone is heard. Hearing the tone in the *better* ear implies that there is a *sensorineural loss* in the poorer ear, whereas hearing the tone in the *poorer* ear suggests a *conductive loss* in that ear. The tone is heard in the middle of the head, "all over," or equally in both ears when the patient has normal hearing, although some patients with sensorineural losses also report such midline lateralizations. If there is a mixed loss, the tone will be lateralized to the better ear if its level is below the poorer ear's bone-conduction threshold. The Weber test will fail to detect the conductive component of a mixed loss in such cases.

The Weber test works for several reasons, all of which are related to the idea that the bone-conduction tone from the tuning fork reaches both cochleae at the same intensity. The tone lateralizes to the better ear with sensorineural losses for either of two reasons: (1) The tone will only be heard in the better ear if its level is lower than the bone-conduction threshold of the poorer ear. (2) The second mechanism is due to the **Stenger effect**, which means that a sound presented to both ears is perceived only in the ear where it is louder. The intensity of the tone from the tuning fork will have a higher sensation level in the better ear than in the impaired ear. Hence, it will be louder in the better ear and will be perceived there. Several factors can explain why a bone-conduction tone would be louder in (and thus lateralized to) the poorer ear. These mechanisms are just briefly mentioned because they are beyond the scope of an introductory text: (1) outer ear obstructions (e.g.,

impacted cerumen) may cause an occlusion effect, (2) mass loading of the middle ear system caused by effusions or ossicular chain interruptions may lower its resonance, and (3) phase advances may be caused by fixations or interruptions of the ossicular chain.

Bing Test

The Bing test is used to determine if closing off the patient's ear canal results in an occlusion effect. The audiometric version of the test has already been discussed. In the traditional Bing test the patient is asked to report whether a tuning fork sounds louder with the ear canal open or closed. The base of a vibrating tuning fork is held against the patient's mastoid process. The tester then presses the tragus down over the entrance of the ear canal to occlude it. The usual technique is to alternately occlude and unocclude the ear canal to help the patient make a reliable louder/softer judgment. It is desirable to make sure that the tuning fork sounds louder when the ear is closed and softer when the ear is open, instead of just asking whether the tone pulses between louder and softer. Unlike the audiometric version, which involves thresholds and thus quantifies the amount of the occlusion effect, the outcome of the tuning fork Bing test is based completely on a subjective judgment of louder versus not louder.

If the occlusion effect is present, covering the ear canal should cause the tuning fork to sound louder. This is called a positive result and implies that the ear is either normal or has a sensorineural hearing loss. A negative result occurs if closing off the ear canal fails to make the tuning fork sound louder, and implies that there is either a conductive or mixed hearing loss.

Rinne Test

The Rinne test is a tuning fork procedure that compares hearing by air-conduction and by bone-conduction; however, the approach used is different from the one used in pure tone audiometry. The Rinne test is based on the idea that the hearing mechanism is normally more efficient by air-conduction than it is by bone-conduction. For this reason, a tuning fork will sound louder by air-conduction than by bone-conduction. However, this air-conduction advantage is lost when there is a conductive hearing loss, in which case the tuning fork sounds louder by bone-conduction than by air-conduction.

Administering the Rinne test involves asking the patient to indicate whether a vibrating tuning fork sounds louder when its base is held against the mastoid process (bone-conduction) or when its prongs are held near the pinna, facing the opening of the ear canal (air-conduction). After striking the fork, the clinician alternates it between these two positions so that the patient can make a judgment about which one is louder. The bone-conduction vibrator is used instead of the tuning fork in the audiometric version of the Rinne test, and the patient indicates whether the vibrator sounds louder on the mastoid or in front of the ear canal. Masking noise must be put into the opposite ear to make sure that the Rinne results are really coming from the test ear.

The outcome of the Rinne test is traditionally called "positive" if the fork is louder by air-conduction, and this finding implies that the ear is normal or has a sensorineural hearing loss. The results are called "negative" if bone-conduction is louder than air-conduction, which is interpreted as revealing the presence of a conductive abnormality. This terminology is confusing because the examiner is often concerned with identifying a conductive loss with this test. Consequently, many clinicians prefer to describe Rinne results as "air better than bone" (AC > BC) versus "bone better than air" (BC > AC). In these terms, AC > BC implies normal hearing or sensorineural impairment, and BC > AC implies a conductive disorder.

Sometimes, the air and bone-conduction signals sound equally loud to the patient (AC = BC). This equivocal outcome can usually be overcome by using the timed Rinne test (Gelfand 1977). This more accurate way to administer the Rinne test involves *timing* how long the patient can hear the tuning fork at the two locations. In this case, the results are (1) positive (AC > BC) when the tone is heard longer by air-conduction, and (2) negative (BC > AC) when it is heard longer by bone-conduction. Another variation of the timed Rinne test involves holding the tuning fork at the mastoid until the tone has faded away, and then moving it to the ear canal (and vice versa). Here, the result is (1) AC > BC if the tone can still be heard by air-conduction after it faded away by bone-conduction, and (2) BC > AC if the tone can still be heard by bone-conduction after it faded away by air-conduction. These timed versions of the Rinne test are well established (Johnson 1970; Sheehy, Gardner, & Hambley 1971). They are more accurate than the loudness comparison method, but are also more cumbersome and time consuming. For this reason, they are not used unless the quicker and easier technique yields equivocal results.

Some Comments on Tuning Fork Tests

Tuning fork tests are quick and easy to administer and do not require special instrumentation, so they can provide general, on-the-spot clinical insights,

and they provide important (albeit limited) diagnostic information, especially when an audiogram is not available. However, tuning fork tests fall short of audiological measures in their ability to assess the patient's hearing status. This is due to the greater precision of audiometric tests made possible by calibrated electronic equipment and systematic testing strategies. Moreover, tuning fork tests are subject to considerable variability in administration and subjectivity in interpretation. Several limitations have already been mentioned with respect to individual tests, and others are worthy of mention. Which frequencies are tested varies among clinicians; some test only at 512 Hz and others use various combinations of frequencies. The intensity of the tone produced by the tuning fork depends on how hard it is struck each time, which causes stimulus levels to be inconsistent. Subjective patient responses can be a confounding variable, especially when dealing with younger children, and when the perception is "not logical" (e.g., when a tone is heard in the bad ear or gets louder when the ear is closed off). Also, tuning fork tests are usually done in examination rooms and clinics that are not sound isolated. Hence, noises that can mask the test signal and/or distract the patient are often a real issue.

It is therefore not surprising that carefully done studies have shown that tuning forks are less accurate than audiometric methods. Wilson and Woods (1975) found that both the Bing and Rinne tests failed to achieve a high level of accuracy in properly identifying conductive versus nonconductive losses. Gelfand (1977) studied the diagnostic accuracy of the Rinne test. All of the tuning fork tests were done with masking of the opposite ear. He found that the Rinne test cannot identify a conductive loss with reasonable accuracy until the size of the air-bone-gap becomes at least 25 to 40 dB wide (**Table 5.5**).

Table 5.5 Minimum air-bone-gaps needed for Rinne test to identify conductive losses with 75% accuracy (Gelfand 1977)

Frequency (Hz)	Air-bone-gaps (dB)
128	25–30
256	5–40
512	55–60
1024	45–50
2048	None[a]

[a]Correct identification of conductive losses failed to reach chance at 2048 Hz, no matter how large the size of the air-bone-gap.

Thus, mild conductive hearing losses that are easily revealed audiometrically are frequently missed by tuning fork tests like the Rinne.

Some tuning fork test problems are exacerbated by how and where the test is done. For example, the need for masking with certain tuning fork tests, particularly the Rinne, is well established in the otological literature (Shambaugh 1967; Johnson 1970; Sheehy et al 1971). However, few physicians actually perform the Rinne test this way.

■ Sound Field Testing

A **sound field** is an environment where sound is present.[3] Testing from *loudspeakers* is called **sound field testing** because the sound is delivered into the air in the test room (the sound field), which then transmits it to the patient's ears. This means that the sound reaching the patient's ears will be affected by the acoustical characteristics of the room and any objects in the room, including the patient himself. Due to the acoustical differences between sounds from earphones and loudspeakers, it is necessary for the earphone and sound field testing systems to be calibrated separately. In addition, because of the nature of standing waves (Chapter 1), (1) pure tones and other very narrow band signals are not appropriate for sound field testing, and (2) the sound levels produced by the loudspeaker may not be the same throughout the test room. In addition, recall from Chapter 4 that different reference levels are used depending on the direction of the loudspeaker relative to the patient's head (ANSI S3.6-2010). The beginning audiology student and those planning to be speech-language pathologists should be aware of these acoustical factors even though they are actually advanced issues.

Once the sound reaches the ear, it follows the air-conduction route that was described for earphones. But here, too, there are at least two major differences between earphone and loudspeaker testing. The first difference is that the ears are uncovered during sound field testing but are covered by the earphones and their cushions during headphone testing. Covering the ears blocks out room noises that can reach the eardrum when the ears are uncovered. This noise can mask, or interfere with the ability to hear, soft sounds. This quieter environment at the eardrum during earphone testing can make it possible to get lower (better) thresholds than could be obtained in the sound field. We encountered this issue when considering the maximum allowable noise levels for audiometric test rooms in Chapter 4.

The second difference between earphone and sound field testing has to do with the ability to test the two ears separately. Earphones allow us to test each ear separately because each ear has its own receiver. In contrast, the sound from a loudspeaker is picked up by both ears, so that they are not being tested separately. This means that a given sound field threshold must be coming from the *better ear* if the ears are different, or from both ears if they are the same. Consider the case of 2-year-old Johnny, who will not put on earphones but responds to sounds as low as 10 dB HL from loudspeakers. Here are the possible choices:

1. The response at 10 dB HL is really from both ears, which are the same. In this case, he is normal in both ears.
2. He really heard the 10 dB HL sound in his right ear. In this case, the right ear is fine, but the left ear could be *anything* from just a bit poorer than the right all the way to completely deaf.
3. He really heard the 10 dB HL sound in his left ear. Here, the left ear is okay, but the right ear could be just a bit worse, completely deaf, or anywhere in between.

The disturbing problem is that we simply do not know which of these alternatives is the right answer. This is why the sound field threshold symbol (S) is described as "ear unspecified" on the audiogram key.

One way to help distinguish between the right and left ears during sound field testing is to "block" one ear at a time. This can be done by (1) putting the earphone headset on the patient's head so that only one ear is covered by one of the earphones and its cushion, and/or (2) inserting an earplug into the ear, or (3) covering one ear with an earphone that also directs a masking noise into that ear. These techniques are used to test one ear at a time in sound field for special purposes, but they would not be much help for cases like little Johnny, who will not put on a headset to begin with.

■ Study Questions

1. Describe how bone-conduction testing differs from air-conduction testing.
2. Describe how pure tone thresholds are obtained using the "up-5 down-10" method.

[3] For informative tutorials on sound field measurements, see ASHA (1991) and Ghent (2005).

3. Explain the major characteristics of a standard audiogram form, including axis labeling and orientation, relative dimensions, and the conventions used for entering symbols.

4. Explain why we test by both air-conduction and bone-conduction.

5. What are the characteristics of a sensorineural hearing loss?

6. What are the characteristics of a conductive hearing loss?

7. What are the characteristics of a mixed hearing loss?

8. Define and explain the implications of the following terms: (a) false-positive responses, (b) occlusion effect, (c) tactile responses, (d) ear canal collapse.

9. What is sensation level (SL), and how is it different from hearing level (HL)?

10. What considerations must be kept in mind when measuring and interpreting sound field thresholds (as opposed to those obtained with earphones)?

References

American National Standards Institute (ANSI). 2004. Methods for Manual Pure-Tone Threshold Audiometry. ANSI S3.21-2004. New York, NY: ANSI

American National Standards Institute (ANSI). 2010. American National Standard Specifications for Audiometers. ANSI S3.6-2010. New York, NY: ANSI

American Speech-Language-Hearing Association (ASHA). 2005. Guidelines for Manual Pure-Tone Threshold Audiometry. Rockville, MD: ASHA

American Speech-Language-Hearing Association (ASHA). Committee on Audiologic Evaluation. Guidelines for audiometric symbols. ASHA Suppl 1990;32(2): 25–30

American Speech-Language-Hearing Association (ASHA). Working Group on Sound Field Calibration of the Committee on Audiologic Evaluation. Sound field measurement tutorial. ASHA Suppl 1991;33(3):25–38

Bekesy G. A new audiometer. Arch Otolaryngol 1947; 35:411–422

Bell I, Goodsell S, Thornton ARD. A brief communication on bone conduction artefacts. Br J Audiol 1980;14(3): 73–75

Burk MH, Wiley TL. Continuous versus pulsed tones in audiometry. Am J Audiol 2004;13(1):54–61

Carhart R, Jerger J. Preferred method for clinical determination of pure-tone thresholds. J Speech Hear Disord 1959;24:330–345

Coles P. External meatus closure by audiometer earphones. J Speech Hear Disord 1967;32:296–297

Dirks D. Factors related to bone conduction reliability. Arch Otolaryngol 1964;79:551–558

Dirks DD, Malmquist GM. Comparison of frontal and mastoid bone-conduction thresholds in various conductive lesions. J Speech Hear Res 1969;12(4):725–746

Eagles EL, Wishik SM, Doerfler LG. Hearing sensitivity and ear disease in children: a prospective study. Laryngoscope 1967;(Suppl):1–274

Fletcher H. 1929. Speech and Hearing in Communication. Princeton, NJ: Van Nostrand Reinhold

Fletcher H. A method of calculating hearing loss for speech from an audiogram. Acta Otolaryngol Suppl 1950;90:26–37

Frank T, Crandell CC. Acoustic radiation produced by B-71, B-72, and KH 70 bone vibrators. Ear Hear 1986;7(5):344–347

Frank T, Klobuka CS, Sotir PJ. Air-bone gap distributions in normal-hearing subjects. J Aud Res 1983;23(4): 261–269

Franklin C, Johnson K, Smith-Olinde L, Nicholson N. The relationship of audiometric thresholds elicited with pulsed, warbled, and pulsed-warbled tones in adults with normal hearing. Ear Hear 2009;30(4):485–487

Gelfand SA. Clinical precision of the Rinne test. Acta Otolaryngol 1977;83(5-6):480–487

Gelfand SA, Silman S. Functional hearing loss and its relationship to resolved hearing levels. Ear Hear 1985; 6(3):151–158

Gelfand SA, Silman S. Functional components and resolved thresholds in patients with unilateral nonorganic hearing loss. Br J Audiol 1993;27:29–34

Ghent RM. A tutorial on complex sound fields for audiometric testing. J Am Acad Audiol 2005;16(1):18–26

Harris JD. Optimum threshold crossings and time-window validation in threshold pure-tone computerized audiometry. J Acoust Soc Am 1979;66(5):1545–1547

Hochberg I, Waltzman S. Comparison of pulsed and continuous tone thresholds in patients with tinnitus. Audiology 1972;11(5):337–342

Hughson W, Westlake H. Manual for program outline for rehabilitation of aural casualties both military and civilian. Trans Am Acad Ophthalmol Otolaryngol 1944;48(Suppl):1–15

Jerger J, Tillman T. A new method for clinical determination of sensorineural acuity level (SAL). Arch Otolaryngol 1960;71:948–953

Johnson EW. Tuning forks to audiometers and back again. Laryngoscope 1970;80(1):49–68

Link R, Zwislocki J. Audiometrische knochenleitungsuntersuchungen. Arch Klin Exp Ohr Nas Kehkopfheik 1951; 160:347–357

Marshall L, Martinez SA, Schlaman ME. Reassessment of high-frequency air-bone gaps in older adults. Arch Otolaryngol 1983;109(9):601–606

Mineau SM, Schlauch RS. Threshold measurement for patients with tinnitus: pulsed or continuous tones. Am J Audiol 1997;6:52–56

Nober EH. Cutile air and bone conduction thresholds of the deaf. Except Child 1970;36(8):571–579

Randolph LJ, Schow RL. Threshold inaccuracies in an elderly clinical population: ear canal collapse as a possible cause. J Speech Hear Res 1983;26(1):54–58

Reiter LA, Silman S. Detecting and remediating external meatal collapse during audiologic assessment. J Am Acad Audiol 1993;4(4):264–268

Shambaugh G. 1967. Surgery of the Ear. Philadelphia, PA: WB Saunders

Sheehy JL, Gardner G Jr, Hambley WM. Tuning fork tests in modern otology. Arch Otolaryngol 1971;94(2): 132–138

Shipton MS, John AJ, Robinson DW. Air-radiated sound from bone vibration transducers and its implications for bone conduction audiometry. Br J Audiol 1980;14(3):86–99

Studebaker GA. Placement of vibrator in bone-conduction testing. J Speech Hear Res 1962;5:321–331

Studebaker GA. Intertest variability and the air-bone gap. J Speech Hear Disord 1967;32(1):82–86

Tyler RS, Wood EJ. A comparison of manual methods for measuring hearing levels. Audiology 1980;19(4): 316–329

Ventry IM, Chaiklin JB, Boyle WF. Collapse of the ear canal during audiometry. Arch Otolaryngol 1961;73: 727–731

Wilson WR, Woods LA. Accuracy of the Bing and Rinne tuning fork tests. Arch Otolaryngol 1975;101(2): 81–85

6 Auditory System and Related Disorders

This chapter gives an overview of the disorders of the auditory system. We will address the nature of various pathologies, where and when they occur, their major signs and symptoms, how hearing is affected, and the ways they are treated. Further coverage of auditory disorders, their diagnosis, and their treatment may be found in many fine otolaryngology texts (e.g., Hughes 1985; Buckingham 1989; Bluestone, Stool, & Kenna 1996; Paparella, Shumrick, Gluckman, & Meyerhoff 1991; Tos 1993, 1995; Hughes & Pensak 2007; Lalwani & Grundfast 1998; Wetmore, Muntz, & McGill 2012; Van De Water & Staecker 2005).[1]

Hearing impairments are caused by abnormalities of structure and/or function in the auditory system, which are often called **lesions**. Using this terminology, a hearing loss may be viewed as one of the manifestations of a lesion somewhere in the ear, as are other symptoms such as pain, ringing in the ears, and dizziness. We are interested in the nature of the lesion, as well as its severity, etiology (cause), location, and time course (including when it began and how it has progressed). Disorders are often called **idiopathic** if a specific underlying cause cannot be identified. The interactions among these various factors can often be important. Consider, for example, the distinction between "congenital" and "hereditary." A disorder is **congenital** if it is present at birth, a matter of timing. On the other hand, a disorder is **hereditary** or **genetic** if it is transmitted by the genetic code that the child inherits from her parents; otherwise it is **acquired**, which is a matter of causation. A congenital disorder may be caused by a genetic problem or other factors that interfere with normal embryological development or occur during the birth process. Similarly, genetic disorders are often present at birth, but others are delayed, mani-

festing themselves long after birth. Moreover, some degree of hereditary predisposition is involved in many acquired disorders.

We are equally interested in the nature, severity, and time course of the hearing impairment itself. Although the nature of a hearing loss goes hand-in-hand with that of the lesion, the same cannot always be said about severity and time course. For example, middle ear infections cause conductive losses, but the magnitude of the hearing loss is not clearly related to the severity of the infection. Similarly, hair cell damage due to noise exposure and/or aging is typically underway long before the patient notices (or at least admits to) a hearing problem. A more dramatic issue has to do with when a severe hearing loss develops in a child and when it is identified and addressed. **Prelingual** impairments occur before the development of speech and language, and have a catastrophic effect on this process, precipitating serious communicative impairments and interference with academic development. **Postlingual losses** develop after speech and language have been established, and have a *relatively* smaller effect. The earlier the onset, and the longer the child is deprived of auditory stimulation, the more the loss will interfere with speech and language development, and hence the more devastating its effect. Conversely, the earlier that a significant hearing impairment is identified, the sooner its effects can be mitigated by appropriate intervention techniques.

■ The Case History

The case history includes information about the patient that provides insight into his auditory status and related factors, and that contributes to the development of a diagnostic impression, a plan for audiological remediation, and appropriate referrals to other professionals. Thus, the clinical case history involves

---

[1] These texts served as references for material used throughout this chapter.

obtaining a complete picture of the patient's auditory and communicative status, historical information about factors known to influence or to be related to auditory functioning, and his pertinent medical and family history. These points should be kept in mind while reading this chapter, and necessitate addressing the issue of case histories at this point.

Exactly how the case history is obtained is often a matter of personal style and interviewing skills. At one extreme is the use of a formal "case history form" that the patient completes in advance, which is then reviewed and discussed with the patient. The other extreme involves conducting an open-ended interview, in effect asking, "What's a nice person like you doing in a place like this?" This method is quite effective in the hands of a "master clinician," but it is easy for those with less experience to lose control of an open-ended interview, or to omit information that would have been obtained with a more structured approach. For this reason, those who prefer the open-ended approach are often well served by completing items on a prepared form during the interview rather than starting with a blank sheet of paper. Many audiologists prefer to use a structured interview in which they ask the patient a predetermined set of questions, and then probe further depending on the answers. Regardless of one's approach to the clinical interview, it is desirable for the evaluation process to include a functional assessment (self-assessment) scale completed by the patient and/or a parent or spouse (see Chapter 16).

A "case history form" is not included here because what is covered in a clinical case history should stem from an integrated knowledge and understanding of the nature, signs, and symptoms of auditory and related disorders. The case history can be meaningful only if one has an integrated knowledge and understanding of normal auditory functioning and the characteristics of auditory and related disorders. Otherwise, one is filling out the form for the sake of filling out the form. The serious student will find that an instructive and useful exercise is to derive a case history outline on the basis of the material in this chapter and elsewhere in the text, particularly Chapters 12 and 13.

■ Conductive, Sensorineural, and Mixed Impairments

Sensorineural lesions involve the cochlea and/or auditory nerve, and may affect sensory receptor (hair) cells, auditory neurons, and/or any of the many structures and processes that enable them to be activated and function properly. The resulting impairment of auditory functioning is called a **sensorineural hearing loss**. *Nerve deafness* and *perceptive loss* are obsolete terms for sensorineural hearing loss, but are occasionally encountered. Using the term *sensorineural* (sometimes *sensori-neural* or *neurosensory*) highlights the anatomical and physiological interdependence of the cochlea and the eighth nerve. In addition, cochlear and auditory nerve lesions cannot be distinguished on the audiogram because both result in threshold shifts that are the same for air and bone-conduction (i.e., no air-bone-gaps). Moreover, sensory and neural lesions can coexist because, for example, the absence of cochlear hair cells can result in degeneration of the auditory neurons associated with them, and an eighth nerve tumor can indirectly damage the cochlea by putting pressure on its blood supply. In spite of these points, it is not uncommon to find that *sensorineural loss* is being used to mean or imply "sensorineural loss of cochlear origin," in which case the intended meaning is usually understood from the context. Disorders of the eighth nerve are often described as being **retrocochlear**, meaning "beyond the cochlea." Let us review some of the more common characteristics of sensorineural losses, which are due to cochlear lesions in the preponderance of cases. We will then go over conductive impairments, so that the student can appreciate the major differences between these two broad categories. The characteristics associated with neural lesions, per se, will be covered later in the section on retrocochlear disorders.

Cochlear disorders result in a loss of hearing sensitivity that is essentially the same for air and bone-conduction. There is a rather systematic relationship between *where a lesion occurs* along the cochlear spiral and *which frequencies* have elevated thresholds on the audiogram: High-frequency hearing losses are associated with damage toward the *base* of the cochlea, and the hearing loss includes successively lower frequencies as the damage to the cochlea extends upward toward the apex. Similarly, lesions affecting the *apical* regions of the cochlea are associated with low-frequency sensorineural hearing losses, and the loss widens to include successively higher frequencies as the cochlear abnormality spreads downward toward the base. The outer hair cells are generally more susceptible to damage than the inner hair cells, and lesions involving the outer hair cells alone are typically associated with mild to moderate degrees of hearing loss. Damage to both the outer and inner hair cells produces more severe losses. Locations along the basilar membrane without functioning inner hair cells (and/or auditory nerve fibers) cannot respond to stimulation, and are known as **dead regions** (Moore 2004). However, it is difficult to establish a clear relationship between the *severity of cochlear damage* and the *amount of hearing loss* it causes.

Unlike the situation for many conductive disorders, medicine and surgery cannot correct sensorineural hearing losses because they are due to cochlear and/or neural damage that is permanent. In effect, missing hair cells and neurons do not regenerate. The student should be aware that hair cell regeneration can occur in birds (Corwin & Cotanche 1988; Ryals & Rubel 1988; Cotanche, Lee, Stone, & Picard 1994; Tsue, Oesterle, & Rubel 1994). This is an avenue of critically important research that might provide hope for the future. However, counseling skill is often needed to help patients be aware (and accept) that while research on hair cell regeneration and related issues is critically important, it is also unrealistic to expect practical benefits for hearing improvement within the foreseeable future.

Sensorineural hearing losses can be of *any* shape and degree, but the most common configurations have thresholds that get worse as frequency increases. In other words, sensorineural impairments often involve a greater loss of hearing sensitivity at higher frequencies than at lower frequencies, so that the audiometric configuration may be described as sloping. This creates a burdensome problem for the hearing-impaired patient because many of the acoustical cues that distinguish speech sounds involve the higher frequencies, and because, on average, the intensity of the speech signal gets weaker as frequency increases.

Most patients with sensorineural hearing losses complain that they can *hear* speech, but that it is *unclear* or *hard to understand,* and that this problem becomes worse when noise or competing sounds are present. These ubiquitous complaints occur for several reasons. Many high-frequency speech cues are rendered inaudible or barely audible by the frequency dependence of many of the sensorineural losses described previously. In addition, speech cues are distorted because inner ear lesions cause a variety of auditory impairments above and beyond elevated thresholds, such as the dulling of fine frequency and temporal distinctions. As a result, the auditory representation of speech cues is less faithfully encoded and noisy. In other words, cochlear lesions impair the clarity of speech due to both **attenuation** and **distortion** (e.g., Plomp 1986; Vermiglio, Soli, Freed, & Fisher 2012).

Patients with cochlear disorders often experience aberrations of pitch and loudness perception, such as diplacusis and loudness recruitment. **Diplacusis** means that more than one pitch (a perception) is heard in response to the same pure tone (i.e., frequency). This phenomenon is called monaural diplacusis when the same tone elicits different pitch sensations within the same ear, and binaural diplacusis when there is a pitch difference for the same tone between the two ears.

Loudness recruitment means that the loudness of a sound (a perception) grows abnormally rapidly as the intensity of the sound (its physical level) is raised above the patient's threshold. For example, suppose a patient has a 50 dB HL cochlear loss in one ear and normal hearing (0 dB HL) in the other ear. A l00 dB HL sound would be l00 dB above the threshold in the normal ear but only 50 dB above threshold in the abnormal ear; yet l00 dB would sound equally loud in both ears. In other words, a 50 dB increment in the impaired ear sounds as loud as the l00 dB increment in the normal ear. As a result, many sounds are either too soft to hear adequately or too loud to hear comfortably. This is why a hearing-impaired patient might ask you to "speak up" and then ask you to "stop shouting" after you comply with the first request. It also creates a dilemma for hearing aid use because the same amount of amplification that makes softer sounds audible also makes more intense sounds too loud.

Patients with severe and profound degrees of sensorineural hearing loss will not be able to hear speech without amplification. The inability of these patients to monitor their own speech can lead to aberrations in vocal pitch and loudness, as well as articulation errors. Along with language disorders, speech production problems are a major issue for patients with prelingual hearing losses, but are less common than once thought among adults with adventitious impairments.

Conductive lesions impair the *transmission* of sound from the environment to the cochlea, so that the signal reaching the sensorineural system is weaker than it should be. A **conductive hearing loss** is the amount by which the signal is attenuated (weakened) due to the disorder, and is expressed by the size of the air-bone-gap (Chapter 5). For example, a 30 dB conductive hearing loss means that the signal reaching the cochlea is 30 dB weaker than it would have been if the conductive mechanism had been normal, resulting in a 30 dB HL hearing loss. Assuming that the patient has a normal sensorineural system (with a bone-conduction threshold of 0 dB HL), this 30 dB conductive loss would cause (1) a 40 dB HL signal to sound softer than normal because the signal reaches the cochlea at 40 − 30 = 10 dB HL, and (2) a 25 dB HL signal to be inaudible because it reaches the cochlea below threshold at 25 − 30 = −5 dB HL.

The size of the conductive hearing loss is not necessarily related to the severity of the underlying disease (e.g., an ear infection), but rather depends on how the lesion impedes the transmission of energy to the cochlea (e.g., by interfering with the middle ear transformer function). In contrast to the sloping configuration of the "typical" sensorineural impairment, conductive losses as a group tend to have *relatively* little variation in the amount of hearing loss from frequency to frequency. Notice that the emphasis is on the word *relatively*, and that conductive audiograms do not have to be "flat" any more than sensorineural audiograms have to be sloping; there are many exceptions to both generalities.

Because conductive disorders affect energy transmission to the cochlea but not the sensory processes within the cochlea, we expect the patient's complaints to reveal that she is experiencing a loss of intensity but not distortions or a loss of clarity; for example, "Speech is too soft but it does sound clear once it's loud enough." However, patients do not necessarily characterize their perceptual experiences using our concepts. Thus, when the patient says something like "Speech sounds *muffled,*" we need to find out what she means by "muffled." Does it mean that speech is *too low* unless people speak loudly (a typical conductive loss complaint) or that speech is *lacking in clarity* even though it is loud enough (often associated with sensorineural loss)?

Relatively intense sounds are generally less bothersome to patients with conductive hearing losses because these sounds are reduced in level before entering the cochlea. In one sense, the conductive loss is like an "ear plug" that lowers sounds by the amount of the air-bone-gap. For example, a 100 dB HL sound will reach the cochlea of a patient with a 40 dB conductive loss (air-bone-gap) at only 60 dB HL (i.e., 100 – 40 = 60). In contrast, the same 100 dB HL sound would reach a normal person's cochlea at 100 dB HL, and thus be very loud. This phenomenon is advantageous when these patients use hearing aids because it permits many sounds to be amplified without becoming too loud. However, this apparent "benefit" of a conductive hearing loss is no larger than the size of the air-bone-gap, and certainly does *not* shield the ear from sounds that are intense enough to cause a tactile sensation or pain.

Patients with conductive losses may report that speech is heard better in a noisy environment than in a quiet one. This phenomenon is the opposite of the normal experience and is called **paracusis willisii**. It occurs for the following reasons: Normal people have no trouble hearing conversational speech in a quiet room, but this speech is too low for the patient with a conductive loss. People talk louder in the presence of a background noise because of the Lombard voice reflex (see Chapter 14). However, the background noise level is still high enough to interfere with the ability to hear the talker's voice for normal-hearing people. In contrast, the background noise is effectively lowered (or even made inaudible) by the conductive hearing loss, while at the same time

the talker's increased vocal effort makes his speech intense enough to become audible above the noise for people with conductive losses. In other words, the noise makes the talker speak louder, and the conductive loss makes the noise sound lower. It is also common (but certainly not universal) to find that patients with conductive losses speak relatively softly. This occurs because the patient hears her own speech loud and clear via bone-conduction (which is normal) but at the same time fails to adjust her vocal level to account for environmental noises that are rendered inaudible or very low due to the hearing loss.

A **mixed hearing loss** is the combination of a sensorineural loss and a conductive loss in the same ear. Mixed losses may be caused by the presence of two separate disorders in the same ear (e.g., noise-induced hearing loss plus otitis media) or by a single disorder that affects the conductive and sensorineural systems (e.g., head trauma or advanced otosclerosis).

■ Tinnitus and Hyperacusis

Tinnitus is the abnormal perception of sounds for which there is no external stimulus (see, e.g., Tyler, 2000 2006; Snow 2004; Henry, Dennis, & Schechter 2005). Tinnitus is typically associated with a wide variety of sensorineural and conductive hearing losses, but it also occurs when hearing is within normal limits. The sensations are often described as ringing in the ears, head noises, or ear noises, and the sounds are variously characterized as tonal, ringing, buzzing, rushing, roaring, hissing, chirping, pulsing, humming, etc. Sounds audible only to the patient are called **subjective tinnitus**, in contrast to **objective tinnitus** (or **somatosounds**), which also can be detected by an examiner, and is much less common. A particular etiology for subjective tinnitus is evident in some cases (e.g., Meniere's syndrome and acoustic neuroma), but an identifiable original source is not clear in most patients with chronic tinnitus. Moreover, while most cases of chronic tinnitus are *initiated* by damage to the cochlea, its *persistence* and the *annoyance* it causes are related to processes and changes in both auditory and nonauditory aspects of the central nervous system (Henry, Roberts, Caspary, & Theodoroff 2014).

Objective tinnitus tends to be associated with sources involving, for example, the vascular system, Eustachian tube, temporomandibular joint, and/or muscular activity. As a result, medical assessment is an important step in the assessment of the patient with tinnitus.

Chronic tinnitus may be the most common health-related complaint, affecting ~ 10 to 15% of the population, and having symptoms severe enough to affect day-to-day living in roughly 1 to 2.5% (e.g., Davis & El Refaie 2000; Henry et al 2005; Shargorodsky, Curhan, & Farwell 2010; Kochkin, Tyler, & Born 2011). To appreciate the impact of clinically significant tinnitus, let us consider some statistics derived from a database by Meikl, Creedon, & Griest SE (2004) on 1630 patients seen for tinnitus management. Sixty-nine percent of their patients reported that their tinnitus caused moderate or greater degrees of discomfort, 74% were uncomfortable in quiet environments, and 92% had difficulty ignoring their tinnitus. Sleep interference was a problem for 71% of their patients, 82% reported irritability or nervousness, 82% had difficulty relaxing, and 79% had difficulty concentrating. Moderate or greater degrees of interference were experienced by 62% for social activities, 52% for work activities, and 72% for overall enjoyment.

As many as 45% of patients with tinnitus also experience hyperacusis (Henry et al 2005); conversely, roughly 86% of those with hyperacusis also experience tinnitus (Anari, Axelsson, Eliasson, & Magnusson 1999), and the evaluation and treatment of these problems are intertwined (see Chapter 15). **Hyperacusis** refers to an *intolerance* for sound in which the patient experiences discomfort, and is often distinguished from misophonia and phonophobia, although these terms are variously defined (e.g., Vernon 1987, 2002; Katzenell & Segal 2001; Jastreboff & Jastreboff 2002; Baguley 2003; Jastreboff & Hazel 2004). **Misophonia** and **phonophobia** implicate *emotional* components in one's reactions to sounds, with the former involving a dislike of sounds and the latter connoting actual fear.

■ Congenital and Hereditary Disorders

Genetic Influences

The information needed to make a particular person (the genetic code) exists in the form of deoxyribonucleic acid (DNA) molecules packaged as chromosomes in every cell. Genes are segments of DNA that occur at fixed locations on the chromosomes, and operate as the biological units of inheritance. In other words, hereditary characteristics (traits) are carried by genes, which are arranged along the chromosomes. Humans have 46 chromosomes arranged in 23 pairs. One pair is different for females (XX) and males (XY), and the other 22 pairs are autosomes, or the same for both sexes. Each parent contributes half of each pair.

A **genetic** or **hereditary disorder** is an abnormal trait that is transmitted by an abnormal gene. Disorders may be the result of single- or multiple-gene abnormalities, or multifactorial inheritance, which is the combined effect of genetic and environmental factors. Hereditary hearing losses can occur alone (**nonsyndromic**) or in combination with other genetic abnormalities (**syndromic**), and may be transmitted by autosomal dominant, autosomal recessive, and X-linked inheritance, and by mitochondrial mutations (e.g., Friedman, Schultz, Ben-Yosef, et al 2003; Fischel-Ghodsian 2003; Nance 2003; Van Laer, Cryns, Smith, & Van Camp 2003; Smith, Shearer, Hildebrand, & Van Camp 2013; Toriello & Smith 2013; Van Camp & Smith 2013; OMIM 2013). Genetic hearing losses occurring alone are called nonsyndromic, and we shall see that they have been associated with a large number of specific genes and/or chromosome locations of the genes in the human genome. (Syndromes involving hearing loss are discussed later in this chapter.)

Autosomal dominant inheritance means that only one abnormal gene is needed in order for the trait to appear (hence, it is dominant). Suppose one parent is hearing impaired due to an autosomal dominant gene and the other parent is normal. It does not make a difference which parent is affected because the sperm and egg each contribute half of every chromosome pair. If the mother is affected, then there will be a 50% chance that a given egg will contain the abnormal gene. If the father is affected, then half of his sperm will carry the abnormal gene and half will not. In either case, the chances are 50-50 for any pregnancy to result in a hearing-impaired child, as illustrated by the pedigree diagram in **Fig. 6.1a**.

The situation is different with **autosomal recessive inheritance** because both genes in the pair must be present for the trait to manifest itself. There are three possibilities with respect to the abnormal recessive gene: (1) One may be altogether free of the abnormal gene. (2) A person with both abnormal genes will have the disorder and will be able to transmit the disorder to an offspring. Such an individual is a **homozygote** because the same (*homo*) kind of abnormal gene was contributed by both parents when the fertilized egg (*zygote*) was produced. (3) An individual may have only one abnormal recessive gene, while the other one in the pair is normal. This person is a **heterozygote** because the two genes in the pair are different (*hetero*). He will not have a hearing loss because he has only one abnormal gene and it is recessive, but he is a **carrier** because he can transmit the abnormal gene to his offspring.

Let's see what happens when both parents are normal-hearing carriers of a certain recessive gene for hearing loss, that is, heterozygotes with one abnor-

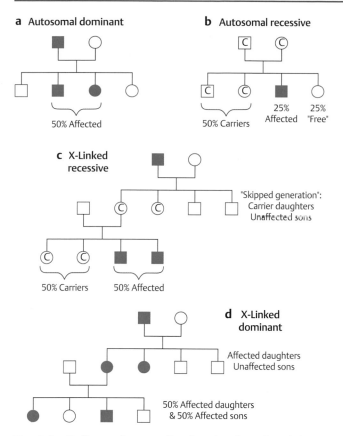

a Autosomal dominant

50% Affected

b Autosomal recessive

50% Carriers   25% Affected   25% "Free"

c X-Linked recessive

"Skipped generation": Carrier daughters Unaffected sons

50% Carriers   50% Affected

d X-Linked dominant

Affected daughters Unaffected sons

50% Affected daughters & 50% Affected sons

Fig. 6.1 Pedigree diagrams for disorders based on **(a)** autosomal dominant, **(b)** autosomal recessive, **(c)** X-linked recessive, and **(d)** X-linked dominant inheritance. Circles, females; squares, males; open symbols, individuals free of the abnormal gene; filled symbols, affected individuals with the abnormal gene; "C," unaffected carriers of the abnormal gene.

X-linked (or **sex-linked**) **inheritance** occurs when the gene is associated with the X chromosome instead of being autosomal. With an *X-linked recessive* disorder (**Fig. 6.1c**), an affected male transmits the abnormal gene to all of his daughters, who become unaffected carriers of the trait, but not to his sons. In turn, a female carrier has a 50% chance of having sons who are affected and a 50% chance of having daughters who are unaffected carriers. In *X-linked dominant* inheritance (**Fig. 6.1d**), an affected male will have all affected daughters and no affected sons. An affected female has a 50% chance of having affected children, whether they are males or females.

In contrast to the DNA in the nucleus, which is inherited from both parents, the 37 genes of the mitochondrial DNA are inherited from the mother alone. **Mitochondrial mutations** cause both syndromic and nonsyndromic deafness, and the latter is often related to aminoglycoside ototoxicity (e.g., Fischel-Ghodsian 2003; Kokotas, Petersen, & Willems 2007; Forli, Passetti, Mancuso, et al 2007; Bindu & Reddy 2008; Pandya 2011; Van Camp & Smith 2013). Ototoxicity is discussed later in this chapter.

Nonsyndromic Hearing Loss

About 50% of prelingual hearing losses ≥ 40 dB are hereditary, of which roughly 70% are nonsyndromic (Smith et al 2013). Approximately 75 to 85% of the nonsyndromic hearing losses are autosomal recessive, 15 to 20% are autosomal dominant, and 1 to 2% are X-linked. Mitochondrial defects account for less than 1% of the cases. To date, at least 26 genes have been linked to autosomal dominant deafness, 36 genes to autosomal recessive deafness, 4 to X-linked deafness, and 7 to mitochondrial losses (Smith et al 2013; Van Camp & Smith 2013; OMIM 2013).[2] These hearing losses are identified by DFN (for "deafness") followed by A for dominant, B for recessive, or X for X-linked, and then a number. For example, DFN1 is an autosomal dominant hearing loss involving the *DIAPH1* gene; DFNB21 is an autosomal recessive hearing loss associated with the *TECTA* gene, and DFNX1 is an X-linked hearing loss related to the *PRPS1* gene.

The most common form of genetic hearing loss is DFNB1, which accounts for half of the autosomal recessive cases (Smith et al 2013; Van Camp & Smith

mal gene and one normal gene (**Fig. 6.1b**). The probability of getting the mother's abnormal gene is 0.5 and the probability of getting the father's abnormal gene is also 0.5. Therefore, the probability of getting *both abnormal genes* is 0.5 × 0.5 = 0.25. In other words, a given pregnancy has a 25% chance of producing a child who has both abnormal genes and is hearing impaired. On the other hand, the probability of getting *both normal genes* is also 0.5 × 0.5 = 0.25, which means a 25% chance that a given pregnancy will result in a child who is altogether free of the abnormal gene. What about the other 50%? These are the two remaining combinations (normal gene from the mother with abnormal from the father, and abnormal from the mother with normal from the father), both of which produce an unaffected carrier of the abnormal gene. Autosomal recessive hearing losses can be very hard to trace because a particular kind of abnormal gene can be transmitted across several generations before two unaffected (and unaware) carriers coincidentally find each other and fail to beat the odds.

[2] Research in this area is progressing very actively. For up-to-date information and links to the current literature, see http://hereditaryhearingloss.org/, http://www.nhgri.nih.gov/, and http://www.omim.org/.

2013). Children born with DFNB1 have prelingual bilateral sensorineural hearing losses that can vary in degree of severity from mild to profound, and are nonprogressive. It is caused by mutations of the *GJB2* and *GJB6* genes, which provide for the expression of proteins in the inner ear called connexin 26 and 30. The connexins form gap junctions, which are channels that permit substances such as ions to flow across cell membranes, and are thus essential for maintaining the required balance and flow of potassium ions and other functions in the inner ear; however, the exact mechanism of the hearing loss is not fully understood (see, e.g., Ortolano et al 2008; Nickel & Forge 2008, 2010; Toriello & Smith 2013).

Syndromic Hearing Loss

Approximately 30% of significant hereditary hearing losses occur in syndromes (Smith et al 2013). A **syndrome** is a pattern of abnormalities and/or symptoms that result from the same cause. Related terms include an **association**, which describes a group of abnormalities that occur together too often to be due to chance; and a **sequence**, which is a group or pattern of abnormalities that result from a primary anomaly. Auditory disorders can be found in a great many syndromes, and extensive listings are readily available (e.g., Northern & Downs 1991; Hall, Prentice, Smiley, & Werkhaven 1995; Friedman et al 2003; Toriello & Smith 2013; Van Camp & Smith 2013; OMIM, 2013). Several representative syndromes known to cause hearing impairments are outlined in **Table 6.1**. Notice that different syndromes are associated with different kinds of hearing loss; some appear to be present at birth (congenital), whereas others are delayed in onset. Other syndromes are discussed elsewhere in the chapter.

Maternal Infections

Fetuses and newborns are adversely affected in various ways by at least 16 viruses and 6 bacteria. The major offenders are called the **TORCH complex**, which includes toxoplasmosis, "other" (including syphilis), rubella, cytomegalovirus, and herpes simplex. Many authorities have replaced TORCH with **STORCH** or **(S)TORCH** to recognize the importance of congenital syphilis in this group.

Syphilis (lues) is a sexually transmitted bacterial infection caused by the spirochete *Treponema pallidum,* which can be passed to the fetus from an infected mother. The number of reported cases of congenital syphilis increased dramatically from only 160 in 1981 to 2867 in 1990 (Shimizu 1992). Congenital syphilis is associated with notched incisor teeth, interstitial keratitis (a chronic inflammation of the cornea with the appearance of ground glass), and sensorineural hearing loss. The hearing loss can develop at any time during childhood or adulthood, even as late as ~ 60 years old. The sensorineural hearing loss is usually bilateral, symmetrical, and progressive, typically becoming severe-to-profound in degree. It is not uncommon for the loss to have a sudden onset or to fluctuate over time. Vertigo and/ or tinnitus can also occur. **Vertigo** is a specific kind of dizziness in which the patient experiences a sensation of *whirling* or *rotation.* It is associated with nystagmus (Chapter 11) and is often accompanied by nausea. The shape of the audiogram is often flat or rising, but any configuration is possible. It is sometimes possible to arrest (and possibly even reverse) the progression of early-onset luetic hearing loss with high doses of penicillin and steroids.

Toxoplasmosis is a parasitic infection caused by the protozoan *Toxoplasma gondii,* and is often contracted from contaminated raw meats and eggs, as well as from contact with cat feces. The disease is transmitted to the developing fetus via the placenta, often from a mother who does not have any symptoms herself. The risk of adverse effects in the infant is great for infections incurred during the first trimester but small during late pregnancy. The incidence of toxoplasmosis is roughly 1.1 in 1000 births. Congenital toxoplasmosis causes a variety of disorders, including central nervous system disorders (e.g., microcephaly, hydrocephaly, intracranial calcifications, and intellectual disability [intellectual developmental disorder][3]), chorioretinitis (inflammation of the choroid and retina) and other eye disorders, and bilateral sensorineural hearing loss that may be moderate to severe and progressive. Hearing losses have been reported in 14 to 26% of children with congenital toxoplasmosis. Optimistically, Stein and Boyer (1994) found no hearing losses in 58 children treated with antiparasitic and sulfonamide drugs for 12 months beginning when they were less than 2.5 months old, although long term follow-up studies of these children are still needed.

Rubella (German measles) is a viral disease transmitted from the mother to the fetus via the placenta. Epidemics in the United States during the 1960s have probably made it the most infamous viral cause of congenital hearing impairment, but the rubella vaccine has reduced the number of congenital rubella

---

[3] The American Psychiatric Association changed the diagnostic term *mental retardation* to *intellectual disability (intellectual developmental disorder)* beginning with the *Diagnostic and Statistical Manual of Mental Disorders,* 5th edition (DSM-5). *Intellectual developmental disorder* is used when the problem arises during the developmental period of life.

cases to ~ 50 per year (Strasnick & Jacobson 1995). Babies affected by congenital rubella may have heart disorders, kidney disorders, intellectual developmental disorder, visual defects, and hearing loss. The risk for congenital rubella is greatest if the fetus is exposed during the first trimester (roughly 50% in the first month, 20% in the second month, and 10% in the third), but the possibility of significant risks extends out to the 16th week. Sensorineural hearing loss is the most frequent sequela, with an incidence of ~ 50% when rubella is contracted during the first trimester and ~ 20% in the second and third trimesters. Congenital rubella is typically associated with bilateral sensorineural hearing losses that are severe to profound in degree, and either flat, bowl-shaped, or sloping in configuration.

Cytomegalovirus (CMV) affects 2 to 3% of live births and is probably the most common viral cause of congenital hearing loss. It is a herpes-type virus often contracted by sexual contact, and is also known to be transmitted by close associations with infected children. Pregnant women can be infected by a new exposure or by the reactivation of latent viruses already present in their bodies, and are usually asymptomatic when they do have the infection. The major consequences of CMV are associated with transmission to the developing fetus; postnatal CMV infections do not seem to present any major risks for an otherwise healthy child.

The severe outcomes of congenital CMV may include death, microcephaly, pneumonia, intellectual developmental disorder, liver disease, dental defects, visual lesions, and sensorineural hearing loss (Stagno 1990; Schildroth 1994; Strasnick & Jacobson 1995). About 10% of CMV infected newborns are *symptomatic,* with one or more manifestations such as a purple rash, jaundice, "blueberry muffin" skin discolorations, and various signs of infection. About 90% are *asymptomatic,* having "silent" CMV infections. Overall, Stagno (1990) reported that 92% of symptomatic newborns have one or more serious sequela (including a 30% death rate) compared with only 6% for asymptomatic infants. About 10 to 15% of the cases eventually have one or more serious complications of congenital cytomegalovirus.

Cytomegalovirus causes a wide variety of sensorineural hearing losses, ranging from mild through profound, which may be bilateral or unilateral, progressive or stable. Overall, ~ 14% of children born with CMV have some degree of sensorineural hearing loss (Schildroth 1994; Grosse, Ross, & Dollard 2008). However, while Schildroth (1994) reported that ~ 88% have severe to profound impairments and 50% have at least one additional disability, Grosse et al (2008) estimated that ~ 3 to 5% of children with CMV have bilateral losses that are moderate to profound.

Herpes simplex is a sexually transmitted viral disease that can be passed from an infected mother to the developing fetus either during pregnancy or during delivery (perinatally). Infected infants are affected by central nervous system problems (e.g., microcephaly and psychomotor disorders), growth deficiencies, retinal dysplasia, and moderate to severe sensorineural hearing loss in one or both ears.

Other Influences in the Maternal Environment

Maternal infections are not the only adverse influences that can cause or contribute to hearing impairments in the developing fetus. Another group of causes includes drugs, chemicals, and other agents in the maternal environment (Strasnick & Jacobson 1995). For example, congenital hearing loss can be caused by the maternal use of certain medications that may be passed to the fetus via the placenta. The most prominent group of drugs are the **aminoglycoside antibiotics**, such as kanamycin, gentamicin, and streptomycin, which are sometimes essential in the treatment of severe infections. Other aspects of the maternal environment that can contribute to congenital hearing impairments and related anomalies include maternal diseases such as toxemia and diabetes, nutritional deficiencies and disturbances, Rh-factor incompatibility between the mother and fetus, exposure to physical agents such as heat and radiation, and use of non-medicinal drugs and chemicals such as alcohol.

Adverse factors that occur just before, during, and immediately after birth include compromise of the oxygen supply (asphyxia, anoxia, hypoxia), trauma during labor and/or delivery, hyperbilirubinemia (jaundice) leading to kernicterus, and infections. Borg (1997) reviewed 20 years of research to clarify the relationship between hearing loss and prenatal hypoxia (oxygen deficiency), ischemia (blood supply deficiency), and asphyxia (indicated by a low Apgar score). He found that the risk of permanent sensorineural hearing loss is greater for ischemia than for hypoxia; the central nervous system (CNS) is more susceptible to these kinds of insults than is the inner ear; and preterm infants are more susceptible than full-term babies. Interestingly, hearing losses were rarely caused by birth asphyxia alone, and hypoxia all by itself appeared to be associated with temporary hearing losses as opposed to permanent ones.

Some elucidation about **hyperbilirubinemia** is desirable because not every newborn with jaundice is at risk. The normal breakdown of spent red blood cells produces bilirubin, which is detoxified by the liver and excreted. Hyperbilirubinemia is a build-up

Table 6.1 Some examples of syndromes that affect hearing[a]

Syndrome	Inheritance (identified genes in italics)	Hearing loss	Characteristics
Alpert syndrome	Autosomal dominant: *FGFR2*	Conductive (congenital)	Craniofacial anomalies affecting the ears, stapes fixation, fused fingers and toes, and spina bifida; associated with conductive hearing loss
Alport syndrome	X-linked: ~ 80%; *COL4A5* Autosomal recessive: ~ 15%; *COL4A3*, *COL4A4* Autosomal dominant: ~ 5%; single mutation of *COL4A3* or *COL4A4*	Sensorineural (delayed onset, progressive)	Varies by type: renal disease, ocular disorders, blood platelet defect, hearing loss
Branchio-oto-renal, syndrome	Autosomal dominant: *EYA1*, *SIX1*, *SIX5*	Sensorineural, conductive, mixed (congenital or delayed onset)	Outer, middle, inner ear deformities (characteristic ear pits), renal disorders, branchial fistulas/cysts, hearing loss
CHARGE syndrome	*CHD7* (> 50% of cases)	Mixed, progressive	Coloboma (malformation of iris giving the pupil a "keyhole" appearance, disk, or retina); congenital heart defects; atresia of the choanae (so posterior nasal airway is obstructed); retarded development and/or growth; ear anomalies and/or hearing loss
Crouzon syndrome	Autosomal dominant: *FGFR2*	Conductive, mixed (congenital)	Prematurely fused cranial sutures, beak-shaped nose, exophthalmos, variable outer/middle ear anomalies, hearing loss
Down (trisomy 21) syndrome	Improper separation of chromosome pairs, causing an extra copy of chromosome 21	Conductive, mixed	Multisystem disorder; intellectual developmental disorder; characteristic facial features (tilted palpebral fissures, epicanthal folds, broad nasal bridge, flattened profile, open mouth with protruding tongue); outer/middle/inner ear hypoplasias have been reported; muscular hypotonia; short hands with simian line; congenital heart disease; frequent upper respiratory infections; recurrent otitis media, hearing loss
Friedreich's ataxia	Autosomal recessive: *FXN*	Sensorineural (delayed onset, progressive)	Ataxia, nystagmus, optic atrophy, hearing loss
Goldenhar syndrome (oculoauriculovertibral dysplasia)	Undetermined	Conductive (congenital)	Facial asymmetry, microtia, atresia, preauricular tags, eye anomalies, oral defects, clubfoot, hemivertebrae, congenital heart disease, abnormal semicircular canals, hearing loss
Klippel-Feil syndrome	Autosomal dominant: *GDF3*, *GDF6*	Sensorineural, conductive (congenital)	Fused cervical vertebrae, short neck, decreased head mobility, low occipital hairline, ossicle abnormalities, hearing loss

Syndrome	Inheritance (identified genes in italics)	Hearing loss	Characteristics
Hunter syndrome (mucopolysaccaridosis II)	X-linked: *IDS*	Sensorineural, conductive, mixed (progressive)	Skeletal deformities, dwarfism, coarse facial features, corneal clouding, cardiovascular disorders, intellectual developmental disorder; mucopolysaccharide accumulations in tissues result in progressive characteristics, hearing loss; males affected only
Hurler syndrome (mucopolysaccaridosis I)	Autosomal recessive: *IDUA*	Sensorineural, conductive, mixed (progressive)	Same features as Hunter syndrome, but may be more severe; affects both sexes
Jervell and Lange-Nielsen syndrome	Autosomal recessive: *KCNE1, KCNQ1*	Sensorineural	Cardiac problems, syncope, sudden death, hearing loss
Osteogenesis imperfecta	Autosomal dominant: *COL1A1, COL1A2*	Sensorineural, conductive, mixed (progressive)	Fragile bones, large skull, triangular facies, hemorrhage tendency, stapes fixation, hearing loss
Pendred syndrome	Autosomal dominant: ~ 50% involve *SLC26a4*	Sensorineural (variable, congenital, progressive)	Hearing loss and thyroid enlargement (goiter), both variable
Stickler/Marshall syndromes	Autosomal dominant: type 1, *COL2A1*; type 2, *COL11A1*; type 3, *COL11A2*	Sensorineural, conductive, mixed	Three types: severe eye disorders (detached retina, myopia) in types 1 and 2, but not in type 3; small lower jaw, hearing loss
Treacher Collins syndrome (mandibulofacial dysostosis)	Autosomal dominant: *TCOF1* (mainly), *POLR1C, POLR1D*	Conductive, mixed (congenital)	Facial anomalies (depressed zygomatics, eyes slant downward laterally, receding mandible, mouth large and fish-like, dental anomalies, cleft palate); outer and middle ear deformities, hearing loss
Usher Syndrome (Vestibulocerbellar ataxia)	Autosomal recessive: type I, *CDH23, MYO7A, PCDH15, USH1C, USH1G*; type II, *USH2A, GPR98*; possibly ≥ 2 others; type III, *CLRN*; ≥ 1 other[s]	Sensorineural (congenital in types I and II)	Type I: retinitis pigmentosa, vestibular dysfunction, profound hearing loss Type II: retinitis pigmentosa, sloping hearing loss (variable degree) Type III: retinitis pigmentosa, vestibular dysfunction; initially normal hearing or mild loss, then hearing loss progresses
Waardenburg syndrome	Autosomal dominant: type I, *PAX3*; type II, *MITF, SNAI2*; type III, *PAX3*; type IV, *EDN3, EDNRB, SOX10* (Some type II & IV cases might be autosomal recessive)	Sensorineural (congenital)	White forelock in hair, prominent root of nose, differently colored eyes, hyperplasia of medial third of eyebrows, medial canthi displaced laterally; inner ear dysplasia, hearing loss Four types identified, differing by abnormalities present and/or genes involved

[a]Compilation based on Nance (2003); Vissers, van Ravenswaaij, Admiraal, et al (2004); Jongmans, Admiraal, van der Donk, et al (2006); Smith et al (2013); Toriello & Smith (2013); Van Camp & Smith (2013); OMIM (2013).

of bilirubin in the blood and is observed as jaundice. Some degree of jaundice is common among newborns, and it is successfully treated by exposing the baby to ultraviolet light (phototherapy). However, **Rh-factor incompatibilities** between the mother (who is Rh-negative) and the fetus (who is Rh-positive) can result in the production of antibodies in the mother's blood, which can attack and break down red blood cells in the fetus. This disorder is called **erythroblastosis fetalis** or **hemolytic disease** of the neonate, and usually occurs in subsequent pregnancies where the fetus is Rh-positive. The concentration of bilirubin in the blood of the fetus can become high enough to cross the blood-brain barrier, causing **kernicterus**, or the deposit of bilirubin in the brain. Kernicterus causes brain damage because bilirubin is toxic to neural tissue. It can be widespread, but particularly affects the basal ganglia. Typical sequelae include athetoid cerebral palsy, intellectual developmental disorder, and hearing impairment. Blood transfusions (exchange transfusions) are used to avert or minimize these effects in newborns with high bilirubin levels. A variety of sensorineural losses are found in ~ 4% of babies with hemolytic disease or hyperbilirubinemia (Hyman, Keaster, Hanson, et al 1969). However, whether hearing losses in kernicterus patients come from damage to the brainstem centers (such as the cochlear nuclei) and/or to coincidental peripheral impairments seems to be an unresolved issue.

Congenital Anomalies of the Ear

Outer and Middle Ear

Dysplasia means an abnormality in the development of an anatomical structure. These congenital anomalies can affect the outer, middle, and/or inner ear, and can occur alone or as part of syndromes. The conductive system anomalies span a range of severity, from barely noticeable cosmetic aberrations to a complete lack of development **(aplasia)**. Outer and middle ear anomalies may occur alone or together, as well as in combination with inner ear dysplasia, especially in more severe cases.

The major external ear anomalies are microtia and atresia, which often occur together. **Microtia** means an abnormally small pinna, but it actually refers to a wide range of auricle deformities. *Type I microtias* have recognizable parts, and can be more or less well formed except for their size. Pinnas that are only partially formed, generally resembling a curved or straight ridge, are *type II microtias*. A *type III microtia* is a tissue mass that does not resemble a pinna. Finally, the auricle may be completely absent, which is called **agenesis** (or **aplasia**) of the pinna, or **anotia**. Microtias are

a major cosmetic problem, but do not cause substantial hearing losses in and of themselves. (This is not to undervalue the important auditory role of the pinna in such processes as directional hearing.) In contrast, considerable degrees of hearing loss can be produced by **aural atresia**, which is the absence of an external auditory meatus. If the canal opening is abnormally narrow, then the condition is called **aural stenosis**.

Many kinds of congenital middle ear anomalies are possible, such as these:

1. The middle ear cavity and antrum may be grossly malformed, slit-like, or altogether absent.
2. The tympanic membrane may be rudimentary or absent.
3. Ossicles may be abnormally formed; for example, the malleus and incus are often conglomerated into a unit.
4. Ossicles may be missing.
5. Ossicles may be attached to the abnormally formed middle ear cavity either directly or via bony bridges.
6. Facial nerve abnormalities are also frequently encountered.

Outer and middle ear anomalies produce a conductive hearing loss, provided the inner ear is not also affected. The degree of the conductive loss depends on the nature and extent of the abnormalities and is often ~ 60 dB. Surgical reconstruction of the conductive mechanism is generally possible, provided there is a serviceable cochlea behind the abnormal conductive mechanism. Depending on the nature of the abnormal anatomy, it is often possible to reduce the conductive loss to the 30 dB range, which is a considerable degree of improvement. Surgical reconstruction for the microtia provides the child with cosmetic improvements, the importance of which should not be underestimated.

Inner Ear

The congenital anomalies of the inner ear also exist along a continuum of severity from slight to complete. The worst case is the total absence of any inner ear structures, known as **Michel's aplasia**. It is possible for this to occur even with a normal conductive mechanism. Incomplete anomalies and developmental failures of the bony and membranous ducts of the inner ear are known as **Mondini's dysplasia** and vary widely in severity. The most common abnormality is dysplasia of the membranous ducts of the cochlea and saccule, and is called **Scheibe's aplasia**. It is generally believed that Michel's and Mondini's anomalies are caused by autosomal dominant traits, and that Scheibe's aplasia is transmitted by the autosomal recessive route. **Alexander's aplasia** refers to congenital abnormalities of the cochlear duct, especially affecting the basal turn (high-frequency region) of the cochlea.

Acquired Disorders

Head Trauma

Traumatic head injuries can cause conductive, sensorineural, and mixed hearing losses, depending on the nature and extent of the injuries. Head trauma causes a conductive hearing loss by such mechanisms as injuries to the eardrum and/or ossicles, accumulations of blood and debris in the ear canal and middle ear, and temporal bone fractures. Traumatic sensorineural losses are typically caused by concussion to the inner ear and fractures of the temporal bone directly injuring the inner ear structures.

Temporal bone fractures are classified according to whether the fracture line is in the same direction as the axis of the petrous pyramid (longitudinal) or across it (transverse). The relationships of these fractures to the structures of the ear are shown in **Fig. 6.2**. **Longitudinal fractures** go through the ear canal and middle ear and usually bypass the inner ear structures, so that they are most likely to produce conductive losses. About 80% of temporal bone fractures are longitudinal. In addition, concussion to the cochlea can result in a sensorineural loss (generally high-frequency) even though the inner ear structures are not directly involved in the longitudinal fracture. In contrast, **transverse fractures** cut through the inner ear, often resulting in profound sensorineural hearing loss and vertigo. Facial nerve paralysis occurs in ~ 50% of patients with transverse fractures. Mixed fractures are also common.

Outer Ear Disorders

Impacted Cerumen

Cerumen is a waxy substance that is supposed to be in the ear canal, where it serves lubricating and cleansing functions and also helps to protect the ear from bacteria, fungi, and insects. The cerumen is produced by glands in the cartilaginous portion of the ear canal and migrates out over time. Small amounts of cerumen often accumulate in normal ears, typically seen as yellow to brown globs that do not obstruct the ear canal. **Impacted cerumen** is an accumulation of wax in the ear canal that interferes with the flow of sound to the eardrum. Impacted cerumen occurs naturally in many patients who produce excessive amounts of cerumen, which builds up over time. It is also the fate of many Q-tip-wielding patients who inadvertently pack cerumen farther back into the canal (and frequently against the eardrum) in an ironic attempt to clean their ears.

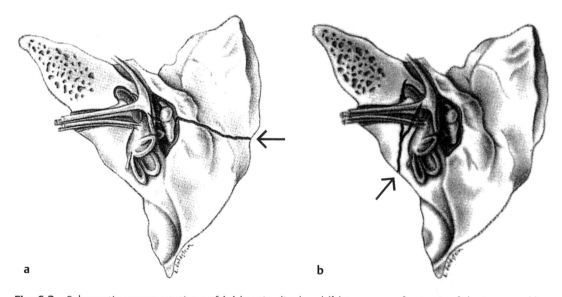

Fig. 6.2 Schematic representations of **(a)** longitudinal and **(b)** transverse fractures of the temporal bone and how they relate to ear structures. (Adapted from Swartz and Harnsberger [1998], with permission.)

Impacted cerumen commonly produces conductive hearing loss, itching, tinnitus, vertigo, and external otitis. The hearing loss gradually worsens as the cerumen builds up, and can reach ~ 45 dB when the canal is completely occluded. Some patients may experience a "sudden" hearing loss in the shower or swimming pool if they have a small opening in the cerumen plug that is abruptly closed by the water.

The treatment for excessive cerumen is to remove it. **Cerumen management** procedures (e.g., Ballachanda & Peers 1992; Roeser & Wilson 2000; Roland, Smith, Schwartz, et al 2008) are undertaken only after an otoscopic examination and a complete history are taken. Cerumen removal may be preceded by the use of a wax softening product, and is accomplished by one technique or a combination of techniques including irrigation of the ear with water, removal with a blunt curette designed for this purpose, and suction. Cerumen management is within the scope of audiological practice (e.g., ASHA 2004, 2006), with ~ 69% of audiologists overall (and ~ 87% of private practitioners) providing this service as of 2011 (Johnson, Danhauer, Rice, & Fisher 2013).

Foreign Bodies

A seemingly endless assortment of **foreign bodies** can get into the ear. Some of these may get pushed into the ear where they can produce traumatic injuries to the canal wall, tympanic membrane, and middle ear structures. Others get stuck in the canal. Others do both. Foreign bodies that get stuck in the canal may be inorganic or organic, including live insects, and can produce the same effects as impacted cerumen *plus* traumatic injuries and/or infection depending on the nature of the object. Foreign objects in the ear should be removed by an otologist.

Growths and Tumors

The outer ear can be the site of cysts as well as benign and malignant tumors that should be addressed medically. Hearing becomes a factor if the ear canal is obstructed. **Exostoses** are the most common tumors of the ear canals, and are regularly encountered audiologically. These are benign, skin-covered bony growths from the canal walls that are smooth and rounded. They are usually found bilaterally. The development of exostoses is encouraged by repeated encounters with cold water and are common among swimmers. It is uncommon to find exostoses that will fully occlude the external auditory meatus by themselves, but their presence makes it easier for the canal to be blocked by cerumen or debris in the canal.

Infections

External otitis (otitis externa) is a diffuse infection of the external auditory meatus usually caused by pseudomonas (and less often by staphylococcus) bacteria. It is occasionally known as "swimmer's ear" because of its association with swimming in inadequately maintained pools. External otitis produces a considerable amount of pain, as well as edema (swelling), discharge, itching, and a conductive hearing loss if the canal is occluded by the swelling and debris. It is treated with antibiotic drops or creams that are frequently mixed with hydrocortisone to help reduce the edema. When there is considerable edema a gauze wick may be impregnated with the antibiotic/cortisone cream and gently pushed into the swollen ear canal to act as a medication applicator.

Otitis externa can develop into an aggressive and life-threatening form of the infection called **necrotizing (malignant) external otitis** in diabetics and other susceptible patients, and requires extensive antibiotic and other medical treatment.

The **furuncle** is an example of a more circumscribed outer ear infection. It is a staphylococcus infection of a hair follicle in the cartilaginous portion of the ear canal. Furuncles are treated with oral antibiotics, the placement of an alcohol-soaked wick in the ear canal until it spontaneously opens and drains, and/or incision and drainage of the furuncle under local anesthesia.

■ Middle Ear Disorders

Bullus myringitis is a very painful viral infection seen as inflamed, fluid-filled blebs or blister-like sacs on the tympanic membrane and nearby ear canal walls. It often occurs in association with upper respiratory infections as well as with otitis media. Very little hearing loss is associated with this condition even though it does impair the mobility of the tympanic membrane to some extent. Bullus myringitis is usually self-limiting, and a thin fluid (perhaps with blood) is discharged when the blebs rupture. Antibiotics are often used to avoid secondary infections.

Tympanosclerosis refers to a variety of tissue changes that occur as the result of repeated middle ear infections. It is often seen as chalky white calcium plaques and scar tissue on the pars tensa of the eardrum, which has little if any effect on hearing sensitivity. Tympanosclerosis also affects the other structures of the middle ear, and can affect hearing if the calcification or other changes impair the mobility of the ossicular chain.

Perforations of the tympanic membrane can be caused by ear infections and various kinds of traumatic insults. Typical traumatic causes include (1) punctures; (2) chemical injuries; and (3) forceful pressure changes due to an explosion, a slap to the ear, intense sound (**acoustic trauma**), and sudden changes in air pressure while flying or in water pressure while diving (**barotrauma**). As illustrated in **Fig. 6.3**, the opening is described as a central, marginal, or attic perforation, according to its location on the eardrum. Attic perforations involve the pars flaccida and are often associated with cholesteatoma, as discussed below. Eardrum perforations produce conductive hearing losses because they (1) reduce the size of the drum's vibrating surface area, which reduces the eardrum-to-oval-window area advantage; (2) impair the coupling of the eardrum to the ossicular chain so that signal transmission is reduced; and (3) interfere with the proper phase relationship at the oval and round windows by allowing sound to impact upon the round window. In general, the magnitude of the conductive hearing loss gets worse as the size of the perforation increases.

Many tympanic membrane perforations heal spontaneously. Healed perforations are associated with the development of *scar tissue* and thin areas that do not have a fibrous middle layer, which are sometimes called *monomeric membranes*. Larger perforations and those associated with chronic middle ear infections generally do not heal on their own, and require a surgical repair of the eardrum called a **myringoplasty**.

Otitis Media and Associated Pathologies

Inflammations of the middle ear are called **otitis media**, and constitute the most common cause of conductive hearing losses. Otitis media affects people of all ages, but the incidence among children is particularly high. For example, incidence figures have been reported at over 50% by age 1 and 60% by age 2, ~ 33% for at least three episodes by age 3, roughly 80% for children in day care centers, and ~ 90% by the time a child reaches school age (e.g., Denny 1984; Teele, Klein, & Rosner 1984; Prellner, Kalm, & Harsten 1992; AAP 2004).

The implications of otitis media in children go beyond the medical ramifications of the pathology and the direct interference with communication caused by the conductive hearing loss. Young children with **recurrent otitis media** are subjected to frequent and sustained periods of conductive hearing impairment during critical learning periods. For example, Gravel and Wallace (2000) found that during years 1 through 3, children who had otitis media with effusion (OME) had consistently poorer hearing

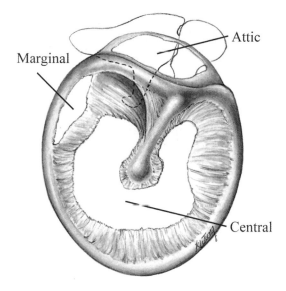

Fig. 6.3 Examples of central, marginal, and attic perforations of the tympanic membrane. (Adapted from Hughes [1985], with permission.)

thresholds than their OME-free counterparts. For this reason, it is not surprising that recurrent otitis media in young children has been associated with deficits affecting auditory processing, language development, cognitive and academic skills (e.g., Jerger, Jerger, Alford, & Abrams 1983; Friel-Patti & Finitzo 1990; Menjuk 1992; Gravel & Wallace 1992; Brown 1994; Downs 1995; Schwartz, Mody, & Petinou 1997; Mody, Schwartz, Gravel, & Ruben 1999). It is interesting to note here that the temporal characteristics of auditory cortex activity were changed by 1 to 2 weeks of experimentally induced conductive hearing losses in developing gerbils (Xu, Kotak, & Sanes 2007).

Otitis media can take several forms depending on such factors as the development and time course of the disease, whether a bacterial infection is present, the nature of the fluid in the middle ear space, and the kinds of complications that exist. One way to address these issues is to trace the course that the disease might follow.

A properly functioning Eustachian tube provides the middle ear with ventilation and drainage, and maintains the same amount of pressure on both sides of the tympanic membrane. Recall from Chapter 2 that the Eustachian tube is normally closed, and that it is opened by the tensor palatini muscle during activities such as chewing and yawning; and we shall soon see that problems with this process can lead to an accumulation of fluid in the middle ear and the possible development of more serious disease. It is interesting to note in this context that middle ear fluid was found to be significantly less common among 2- to 6-year olds who regularly chew gum compared with those who do not (Kouwen & DeJonckere 2007).

Eustachian Tube Dysfunction

Eustachian tube dysfunction exists when the tube does not open properly, is not patent, or is blocked in one way or another. The tube might be blocked by edema (swelling) and/or fluid caused by an upper respiratory infection, sinusitis, inflamed adenoids, or allergies; obstruction by hypertrophic (enlarged) adenoids; or obstruction or encroachment by a nasopharyngeal tumor or other growth. The Eustachian tube may also fail to open appropriately (e.g., upon swallowing or yawning) due to structural or functional abnormalities affecting the tensor palatini muscle. This problem is common among cleft palate patients.

Unlike the adult Eustachian tube, which tilts downward by ~ 45°, infants and young children have almost horizontal Eustachian tubes (**Fig. 6.4**), which are also relatively shorter and wider, in addition to which their tensor palatini muscles operate less efficiently. These factors increase the chances of Eustachian tube dysfunction and middle ear disease among infants and young children with growth and development by age 6 or 7 (Rovers, Schilder, Zielhuis, & Rosenfeld 2004).

Eustachian tube dysfunction prevents the middle ear from being ventilated, causing the air within the middle ear cavity to become stagnant. Part of the stagnant air is then absorbed by the tissues of the middle ear. As a result, the air pressure will be lower inside the middle ear than it is outside in the surrounding atmosphere. This situation is called **negative pressure** in the middle ear.[4] This pressure difference on the two sides of the tympanic membrane (higher outside, lower inside) causes it to be drawn inward, or **retracted.** The same nonpatency of the Eustachian tube that caused the air to be trapped within the middle ear cavity also prevents ventilation of the middle ear that would re-equalize the pressure and "unclog" the ear. If this problem is caused by an abrupt pressure change, it is called **aerotitis** or **barotrauma.** Aerotitis is usually caused by the abrupt air pressure increase of an airplane descent, which causes the tympanic membrane to retract and prevents the Eustachian tube from opening.

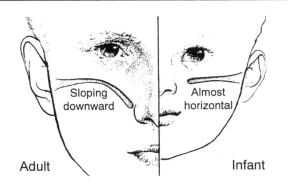

Fig. 6.4 The Eustachian tube slopes downward in adults but is closer to being horizontal in infants and young children. (Adapted from Pulec and Horwitz [1973], with permission.)

Otitis Media with Effusion

Fluid might accumulate in the middle ear, typically because it was drawn from the middle ear tissues by negative pressure caused by Eustachian tube dysfunction or allergies, or as an inflammatory response after an acute infection (e.g., Gates, Klein, Lim, et al 2002; AAP 2004). The presence of this fluid (effusion) in the middle ear in the absence of an acute infection is called **otitis media with effusion (OME)** (e.g., Stool, Berg, Berman, et al 1994; AAP 2004). Not surprisingly, otitis media is associated with conductive hearing loss. Since the effusion contains **serous fluid**, which is a watery and clear transudate that is free of cells and other materials, the condition is often called **serous otitis media.** The term **middle ear effusion (MEE)** is often used here as well, but different kinds of fluids may also accumulate in the middle ear. Continuation of the disease process may involve **mucoid fluid** from secretory (goblet) cells in the middle ear mucosa. This cloudy exudate is thicker and more viscous than serous fluid, containing white blood cells and other cellular material. At this stage the condition might be described as **secretory otitis media,** and the term **mucoid otitis media** may eventually be applied with the continued thickening of the effusion. Because serous fluid is absorbed by the middle ear mucosa over time, it is possible for the effusion can become progressively thicker and more viscous, eventually leading to **adhesive otitis media** or "**glue ear**," preventing motion of the ossicles. Blood in the middle ear is called **hemotympanum.**

Middle ear fluid can sometimes be detected otoscopically by seeing a fluid line or **meniscus** or by the presence of bubbles. It is often not possible to distinguish between the presence versus absence of effusion if the tympanum is completely filled

---

[4] The nonpatent Eustachian tube explanation appears to account for negative pressures up to only about -100 daPa (Cantekin et al, 1980; Yee & Cantekin, 1986), so that other mechanisms may also be involved in creating abnormally negative middle ear pressures.

with serous fluid. The diagnosis of middle ear effusion involves the use of a **pneumatic (Siegel) otoscope** (AAP 2004), which has a rubber bulb and tube that allows the examiner to change the air pressure against the eardrum (by squeezing the bulb). Middle ear fluid is indicated if the air pressure fails to cause observable eardrum movement.

Acute Otitis Media

So far we have been assuming that the patient has a middle ear effusion that is **nonsuppurative** or **nonpurulent**, which means that it is free of bacterial infection. However, infections can readily develop once microbes gain access to the middle ear, usually from the nasopharynx via the Eustachian tube. Otitis media becomes **suppurative** or **purulent** when bacteria invade the middle ear system. **Acute (purulent or suppurative) otitis media** typically occurs during or soon after an upper respiratory infection. The most common bacteria responsible for acute suppurative or purulent otitis media are *Streptococcus pneumoniae, Haemophilus influenzae,* and *Branhamella catarrhalis.*

The typical course of events often begins with **hyperemia** (engorgement of the tissues with blood), often seen as reddening on the tympanic membrane, accompanied by **otalgia** (ear pain) and possibly fever. This may be followed by **exudation**, in which the middle ear space is filled with fluid containing white blood cells, red blood cells, mucus, and other materials. The eardrum is red and thickened so that landmarks cannot be seen, and it bulges due to pressure from the exudate in the middle ear. This comes with increased pain, fever, and a conductive hearing loss. Building pressure can cause the eardrum to rupture, resulting in the drainage of pus and other materials from the infected middle ear. Such a purulent discharge from the ear is called **otorrhea**. It is often preferable for the drainage to be effected by a small surgical incision of the eardrum (called a myringotomy, which is discussed below). Drainage relieves the pressure and pain, and there is often spontaneous healing of the tympanic membrane.

Ongoing or repeated episodes of acute otitis media are called **chronic otitis media**, which is often associated with a perforated tympanic membrane. However, ongoing ear pathology can occur even without a perforation. Hence, the distinction between acute and chronic otitis media may also be made on the basis of how long the disease lasts. For example, a case of otitis media might be called **acute** if it lasts up to 3 weeks, chronic if it lasts more than 12 weeks, and subacute for intermediate durations. Some cases of chronic otitis media with intact eardrums are not detected clinically and may even be undetectable, and have been termed *silent otitis media* (Paparella, Goycoolea, Bassiouni, & Koutroupas 1986). As one might expect, patients who experience repeated episodes over time are said to have **recurrent otitis media**.

Complications and Sequelae of Otitis Media

Otitis media can result in quite a few sequelae and complications of major medical significance, some of which can have life-threatening consequences. Cholesteatoma is a common problem, and is discussed below. Facial paralysis can result if the infection erodes the Fallopian canal and affects the seventh cranial nerve. Spread of the infection to the inner ear results in labyrinthitis. Recall that the tympanum communicates with the mastoid antrum and air cell system, so that otitis media can spread to infect the mastoid, producing **mastoiditis**. Mastoiditis can lead to the further spread of the infection to the central nervous system, as well as to other sites.

Conductive hearing loss is certainly the effect with which we are most directly concerned. Any amount of conductive loss can occur with otitis media, and fluctuation is common. These audiograms tend to be reasonably flat, but it is not uncommon to find losses that are poorer in the low frequencies, and others that are somewhat tent-shaped (**Fig. 6.5**). Otitis media can also cause a sensorineural loss, particularly in the high frequencies. The sensorineural component may be caused by the transmission of toxins to the perilymph via the round window. However, conductive lesions can affect bone-conduction thresholds, which might account for some of the sensorineural components seen in these patients, at least in part (see Chapter 5, and the section on otosclerosis in this chapter).

Otitis media can lead to a continuing conductive hearing loss by causing such conditions as (1) perforated eardrums; (2) adhesions, tympanosclerosis, and glue ear, which restrict or prevent motion of the ossicles; and (3) ossicular chain discontinuities that occur when the infective process causes part of the chain to be eroded away.

A **cholesteatoma** is a cyst made of layers of keratin producing squamous epithelium filled with an accumulation of keratin and cellular debris. It is also known as a **keratoma** or an **epidermoid inclusion cyst**. Even though *keratoma* is the less popular term, it is actually more appropriate because cholesteatomas contain considerable amounts of keratin but little if any cholesterol.

Cholesteatomas are usually associated with chronic otitis media, and with perforated and retracted tym-

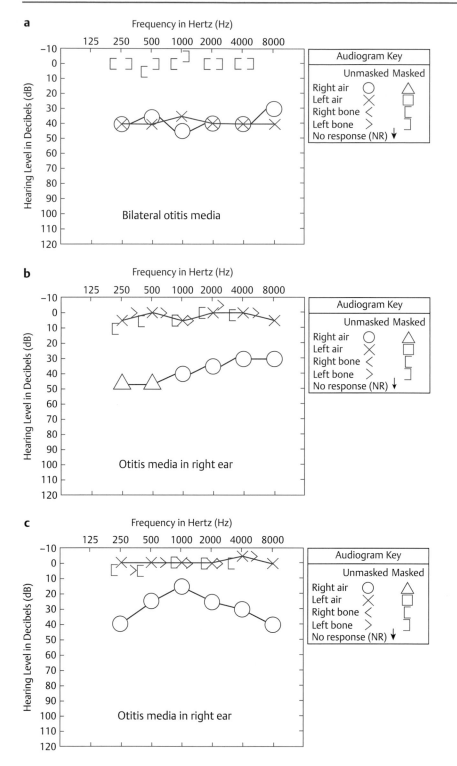

Fig. 6.5 (a–c) Audiograms from three patients with otitis media.

panic membranes. They also occur spontaneously in a small percentage of patients and can develop in the middle ear, eardrum, or petrous portion, and even intracranially. The most common sites for cholesteatoma formation are pars flaccida and marginal perforations. Let us consider the development of an attic cholesteatoma, which is a very common type. The cholesteatoma might begin as a small retracted pouch (retraction pocket) in the pars flaccida, often encouraged by ongoing negative pressure in the middle ear. The sac retains keratin and debris. Inflammation of the sac causes it to swell and expand. The cholesteatoma may lie dormant for some time, or it may grow slowly or quickly. The invasion route begins in the epitympanic recess, or attic, as shown in **Fig. 6.6**. Notice in the figure that a cholesteatoma that appears tiny when viewed from the outside can actually be quite large. The expanding cholesteatoma destructively encroaches upon the middle ear space and structures. As it continues to grow, the cholesteatoma has the potential to invade other locations, such as the mastoid, labyrinth, and cranium. This aggressive capability makes the cholesteatoma a potentially life-threatening lesion that must be removed surgically.

Infections (as well as traumatic injuries) can also result in various kinds of middle ear defects, such as **ossicular discontinuities**, which are interruptions in the ossicular chain, and other disorders that prevent the ossicular chain from vibrating effectively or at all, such as extensive tympanosclerosis or adhesions. **Fig. 6.7** compares a normal conductive system to a simple perforation, a perforation with an ossicular chain interruption involving the malleus, and an ossicular discontinuity with an intact eardrum.

Management of Otitis Media and Related Pathologies

The recommended management of otitis media with effusion (AAP 2004) initially involves a 3-month period of *watchful waiting* (monitoring without intervention) in children between 2 months and

Fig. 6.6 Example of a large attic cholesteatoma. Notice that only a tiny portion of the cholesteatoma is visible outside the tympanic membrane. (Adapted from Hughes [1985], with permission.)

12 years old who are free of risk factors for speech-language-hearing, learning, or developmental disorders. Watchful waiting is recommended because OME often resolves spontaneously over time, and to avoid the negative effects of unnecessary treatment. If the OME persists, monitoring might continue at 3- to 6-month intervals until the effusion resolves or there is a need for intervention. Antihistamines and decongestants have not been found to be effective

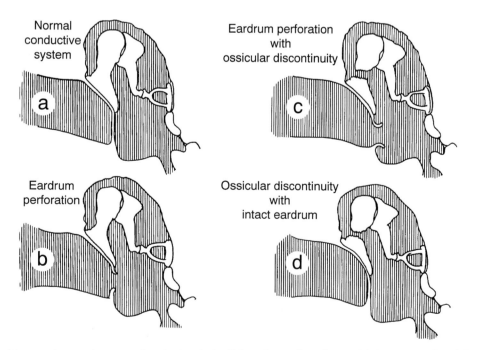

Fig. 6.7   **(a)** Normal tympanic membrane and ossicular chain; **(b)** perforated eardrum with intact ossicles; **(c)** perforated eardrum with interrupted ossicular chain due to eroded malleus; **(d)** intact eardrum with interrupted ossicular chain due to eroded malleus. (Adapted from Hughes [1985], with permission.)

treatments for OME; and the antibiotics and corticosteroids are not recommended as routine treatments for OME because they do not provide long-term benefits. Should it become necessary, the recommended treatment for OME involves the surgical insertion of a pressure equalization tube in the eardrum. For patients requiring additional surgical treatment because OME recurs, then an adenoidectomy along with a myringotomy are recommended. These and other surgical treatments are discussed in more detail below.

Acute otitis media is generally treated with oral antibiotics. Treating just the symptoms (e.g., pain, fever) without antibiotics for 48 to 72 hours is also considered for otherwise healthy children between 2 months and 12 years old providing certain conditions are met,[5] after which antibiotics are introduced if needed (AAP 2004). Typical antibiotics used to treat acute otitis media include amoxicillin, ampicillin, erythromycin, trimethoprim-sulfa preparations, and cephalosporins, depending on the microbe and the patient's drug sensitivities. The effectiveness of antihistamines and decongestants is questionable, unless the underlying problem is allergic.

Several mechanical methods can also be used to ventilate clogged ears by opening the patient's nonpatent Eustachian tubes. Patients can use the **Valsalva maneuver**, provided they do not have an upper respiratory infection that could be spread to the middle ear. This method involves forcing the Eustachian tube open by blowing forcefully with the mouth closed tightly and the nose pinched closed. The middle ear can also be ventilated by **politzerization**. This procedure uses a rubber tube with a compressible rubber bulb. The physician places the free end of the tube into one nostril (with the other one pinched closed) and air is forced in by squeezing the bulb. Other air pressure sources can also be used. An effective but thoroughly unpleasant method for ventilating the middle ear involves forcing air directly into the Eustachian tube orifice in the nasopharynx through a catheter inserted into the nose.

Adenoidectomy (removal of the adenoids) is considered a treatment for recurrent otitis media with effusion in children when the problem can be attributed to a blockage of the Eustachian tube by hypertrophic adenoids. Children with middle ear effusion may be helped by adenoidectomy, but adding a **tonsillectomy** (removal of the tonsils) does not provide any benefit (e.g., Mau 1984; AAP 2004).

A **myringotomy** or **paracentesis** is a surgical incision in the tympanic membrane usually performed for the purpose of draining the middle ear. Myringotomies are commonly done in children who have persistent or recurrent middle ear effusions to remove the fluid, thereby alleviating the conductive hearing loss, and helping prevent recurrences by keeping the middle ear ventilated. In cases of acute otitis media, myringotomies may be performed to prevent the rupturing of a markedly distended eardrum, and when there is severe pain, high fever, toxicity, evidence of medical complications, or poor responsiveness to antibiotics.

The myringotomy procedure is straightforward (**Fig. 6.8**): A small incision is made in the eardrum, which is commonly placed in the anteroinferior quadrant. The fluid is then aspirated (removed with suction) from the middle ear. Finally, a **pressure equalization (PE)**, **tympanostomy**, or **ventilation tube** (or **grommet**) is usually inserted into the incision to keep it open. These tubes are made of many different kinds of materials and come in a wide variety of designs. The purpose of the PE tube becomes apparent when we realize that removing the fluid does not fix the Eustachian tube problem, which is usually the underlying culprit. Pressure equalization tubes help prevent the recurrence of effusions by keeping the middle ear ventilated and preventing the development of negative pressure, and also provide a route for any continued drainage. In effect, ventilation tubes replace the functions of a dysfunctional Eustachian tube. Ventilation tubes are usually left in place for several months or until they are naturally extruded by the eardrum.

The overall efficacy of PE tubes is well established (e.g., Valtonen, Tuomilehto, Qvarnberg, & Nuutinen 2005a,b), but one must still be alert to the development of problems and complications associated with their use. The major concerns are (1) clogging or premature extrusion of the tubes; (2) water getting into the middle ear through the tubes; (3) persistence of the Eustachian tube blockage, leading to recurrence of the disease once the tubes are out; and (4) medical complications such as otorrhea, tympanosclerosis, and cholesteatoma.

At least three kinds of audiological services are important for patients with ventilation tubes: (1) Custom-made earplugs often called "swimming earmolds" are needed to prevent water from entering the middle ear via the PE tubes when the patient swims, showers, and engages in similar activities. (2) Periodic monitoring with acoustic immittance tests (Chapter 7) is needed to determine if the PE tube is still in place and patent, or if it has become clogged or dislodged. (3) Audiological assessments are neces-

---

[5] The principal conditions are an uncertain diagnosis of acute otitis media and less than severe illness for 6–24-month-olds; uncertain diagnosis or less than severe illness for those who are at least 2 years old; and confidence that the child will promptly be returned for follow-up evaluation and treatment (AAP, 2004).

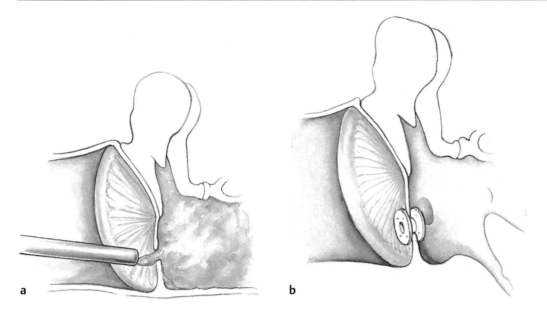

Fig. 6.8 **(a)** Myringotomy with aspiration of middle ear fluid and **(b)** placement of a pressure equalization tube in the eardrum. (Adapted from Hughes [1985], with permission.)

sary so that residual hearing impairments or changes in hearing over time can be identified and addressed. Notice that the first two activities address medical concerns and the status of the PE tube. The third directly addresses the patient's auditory status.

Surgery for more severe cases of otitis media and mastoiditis is less common than in the past when antibiotics were unavailable. However, surgery is still necessary for chronic conditions, when antibiotics are not fully effective, and when the infection becomes sufficiently severe, such as when it invades bone tissue. Cholesteatomas must always be removed unless the patient has general medical/surgical contraindications for surgery. Usage varies, but the term **mastoidectomy** generally describes the surgical removal of disease, and **tympanoplasty** often refers to the surgical reconstruction of the eardrum and middle ear structures. The two may be done in one combined procedure, or surgical reconstruction may be attempted at a later time, after the disease has been alleviated. A **radical mastoidectomy** is done when the disease is so widespread, severe, or aggressive that the surgeon must remove much or all of the mastoid along with the entire contents of the middle ear. As expected from the description of what is removed, a radical mastoidectomy leaves the patient with a structural defect called a mastoidectomy cavity and a very large conductive hearing loss. Thus, it is important for the patient to understand that the purpose of this kind of surgery is to preserve life rather than to address a hearing loss.

A **modified radical mastoidectomy** involves the surgical removal of the pathological tissue and alleviation of the disease process without sacrificing the eardrum and ossicles. An optimal result does not necessarily worsen the hearing loss, and might even improve hearing to some extent by removing a lesion that interferes with sound transmission or by being done in combination with a tympanoplasty. This approach is often used when there is a cholesteatoma in locations such as the attic or antrum. A **simple mastoidectomy** removes diseased tissue in the mastoid without "breaking through" the posterior canal wall (which would constitute a modified radical mastoidectomy). Surgery to reconstruct the sound transmission system and restore hearing is covered later in this chapter.

Otosclerosis

Otosclerosis is a disease of the temporal bone in which normal bone is progressively resorbed and replaced with *spongy* bone that may harden to become sclerotic. Many authorities prefer to call the disorder **otospongiosis** because of the spongy nature of the otosclerotic deposits. Otosclerosis develops at isolated locations and usually affects the oval window and stapedial footplate **(stapedial otosclerosis)**. Otoscerlosis is usually bilateral, but often progresses at different rates for the two ears. **Clinical otosclerosis** exists when the patient begins to experience a hearing problem due to the disorder. This occurs because the otosclerotic material interferes with the normal motion of the stapedial footplate at the oval window, eventually resulting in complete **ankylosis** or **fixation** (Fig. 6.9). The progressive and eventually complete impediment of the ossicular chain's ability to effectively transmit signals to the cochlea produces a progressive conductive hearing loss. **Cochlear otosclerosis** may occur in advanced cases, in which case the disease process encroaches upon the inner ear, adding a sensorineural component to the hearing loss. Stapedial fixation that occurs in association with fragile, easily fractured bones (**osteogenesis imperfecta tarda**) and a bluish tint to the whites of the eyes (**blue sclerae**) is known as **van der Hoeve's syndrome**, and may be related to otosclerosis.

Patients with otosclerosis usually complain about a slowly progressive *hearing loss* that is frequently accompanied by *tinnitus,* and they often typify the characteristics of conductive losses that were outlined earlier in the chapter. Assuming that otosclerosis is the only problem, these patients generally have no other otologic or related complaints and are otoscopically normal. However, it is sometimes possible to see a reddish/pinkish coloration of the cochlear promontory through the eardrum called **Schwartze's sign**, which is due to vascularization associated with active otosclerosis. Several generalities about otosclerosis can be helpful when assessing a patient's case history: (1) Otosclerosis tends to run in families; (2) it typically begins to show up clinically during the second to fourth decades of life; (4) it is

about twice as common in women than in men; and (4) progression is often noticed in association with hormonally active periods like pregnancy and menopause. These characteristics reveal that otosclerosis has hereditary as well as nonhereditary components, and it is noteworthy that it has been linked to at least eight genetic sites (Tomek, Brown, Mani, et al 1998; Chen Campbell, Green, et al 2002; Van Den Bogaert, De Leenheer, Chen, et al 2004; Brownstein, Goldfarb, Levi, et al 2006; Thys, Van Den Bogaert, Iliadou, et al 2007; Schrauwen, Weegerink, Fransen, et al 2011).

The audiological picture of otosclerosis involves a conductive hearing loss in the affected ear(s). The size of the loss depends on the degree of progression of the disease at the time of testing and can be anywhere from mild to as severe as 65 to 70 dB HL. The loss tends to be somewhat worse in the lower frequencies, at least initially (**Fig. 6.10a**), and becomes flatter as the loss progresses. In addition, there is often an elevation of the bone-conduction threshold at 2000 Hz, called **Carhart's notch** (Carhart 1950). However, this does not reflect a true sensorineural component of the disorder. Instead, Carhart's notch is thought to occur because the mechanical advantage provided by the 2000 Hz resonance of the ossicular chain is altered by the ankylosis, which prevents the ossicles from vibrating normally. Moreover, it can be alleviated by surgery that restores normal ossicular chain vibration. This should not be altogether surprising. Recall from Chapter 5 that it is not unusual for conductive impairments to affect bone-conduction thresholds. In more advanced cases the

anterior

posterior

Fig. 6.9   Left panel: Otosclerotic involvement affecting various parts of the stapedial footplate (**a–d**) as well as complete obliteration of the oval window (**e**). Right panel: Otosclerosis fixating the stapes in the oval window. (Adapted from Hughes [1985], with permission.)

presence of cochlear otosclerosis will add a sensori-neural component to the conductive loss produced by stapedial otosclerosis, resulting in a mixed loss (**Fig. 6.10b**). The typical acoustic immittance characteristics of otosclerosis include essentially normal tympanometric peak pressure, abnormally low static acoustic admittance, and absent acoustic reflexes.

Surgery is often considered the treatment of choice for otosclerosis that produces a clinically significant hearing impairment because it is the only available means to ameliorate the conductive loss. Hearing aids are a viable alternative, particularly when surgery is not indicated, but of course cannot reverse the loss or arrest its progression. Shambaugh and Causse (1974) found that medical treatment with sodium fluoride was successful in arresting the progression of otosclerosis in 80% of 4000 patients, but yielded some degree of improvement in only 3%. A "good candidate" for otosclerosis surgery should

be medically appropriate for elective surgery and the risks it entails, and should have a substantial conductive hearing loss (air-bone-gap), normal or near-normal bone-conduction thresholds, and a relatively good speech recognition score for the ear in question. The latter two criteria are sometimes referred to as good **"cochlear reserve."**

Surgery to Improve/Restore Hearing

Otosclerosis Surgery

The three general types of operations that have been used to improve hearing in cases of otosclerosis are fenestration (Lempert 1938), stapes mobilization (Rosen 1953), and stapedectomy (Shea 1958). **Fenestration** completely bypasses the fixated stapes and was a popular operation for otosclerosis for

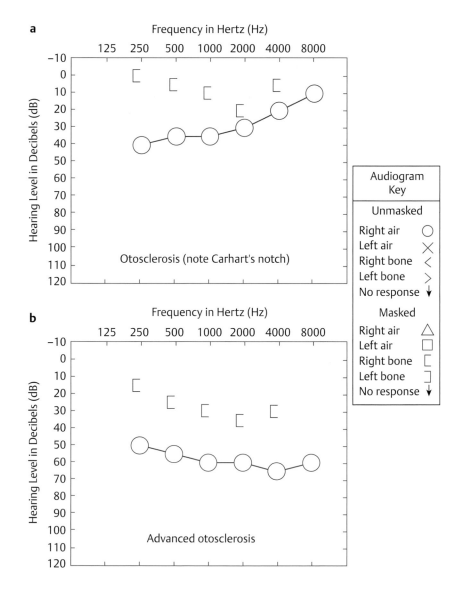

Fig. 6.10 **(a)** Otosclerosis with Carhart's notch. **(b)** Mixed hearing loss due to advanced cochlear and stapedial otosclerosis. (Opposite ears not shown for clarity.)

quite some time. The incus and most of the malleus are excised. The unusable oval window is replaced by a new window (*fenestra*) that is drilled into the lateral semicircular canal and covered with a soft tissue flap derived from the tympanic membrane. The new fenestra enables sound to be transmitted to the cochlea by taking advantage of the shared perilymph system of the hearing and balance parts of the inner ear, provided that the round window is still compliant. Fenestrations successfully reduce the size of large conductive losses to ~ 25 to 30 dB, but do not completely eliminate air-bone-gaps because they do not restore the middle ear transformer mechanism.

Stapes mobilization directly addresses the fixated stapes by palpating the incus, incudostapedial joint, and/or stapes until the footplate essentially breaks free of its fixation by the otosclerotic growth and is again mobilized in the oval window. Compared with fenestration, the surgery involved in stapes mobilization is far less extensive and invasive, and has fewer complications. It also effectively reestablishes the normal physiologic activity of the ossicular chain. However, refixation of the stapes often occurs over time, which of course comes with recurrence of the hearing loss.

Stapes mobilizations and fenestrations have been almost completely replaced by the **stapedectomy** operation and its variations. A total stapedectomy involves removing the ankylosed stapes and footplate, and sealing the oval window with a connective tissue or vein graft, or some other suitable material. The stapes is then replaced with a **prosthesis** that connects the incus to the oval window, and thus reestablishes the ability of the ossicular chain to transmit signals to the cochlea via the normal route. The prosthesis itself may be a wire, strut, or piston made of a synthetic material, metal, cartilage, etc. The procedure is illustrated in **Fig. 6.11a,b**. A **partial stapedectomy** may be done if only the anterior aspect of the stapes is fixated (the most common site). It involves removing only the anterior footplate and anterior crus, leaving the posterior crus to transmit signals to the cochlea. **Stapedotomy** (Fisch 1980; Lesinski 1989) is a modification of the stapedectomy in which the fixated stapedial footplate is left in the oval window. A hole (fenestra) is then bored through the footplate using either a drill or a laser. One end of a piston prosthesis is then inserted into the fenestra and the other end is attached to the incus, completing the connection between the oval window and the ossicular chain (**Fig. 6.11c,d**). Assuming a normal cochlea, stapedectomies tend to result in normal or near-normal hearing in ~ 80 to 90% of cases, with a 1 to 3% risk of deafness. Stapedotomy outcomes appear

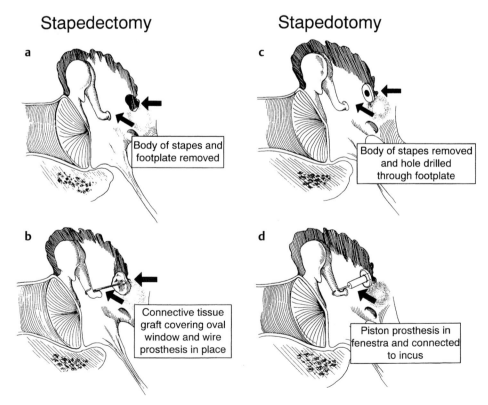

Stapedectomy

a

Body of stapes and footplate removed

b

Connective tissue graft covering oval window and wire prosthesis in place

Stapedotomy

c

Body of stapes removed and hole drilled through footplate

d

Piston prosthesis in fenestra and connected to incus

Fig. 6.11   Stapedectomy **(a,b)** and stapedotomy **(c,d)** procedures for otosclerosis. (Adapted from Hughes [1985], with permission.)

to be at least comparable to those obtained by stapedectomy (McGee 1981; Levy, Shvero, & Hadar 1990). Success rates are low and complication rates are higher for revision stapedectomies, that is, when an ear is operated on again due to progression of the otosclerosis or complications. When surgery is planned for both ears it is desirable to operate on one ear first (the poorer one if there is a difference) and to defer the second procedure for at least several months to ensure that the initial result has been successful and that no delayed complications have arisen.

Tympanoplasty

Structural defects of the conductive system may be the result of a congenital anomaly, injury, or disease. The surgical repair and reconstruction of the tympanic membrane and/or middle ear is known as a **tympanoplasty**, and is intended to resolve (or at least minimize) the conductive hearing loss due to structural deficits. These procedures may be done along with operations used to eradicate the ear disease (e.g., mastoidectomy) or at a later time, depending on what is medically and surgically appropriate.

Traditional tympanoplasty procedures are classified by type from I to V. We will outline the traditional classifications, but one should be aware that quite a few classification systems have been proposed (e.g., Farrior 1968; Bellucci 1973; Kley 1982; Wullstein & Wullstein 1990; Tos 1993). According to the classical approach, a simple perforated eardrum is repaired with a *type I tympanoplasty* or **myringoplasty**, which typically results in normal or near-normal hearing. It involves patching the eardrum defect with a graft made of various materials, such as muscle facie, perichondrium, and homografts (transplanted material). Types II to IV are used when there is an ossicular discontinuity, provided that the remaining segments of the ossicular chain leading to the oval window are mobile so that they can transmit vibrations to the cochlea. Depending on what is missing, the eardrum graft may be attached to the incus (*type II*), head of the stapes (*type III*), or even the stapes footplate (*type IV*). The *type V* tympanoplasty is used when the stapes footplate is fixated rather than mobile. In the traditional procedure (*type Va*) the fixated footplate is ignored, and a new window (fenestra) is drilled into the horizontal semicircular canal, to which the eardrum graft is connected. Sizable air-bone-gaps can remain after these procedures because they do not fully restore the middle ear transformer mechanism (especially in types IV and V). The traditional approaches have largely been superseded by ossicular reconstruction methods that bridge the gap in the ossicular chain with a bone or cartilage graft, or by

substituting the missing structures with a homograft or a prosthesis. The traditional type Va tympanoplasty has largely been replaced by the *type Vb* procedure, which uses a prosthesis to bridge the missing ossicles and to transmit signals to the oval window, as in the stapedectomy operation for otosclerosis.

Growths and Tumors

Benign and malignant tumors can occur anywhere in the temporal bone, including the tympanum, although middle ear tumors are relatively rare. **Glomus tumors** (paragangliomas or chemodectomas) are particularly relevant audiologically (Woods, Strasnick, & Jackson 1993; Baguley, Irving, Hardy, et al 1994). Glomus tumors are highly vascular tumors that arise from glomus bodies (which serve as chemoreceptors) that are associated with branches of the glossopharyngeal and vagus (ninth and tenth cranial) nerves that course through the temporal bone, as well as elsewhere in the body. They are called **glomus tympanicum tumors** when they develop within the middle ear cavity and **glomus jugulare tumors** when they develop from the crest of the jugular bulb under the floor of the middle ear. Glomus tumors invade the middle ear and other parts of the temporal bone, and can also extend intracranially. They are usually unilateral and are more common in women than in men by a ratio of roughly 3 to 1. The most common characteristics of patients with glomus tumors are pulsing tinnitus that is synchronized to the patient's vascular pulse and a conductive or mixed hearing loss, which is unilateral in a wide majority of cases. Bleeding from the ear occurs in some cases, and patients may also experience a feeling of pressure in the ear. Other complaints may also occur but are highly variable. Glomus tumors are usually seen as a reddish mass behind the tympanic membrane, often with a "rising sun" appearance; one might also see it pulsating, and possibly causing the eardrum to bulge. Glomus tumors are treated surgically.

■ Cochlear Disorders

Noise-Induced Hearing Loss

High sound levels can produce both temporary and permanent hearing losses due to overstimulation and/or mechanical trauma (Miller 1974; Schmiedt 1984; Henderson & Hamernik 1986; Saunders, Dear, & Schneider 1985; Boettcher, Henderson, Gratton, et al 1987; Clark 1991; Hamernik & Hsueh 1991;

Hamernik, Ahroon, & Hsueh 1991; Melnick 1991; Saunders, Cohen, & Szymko 1991; Ward 1991). A sensorineural hearing loss produced by the damaging effects of overstimulation by high sound levels, usually over a long period of time, is called a **noise-induced hearing loss.** In contrast, the term **acoustic trauma** usually refers to the hearing loss produced by extremely intense and impulsive sounds like explosions or gunshots. They can mechanically traumatize the eardrum, middle ear, and/or cochlear structures in addition to producing damage by overstimulation, and often from a single insult.

Almost everybody has experienced temporary hearing difficulty (often with tinnitus) after being exposed to high sound levels of one kind or another, such as loud music, construction noise, lawn mowers, subways, etc. This short-term decrease in hearing sensitivity is sensorineural in nature and is called a **temporary threshold shift (TTS)**. In general, a TTS can be produced by sound levels greater than ~ 80 dB sound pressure level (SPL). As the intensity and/or duration of the offending sound increases, the size of the TTS gets bigger and the time it takes for recovery gets longer. A **permanent threshold shift (PTS)** exists when the TTS does not recover completely, that is, when hearing sensitivity does not return to normal. Because PTS could refer to just about any permanent hearing loss, we generally lengthen the term to **noise-induced permanent threshold shift (NIPTS)** for clarity. The nature and severity of a NIPTS is determined by the intensity, spectrum, duration, and time course of the offending sounds; the overall duration of the exposures over the years; and the patient's individual susceptibility to the effects of noise. In addition, the amount of hearing loss produced by noise exposure is exacerbated if vibration is also present, and by the use of potentially ototoxic drugs.

The kinds of anatomical and physiological abnormalities caused by noise exposure range from the most subtle disruptions of hair cell metabolic activities and losses of stereocilia rigidity (leading to "floppy cilia") to the complete degeneration of the organ of Corti and the auditory nerve supply. Both outer and inner hair cells are damaged by noise, but outer hair cells are more susceptible. Some of the abnormalities include metabolic exhaustion of the hair cells, structural changes and degeneration of structures within the hair cells, morphological changes of the cilia (so that they become fused and otherwise distorted), ruptures of cell membranes, and complete degeneration and loss of hair cells, neural cells, and supporting cells. Mild metabolic disruptions and floppy cilia can be reversible, and are thought to be related to TTS. It should be noted in this context that oxidative stress associated with accumulations of free radicals has been identified as

a factor in noise-induced hearing loss (Henderson, Bielefeld, Harris, & Hu 2006).[6] Greater amounts of interference and damage are associated with permanent hearing losses.

Unfortunately, noise exposures capable of producing *temporary* hearing loss can also cause *permanent* neural degeneration. Specifically, Kujawa and Liberman (2009) demonstrated that noise exposures that produced a 40 dB TTS quickly resulted in a loss of synaptic terminals followed by a delayed and permanent degeneration of the auditory nerve cells even though the TTS was completely resolved and there was no loss of hair cells.

Noise-induced impairments are usually associated with a notch-shaped high-frequency sensorineural loss that is worst at 4000 Hz (**Fig. 6.12**), although the notch often occurs at 3000 or 6000 Hz as well. The reason for the notch in this region is not definitively established. One explanation is that this region is most susceptible to damage due to the biology and mechanics of the cochlea. Another rationale is that commonly encountered noises have broad spectra that reach the cochlea with a boost in the 2000 to 4000 Hz region because of the resonance characteristics of the outer and middle ear. Noise-induced losses tend to be bilateral and more or less symmetrical; however, there are many exceptions, especially when one ear has been subjected to more noise than the other.

Not all "noise-induced" audiograms conform to the idealized picture in **Fig. 6.12**. Analyses of the progression of noise-induced hearing losses across many studies have revealed that the general audiometric pattern of noise-induced hearing loss evolves as noise exposure continues over the course of many years (Passchier-Vermeer 1974; Rösler 1994). The hearing loss typically begins as a notch at 4000 Hz. As noise exposure continues, the notch widens to include a wider range of frequencies, but continues to progress most noticeably at 4000 Hz. After perhaps 10 to 15 years of exposure, the progression of the loss at 4000 Hz often slows down, and progression now becomes more apparent at other frequencies, such as 2000 Hz.

Meniere's Disease

Meniere's disease or **syndrome (endolymphatic hydrops)** is an inner ear disease attributed to excessive endolymphatic fluid pressure in the mem-

---

[6] Free radicals also have been implicated in ototoxicity (e.g., Priuska & Schacht 1995; Rybak, Whitworth, Mukherjea, & Ramkumar 2007) and presbycusis (e.g., Jiang, Talaska, Schacht, & Sha 2007).

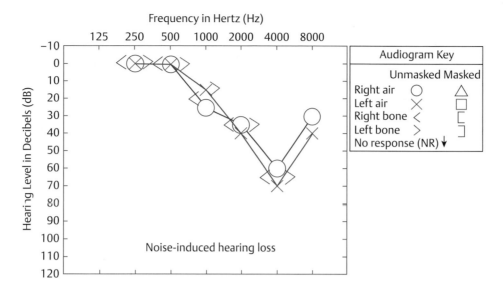

Fig. 6.12 The audiogram of a patient with a bilateral sensorineural hearing loss due to noise exposure.

branous labyrinth, causing Reissner's membrane to become distended. Many causes have been proposed, and it is generally thought to be associated with problems regulating the production of endolymph or a blockage of the endolympathic duct and sac, but the etiology of Meniere's disease is not fully established (Gates 2006; Ghossaini & Wazen 2006). Meniere's disease has been attributed to may different causes, such as food allergies, hypothyroidism, adrenal and pituitary gland insufficiencies, autoimmune disorders, vascular diseases, stenosis of the internal auditory meatus, trauma, syphilis, viral infections, and genetic origins. It is interesting to note here that Klar and colleagues (2006) were able to link Meniere's disease to chromosome 12p in several Swedish families. However, Meniere's disease is often viewed as an idiopathic disorder because precise etiologies are difficult to establish.

Clinically, Meniere's disease is characterized by episodic attacks of (1) vertigo, (2) hearing loss, (3) tinnitus, and (4) a feeling of fullness or pressure in the ear. Attacks last for as little as 20 minutes or as long as several hours. The tinnitus is usually described as roaring or as a low-pitch noise, but this can vary. The vertigo can be extremely severe and debilitating and is the principal problem for most patients. Endolymphatic hydrops commonly produces a low-frequency (rising) sensorineural hearing loss (**Fig. 6.13**), but the loss often extends to include the higher frequencies so that there is often a flat configuration as the disease progresses.

Meniere's disease has also been associated with thresholds that are poorer at the higher and lower frequencies, with relatively better sensitivity at the frequencies between them (Paparella, McDermott, & deSousa 1982; Lee, Paparella, Margolis & Le 1995; Ries, Rickert, & Schlauch 1999). These peak-shaped audiograms can be due to the endolymphatic hydrops itself or to the combination of a low-frequency loss from Meniere's disease with a high-frequency loss from, for example, noise or aging.

The impairment fluctuates because the hearing loss and tinnitus often improve between attacks, and may even resolve between attacks in the early stages of the disease. However, the long-term trend is in the direction of constant hearing loss and tinnitus that worsens during attacks, and it is possible for the loss to eventually become profound.

Two variants of the classical disorder are also recognized. These are identified as **cochlear Meniere's disease** when the symptoms do not include vertigo, and as **vestibular Meniere's disease** when there is no hearing loss. Meniere's disease is unilateral in roughly 70 to 85% of the cases, but the incidence of bilateral cases increases with the duration of the disease, reaching ~ 40% after 15 years (Morrison 1976).

Several treatments are currently available for the treatment of Meniere's disease (Gates 2006; Ghossaini & Wazen 2006; Hamill 2006). Medical treatment generally consists of a low-salt diet, diuretics, and the use of vestibular suppressants and sedatives to control the vertigo. (Corticosteroid injections

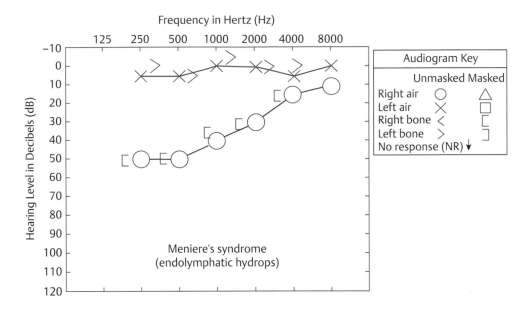

Fig. 6.13 A principally low-frequency sensorineural hearing loss in a patient with Meniere's disease.

into the middle ear have also been tried.) Medical treatment is effective in controlling the vertigo in ~ 70% of patients, but ~ 30% require more invasive approaches, which include both nondestructive and destructive methods.

Nondestructive approaches attempt to control vertigo while preserving hearing. The least aggressive of these invasive approaches uses the *Meniett* device, which directs a series of pressure pulses into the middle ear through a tympanostomy tube in the eardrum. Endolymphatic sac surgery is used to control debilitating vertigo while preserving the patient's hearing. These operations attempt to relieve the hydrops by removing bone to alleviate pressure on the endolymphatic sac (*endolymphatic sac decompression*) or by decompressing the sac and then providing a route for the endolymph to drain into the subarachnoid space or mastoid (*endolymphatic subarachnoid shunt*).

Whether sac surgery works by alleviating the endolymphatic hydrops has been questioned by the recent findings of Chung, Fayad, Linthicum, Ishiyama, and Merchant (2011). They examined the temporal bones of 15 patients who had endolymphatic sac surgery during their lifetimes. They found that only 2 of the patients actually had successfully placed shunts, and neither of them had relief from their vertigo. On the other hand, the sac was either not actually exposed or was not actually reached by the shunt in 13 cases; yet, 8 of them did experience relief from their vertigo. These findings suggest that

although endolymphatic sac surgery does relieve vertigo symptoms in some patients with Meniere's syndrome, it accomplishes this by some unknown mechanism instead of by actually relieving the endolymphatic hydrops itself.

Destructive approaches can also be used to control intractable vertigo. However, destructive techniques are usually reserved for cases where there is no serviceable hearing in the affected ear because they result in deafness. The two surgical approaches involve removing or destroying the diseased labyrinth (*labyrinthectomy*), and cutting the vestibular nerve (*vestibular neurectomy*). Injecting *gentamicin* into the middle ear (typically through the eardrum) is the least invasive destructive approach for controlling debilitating vertigo. Gentamicin is a drug that is toxic to the inner ear and affects the vestibular end organs more than the cochlea. Thus, *gentamicin injections* constitute a "chemical labyrinthectomy." In fact, this may be the treatment of choice for ears without usable hearing, but it can also be used in ears that have serviceable hearing, in which case the chances of causing a hearing loss average ~ 30%.

Ototoxicity

Ototoxicity means damage to the ear due to the toxic effects of various chemical agents, especially drugs. The most ototoxic medications belong to a class of antibiotics called **aminoglycosides**, such as amikacin, dihydrostreptomycin (no longer used), gentamicin, kanamycin, neomycin, netilmicin, streptomycin, and tobramycin. Aminoglycosides are generally administered in cases of very severe or life-threatening infections, and to newborns who are in a state of sepsis. Other kinds of antibiotics can also be ototoxic, such as capreomycin, vancomicin, and even erythromycin. However, the suffix *mycin* does not necessarily mean a drug is ototoxic; for example, clindamycin, Terramycin, and Vibramycin are not ototoxic (although they do involve other adverse reactions). Among the other kinds of ototoxic drugs are cisplatinum, an antineoplastic, and quinine, which was popular in the treatment of malaria. Salicylates (aspirin) are ototoxic in large doses, but the hearing loss is usually reversible.

Loop diuretics such as bumetanide (Bumex), ethacrynic acid (Edecrin), and furosemide (Lasix) are also ototoxic, although the effect can be reversible. Diuretics are commonly used in the treatment of congestive heart disease and other edematous disorders. In addition, sudden hearing loss has occurred in some patients using sildenafil (Viagra), tadafil (Cialis), and vardenafil (Livitr) for erectile dysfunction, and sildenafil (Revatio) for pulmonary arterial hypertension (FDA 2007).

It is not yet clear whether the anti-retroviral drugs used to treat human immunodeficiency virus (HIV) have ototoxic effects. Some studies have reported an association between hearing loss and some of these agents, such as human immunodeficiency virus (HIV) (Marra et al 1997; Vieira, Greco, Teóphyllo & Gonçalves 2008). However, this association was not found in a prospective study involving 32 weeks of treatment with anti-retroviral drugs (Schouten, Lockhart, Rees, Collier, & Marra 2006).

Typical ototoxic chemicals include heavy metals (such as lead and mercury, and probably germanium and tin compounds, as well), tetrachlorocarbon and sulfur compounds, organic phosphates and solvents (such as styrene and toluene), and carbon monoxide, among others. Toxicity from agents such as these also affects other body organs, and exposures to one or more of them are possible in several industries and in homes (see, e.g., Fuente & McPherson 2006; Campo, Maguin, Gabriel et al 2009; Nies 2012).

Most ototoxic drugs affect both the cochlear and vestibular parts of the inner ear. However, some are relatively more cochleotoxic (e.g., neomycin) and others are more vestibulotoxic (e.g., streptomycin). Ototoxic drugs cause hearing losses by affecting the cochlear hair cells and the stria vascularis. The outer hair cells are usually affected before the inner hair cells, and damage usually begins in the basal part of the cochlea. As a result, the hearing loss usually begins in the high frequencies and then proceeds to include successively lower frequencies. The hearing loss is usually bilateral, but can be unilateral as well. Tinnitus usually accompanies or precedes the hearing loss, but not always. Vestibulotoxicity can produce symptoms such as vertigo, general unsteadiness or disequilibrium, and/or ataxia. Most ototoxic effects occur during or soon after administration, but hearing losses due to aminoglycoside ototoxicity can develop or continue for many months after treatment has ended, depending on the drug.

The major factors affecting the risk of ototoxicity include dosage, duration of treatment, the adequacy of the patient's renal (kidney) functioning, and whether other potentially ototoxic agents are also being used. The ototoxic effects of aminoglycosides are substantially greater when the patient is also receiving diuretics. Ototoxic drugs also interact with noise to produce greater amounts of hearing loss (e.g., Boettcher, Henderson, Gratton, Danielson, & Byrne 1987). A further complication is that many ototoxic drugs are also toxic to the kidneys.

To minimize the risk of hearing loss, it is important to closely monitor those patients receiving ototoxic drugs for renal functioning, drug levels in their blood, and hearing status throughout the treatment period. A baseline audiological evaluation should be obtained as soon as possible, although the degree of illness often makes a preadministration baseline unrealistic. It is important to keep in mind that the decision to use ototoxic medications depends on the nature and severity of the patient's illness, and that it is sometimes necessary to continue their use even if a hearing loss develops. Because of the risk of delayed onset and/or progression of hearing loss, periodic audiological monitoring should continue for quite some time after treatment is over.

Perilymphatic Fistulas

A **perilymphatic fistula** is a leak of perilymph from a rupture of the oval and/or round window, and is a common cause of sudden hearing loss. The fistula itself can be quite small and even microscopic. Oval and round window fistulas can result from explosions, barotrauma, and increased intracranial pressure due to straining or physical exertion, sneezing, coughing, Valsalva maneuvers, and other precipitating events. Fistulas may also be the result of bone erosion due to a cholesteatoma or infection, and of untoward outcomes of stapes surgery.

The **fistula test** is usually administered to a patient who is suspected of having a perilymphatic fistula. Air is pumped into the ear canal by squeezing the bulb of a Siegel (pneumatic) otoscope or using the pressure pump of an acoustic immittance device

(Chapter 7). The positive pressure is expected to cause a considerable amount of vertigo and nystagmus if the patient has a perilymphatic fistula. Here is why: The air pressure causes an inward displacement of the tympanic membrane that is transmitted to the stapes footplate, which in turn presses in on the perilymph. There will be an abnormally large amount of fluid displacement because the fistula acts like an open valve. The excessive fluid displacement overstimulates the receptors in the semicircular canals, resulting in vertigo and nystagmus. Positive outcomes are highly suggestive of a fistula. However, false negative outcomes occur in about half the cases (e.g., Goodhill 1981), so that a negative test result does not rule out a fistula.

Once a perilymphatic fistula is diagnosed, the otologist might choose to treat it conservatively, or to perform a surgical exploration of the middle ear (tympanotomy) to find and repair the fistula. The conservative approach might include bed rest with the head elevated and avoidance of straining. The surgical repair of a fistula involves patching it with materials such as perichondrium, a vein graft, or fat. Successful surgery can arrest the progression of hearing loss or even improve hearing to some extent if performed soon enough.

Superior Canal Dehiscence

Superior canal dehiscence (SCD) is an inner ear disorder in which a section of the bone enclosing the superior semicircular canal is open or extremely thin, resulting in vestibular and or auditory symptoms that are caused by sound and/or pressure (e.g., Minor, Solomon, Zinreich, & Zee 1998; Minor 2000, 2005; Brantberg et al 2001; Belden, Weg, Minor, & Zinreich 2003; Cox, Lee, Carey, & Minor 2003; Banerjee, Whyte, & Atlas 2005; Zhou, Gopen, & Poe 2007; Merchant & Rosowski 2008). To understand why this happens, recall that the labyrinth has compliant locations at the round window and to a lesser extent at the oval window. The open or very thin bone in the superior semicircular canal provides another compliant location. This abnormal "third window" makes it possible for sound and/or pressure to displace the inner ear fluids, which in turn precipitates the vestibular and auditory symptoms.

The vestibular problems are the most disturbing symptoms of SCD. They include episodes of vertigo, nystagmus, and oscillopsia (an oscillating visual field) that are induced by sound and/or pressure events like nose blowing, straining to lift heavy objects, flying, etc. (Vertigo and nystagmus caused by pressure in the ear canal is called the *Hennebert sign*, and the *Tullio effect* when it is due to sound stimula-

tion.) In addition, patients often experience ongoing problems with imbalance or unsteadiness as well tolerating motion.

The hearing loss typically associated with superior canal dehiscence is *conductive* in nature with air-bone-gaps in the low to mid-frequencies, but other kinds of hearing loss are possible and sensorineural losses have also been reported. The air-bone-gaps involved in SCD often include better-than-expected bone-conduction thresholds (sometimes called *conductive hyperacousis*) in addition to elevated air-conduction thresholds. In addition, a notable feature of SCD is the tendency for there to be normal tympanograms and present acoustic reflexes in spite of the air-bone-gap. This contrasts with the abnormal admittance findings associated with disorders of the conductive system, as we shall see in Chapter 7. Pulsatile tinnitus and the hyper-perception of the sounds produced by one's own body (*autophony*) are also common.

A diagnosis of SCD is confirmed with computerized tomography (CT). Treatment options range from counseling patients about avoiding stimuli that trigger the symptoms in milder cases to surgically repairing the canal in severe cases, such as when the symptoms are debilitating.

■ Retrochochlear Disorders

Retrocochlear disorders involve the structures that are medial to the cochlea. In the broadest sense, this includes any problem that involves the vestibuloacoustic (eighth cranial) nerve or any part of the central auditory nervous system. In practice, however, **retrocochlear** usually refers to a disorder involving the **eighth cranial nerve** and/or the **cerebellopontine angle (CPA)**. Disorders are generally classified as **central** when the abnormality is in the central nervous system. Particularly when dealing with brainstem disorders, the term **extra-axial** is often used to describe a lesion that is located *outside* the brainstem (e.g., a CPA tumor that is pressing on the brainstem from without), and the term **intra-axial** is used when the lesion is actually *inside* the brainstem itself.

Eighth Cranial Nerve and Cerebellopontine Angle Tumors

Tumors affecting the eighth cranial are often referred to as **eighth nerve tumors, acoustic neuromas, acoustic neurilemomas, acoustic neurinomas,** and **acoustic tumors.** However, the technically preferred term is **vestibular schwannomas** because most eighth cranial nerve tumors actually involve the Schwann cells of the vestibular division of the nerve rather than its auditory branch (NIH 1991). Almost everybody uses these terms interchangeably (as we will in this text), but it is important to remember that the primary site is usually the vestibular branch of the nerve.

Vestibular schwannomas are relatively uncommon, with modern prevalence estimates ranging from as low as ~ 0.001% (Tos, Stangerup, Cayé-Thomasen, Tos, & Thomsen 2004) to between roughly 0.02% (Lin, Hegarty, Fischbein, & Jackler 2005) and 0.07% (Anderson, Loevner, Bigelow, & Mirza 2000). They can occur anywhere along the eighth nerve, either within the internal auditory meatus or medial to it in the cerebellopontine angle. The great majority of them are unilateral. However, ~ 5% of them are bilateral and are associated with a genetic syndrome called **neurofibromatosis type 2**. Acoustic tumors located in (or expanding into) the CPA are also called cerebellopontine angle or posterior fossa tumors. Acoustic tumors inside the internal auditory meatus erode the bony walls of the canal as they grow, and often expand medially into the CPA because this is the road of least resistance. The eighth nerve is compressed, deformed, and displaced by the growing tumor. Pressure from the tumor can also interfere with the blood supply to the cochlea, which is probably why many "retrocochlear patients" have "cochlear findings" such as loudness recruitment. As tumor size increases, pressure can also be exerted on other cranial nerves, especially the facial (seventh) and trigeminal (fifth), and can even displace the brainstem. As a result, vestibular schwannomas can produce extensive and even life-threatening consequences even though they are benign and usually slow growing. In addition to vestibular schwannomas, other kinds of space-occupying lesions of the CPA are also encountered, such as neurilemomas, meningiomas, and cholesteatomas.

The presenting complaints of patients with eighth nerve tumors vary widely, depending largely on the size and location of the lesion. Even though impressive neurological complaints are mentioned in the traditional literature, these are no longer as common because retrocochlear lesions now tend to be identified before tumors grow large enough for many of these symptoms to occur. The most common complaint is a hearing disturbance in one ear. It is usually slowly progressive but can be sudden. Other complaints include tinnitus, dizziness and/ or imbalance, facial numbness, gait disturbances, and headaches. It might seem odd that hearing disturbances are the preponderant complaint when most eighth-nerve tumors originate on the vestibular branch. The most likely reason is that the slowly developing vestibular problem is offset by central compensation. The majority of these patients have at least some degree of high-frequency loss, but their audiograms vary greatly, so that any audiometric configuration is possible, varying from normal thresholds to profound sensorineural hearing losses (e.g., Johnson 1977; Matthies & Samii 1997; Gimsing 2010; Suzuki, Hashimoto, Kano, & Okitsu 2010). The retrocochlear indications of audiological tests are covered in Chapters 8, 10, and 11, but the importance of physiological tests such as the auditory brainstem response and acoustic reflexes should be highlighted. The diagnosis of acoustic tumors and related lesions depends on the use of radiological techniques, and magnetic resonance imaging (MRI) with gadolinium enhancement is accepted as the "definitive" test.

The traditional treatment for acoustic tumors is surgical removal. The tumor may be approached surgically by three general routes, as shown by the arrows in **Fig. 6.14**. The *suboccipital* or *retrosigmoid* route can be used for both large and small lesions and is the major neurosurgical approach for acoustic tumor surgery. The *middle fossa* approach is usable for small tumors. These approaches make it possible for the patient's hearing to be preserved (at least for many small tumors) because they do not involve dissecting the inner ear structures. The *translabyrinthine* route is the otologic approach to the acoustic tumor by dissection through the temporal bone. By approaching the tumor laterally via the temporal bone, the translabyrinthine approach avoids manipulating brain tissue and also allows the surgeon to identify and protect the integrity of the seventh cranial (facial) nerve. On the other hand, it results in deafness on the operated side because the route to the tumor involves drilling through the labyrinth. Combined neurologic-otologic approaches are also used.

Radiological techniques such as *stereotactic radiosurgery* (using gamma knife or linear accelerator technologies) provide another treatment option available for patients who cannot or will not have traditional surgery. Although disagreements exist, considerable experience is accumulating on the use of radiosurgery as a treatment for acoustic tumors (e.g., Perks, St. George, El Hamri, Blackburn, & Plowman 2003; Hasegawa et al 2005; Likhterov, Allbright, & Selesnick 2007; Mathieu, Kondziolka, Flickinger, et al 2007).

The treatment choice for acoustic tumor must consider whether the patient has usable preoperative hearing in the pathological ear, as well as the size and location of the tumor, and general medical/ surgical issues. The hearing ability of the opposite ear must also be considered in eighth-nerve tumor management. For example, using a technique that is more likely to preserve hearing becomes a major consideration when the patient already has a significant hearing impairment in the opposite ear.

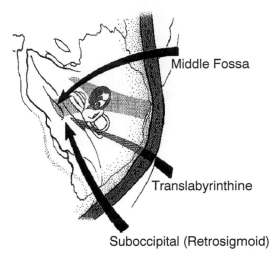

Middle Fossa

Translabyrinthine

Suboccipital (Retrosigmoid)

Fig. 6.14 The three arrows show the major approaches used in acoustic tumor surgery. (Adapted from Buckingham et al [1989], with permission.)

Neurofibromatosis

Bilateral acoustic tumors are commonly associated with a hereditary disease known as neurofibromatosis. However, neurofibromatosis actually refers to two different disorders that have different characteristics and genetic origins (NIH 1991; Pikus 1995). **Neurofibromatosis type 1 (NF1)**, or **von Recklinghausen's disease**, is an autosomal dominant syndrome associated with chromosome 17. Individuals with NF1 typically have neurofibromas involving the skin, CNS tumors, skeletal deformities including macrocephaly, visual system disorders, and characteristic *café-au-lait* spots (coffee-with-milk colored blotches). These stigmata are observed in early childhood and increase with age.

Neurofibromatosis type 2 (NF2) is an autosomal dominant syndrome associated with chromosome 22. It is characterized by *bilateral* eighth nerve tumors, and the possibility of other tumors of the brain and/or spinal cord, but not the dramatic outward characteristics of NF1. Thus, bilateral eighth-nerve tumors are virtually the hallmark of neurofibromatosis type 2, but are rare in type 1. This important distinction is missed by the old notion that von Recklinghausen's disease was a singular, unified syndrome, which permeates the traditional literature. Diagnostic criteria for NF1 and NF2 (NIH 1991) are enumerated in **Table 6.2** for ready reference.

Table 6.2 Diagnostic criteria for neurofibromatosis type 1 (NF1) and neurofibromatosis type 2 (NF2) based on NIH (1991)

NF1 is revealed by the presence of ≥ 2 of the following characteristics:
≥ 6 café-au-lait spots that are
> 5 mm in diameter before puberty
> 15 mm in diameter after puberty
≥ 2 neurofibromas of any type, even 1 plexiform fibroma
Freckling in the axillary (armpit) region or inguinal (groin) region
Optic glioma
≥ 2 Lisch nodules (pigmented iris hamartomas)
Having a parent/sibling/child with NF1 (based on the above criteria)
NF2 is revealed by the presence of any of the following characteristics:
– Bilateral eighth-nerve tumors
– Having a parent/sibling/child with NF2 *and either* a unilateral eighth-nerve tumor
or any one of the following:
– Neurofibroma
– Meningioma
– Glioma
– Schwannoma
– Posterior capsular cataract or opacity at any early age

Other Retrocochlear Disorders

Although the issue of retrocochlear pathology usually focuses on eighth nerve and cerebellopontine angle tumors of one type or the other, these are certainly not the only kinds of retrocochlear disorders. For example, as mentioned earlier, hair cell destruction (a cochlear lesion) leads to the retrograde degeneration of auditory nerve fibers (a retrocochlear lesion), and this effect can be quite extensive when the cochlear impairment is severe or profound. Neural presbycusis is a form of age-associated hearing impairment characterized by a loss of auditory neurons. Bone pathologies such as Paget's disease and temporal bone tumors can interfere with the eighth nerve. The eighth nerve can also be compressed by a vascular loop of the anterior inferior cerebellar artery. Neural degeneration or viral infection of the vestibular branch of the eighth nerve can produce acute or chronic vertigo, nausea, and vomiting, known as **vestibular neuronitis**. The eighth nerve can also be affected by such diverse diseases as multiple sclerosis and syphilis.

Auditory Neuropathy Spectrum Disorder

Auditory neuropathy spectrum disorder (ANSD) refers to auditory disorders in which abnormal results are found on physiological tests sensitive to eighth cranial functioning, and normal results are obtained on physiological measures sensitive to outer hair cell functioning. It is also known as **auditory neuropathy** or **auditory dys-synchrony**, but ANSD is the preferred term, largely because it does not always stem from a problem with the auditory nerve itself (Guidelines Development Conference 2008). More specifically, ANSD can be the result of abnormalities of the auditory nerve, the inner hair cells (IHCs), and/or the synapses between the IHCs and the auditory neurons (e.g., Starr, Zeng, & Michalewski 2008). However, the *outer* hair cells are working normally.

Auditory neuropathy spectrum disorder has been described and studied in detail (e.g., Sininger, Hood, Starr, Berlin, & Picton 1995; Starr, Picton, Sininger, Hood, & Berlin 1996; Stein et al 1996; Berlin, Bordelon, & St. John 1998; Berlin, Hood, & Rose 2001; Madden, Rutter, Hilbert, Greinwald, & Choo 2002; Shivashankar, Satishchandra, Shashikala, & Gore 2003; Rance 2005; Rance, McKay, & Grayden 2004; Rance et al 2007; Guidelines Development Conference 2008; Starr et al 2008; Berlin, Hood, Morlet, et al 2005, 2010). Patients with ANSD can have sensorineural hearing losses of any degree from quite mild through profound. The hallmark of the disorder is the combination of very *abnormal or absent auditory brainstem responses (ABR)* along with *normally functioning outer hair cells* shown by *normal otoacoustic emissions* and/or *cochlear microphonics*. In addition, acoustic reflexes are elevated or absent in patients with ANSD, and they fail to have efferent suppression of their otoacoustic emissions. The majority of ANSD cases are binaural, but unilateral ANSD also occurs. The speech recognition ability of ANSD patients is impaired for listening in noise, but may or may not be affected in quiet; and their performance on tests of temporal resolution is often impaired.

Auditory neuropathy spectrum disorder occurs in roughly 10% of children with sensorineural hearing impairments (e.g., Rance 2005; Berlin et al 2010; Ching, Scollie, Dillon, et al 2013) and has been identified in as many as 10% of normal newborns and ~ 40% of those in neonatal intensive care units (Rea & Gibson 2003). It has been associated with a host of risk factors, such as prematurity, ototoxic drugs, hyperbilirubinemia, and hypoxia. In addition, ANSD has been linked to genetic etiologies, such as nonsyndromic genetic origins with both autosomal dominant (e.g., Kim et al 2004) and autosomal recessive (e.g., Varga, Avenarius, Kelly, et al 2006) transmission, as well as syndromes involving peripheral neuropathies (Kovach, Campbell, Herman, et al 2002; Postelmans & Stokroos 2006).

Hearing aids and cochlear implants have been used with ANSD patients, in addition, of course, to the very important early intervention efforts addressing speech-language and communication development (Fabry 2000; Sininger & Trautwein 2002; Trautwein, Sininger, & Nelson 2000; Shallop,Peterson, Facer, Fabry, & Driscoll 2001; Madden et al 2002; Peterson, Shallop, Driscoll, et al 2003; Postelmans & Stokroos 2006; Zeng & Liu 2006; Guidelines Development Conference 2008; Berlin et al 2010; Rance, Cone-Wesson, Wundelich, & Dowell 2002; Roush, Frymark, Venediktov, & Wang 2011; Ching et al 2013). Patients with ANSD typically do not benefit from conventional amplification, but hearing aids still should be tried because there are ANSD patients who do benefit from them. Fortunately, many patients with ANSD have benefited from cochlear implantation.

(Central) Auditory Processing Disorders

Disorders of the auditory central nervous system and of auditory perceptual functioning are variously referred to as **central auditory processing disorders** (**CAPD**; e.g., AAA 2010), **auditory processing disorders** (**APD**; e.g., Jerger & Musiek 2000), and **(central) auditory processing disorders** (**(C)APD**; e.g., ASHA 2005). Auditory processing disorders can be caused by a wide variety of factors, such as age-related deterioration, congenital and/or hereditary disorders, degenerative and demyelinating diseases, developmental disorders, chemical or drug-induced problems, head trauma, infections (e.g., encephalitis, meningitis), tumors, kernicterus, metabolic disturbances, vascular diseases, and even surgically induced lesions (e.g., sectioning of the corpus callosum). However, a great many if not most patients with (C)APDs experience auditory perceptual difficulties that are not attributable to identifiable brain lesions or disease processes; and auditory processing deficits also have been associated with chronic middle ear effusion and auditory deprivation. In addition, many (C)APDs coexist with other (comorbid) issues such as speech-language and learning disorders, and attention deficit hyperactivity disorder (ADHD), among many others, especially in children.

Disorders of the central auditory nervous system do not produce a hearing loss per se, because information from each ear is represented very redundantly in both the right and left auditory pathways. Instead, patients with auditory processing disorders typically experience one or more of the following problems with the perceptual processing of auditory information (e.g., Jerger & Musiek 2000; ASHA 2005; AAA 2010): Disturbances of speech perception are often experienced when there is noise, reverberation, or competing signals, as well as when the signal is degraded in some way. There may be impairments of auditory discrimination, pattern recognition, and various binaural processes, such as directional hearing (localization and lateralization), dichotic listening, spatial orientation, masking level differences, and the ability to put together signals that have been presented to the two ears (often described as binaural fusion or resynthesis). Further, there may be problems with aspects of hearing involving the time domain, such as temporal integration, temporal resolution or discrimination, temporal masking, and temporal ordering, among others.

There is considerable ongoing controversy about (C)APD, involving issues at every level from its very definition to its assessment and management.[7] Some of the most prominent points of contention involve comorbid disorders, shared features with other clinical entities, and modality specificity. The comorbidity of (C)APD and other disorders has already been mentioned, and makes it very difficult to separate auditory processing problems and other deficits, such as speech and language impairments or ADHD, especially in children. A related diagnostic challenge is that many of the manifestations of (C)APD are also encountered among patients with language impairments, ADHD, learning disabilities, autistic spectrum disorders, dyslexia, and ANSD, as well as in those with difficulties with memory, attention, and other cognitive functions. Moreover, there is consid-

erable controversy about whether deficits must be limited to the auditory realm (*modality specificity*) as opposed to occurring in other modalities as well (see, e.g., Cacace & McFarland 2005a,b, 2013; Katz & Tillery 2005; Musiek, Bellis, & Chermak 2005; Rosen 2005). The degree to which modality specificity should be addressed and/or tested also varies widely, from considering attention and cognitive problems when auditory test findings disagree, to multidisciplinary assessment, to the use of specially designed testing techniques that compare performance on analogous auditory versus nonauditory (e.g., visual) tasks (see, e.g., AAA 2010; Bellis & Ross 2011; Bellis, Billiet, & Ross 2011; Cacace & McFarland 2013; Weihing, Bellis, Chermak, & Musiek 2013). While a clear consensus is certainly lacking, it is probably fair to say that absolute modality specificity probably is not a viable requirement, so that (C)APD is an appropriate diagnosis when the patient's problems are primarily involved with the processing of auditory material (e.g., ASHA 2005).

It is interesting to note in this context that the term **obscure auditory dysfunction (OAD)** has been used to describe complaints about hearing difficulty, particularly in noisy and other difficult listening situations, in spite of essentially normal hearing thresholds and no disorders that could explain the problem (Saunders & Haggard 1989, 1992; Saunders, Field, & Haggard 1992; Baran & Musiek 1994; Higson, Haggard, & Field 1994). These complaints may reflect one or a combination of disorders of the peripheral ear and/or central auditory system, cognitive dysfunctions, psychosocial factors, changing acoustical environments or communicative demands, linguistic factors, and age-related effects.[8] Disproportionately severe auditory complaints should be assessed to rule out significant pathology and provide for appropriate referrals and counseling. Using an OAD test battery by Saunders and Haggard (1989, 1992), Higson, Haggard, and Field (1994) found performance deficits in 81% of OAD patients, and were able to categorize 73% of the patients on the basis of auditory, cognitive, and/or personality factors.

Aphasia is the general term used to describe a variety of central speech and language disorders resulting from lesions affecting the language-dominant hemisphere of the brain. **Auditory agnosia** is the inability to recognize sound that has been heard, and **verbal agnosia** is the inability to recognize linguistic material, often called **word deafness.** However, pure word deafness in the absence of aphasia

---

[7] Interested students will find several contemporary perspectives on controversial (C)APD issues (e.g., Katz & Tillery 2005; Cacace & McFarland 2005a,b, 2008, 2013; Jerger & Musiek 2000; Musiek, Bellis, & Chermak 2005; Rosen 2005; DeBonis & Moncrieff 2008; Kamhi 2011; Medwetsky 2011; Miller 2011; Moore 2011; Geffner & Ross-Swain 2013; Weihing, Bellis, Chermak, & Musiek 2013).

---

[8] Although Saunders and Haggard (1989) applied the term *OAD* to those who are <55 years old.

is extremely rare. Cases of central deafness resulting from bilateral temporal lobe damage have been reported from time to time (e.g., Landau, Goldstein, & Kleffner 1960; Jerger, Weikers, Sharbrough, & Jerger 1969; Tramo, Bharucha, & Musiek 1990). For an exhaustive coverage of this rare disorder, see the 20-year longitudinal case study by Hood, Berlin, and Allen (1994).

■ Sudden Hearing Loss

Sudden hearing loss means the rapid onset of a hearing loss, which might develop instantaneously, overnight, or over the course of a few days. The hearing loss is usually unilateral, but it can be bilateral, and any degree of severity is possible. It is almost always accompanied by tinnitus, and a feeling of pressure or fullness in the affected ear(s) is also very common; vertigo may or may not be present.

The possible etiologies that must be considered as the cause of sudden hearing loss include a variety of viral infections; various autoimmune disorders; perilymphatic fistula; interference with the cochlear blood supply due to, for example, vascular disease, blood disorders (e.g., sickle cell), embolisms, and vascular spasms; perilymph hypertension; rupturing of Reissner's membrane; Meniere's disease; multiple sclerosis; acoustic tumor and other neoplasms; and others. Recent head trauma, ear surgery, acoustic trauma, and exposure to ototoxic drugs (including sildenafil and similar medications) should not be overlooked. Finally, we cannot forget that impacted cerumen as well as acute Eustachian tube occlusion can also lead to sudden hearing losses. It is true that these conductive disorders are not what we usually have in mind here, but we do not know the cause until after the patient has been seen. No matter what the etiology eventually turns out to be, *a current complaint of sudden hearing loss constitutes a medical emergency.*

The expected course of sudden hearing loss is difficult to project because it depends on the underlying cause of the symptoms. Some of these losses resolve spontaneously. Some cases are responsive to medical or surgical treatment, which may have to be initiated quickly to avert a permanent hearing loss. Others are permanent, and others still may be progressive. The treatment for sudden hearing loss is usually medical, and might consist of corticosteriods, vasodilators, anticoagulants, rebreathing of 95% oxygen/5% carbon dioxide, diuretics, and/or a low-sodium diet, depending on the diagnosis. Outcomes run the gamut from no effect to dramatic improvement. Unfortunately, however, the effectiveness of medical treatments for sudden sensorineural hearing loss (including the use of corticosteroids) has not been confirmed by randomized controlled studies (Kitajiri, Tabuchi, Hiraumi, & Hirose 2002; Conlin & Parnes 2007a,b).

■ Presbycusis

The aging process comes with some degree of deterioration at most and probably all levels of the auditory system, resulting in age-related auditory impairments that are collectively known as **presbycusis**. There is a general consensus that presbycusis is the result of various kinds of physiological degeneration due to the normal aging process (theoretically "pure presbycusis") plus the accumulated effects of noise exposure, ototoxicity, medical disorders and their treatment, and genetic components (Gates, Couropmitree, & Myers 1999; Johnson, Zheng, & Erway 2000; Fischel-Ghodsian 2003; Garringer, Pankratz, Nichols, & Reed 2006).

Presbycusis is often described in terms of how hearing thresholds change with increasing age (Corso 1963; Spoor 1967; Robinson & Sutton 1979; Marshall 1981; Kryter 1983; Mościcki, Elkins, Baum, & McNamara 1985; Robinson 1988; Gates, Cooper, Kannel, & Miller 1990; Brant & Fozard 1990; Weinstein 2000; Echt, Smith, Burridge, & Spiro 2010; ISO 2013). Differences exist among presbycusis curves, reflecting differences between the populations sampled, degrees of exposure to social and/or occupational noises, and the extent to which people with otological disorders were excluded from the samples. Representative curves are shown in **Fig. 6.15**. Notice that (1) age-related threshold shifts are greater and begin sooner for the higher frequencies, suggesting greater involvement toward the base of the cochlea; and (2) males are affected more than females, presumably reflecting more exposure to occupational and recreational noises. **Fig. 6.16** shows the audiogram of a typical patient with presbycusis, showing a sloping sensorineural hearing loss that is essentially symmetrical in the two ears.

Difficulty with speech recognition is the most common complaint of presbycusics. There is a general trend for speech recognition scores in quiet to decrease with age, but there is also considerable variability, and it has been suggested that the performance of the elderly is comparable to that of young persons with similar audiograms when they are tested at adequate intensity levels (Marshall 1981). Gates et al (1990) found that only 3 out of 1026 elderly subjects (0.3%) had disproportionately low speech recognition scores with respect to their

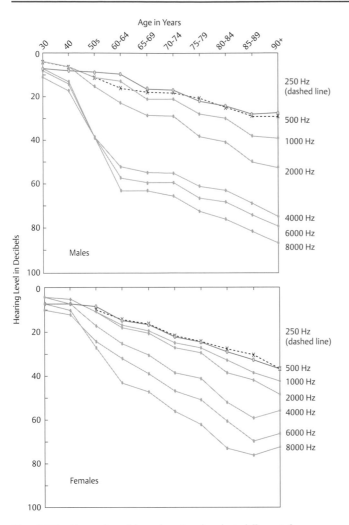

Fig. 6.15 Examples of how hearing level at different frequencies changes as a function of age (presbycusis curves) among males and females. (Based on values from several sources: 30 and 40 [medians (ISO 2013)]; 50s [right ear means for 48–59-year-olds 60 and older (Gates et al 1990)].)

audiograms. In contrast, it is clear that speech intelligibility decreases with aging for speech that is presented under difficult listening conditions (noise, competition, reverberation, time compression, interruptions, etc.). In fact, age-related declines appear to emerge earlier than one might expect. In 1980, Bergman reported that the presbycusic effect for degraded speech becomes evident as early as the fifth decade of life (years 40–49). Since then, a growing body of literature has shown that middle-age listeners (even those with essentially normal hearing thresholds) perform more poorly than younger adults on measures of speech perception under challenging listening conditions, as well as other kinds of auditory performance, such as gap detection,

masking level differences, localization and difference limens (Wilson, Civitello, & Margolis 1985; Abel, Giguère, Consoli, & Papsin 2000; Babkoff, Muchnik, Ben-David, Furst, & Even-Zohar 2002; Grose, Hall, & Buss 2006; Helfer & Vargo 2009; Grose & Mamo 2010; Leigh-Paffenroth & Elangovan 2011).

Various histological types of presbycusis have been described, as illustrated in **Fig. 6.17**. However, the student should be aware that many patients have more than one kind of histological deterioration, and that not all of the idealized types of presbycusis have been observed by all investigators. The four classical types of presbycusis were based on a combination of clinical and histological findings by Schuknecht (1955, 1964, 1974): **Sensory presbycusis** is due to the degeneration of the sensory hair cells and supporting cells mainly toward the basal turn of the cochlea, and can also include atrophy of the associated neurons as a secondary effect. It is associated with a sloping (often steeply) high-frequency sensorineural hearing loss and speech recognition scores that are consistent with the nature of the audiogram. **Neural presbycusis** is related to primary degeneration of the auditory neurons. The reduced neuronal population is characterized clinically by speech recognition scores that are lower than what would be expected from the audiogram. Atypically poor speech recognition in presbycusis is sometimes called *phonemic regression* (Gaeth 1948), but this phenomenon appears to be rare (Gates et al 1990).

Metabolic or **strial presbycusis** is caused by degeneration of the stria vascularis, causing a relatively flat sensorineural hearing loss with speech recognition scores that are in line with the audiogram. **Mechanical** or **cochlear conductive presbycusis** is attributed to structural changes in the basilar membrane, affecting its mass and stiffness, which would in turn affect the mechanics of the cochlea and produce a sloping sensorineural hearing loss. This kind of presbycusis may be hypothetical.

Two additional forms of presbycusis have also been identified (Johnsson & Hawkins 1979; Hawkins & Johnsson 1985): **Vascular presbycusis** is associated with deterioration of the blood supply to the lateral wall of the cochlear duct and the spiral lamina, and may play a part in the deterioration of the stria vascularis and spiral ligament (Johnsson & Hawkins 1972; Johnsson 1973). **Hyperostotic presbycusis** occurs when abnormal bone growth (hyperostosis) in the modiolus or internal auditory meatus compresses auditory nerve cells so that they degenerate (Krmpotić-Nemanić 1969; Krmpotić-Nemanić, Nemanić, & Kostović 1972; Hawkins & Johnsson 1985).

Central presbycusis refers to deficits in auditory perception that are due to age-related changes in the central auditory system (e.g., CHABA 1988;

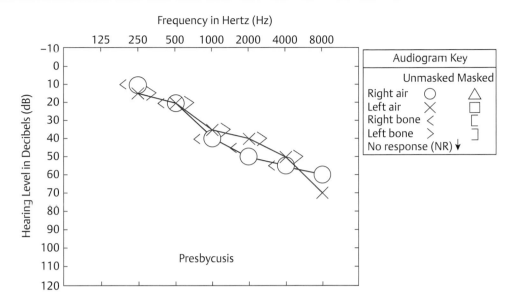

Fig. 6.16 The audiogram of a typical patient with an essentially symmetrical bilateral sloping sensorineural hearing loss associated with presbycusis.

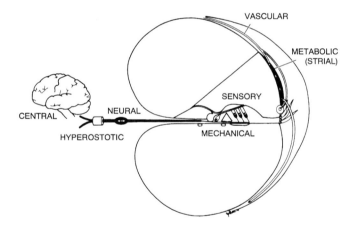

Fig. 6.17 Schematic representation of the various kinds of presbycusis described in the text. (Adapted from Johnsson & Hawkins [1979]. Age-related degeneration of the inner ear. In: Han SS, Coons DH, eds. *Special Senses in Aging.* Ann Arbor: Institute of Gerontology, University of Michigan, 119–135, with permission.)

Humes, Dubno, Gordon-Salant, et al 2012). An extensive systematic by Humes et al (2012) revealed that the existing research could not confirm the idea of central presbycusis as a pure or stand-alone entity; rather, it appears to involve the overlapping effects of peripheral auditory, central auditory, and nonauditory cognitive factors. As they pointed out, research still is needed to fully understand the nature of these age-related deficits.

■ Other Diseases and Influences

In other to give the student a more comprehensive perspective, this section reviews several more general disorders and influences that are capable of causing or complicating hearing loss. In particular, we discuss the hearing effects of several infections, diabetes, and Paget's disease, and well as the implications of general surgery and anesthesia.

Infections

Herpes zoster oticus, also known as **Ramsay Hunt syndrome**, is observed as a painful chicken pox– or shingles-like rash involving the pinna and ear canal, and often appears over portions of the face and neck. This viral infection typically occurs in adults and can cause sensorineural hearing loss, vertigo, and facial palsy.

Syphilis is an infection that was discussed earlier in the context of congenital infections. Acquired syphilis can also cause sensorineural hearing impairments and is known for its ability to mimic other disorders, such as Meniere's disease.

Several kinds of infections commonly cause hearing losses even though they are not ear diseases per se. Many of these diseases are typically associated with infancy and childhood, but are not limited to those years. Sensorineural hearing loss can be a complication of the common viral illnesses of childhood—measles, chicken pox, and mumps—as well as influenza. Measles and mumps are particularly noteworthy. **Measles** has been known to produce sudden-onset bilateral sensorineural hearing losses that are severe in degree and sloping in configuration in ≥ 5% of cases. **Mumps** is probably the most common cause of acquired unilateral sensorineural hearing loss in children. Mumps has been known to cause various degrees of sensorineural hearing loss ranging from a mild high-frequency impairment to deafness on the side of the infection, and profound losses are the most common. The hearing loss usually has a sudden onset and has been known to occur even in cases where there was no apparent swelling of the parotid gland. It is reasonable to expect that the use of vaccines for these common illnesses should reduce the incidence of acquired sensorineural hearing losses among children.

Bacterial meningitis is an acute central nervous system infection that can result in brain damage and hearing loss among those who survive the disease. Historically, ~ 70% of the cases were caused by the *Haemophilus influenzae* type b (Hib) bacteria, and the rest were meningococcal, pneumococcal, and streptococcal infections. However, there has been a substantial decrease in the incidence of Hib infections since the introduction of anti-Hib vaccines in the late 1980s.

A severe-to-profound sensorineural hearing loss is the most common permanent sequela of bacterial meningitis, and occurs when the cochlea is invaded by the infection. Transitory conductive losses have also been reported. The prevalence of sensorineural hearing loss due to bacterial meningitis is variable due to differences in the underlying pathogens and in how the disease is treated. For example, the incidence of hearing loss is between 3 and 16% for Hib meningitis, compared with 10.5% for meningococcal, and between 31 and 50% for pneumococcal infections (Dodge, Davis, Feigin, et al 1984; Stein & Boyer 1994). There appears to be a reduction in hearing losses suffered by those who do contract the disease when they are treated with several newer cephalosporin antibiotics and corticosteroids.

Diabetes

Glucose is the power source for the cells of the body, and the hormone that enables the glucose to enter cells is insulin. In **diabetes mellitus**, the pancreas fails to produce enough insulin, or any at all, and/or the tissues of the body fail to make use of the insulin that is produced (insulin resistance). **Type 1 diabetes** is an autoimmune disease that destroys the insulin-producing β cells of the pancreas, leaving the patient permanently dependent on insulin therapy, and usually develops by early adulthood. However, ~ 95% of diabetes patients have **type 2 diabetes**, in which

there is reduced insulin production in the pancreas and insulin resistance. What results is an accumulation of glucose in the blood (hyperglycemia) while the cells are starved for fuel, leading to a wide variety of serious outcomes and complications; and sensorineural hearing loss is among them.

Lisowska, Namyslowski, Morawski, and Strojek (2001) found that young adults with type 1 diabetes had abnormal physiological test results for the cochlea through the auditory brainstem even though their audiometric thresholds were within normal limits. Compared with age-matched nondiabetics, Frisina, Mapes, Kim, Frisina, and Frisina (2006) found that 59- to 92-year-old patients with type 2 diabetes had poorer results on a variety of measures, particularly those sensitive to cochlear disorders, such as otoacoustic emissions and pure tone thresholds (especially in the lower frequencies); as well as a tendency for the right ear to be affected more than the left. Temporal bone studies have shown degeneration of the stria vascularis and outer hair cells in young adults who had type 1 diabetes as well as in 44- to 65-year-old patients who had type 2 diabetes (Fukushima, Cureoglu, Schachern, et al 2005, 2006).

A review of many thousands of veterans' medical records revealed that sensorineural hearing loss was more common among diabetics than age-matched nondiabetic patients, and that worsening of the diabetes was associated with increasing hearing loss (Kakarlapudi, Sawyer, & Staecker 2003). Cheng et al (2009) found that the prevalence of hearing loss (≥ 26 dB HL) among 25- to 69-year-old adults *with diabetes increased* from 46.4% during 1971 to 1973 to 48.5% during 1999 to 2004, compared with a *decrease* from 27.9 to 19.1% for those *without diabetes*.

Paget's Disease

Paget's disease (osteitis deformans) is a chronic and progressive skeletal disease in which bone is resorbed and replaced with dystrophic bone tissue that is often enlarged and prone to fracture and other complications. Typical sites of the disease include the pelvis, spine, legs, and skull. Paget's disease is generally not diagnosed before the fifth decade, often as an incidental finding. Involvement of the temporal bone affects all parts of the ear.

Paget's disease is often thought of in the context of conductive disorders, but it usually produces hearing losses that are mixed or sensorineural, probably including a sizable presbycusic component. Harner, Rose, and Facer (1978) reviewed a large sample of Paget's disease patients with known audiograms. About 4% of their sample also had otosclerosis. **Fig. 6.18** shows that most of the hearing losses were

Fig. 6.18   Percentages of ears with normal hearing and with conductive, sensorineural (SNHL), and mixed hearing losses for a large sample of patients with Paget's disease and a subgroup with Paget's disease of the skull. (Recalculated from data by Harner, Rose, & Facer [1978].)

sensorineural or mixed, and that less than 2% of the losses were purely conductive regardless of whether the disease affected the skull. However, the percentage of mixed losses was greater when the disease also affected the skull.

Calcitonin has been used to treat hearing loss in Paget's disease with disappointing or inconclusive results. For example, even though Solomon, Evanson, Canty, and Gill (1977) found that hearing improved in calcitonin-treated patients and deteriorated in untreated control subjects, Walker, Evenson, Canty, and Gill (1979) found no differences between subjects from the two groups when they were retested after 3 years.

General Surgery and Anesthesia

The association of hearing loss with general surgery and anesthesia has received considerable attention (Sprung, Bourke, Contreras, Warner, & Findlay 2003). General anesthesia using nitrous oxide has been associated with conductive and sensorineural hearing losses due to pressure changes produced in the middle ear and/or labyrinth. However, hearing losses occurring after patients have been under general anesthesia are more often associated with surgical issues (e.g., emboli) and/or ototoxic agents. The incidence of hearing loss related to heart surgery reaches ~ 0.2%. These are usually permanent unilateral sensorineural hearing losses and are believed to result from microscopic emboli affecting the inner ear. On the other hand, hearing losses following most other forms of general surgery are quite rare.

In contrast to general anesthesia, 10 to 50% of patients receiving spinal anesthesia (as well as spinal taps) experience low-frequency sensorineural hearing losses, usually attributed to drops in cerebrospinal fluid pressure. Fortunately, many of these cases are subclinical, and most of them tend to recover fully.

■ Nonorganic Hearing Loss

It is possible for a patient to have a hearing disturbance that is not attributable to a structural abnormality, or that manifests itself in one or more ways that do not occur with organically based hearing losses. These kinds of apparent hearing problems are variously described as nonorganic, functional, psychogenic, feigned, or exaggerated hearing losses, or as malingering or pseudo-hypacusis. The topic of nonorganic hearing loss is covered in Chapter 14.

■ Study Questions

1. Define autosomal dominant, autosomal recessive, X-linked, and mitochondrial transmission with respect to genetic hearing loss.
2. Define and explain the principal characteristics of Eustachian tube dysfunction, otitis media, cholesteatoma, and otosclerosis.
3. Define tinnitus and describe its implications.
4. Define and explain the principal characteristics of noise-inducted hearing loss.
5. Define ototoxicity and give three examples of commonly encountered ototoxic agents.
6. Define and explain the principal characteristics of Meniere's disease.
7. Define and explain the principal characteristics of acoustic tumor.
8. Define and explain the principal characteristics of presbycusis.
9. Define and explain the principal characteristics of auditory neuropathy syndrome disorder.
10. What do we mean by the term *(central) auditory processing disorder*?

References

Abel SM, Giguère C, Consoli A, Papsin BC. The effect of aging on horizontal plane sound localization. J Acoust Soc Am 2000;108(2):743–752

American Academy of Audiology (AAA). 2010. Clinical Practice Guidelines: Diagnosis, Treatment and Management of Children and Adults with Central Auditory Processing Disorder. Available at: http://www.audiology.org/resources/documentlibrary/documents/capd%20guidelines%208-2010.pdf

American Academy of Family Physicians (AAFP); American Academy of Otolaryngology–Head and Neck Surgery; American Academy of Pediatrics, Subcommittee on Otitis Media with Effusion. Otitis media with effusion. Pediatrics 2004;113(5):1412–1429

American Academy of Pediatrics, Subcommittee on Management of Acute Otitis Media. Diagnosis and management of acute otitis media. Pediatrics 2004; 113(5):1451–1465

American Speech-Language-Hearing Association (ASHA). (2004). Scope of Practice in Audiology. Rockville Pike, MD: ASHA

American Speech-Language-Hearing Association (ASHA). (2005). (Central) Auditory Processing Disorders. Rockville Pike, MD: ASHA

American Speech-Language-Hearing Association (ASHA). (2006). Preferred Practice Patterns for the Profession of Audiology. Rockville Pike, MD: ASHA

Anari M, Axelsson A, Eliasson A, Magnusson L. Hypersensitivity to sound—questionnaire data, audiometry and classification. Scand Audiol 1999;28(4):219–230

Anderson TD, Loevner LA, Bigelow DC, Mirza N. Prevalence of unsuspected acoustic neuroma found by magnetic resonance imaging. Otolaryngol Head Neck Surg 2000;122(5):643–646

Babkoff H, Muchnik C, Ben-David N, Furst M, Even-Zohar S, Hildesheimer M. Mapping lateralization of click trains in younger and older populations. Hear Res 2002;165(1-2):117–127

Baguley DM. Hyperacusis. J R Soc Med 2003;96(12): 582–585

Baguley DM, Irving RM, Hardy DG, Harada T, Moffat DA. Audiological findings in glomus tumours. Br J Audiol 1994;28(6):291–297

Ballachanda BB, Peers CJ. Cerumen management: instruments and procedures. ASHA 1992;34(2):43–46

Banerjee A, Whyte A, Atlas MD. Superior canal dehiscence: review of a new condition. Clin Otolaryngol 2005;30(1):9–15

Baran DJ, Musiek FE. Evaluation of the adults with hearing complaints and normal audiograms. Hear Today 1994;6:9–11

Belden CJ, Weg N, Minor LB, Zinrech SJ. CT evaluation of bone dehiscence of the superior semicircular canal as a cause of sound- and/or pressure-induced vertigo. Radiology 2003;226(2):337–343

Bellis TJ, Billiet C, Ross J. The utility of visual analogs of central auditory tests in the differential diagnosis of (central) auditory processing disorder and attention deficit hyperactivity disorder. J Am Acad Audiol 2011;22(8):501–514

Bellis TJ, Ross J. Performance of normal adults and children on central auditory diagnostic tests and their corresponding visual analogs. J Am Acad Audiol 2011;22(8):491–500

Bellucci RJ. Dual classification of tympanoplasty. Laryngoscope 1973;83(11):1754–1758

Bergman M. 1980. Aging and the Perception of Speech. Baltimore, MD: University Park Press

Berlin CI, Bordelon J, St John P, et al. Reversing click polarity may uncover auditory neuropathy in infants. Ear Hear 1998;19(1):37–47

Berlin CI, Hood L, Rose K. On renaming auditory neuropathy as auditory dys-synchrony. Audiol Today 2001;13(6):15–17

Berlin CI, Hood LJ, Morlet T, et al. Multi-site diagnosis and management of 260 patients with auditory neuropathy/dys-synchrony (auditory neuropathy spectrum disorder). Int J Audiol 2010;49(1):30–43

Berlin CI, Hood LJ, Morlet T, et al. Absent or elevated middle ear muscle reflexes in the presence of normal otoacoustic emissions: a universal finding in 136 cases of auditory neuropathy/dys-synchrony. J Am Acad Audiol 2005;16(8):546–553

Bindu LH, Reddy PP. Genetics of aminoglycoside-induced and prelingual non-syndromic mitochondrial hearing impairment: a review. Int J Audiol 2008;47(11): 702–707

Bluestone CD, Stool SE, Kenna MA, eds. 1996. Pediatric Otolaryngology, 3rd ed. Philadelphia, PA: WB Saunders

Boettcher FA, Henderson D, Gratton MA, Danielson RW, Byrne CD. Synergistic interactions of noise and other ototraumatic agents. Ear Hear 1987;8(4):192–212

Borg E. Perinatal asphyxia, hypoxia, ischemia and hearing loss. An overview. Scand Audiol 1997;26(2):77–91

Brant LJ, Fozard JL. Age changes in pure-tone hearing thresholds in a longitudinal study of normal human aging. J Acoust Soc Am 1990;88(2):813–820

Brantberg K, Bergenius J, Mendel L, Witt H, Tribukait A, Ygge J. Symptoms, findings and treatment in patients with dehiscence of the superior semicircular canal. Acta Otolaryngol 2001;121(1):68–75

Brown DP. Speech recognition in recurrent otitis media: results in a set of identical twins. J Am Acad Audiol 1994;5(1):1–6

Brownstein Z, Goldfarb A, Levi H, Frydman M, Avraham KB. Chromosomal mapping and phenotypic characterization of hereditary otosclerosis linked to the OTSC4 locus. Arch Otolaryngol Head Neck Surg 2006; 132(4):416–424

Buckingham RA, Becker W, Naumann HH, Pfaltz CR, eds. 1989. Ear, Nose and Throat Diseases. New York, NY: Thieme

Cacace AT, McFarland DJ. The importance of modality specificity in diagnosing central auditory processing disorder. Am J Audiol 2005a;14(2):112–123

Cacace AT, McFarland DJ. Response to Katz and Tillery (2005), Musiek, Bellis, and Chermak (2005), and Rosen (2005). Am J Audiol 2005b;14:143–150

Cacace AT, McFarland DJ, eds. 2008. Current Controversies in Central Auditory Processing Disorder. San Diego, CA: Plural

Cacace AT, McFarland DJ. Factors influencing tests of auditory processing: a perspective on current issues and relevant concerns. J Am Acad Audiol 2013;24(7): 572–589

Campo P, Maguin K, Gabriel S, et al. 2009. Combined Exposure to Noise and Ototoxic Substances. European Agency for Safety and Health at Work. Available at https://osha.europa.eu/en/publications/literature_reviews/combined-exposure-to-noise-and-ototoxic-substances

Cantekin EI, Doyle WJ, Phillips DC, Bluestone CD. Gas absorption in the middle ear. Ann Otol Rhinol Laryngol Suppl 1980;89(3 Pt 2, suppl 68):71–75

Carhart R. Clinical application of bone conduction audiometry. Arch Otolaryngol 1950;51(6):798–808

Chen W, Campbell CA, Green GE, et al. Linkage of otosclerosis to a third locus (OTSC3) on human chromosome 6p21.3-22.3. J Med Genet 2002;39(7):473–477

Cheng YJ, Gregg EW, Saaddine JB, Imperatore G, Zhang X, Albright AL. Three decade change in the prevalence of hearing impairment and its association with diabetes in the United States. Prev Med 2009;49(5):360–364

Ching TY, Dillon H, Marnane V, et al. Outcomes of early- and late-identified children at 3 years of age: findings from a prospective population-based study. Ear Hear 2013;34(5):535–552

Ching TYC, Johnson EE, Hou S, Dillon H, Zhang V,Burns L, van Buynder P, Wong A, Flynn C. A comparison of NAL and DSL prescriptive methods for paediatric hearing-aid fitting: Predicted speech intelligibility and loudness. Intl J Audiol 2013; 52; S29–S38

Chung JW, Fayad J, Linthicum F, Ishiyama A, Merchant SN. Histopathology after endolymphatic sac surgery for Ménière's syndrome. Otol Neurotol 2011;32(4):660–664

Clark WW. Recent studies of temporary threshold shift (TTS) and permanent threshold shift (PTS) in animals. J Acoust Soc Am 1991;90(1):155–163

Committee on Hearing, Bioacustics and Biomechanics Working Group on Speech Understanding and Aging (CHABA). Speech understanding and aging. J Acoust Soc Am 1988;83(3):859–895

Conlin AE, Parnes LS. Treatment of sudden sensorineural hearing loss: II. A Meta-analysis. Arch Otolaryngol Head Neck Surg 2007a;133(6):582–586

Conlin AE, Parnes LS. Treatment of sudden sensorineural hearing loss: I. A systematic review. Arch Otolaryngol Head Neck Surg 2007b;133(6):573–581

Corso JF. Age and sex differences in pure-tone thresholds: survey of hearing levels from 18 to 65 years. Arch Otolaryngol 1963;77:385–405

Corwin JT, Cotanche DA. Regeneration of sensory hair cells after acoustic trauma. Science 1988;240(4860):1772–1774

Cotanche DA, Lee KH, Stone JS, Picard DA. Hair cell regeneration in the bird cochlea following noise damage or ototoxic drug damage. Anat Embryol (Berl) 1994; 189(1):1–18

Cox KM, Lee DJ, Carey JP, Minor LB. Dehiscence of bone overlying the superior semicircular canal as a cause of an air-bone gap on audiometry: a case study. Am J Audiol 2003;12(1):11–16

Davis A, El Refaie A. 2000. Epidemiology of tinnitus. In: Tyler RS, ed. Tinnitus Handbook. San Diego, CA: Singular; 1–21

DeBonis DA, Moncrieff D. Auditory processing disorders: an update for speech-language pathologists. Am J Speech Lang Pathol 2008;17(1):4–18

Denny F. Otitis media. Pediatr News 1984;18:38

Dodge PR, Davis H, Feigin RD, et al. Prospective evaluation of hearing impairment as a sequela of acute bacterial meningitis. N Engl J Med 1984;311(14):869–874

Downs MP. 1995. Contribution of mild hearing loss to auditory language learning problems. In: Roeser R, ed. Auditory Disorders in School Children, 3rd ed. New York, NY: Thieme; 188–200

Echt KV, Smith SL, Burridge AB, Spiro A III. Longitudinal changes in hearing sensitivity among men: the Veterans Affairs Normative Aging Study. J Acoust Soc Am 2010;128(4):1992–2002

Fabry L. 2000. Identification and management of auditory neuropathy: a case study. In: Seewald RC, ed. A Sound Foundation through Early Amplification: Proceedings of an International Conference. Switzerland: Phonak; 237–246

Farrior B. 1968. Tympanoplasty in 3-D. Tampa, FL: American Academy of Ophthamology and Otolaryngology

FDA. 2007. Information for Healthcare Professionals: Sildenafil (marketed as Viagra and Revatio) Vardenafil (marketed as Levitra) Tadalafil (marketed as Cialis). Available at http://www.fda.gov/cder/drug/InfoSheets/HCP/ED_HCP.htm

Fisch U. 1980. Tympanoplasty and Stapedotomy. A Manual of Techniques. New York, NY: Thieme-Stratton

Fischel-Ghodsian N. Mitochondrial deafness. Ear Hear 2003; 24(4):303–313

Forli F, Passetti S, Mancuso M, et al. Mitochondrial syndromic sensorineural hearing loss. Biosci Rep 2007;2 7(1-3):113–123

Friedman TB, Schultz JM, Ben-Yosef T, et al. Recent advances in the understanding of syndromic forms of hearing loss. Ear Hear 2003;24(4):289–302

Friel-Patti S, Finitzo T. Language learning in a prospective study of otitis media with effusion in the first two years of life. J Speech Hear Res 1990;33(1):188–194

Frisina ST, Mapes F, Kim S, Frisina DR, Frisina RD. Characterization of hearing loss in aged type II diabetics. Hear Res 2006;211(1-2):103–113

Fuente A, McPherson B. Organic solvents and hearing loss: the challenge for audiology. Int J Audiol 2006; 45(7):367–381

Fukushima H, Cureoglu S, Schachern PA, et al. Cochlear changes in patients with type 1 diabetes mellitus. Otolaryngol Head Neck Surg 2005;133(1):100–106

Fukushima H, Cureoglu S, Schachern PA, Paparella MM, Harada T, Oktay MF. Effects of type 2 diabetes mellitus on cochlear structure in humans. Arch Otolaryngol Head Neck Surg 2006;132(9):934–938

Gaeth JH. 1948. Study of phonemic regression in relation to hearing loss. Unpublished dissertation. Evanston, IL: Northwestern University

Garringer HJ, Pankratz ND, Nichols WC, Reed T. Hearing impairment susceptibility in elderly men and the DFNA18 locus. Arch Otolaryngol Head Neck Surg 2006;132(5):506–510

Gates GA, Cooper JC Jr, Kannel WB, Miller NJ. Hearing in the elderly: the Framingham cohort, 1983–1985. Part I. Basic audiometric test results. Ear Hear 1990;11(4):247–256

Gates GA, Couropmitree NN, Myers RH. Genetic associations in age-related hearing thresholds. Arch Otolaryngol Head Neck Surg 1999;125(6):654–659

Gates GA. Ménière's disease review 2005. J Am Acad Audiol 2006;17(1):16–26

Gates GA, Klein JO, Lim DJ, et al. Recent advances in otitis media. 1. Definitions, terminology, and classification of otitis media. Ann Otol Rhinol Laryngol Suppl 2002;188:8–18

Geffner D, Ross-Swain D, eds. 2013. Auditory Processing Disorders: Assessment, Management, and Treatment, 2nd ed. San Diego, CA: Plural

Ghossaini SN, Wazen JJ. An update on the surgical treatment of Ménière's diseases. J Am Acad Audiol 2006; 17(1):38–44

Gimsing S. Vestibular schwannoma: when to look for it? J Laryngol Otol 2010;124(3):258–264

Goodhill V. Leaking labyrinthine lesions, deafness, tinnitus and dizziness. Ann Otol Rhinol Laryngol 1981; 90:99–106

Gravel JS, Wallace IF. Listening and language at 4 years of age: effects of early otitis media. J Speech Hear Res 1992;35(3):588–595

Gravel JS, Wallace IF. Effects of otitis media with effusion on hearing in the first 3 years of life. J Speech Lang Hear Res 2000;43(3):631–644

Grose JH, Hall JW III, Buss E. Temporal processing deficits in the pre-senescent auditory system. J Acoust Soc Am 2006;119(4):2305–2315

Grose JH, Mamo SK. Processing of temporal fine structure as a function of age. Ear Hear 2010;31(6):755–760

Grosse SD, Ross DS, Dollard SC. Congenital cytomegalovirus (CMV) infection as a cause of permanent bilateral hearing loss: a quantitative assessment. J Clin Virol 2008;41(2):57–62

Guidelines Development Conference (GDC). 2008. Guidelines for Identification and Management of Infants and Young Children with Auditory Neuropathy Spectrum Disorder. Como, Italy. Monograph available at http://www.childrenscolorado.org/pdf/ANSD%20Monograph%20Bill%20Daniels%20Center%20for%20Childrens%20Hearing.pdf

Hall JW III, Prentice CH, Smiley G, Werkhaven J. Auditory dysfunction in selected syndromes and patterns of malformations: review and case findings. J Am Acad Audiol 1995;6(1):80–92

Hamernik RP, Ahroon WA, Hsueh KD. The energy spectrum of an impulse: its relation to hearing loss. J Acoust Soc Am 1991;90(1):197–204

Hamernik RP, Hsueh KD. Impulse noise: some definitions, physical acoustics and other considerations. J Acoust Soc Am 1991;90(1):189–196

Hamill TA. Evaluating treatments for Ménière's disease: controversies surrounding placebo control. J Am Acad Audiol 2006;17(1):27–37

Harner SG, Rose DE, Facer GW. Paget's disease and hearing loss. Otolaryngology 1978;86(6 Pt 1):ORL-869–ORL-874

Hasegawa T, Kida Y, Kobayashi T, Yoshimoto M, Mori Y, Yoshida J. Long-term outcomes in patients with vestibular schwannomas treated using gamma knife surgery: 10-year follow up. J Neurosurg 2005;102(1):10–16

Hawkins JE, Johnsson L-G. Otopathological changes associated with presbycusis. Semin Hear 1985;6:115–133

Helfer KS, Vargo M. Speech recognition and temporal processing in middle-aged women. J Am Acad Audiol 2009;20(4):264–271

Henderson D, Hamernik RP. Impulse noise: critical review. J Acoust Soc Am 1986;80(2):569–584

Henderson D, Bielefeld EC, Harris KC, Hu BH. The role of oxidative stress in noise-induced hearing loss. Ear Hear 2006;27(1):1–19

Henry JA, Roberts LE, Caspary DM, Theodoroff SM, Salvi RJ. Underlying mechanisms of tinnitus: review and clinical implications. J Am Acad Audiol 2014;25(1):5–22, quiz 126

Henry JA, Dennis KC, Schechter MA. General review of tinnitus: prevalence, mechanisms, effects, and management. J Speech Lang Hear Res 2005;48(5):1204–1235

Higson JM, Haggard MP, Field DL. Validation of parameters for assessing obscure auditory dysfunction—robustness of determinants of OAD status across samples and test methods. Br J Audiol 1994;28(1):27–39

Hood LJ, Berlin CI, Allen P. Cortical deafness: a longitudinal study. J Am Acad Audiol 1994;5(5):330–342

Hughes GB, ed. 1985. Textbook of Clinical Otology. New York, NY: Thieme-Stratton

Hughes GB, Pensak ML, eds. 2007. Clinical Otology, 3rd ed. New York, NY: Thieme

Humes LE, Dubno JR, Gordon-Salant S, et al. Central presbycusis: a review and evaluation of the evidence. J Am Acad Audiol 2012;23(8):635–666

Hyman C, Keaster V, Hanson V, et al. CNS abnormalities after hymolyte disease or hyperbilirubinemia: a prospective study of 405 patients. Am J Dis Child 1969;117:395–405

International Standards Organization (ISO). 2013. Acoustics—Estimation of Noise-Induced Hearing Loss (ISO-1999). Geneva: ISO.Jastreboff MM, Jastreboff PJ. Decreased tolerance and tinnitus retraining therapy (TRT). Aust N Z J Audiol 2002;24:74–81

Jastreboff PJ, Hazel JWP. 2004. Tinnitus Retraining Therapy: Implementing the Tinnitus Retraining Model. New York, NY: Cambridge University Press

Jerger J, Musiek F. Report of the consensus conference on the diagnosis of auditory processing disorders in school-aged children. J Am Acad Audiol 2000;11(9):467–474

Jerger J, Weikers NJ, Sharbrough FW III, Jerger S. Bilateral lesions of the temporal lobe. A case study. Acta Otolaryngol Suppl 1969;258(suppl):1–51

Jerger S, Jerger J, Alford BR, Abrams S. Development of speech intelligibility in children with recurrent otitis media. Ear Hear 1983;4(3):138–145

Jiang H, Talaska AE, Schacht J, Sha SH. Oxidative imbalance in the aging inner ear. Neurobiol Aging 2007; 28(10):1605–1612

Johnson CE, Danhauer JL, Rice EN, Fisher SK. Survey of audiologists and cerumen management. Am J Audiol 2013;22(1):2–13

Johnson EW. Auditory test results in 500 cases of acoustic neuroma. Arch Otolaryngol 1977;103(3):152–158

Johnson KR, Zheng QY, Erway LC. A major gene affecting age-related hearing loss is common to at least ten inbred strains of mice. Genomics 2000;70(2):171–180

Johnsson L-G. Vascular pathology in the human inner ear. Adv Otorhinolaryngol 1973;20:197–220

Johnsson L-G, Hawkins JE Jr. Vascular changes in the human inner ear associated with aging. Ann Otol Rhinol Laryngol 1972;81(3):364–376

Johnsson L-G, Hawkins JH. 1979. Age-related degeneration of the inner ear. In: Han SS, Coons DH, eds. Special Senses in Aging. Ann Arbor, MI: Institute of Gerontology, University of Michigan; 119–135

Jongmans MC, Admiraal RJ, van der Donk KP, et al. CHARGE syndrome: the phenotypic spectrum of mutations in the CHD7 gene. J Med Genet 2006;43(4):306–314

Kakarlapudi V, Sawyer R, Staecker H. The effect of diabetes on sensorineural hearing loss. Otol Neurotol 2003;24(3):382–386

Kamhi AG. What speech-language pathologists need to know about auditory processing disorder. Lang Speech Hear Serv Sch 2011;42(3):265–272

Katz J, Tillery KL. Can central auditory processing tests resist supramodal influences? Am J Audiol 2005;14(2):124–127, discussion 143–150

Katzenell U, Segal S. Hyperacusis: review and clinical guidelines. Otol Neurotol 2001;22(3):321–326, discussion 326–327

Kim TB, Isaacson B, Sivakumaran TA, Starr A, Keats BJ, Lesperance MM. A gene responsible for autosomal dominant auditory neuropathy (AUNA1) maps to 13q14-21. J Med Genet 2004;41(11):872–876

Kitajiri S, Tabuchi K, Hiraumi H, Hirose T. Is corticosteroid therapy effective for sudden-onset sensorineural hearing loss at lower frequencies? Arch Otolaryngol Head Neck Surg 2002;128(4):365–367

Klar J, Frykholm C, Friberg U, Dahl N. A Meniere's disease gene linked to chromosome 12p12.3. Am J Med Genet B Neuropsychiatr Genet 2006;141B(5):463–467

Kley W. 1982. Surgical treatment of chronic otitis media. In: Naumann, HH, ed. Head and Neck Surgery, Vol. 3: Ear. Stuttgart, Germany: Thieme

Kochkin S, Tyler R, Born J. Mark VIII: The prevalence of tinnitus in the United States and the self-reported efficacy of various treatments. Hear Rev 2011;18(12):10–26

Kokotas H, Petersen MB, Willems PJ. Mitochondrial deafness. Clin Genet 2007;71(5):379–391

Kouwen HB, DeJonckere PH. Prevalence of OME is reduced in young children using chewing gum. Ear Hear 2007;28(4):451–455

Kovach MJ, Campbell KC, Herman K, et al. Anticipation in a unique family with Charcot-Marie-Tooth syndrome and deafness: delineation of the clinical features and review of the literature. Am J Med Genet 2002;108(4):295–303

Krmpotić-Nemanić J. Presbycusis and retrocochlear structures. Int Audiol 1969;8:210–220

Krmpotić-Nemanić J, Nemanić D, Kostović I. Macroscopical and microscopical changes in the bottom of the internal auditory meatus. Acta Otolaryngol 1972;73(2):254–258

Kryter KD. Addendum and erratum: "presbycusis, sociocusis, and nosocusis" [J. Acoust. Soc. Am. 73, 1897-1919 (1983)]. J Acoust Soc Am 1983;74(6):1907–1909 [and addendum/erratum, J Acoust Soc Am 74, 1907–1909]

Kujawa SG, Liberman MC. Adding insult to injury: cochlear nerve degeneration after "temporary" noise-induced hearing loss. J Neurosci 2009;29(45):14077–14085

Lalwani AK, Grundfast KM. 1998. Pediatric Otology and Neurotology. Philadelphia, PA: Lippincott Raven

Landau WM, Goldstein R, Kleffner FR. Congenital aphasia. A clinicopathologic study. Neurology 1960;10:915–921

Lebo CP, Reddell RC. The presbycusis component in occupational hearing loss. Laryngoscope 1972;82(8):1399–1409

Lee CS, Paparella MM, Margolis RH, Le C. Audiological profiles and Menière's disease. Ear Nose Throat J 1995;74(8):527–532

Leigh-Paffenroth ED, Elangovan S. Temporal processing in low-frequency channels: effects of age and hearing loss in middle-aged listeners. J Am Acad Audiol 2011;22(7):393–404

Lempert J. Improvement of hearing in cases of otosclerosis. Arch Otolaryngol 1938;28:42–97

Lesinski SG, Stein JA. CO_2 laser stapedotomy. Laryngoscope 1989;99(6 Pt 2, Suppl 46):20–24

Levy R, Shvero J, Hadar T. Stapedotomy technique and results: ten years' experience and comparative study with stapedectomy. Laryngoscope 1990;100(10 Pt 1):1097–1099

Likhterov I, Allbright RM, Selesnick SH. LINAC radiosurgery and radiotherapy treatment of acoustic neuromas. Otolaryngol Clin North Am 2007;40(3):541–570, ix

Lin D, Hegarty JL, Fischbein NJ, Jackler RK. The prevalence of "incidental" acoustic neuroma. Arch Otolaryngol Head Neck Surg 2005;131(3):241–244

Lisowska G, Namysłowski G, Morawski K, Strojek K. Early identification of hearing impairment in patients with type 1 diabetes mellitus. Otol Neurotol 2001;22(3):316–320

Madden C, Rutter M, Hilbert L, Greinwald JH Jr, Choo DI. Clinical and audiological features in auditory neuropathy. Arch Otolaryngol Head Neck Surg 2002;128(9):1026–1030

Marra CM, Wechkin HA, Longstreth WT Jr, Rees TS, Syapin CL, Gates GA. Hearing loss and antiretroviral therapy in patients infected with HIV-1. Arch Neurol 1997;54(4):407–410

Marshall L. Auditory processing in aging listeners. J Speech Hearing Dis 1981; 46: 226-240

Mathieu D, Kondziolka D, Flickinger JC, et al. Stereotactic radiosurgery for vestibular schwannomas in patients with neurofibromatosis type 2: an analysis of tumor control, complications, and hearing preservation rates. Neurosurgery 2007;60(3):460–468

Matthies C, Samii M. Management of 1000 vestibular schwannomas (acoustic neuromas): clinical presentation. Neurosurgery 1997;40(1):1–9

Mau A. 1984. Chronic otitis media with effusion and adenotonsilectomy: A prospective randomized controlled study. In: Lim DJ et al, eds. Recent Advances in Otitis Media with Effusion. Philadelphia, PA: Decker; 299–302

McGee TM. Comparison of small fenestra and total stapedectomy. Ann Otol Rhinol Laryngol 1981;90(6 Pt 1): 633–636

Medwetsky L. Spoken language processing model: bridging auditory and language processing to guide assessment and intervention. Lang Speech Hear Serv Sch 2011;42(3):286–296

Meikle MB, Creedon TA, Griest SE. Tinnitus Archive. 2004. Available at http://www.tinnitusarchive.org. Accessed Sept. 29, 2007

Melnick W. Human temporary threshold shift (TTS) and damage risk. J Acoust Soc Am 1991;90(1):147–154

Menjuk P. 1992. Relationship of otitis media to speech and language development. In: Katz J, Stecker N, Henderson D, eds. Central Auditory Processing: A Transdisciplinary Approach. St. Louis, MO: Mosby; 187–197

Merchant SN, Rosowski JJ. Conductive hearing loss caused by third-window lesions of the inner ear. Otol Neurotol 2008;29(3):282–289

Miller CA. Auditory processing theories of language disorders: past, present, and future. Lang Speech Hear Serv Sch 2011;42(3):309–319

Miller JD. Effects of noise on people. J Acoust Soc Am 1974;56(3):729–764

Minor LB. Superior canal dehiscence syndrome. Am J Otol 2000;21(1):9–19

Minor LB. Clinical manifestations of superior semicircular canal dehiscence. Laryngoscope 2005;115(10): 1717–1727

Minor LB, Solomon D, Zinreich JS, Zee DS. Sound- and/or pressure-induced vertigo due to bone dehiscence of the superior semicircular canal. Arch Otolaryngol Head Neck Surg 1998;124(3):249–258

Mody M, Schwartz RG, Gravel JS, Ruben RJ. Speech perception and verbal memory in children with and without histories of otitis media. J Speech Lang Hear Res 1999;42(5):1069–1079

Moore BCJ. Dead regions in the cochlea: conceptual foundations, diagnosis, and clinical applications. Ear Hear 2004;25(2):98–116

Moore DR. The diagnosis and management of auditory processing disorder. Lang Speech Hear Serv Sch 2011;42(3):303–308

Morrison AW. The surgery of vertigo: saccus drainage for idiopathic endolymphatic hydrops. J Laryngol Otol 1976;90(1):87–93

Mościcki EK, Elkins EF, Baum HM, McNamara PM. Hearing loss in the elderly: an epidemiologic study of the Framingham Heart Study Cohort. Ear Hear 1985;6(4): 184–190

Musiek FE, Bellis TJ, Chermak GD. Nonmodularity of the central auditory nervous system: implications for (central) auditory processing disorder. Am J Audiol 2005;14(2):128–138, discussion 143–150

Nance WE. The genetics of deafness. Ment Retard Dev Disabil Res Rev 2003;9(2):109–119

National Institutes of Health (NIH). Consensus Statement on Acoustic Neuroma. 1991;9:1–24

Nickel R, Forge A. Gap junctions and connexins in the inner ear: their roles in homeostasis and deafness. Curr Opin Otolaryngol Head Neck Surg 2008;16(5):452–457

Nickel R, Forge AF. 2010. Gap junctions and connexins: the molecular genetics of deafness. eLS. John Wiley & Sons Ltd, Chichester. Available at: http://www.els.net

Nies E. Ototoxic substances at the workplace: a brief update. Arh Hig Rada Toksikol 2012;63(2):147–152

Northern JL, Downs MP. 1991. Hearing in Children, 4th ed. Baltimore, MD: Williams & Wilkins

Online Mendelian Inheritance in Man (OMIM). 2013. [Updated 28 Oct. 28, 2013.] Available at http://www.omim.org/

Ortolano S, Di Pasquale G, Crispino G, Anselmi F, Mammano F, Chiorini JA. Coordinated control of connexin 26 and connexin 30 at the regulatory and functional level in the inner ear. Proc Natl Acad Sci U S A 2008;105(48):18776–18781

Pandya A. 2011. Nonsyndromic hearing loss and deafness, mitochondrial. 2004 Oct 22 [Updated Apr. 21, 2011]. In Pagon RA, Adam P, Bird TD, et al (Eds.): GeneReviews [Internet]. Seattle (WA): University of Washington. Available from: http://www.ncbi.nlm.nih.gov/books/NBK1422/

Paparella MM, Goycoolea M, Bassiouni M, Koutroupas S. Silent otitis media: clinical applications. Laryngoscope 1986;96(9 Pt 1):978–985

Paparella MM, McDermott JC, de Sousa LC. Meniere's disease and the peak audiogram. Arch Otolaryngol 1982;108(9):555–559

Paparella MM, Shumrick DA, Gluckman JL, Meyerhoff WL, eds. 1991. Otolaryngology. Philadelphia, PA: WB Saunders

Passchier-Vermeer W. Hearing loss due to continuous exposure to steady-state broad-band noise. J Acoust Soc Am 1974;56(5):1585–1593

Perks JR, St George EJ, El Hamri K, Blackburn P, Plowman PN. Stereotactic radiosurgery XVI: Isodosimetric comparison of photon stereotactic radiosurgery techniques (gamma knife vs. micromultileaf collimator linear accelerator) for acoustic neuroma—and potential clinical importance. Int J Radiat Oncol Biol Phys 2003;57(5):1450–1459

Peterson A, Shallop J, Driscoll C, et al. Outcomes of cochlear implantation in children with auditory neuropathy. J Am Acad Audiol 2003;14(4):188–201

Pikus AT. Pediatric audiologic profile in type 1 and type 2 neurofibromatosis. J Am Acad Audiol 1995;6(1): 54–62

Plomp R. A signal-to-noise ratio model for the speech-reception threshold of the hearing impaired. J Speech Hear Res 1986;29(2):146–154

Postelmans JT, Stokroos RJ. Cochlear implantation in a patient with deafness induced by Charcot-Marie-Tooth disease (hereditary motor and sensory neuropathies). J Laryngol Otol 2006;120(6):508–510

Prellner K, Kalm O, Harsten G. Middle ear problems in childhood. Acta Otolaryngol Suppl 1992;493:93–98

Priuska EM, Schacht J. Formation of free radicals by gentamicin and iron and evidence for an iron/gentamicin complex. Biochem Pharmacol 1995;50(11): 1749–1752

Pulec JL, Horwitz MJ. 1973. Diseases of the Eustachian tube. In: Paparella MM, Shumrick A, eds. Otolaryngology, Vol. 2: Ear. Philadelphia, PA: WB Saunders; 75–92

Rance G. Auditory neuropathy/dys-synchrony and its perceptual consequences. Trends Amplif 2005;9(1): 1–43

Rance G, Barker E, Mok M, Dowell R, Rincon A, Garratt R. Speech perception in noise for children with auditory neuropathy/dys-synchrony type hearing loss. Ear Hear 2007;28(3):351–360

Rance G, Cone-Wesson B, Wunderlich J, Dowell R. Speech perception and cortical event related potentials in children with auditory neuropathy. Ear Hear 2002;23(3):239–253

Rance G, McKay C, Grayden D. Perceptual characterization of children with auditory neuropathy. Ear Hear 2004;25(1):34–46

Rea PA, Gibson WP. Evidence for surviving outer hair cell function in congenitally deaf ears. Laryngoscope 2003;113(11):2030–2034

Ries DT, Rickert M, Schlauch RS. The peaked audiometric configuration in Meniere's disease: disease related? J Speech Lang Hear Res 1999;42(4):829–843

Robinson DW. Threshold of hearing as a function of age and sex for the typical unscreened population. Br J Audiol 1988;22(1):5–20

Robinson DW, Sutton GJ. Age effect in hearing—a comparative analysis of published threshold data. Audiology 1979;18(4):320–334

Roeser RJ, Wilson PL. 2000. Cerumen management. In: Hosford-Dunn H, Roeser RJ, Valente M, eds. Audiology Practice Management. New York, NY: Thieme; 273–290

Roland PS, Smith TL, Schwartz SR, et al. Clinical practice guideline: cerumen impaction. Otolaryngol Head Neck Surg 2008; 139(3, Suppl 2):S1–S21

Rosen S. Mobilization of the stapes to restore hearing in otosclerosis. N Y State J Med 1953;53(22): 2650–2653

Rosen S. "A riddle wrapped in a mystery inside an enigma": defining central auditory processing disorder. Am J Audiol 2005;14(2):139–142, discussion 143–150

Rösler G. Progression of hearing loss caused by occupational noise. Scand Audiol 1994;23(1):13–37

Roush J, Ed. 1985. Aging and hearing impairment. Sem Hear 6, 99–219

Roush P, Frymark T, Venediktov R, Wang B. Audiologic management of auditory neuropathy spectrum disorder in children: a systematic review of the literature. Am J Audiol 2011;20(2):159–170

Rovers MM, Schilder AGM, Zielhuis GA, Rosenfeld RM. Otitis media. Lancet 2004;363(9407):465–473

Ryals BM, Rubel EW. Hair cell regeneration after acoustic trauma in adult Coturnix quail. Science 1988; 240(4860):1774–1776

Rybak LP, Whitworth CA, Mukherjea D, Ramkumar V. Mechanisms of cisplatin-induced ototoxicity and prevention. Hear Res 2007;226(1-2):157–167

Saunders GH, Field DL, Haggard MP. A clinical test battery for obscure auditory dysfunction (OAD): development, selection and use of tests. Br J Audiol 1992;26(1): 33–42

Saunders GH, Haggard MP. The clinical assessment of obscure auditory dysfunction—1. Auditory and psychological factors. Ear Hear 1989;10(3):200–208

Saunders GH, Haggard MP. The clinical assessment of "Obscure Auditory Dysfunction" (OAD) 2. Case control analysis of determining factors. Ear Hear 1992; 13(4):241–254

Saunders JC, Cohen YE, Szymko YM. The structural and functional consequences of acoustic injury in the cochlea and peripheral auditory system: a five year update. J Acoust Soc Am 1991;90(1):136–146

Saunders JC, Dear SP, Schneider ME. The anatomical consequences of acoustic injury: A review and tutorial. J Acoust Soc Am 1985;78(3):833–860

Schildroth AN. Congenital cytomegalovirus and deafness. Am J Audiol 1994;3:27–38

Schmiedt RA. Acoustic injury and the physiology of hearing. J Acoust Soc Am 1984;76(5):1293–1317

Schouten JT, Lockhart DW, Rees TS, Collier AC, Marra CM. 2006. A prospective study of hearing changes after beginning zidovudine or didanosine in HIV-1 treatment-naïve people. BMC Infectious Diseases 6, 28–33. (Available as http://www.biomedcentral. com/1471-2334/6/28)

Schrauwen I, Weegerink NJ, Fransen E, et al. A new locus for otosclerosis, OTSC10, maps to chromosome 1q41-44. Clin Genet 2011;79(5):495–497

Schuknecht HF. Presbycusis. Laryngoscope 1955;65(6): 402–419

Schuknecht HF. Further observations on the pathology of presbycusis. Arch Otolaryngol 1964;80:369–382

Schuknecht F. 1974. Pathology of the Ear. Cambridge: Harvard University Press

Schwartz RG, Mody M, Petinou K. 1997. Phonological acquisition and otitis media: speech perception and speech production. In: Roberts J, Wallace I, Henderson F, eds. Otitis Media in Young Children: Medical, Developmental and Educational Considerations. Baltimore, MD: Brookes

Shallop JK, Peterson A, Facer GW, Fabry LB, Driscoll CLW. Cochlear implants in five cases of auditory neuropathy: postoperative findings and progress. Laryngoscope 2001;111(4 Pt 1):555–562

Shambaugh GE Jr, Causse J. Ten years experience with fluoride in otosclerotic (otospongiotic) patients. Ann Otol Rhinol Laryngol 1974;83(5):635–642

Shargorodsky J, Curhan GC, Farwell WR. Prevalence and characteristics of tinnitus among US adults. Am J Med 2010;123(8):711–718

Shea JJ Jr. Fenestration of the oval window. Ann Otol Rhinol Laryngol 1958;67(4):932–951

Shimizu H. Childhood hearing impairment. AAS Bull 1992;17:15–37

Shivashankar N, Satishchandra P, Shashikala HR, Gore M. Primary auditory neuropathy—an enigma. Acta Neurol Scand 2003;108(2):130–135

Sininger YS, Hood LJ, Starr A, Berlin CI, Picton TW. Hearing loss due to auditory neuropathy. Audiol Today 1995;7:10–13

Sininger YS, Trautwein P. Electrical stimulation of the auditory nerve via cochlear implants in patients with auditory neuropathy. Ann Otol Rhinol Laryngol Suppl 2002;189:29–31

Smith RJH, Shearer AE, Hildebrand MS, Van Camp G. 2013. Deafness and hereditary hearing loss overview. [Jan. 3, 2013 revision.] In Pagon RA, Adam MP, Bird TD, Dolan CR, Fong C-T, Karen Stephens K (Eds.): GeneReview [Internet]. Seattle, WA: University of Washington. Available at: http://www.ncbi.nlm.nih.gov/books/NBK1434/

Snow J, ed. 2004 Tinnitus: Theory and Management. Hamilton, Canada: BC Decker

Solomon LR, Evanson JM, Canty DP, Gill NW. Effect of calcitonin treatment on deafness due to Paget's disease of bone. BMJ 1977;2(6085):485–487

Spoor A. Presbycusis values in relation to noise induced hearing loss. Int Audiol 1967;6:48–57

Sprung J, Bourke DL, Contreras MG, Warner ME, Findlay J. Perioperative hearing impairment. Anesthesiology 2003;98(1):241–257

Stagno S. 1990. Cytomegalovirus. In: Remington J, Klein J, eds. Infectious Diseases of the Fetus and Newborn Infant, 3rd ed. Philadelphia, PA: WB Saunders; 240–281

Starr A, Picton TW, Sininger Y, Hood LJ, Berlin CI. Auditory neuropathy. Brain 1996;119(Pt 3):741–753

Starr A, Zeng FG, Michalewski HJ. 2008. Perspectives on auditory neuropathy: disorders of inner hair cell, auditory nerve, and their synapse. In: Dallos P, Oertel D, eds. The Senses: A Comprehensive Reference, Vol. 3: Audition; 397–142. Available at: http://www.healthaffairs.uci.edu/hesp/publications/The%20Senses_AN.pdf

Stein L, Tremblay K, Pasternak J, Banerjee S, Lindemann K, Kraus N. Brainstem abnormalities in neonates with normal otoacoustic emissions. Semin Hear 1996; 17:197–213

Stein LK, Boyer KM. Progress in the prevention of hearing loss in infants. Ear Hear 1994;15(2):116–125

Stool SE, Berg AO, Berman S, et al. 1994. Otitis Media with Effusion in Young Children: Clinical Practice Guideline. AHCPR publ. no. 94-0622. Rockville, MD: Agency for Health Care Policy & Research, Public Health Service, U.S. Department of Health & Human Services

Strasnick B, Jacobson JT. Teratogenic hearing loss. J Am Acad Audiol 1995;6(1):28–38

Suzuki M, Hashimoto S, Kano S, Okitsu T. Prevalence of acoustic neuroma associated with each configuration of pure tone audiogram in patients with asymmetric sensorineural hearing loss. Ann Otol Rhinol Laryngol 2010;119(9):615–618

Swartz JD, Harnsberger HR, eds. 1998. Imaging of the Temporal Bone, 3rd ed. New York, NY: Thieme

Teele DW, Klein JO, Rosner BA. Otitis media with effusion during the first three years of life and development of speech and language. Pediatrics 1984;74(2):282–287

Thys M, Van Den Bogaert K, Iliadou V, et al. A seventh locus for otosclerosis, OTSC7, maps to chromosome 6q13-16.1. Eur J Hum Genet 2007;15(3):362–368

Tomek MS, Brown MR, Mani SR, et al. Localization of a gene for otosclerosis to chromosome 15q25-q26. Hum Mol Genet 1998;7(2):285–290

Toriello HV, Smith SD, eds. 2013. Smith Hereditary Hearing Loss and Its Syndromes, 3rd ed. Oxford: Oxford University Press

Tos M. 1995. Manual of Middle Ear Surgery, Vol. 2: Mastoid Surgery and Reconstructive Procedures. Stuttgart, Germany: Thieme Medical Publishers

Tos M. 1993. Manual of Middle Ear Surgery, Vol. 1: Approaches, Myringoplasty, Ossiculoplasty, and Tympanoplasty. Stuttgart, Germany: Thieme

Tos M, Stangerup SE, Cayé-Thomasen P, Tos T, Thomsen J. What is the real incidence of vestibular schwannoma? Arch Otolaryngol Head Neck Surg 2004;130(2): 216–220

Trautwein PG, Sininger YS, Nelson R. Cochlear implantation of auditory neuropathy. J Am Acad Audiol 2000; 11(6):309–315

Tramo MJ, Bharucha JJ, Musiek FE. Music perception and cognition following bilateral lesions of auditory cortex. J Cogn Neurosci 1990;2(3):195–212

Tsue TT, Oesterle EC, Rubel EW. Hair cell regeneration in the inner ear. Otolaryngol Head Neck Surg 1994;111(3 Pt 1):281–301

Tyler RS, ed. 2000. Handbook of Tinnitus. San Diego, CA: Singular

Tyler RS, ed. 2006. Tinnitus Treatments: Clinical Protocols. New York, NY: Thieme

Valtonen H, Tuomilehto H, Qvarnberg Y, Nuutinen J. A 14-year prospective follow-up study of children treated early in life with tympanostomy tubes. Part 1: Clinical outcomes. Arch Otolaryngol Head Neck Surg 2005a;131(4):293–298

Valtonen H, Tuomilehto H, Qvarnberg Y, Nuutinen J. A 14-year prospective follow-up study of children treated early in life with tympanostomy tubes. Part 2: Hearing outcomes. Arch Otolaryngol Head Neck Surg 2005b;131(4):299–303

Van Camp G, Smith RJH. 2013. The Hereditary Hearing Loss Homepage. [Oct. 18, 2013 update.] Available at http://hereditaryhearingloss.org/

Van De Water TR, Staecker H, eds. 2005. Otolaryngology: Basic Science and Clinical Review. New York, NY: Thieme

Van Den Bogaert K, De Leenheer EM, Chen W, et al. A fifth locus for otosclerosis, OTSC5, maps to chromosome 3q22-24. J Med Genet 2004;41(6):450–453

Van Laer L, Cryns K, Smith RJH, Van Camp G. Nonsyndromic hearing loss. Ear Hear 2003;24(4):275–288

Varga R, Avenarius MR, Kelley PM, et al. OTOF mutations revealed by genetic analysis of hearing loss families including a potential temperature sensitive auditory neuropathy allele. J Med Genet 2006;43(7):576–581

Vermiglio AJ, Soli SD, Freed DJ, Fisher LM. The relationship between high-frequency pure-tone hearing loss, hearing in noise test (HINT) thresholds, and the articulation index. J Am Acad Audiol 2012;23(10):779–788

Vernon JA. Pathophysiology of tinnitus: a special case—hyperacusis and a proposed treatment. Am J Otol 1987;8(3):201–202

Vernon JA. Hyperacusis: testing, treatments and a possible mechanism. Aust N Z J Audiol 2002;24:68–73

Vieira AB, Greco DB, Teófilo MM, Gonçalves DU. Manifestações otoneurológicas associadas à terapia anti-retroviral. Rev Soc Bras Med Trop 2008;41(1):65–69

Vissers LE, van Ravenswaaij CM, Admiraal R, et al. Mutations in a new member of the chromodomain gene family cause CHARGE syndrome. Nat Genet 2004;36(9):955–957

Walker GS, Evanson JM, Canty DP, Gill NW. Effect of calcitonin in deafness due to Paget's disease of skull. BMJ 1979;2(6186):364–365

Ward WD. The role of intermittence in PTS. J Acoust Soc Am 1991;90(1):164–169

Weihing J, Bellis TJ, Chermak GD, Musiek FE. 2013. Current issues in the diagnosis and treatment of CAPD in children. In Geffner D, Ross-Swain D, eds. Auditory Processing Disorders: Assessment, Management, and Treatment, 2nd ed. San Diego, CA: Plural; 3–32

Weinstein B. 2000. Geriatric Audiology. New York: Thieme.

Wetmore RF, Muntz HR, McGill TJ, eds. 2012. Pediatric Otolaryngology: Principles and Practice Pathways, 2nd ed. New York, NY: Thieme

Wilson RH, Civitello BA, Margolis RH. Influence of interaural level differences on the speech recognition masking level difference. Audiology 1985;24(1):15–24

Woods CI, Strasnick B, Jackson CG. Surgery for glomus tumors: the Otology Group experience. Laryngoscope 1993;103(11 Pt 2, Suppl 60):65–70

Wullstein HL, Wullstein S. 1990. Tympanoplasty: Osteoplastic Epitympanoplasty. Stuttgart, Germany: Thieme

Xu H, Kotak VC, Sanes DH. Conductive hearing loss disrupts synaptic and spike adaptation in developing auditory cortex. J Neurosci 2007;27(35):9417–9426

Yee AL, Cantekin EI. Effect of changes in systemic oxygen tension on middle ear gas exchange. Ann Otol Rhinol Laryngol 1986;95(4 Pt 1):369–372

Zeng FG, Liu S. Speech perception in individuals with auditory neuropathy. J Speech Lang Hear Res 2006;49(2):367–380

Zhou G, Gopen Q, Poe DS. Clinical and diagnostic characteristics of canal dehiscence syndrome: a great otologic mimicker. Otol Neurotol 2007;28:920–926

7 Acoustic Immittance Assessment

■ Immittance

We learned in Chapter 1 that **acoustic immittance** is the general term used to describe the various aspects of acoustic impedance and admittance. Let us quickly review the major terms. **Acoustic impedance** (Z_a) is the opposition to the flow of sound energy, measured in ohms. Acoustic impedance is the ratio of sound pressure (P) to sound flow, or volume velocity (U); or

$$Z_a = P / U$$

The reciprocal of acoustic impedance is **acoustic admittance** (Y_a), expressed in acoustic **millimhos (mmhos)**. Acoustic admittance is the ease of sound flow, or

$$Y_a = U / P$$

Acoustic impedance is composed of (1) a frictional component called **acoustic resistance** (R_a), (2) a stiffness component called **negative (stiffness) acoustic reactance** ($-X_a$), and (3) a mass component called **positive (mass) acoustic reactance** ($+X_a$). Their reciprocals are respectively the components of acoustic admittance: (1) **acoustic conductance** (G_a), (2) **positive (compliant or stiffness) acoustic susceptance** ($+B_a$), and (3) **negative (mass) acoustic susceptance** ($-B_a$).

The immittance of the ear is derived from its various sources of mechanical and acoustical springiness, mass, and resistance (Van Camp, Margolis, Wilson, Creten, & Shanks 1986): (1) The *stiffness (springiness) components* come from the volumes of air in the outer ear and middle ear spaces, the tympanic membrane, and the tendons and ligaments of the ossicles. (2) The *mass components* are due to the ossicles, the pars flaccida of the eardrum, and the perilymph. (3) *Resistance (friction)* is introduced by the perilymph, the mucous membrane linings of the middle ear spaces, the narrow passages between the middle ear and mastoid air cavities, and also by the tympanic membrane and the various middle ear tendons and ligaments. Contractions of the middle ear muscles also change the immittance of the ear, usually by increasing the stiffness component. Various pathologies cause changes in the admittance characteristics of the ear that can help us to detect their presence and to distinguish among them. This is why we use acoustic immittance testing in clinical audiology. Admittance measurements are employed clinically because they are more straightforward than those using impedance. The acoustic admittance characteristics of the ear can be assessed using a device such as the one described in **Fig. 7.1**.

The acoustic immittance of the ear is measured by inserting an ear piece called a **probe tip** into the ear canal. The probe tip is encased in a flexible plastic cuff to create an airtight connection between the ear canal and the probe tip, called a **hermetic seal**. The probe tip includes four tubes. One tube is connected to a **receiver** (loudspeaker), which is used to deliver a tone into the ear canal. This sound is called the **probe tone**. The second tube is connected to a measuring **microphone** and is used to monitor the probe sound within the ear canal. The third tube is connected to an air **pressure pump** and **manometer** (pressure meter), and the fourth tube connects to another receiver used to present stimuli for testing the acoustic reflex. In addition to the probe tip in one ear, a second earphone goes to the opposite ear and is used for acoustic reflex tests. The latter earphone may be a standard audiometric earphone or an insert receiver, depending on the device being used. The acoustic admittance (in mmhos or ml) measured with such a device is displayed on a video screen or meter and is usually plotted on paper. **Fig. 7.2** shows a photograph of a typical clinical acoustic immittance instrument.

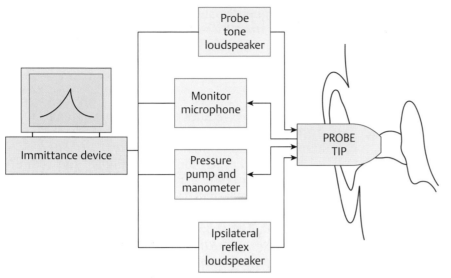

Fig. 7.1 Block diagram of the major components of a clinical acoustic immittance device.

The process of measuring the ear's admittance employs the first two tubes just described, i.e., those connected to the receiver that produces the probe tone, and to the measuring microphone. The basic approach is to introduce an 85 dB sound pressure level (SPL) probe tone into the ear canal, where it will be affected by the admittance properties of the ear. This will be revealed as an increase or decrease in the level of the probe tone as it is monitored by the measuring microphone. The details of immittance device technology are beyond the scope of this book, but the beginning student should be aware that instruments called **bridges** involve a manual intensity adjustment to bring the probe level in the ear to 85 dB SPL, whereas those referred to as **meters** use an automatic volume control to keep the probe level at 85 dB SPL. In addition to measuring overall admittance (Y), most admittance meters also provide separate measurements of susceptance (B) and conductance (G). This is done by analyzing the monitored signal in terms of in-phase (for G) and out-of-phase (for B) components. The characteristics and calibration of acoustic immittance devices are given in the ANSI S3.39 (2012) standard.

Most routine immittance tests use a 226 Hz (or a 220 Hz) probe tone. Low-frequency probe tones such as these were originally chosen because they are sensitive to changes in stiffness reactance, comprising a major part of the normal ear's impedance. In addition, admittance devices are calibrated in terms of the admittance of an **equivalent volume** of air. In other words, when the meter indicates that the admittance of an ear is 1.8 mmhos at 226 Hz, it means that the admittance of the ear corresponds to that of a 1.8 ml (ml) volume of air. Let us see why. Suppose we have

several stainless steel containers (i.e., hard-walled cavities) with various volumes, ranging from perhaps 0.2 to 2.5 ml. The air volume in such a cavity constitutes an acoustical spring, so that its admittance is essentially a compliant susceptance (and its impedance a stiffness reactance). Inserting our probe tip into each of these containers would show that admittance increases (or the impedance decreases) as the volume of the cavity becomes larger. Repeating this experiment with different probe tone frequencies in the same cavity would result in different amounts of admittance at each frequency. This reflects the fact that admittance depends on frequency. We would also find that admittance (in mmhos) is equal to the volume (in ml when the probe tone is 226 Hz). For

Fig. 7.2 An example of a clinical acoustic immittance device.

example, the acoustic admittance (Y_a) at 226 Hz will be 2.0 mmhos for a 2 ml container, 1.2 mmhos for a 1.2 ml container, 0.3 mmho for a 0.3 ml volume, etc. This is why 226 Hz has become the preferred low-frequency probe tone frequency. Higher-frequency probe tones provide other kinds of information and are often used as well.

■ Immittance at the Plane of the Eardrum

For diagnostic purposes we are mainly concerned with the immittance of the middle ear because it provides information about (1) middle ear pathologies and (2) middle ear muscle contractions due to the acoustic reflex. However, the probe tip monitors the immittance of the ear from the perspective of its location, which is in the general vicinity of the ear canal entrance. Thus, the probe tip measures the *total immittance* of the ear, which includes the combined effects of the outer ear and the middle ear. This is a problem because ear canal volume (size) is usually not clinically relevant, yet its influence on the total immittance value (at the probe tip) is often big enough to cloud the effects of the clinically significant middle ear immittance value. For example, a patient with abnormally low middle ear admittance due to a conductive disorder may have a normal total admittance value due to a large ear canal volume. Another individual whose middle ear is normal might seem to have unusually low total admittance because her ear canal volume is quite small. A third patient might have low total admittance due to otitis media when first evaluated. The middle ear problem might be completely resolved (i.e., the middle ear immittance has returned to normal) when she returns for reassessment, but the total Y_a might still be abnormally low simply because her outer ear volume was made to appear smaller by a very deeply inserted probe tip. This can happen because the volume under the probe tip will be different depending on how deeply it has been inserted.

We must remove the outer ear component from the total admittance value at the probe tip to get an undistorted representation of the middle ear's admittance at the eardrum. In other words, removing the effect of the ear canal moves the measurement location from the end of the probe tip to the *plane of the tympanic membrane*. We can achieve this goal by taking advantage of the fact that total admittance (Y_{TOTAL}) is simply the sum of the admittances of the outer ear (Y_{OE}) and the middle ear (Y_{ME})[1]:

$$Y_{TOTAL} = Y_{OE} + Y_{ME}$$

Consequently, subtracting the admittance of the outer ear from the total admittance leaves the middle ear admittance, which is the value that we need:

$$Y_{ME} = Y_{TOTAL} - Y_{OE}$$

This simple, additive relationship is one of the main reasons why we use measurements based on admittance rather than impedance.[2]

The procedure for determining the admittance of the middle ear (i.e., at the plane of the ear drum) is simple and straightforward: The first step is to measure the total admittance (Y_{TOTAL}) of the ear (**Fig. 7.3a**). The second step is to measure the ear's admittance again while pressure is being exerted on the tympanic membrane. This measurement reflects the admittance of the outer ear (or ear canal) alone, and is depicted in **Fig. 7.3b**. The pressure change is accomplished using the pressure pump connected to one of the tubes in the probe tip. The rationale for this tactic is that the heightened air pressure puts the eardrum under so much tension that it acts like a hard wall, so that essentially no sound energy can be transmitted into the middle ear. This strategy prevents the probe tip from measuring the admittance of the middle ear. In this case, we say that the middle ear has been excluded from the measurement. Hence, the admittance obtained under these conditions comes from the outer ear alone.

We now know the total admittance (of the outer and middle ear combined) from the first measurement and the admittance of the outer ear from the second measurement. The third step (**Fig. 7.3c**) is to figure out the previously unknown middle ear admittance (Y_{ME}) by simply subtracting the outer ear admittance (Y_{OE}) from the total admittance (Y_{TOTAL}).

■ Tympanometry

Tympanometry involves measuring the acoustic admittance of the ear with various amounts of air pressure in the ear canal. We can control the amount

---

[1] Y_{ME} can also called Y_{TM}, which stands for the admittance at the plane of the tympanic membrane.

[2] The equivalent impedance formula is more complicated:

$$Z_{ME} = \frac{\left(Z_{OE}\, Z_{TOTAL} \right)}{\left(Z_{OE} - Z_{TOTAL} \right)}$$

where Z_{TOTAL} is the total impedance, Z_{OE} is outer ear impedance, and Z_{ME} is middle ear impedance.

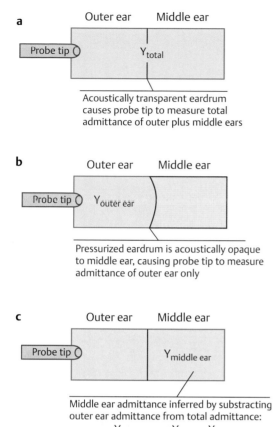

Acoustically transparent eardrum causes probe tip to measure total admittance of outer plus middle ears

Pressurized eardrum is acoustically opaque to middle ear, causing probe tip to measure admittance of outer ear only

Middle ear admittance inferred by substracting outer ear admittance from total admittance:

$$Y_{middle\ ear} = Y_{total} - Y_{outer\ ear}$$

Fig. 7.3 **(a)** Total admittance (Y_{TOTAL}) at the probe tip includes the combined admittances of the outer and middle ear. **(b)** The middle ear is excluded from the admittance measurement by using air pressure to tense the eardrum. The probe tip now registers the admittance of just the outer ear (Y_{OE}). **(c)** Admittance at the plane of the drum, or middle ear admittance (Y_{ME}), is inferred by subtracting Y_{OE} from Y_{TOTAL}.

of air pressure in the ear canal because the probe tip makes an hermetic seal with the ear canal, and one of its tubes is connected to an air pump and manometer. The amount of air pressure is expressed in terms of **dekapascals (daPa)** or of millimeters of water pressure (mm H_2O),[3] relative to the atmospheric pressure in the room where the test is being done. Hence, *0 daPa* implies that the pressure in the ear canal is equal to the atmospheric pressure, *positive pressure* (e.g., +100 daPa) means that the ear canal pressure is greater than atmospheric pressure, and *negative pressure* (e.g., –100 daPa) means it is less than

---

[3] The relationship between these two units of pressure is so close (1 daPa = 1.02 mm H_2O, and 1 mm H_2O = 0.98 daPa) that we can think of them interchangeably for most purposes.

atmospheric pressure. This information is shown on a diagram called a **tympanogram (Fig. 7.4a)**, with admittance in mmhos or (or equivalent volume in ml) on the y-axis, and pressure in daPa (or mm H_2O) on the x-axis. Notice in the figure that atmospheric pressure (0 daPa) is in the middle, with positive pressure increasing to the right and negative pressure increasing to the left.

Because most instruments generate tympanograms automatically, we can concentrate on what is happening and why. (Here, as elsewhere, it is assumed that the ear and related structures have already been inspected.) The first step in tympanometry is to properly insert the probe so that it makes a hermetic seal with the external auditory meatus. The probe tip should face the drum and not the ear canal wall, and the path to the tympanic membrane should not be blocked. Cerumen will be problematic if it gets into the probe tip tubes or completely obstructs the path to the tympanic membrane, but the simple presence of some wax is usually not a problem. The next step is to select the probe frequency and the admittance parameter(s) to be measured. We will measure overall acoustic admittance (Y) with a 226 Hz probe tone. The appropriate button(s) on the immittance device are then pushed to initiate the following tympanometry procedure.

The 226 Hz probe tone is turned on and the pressure in the ear canal is then raised to +200 daPa. This amount of positive pressure is usually assumed to tense the eardrum sufficiently to prevent the admittance of the middle ear from being measured, as described in the previous section and illustrated in **Fig. 7.3b**. A useful analogy is to imagine that the +200 daPa pressure causes the tympanic membrane to become "opaque" to sound, so that the probe cannot "see" the middle ear through it. Thus, the admittance obtained at +200 daPa is assumed to represent just the outer ear. In **Fig. 7.4a**, the admittance at +200 daPa is 1.0 mmho (*point 1*). This means that the acoustic admittance of the outer ear is 1.0 mmho, and that the ear canal volume is 1.0 ml because mmhos equals volume at 226 Hz. The air pressure is then decreased at a steady rate while we continue to measure the admittance. Notice that the tympanogram curve slowly rises as the pressure decreases below +200 daPa. The total admittance rises by ~ 0.1 mmho, to reach 1.1 mmhos, when the pressure is +100 daPa (*point 2*). It then increases more rapidly as the pressure drops further, and achieves 1.75 mmhos at 0 daPa, or at atmospheric pressure (*point 3*).

Why is this happening and what does it mean? As the pressure in the ear canal is steadily reduced, the tension on the tympanic membrane also diminishes. The middle ear is no longer being completely blocked from the view of the probe tip. Instead, the probe tip

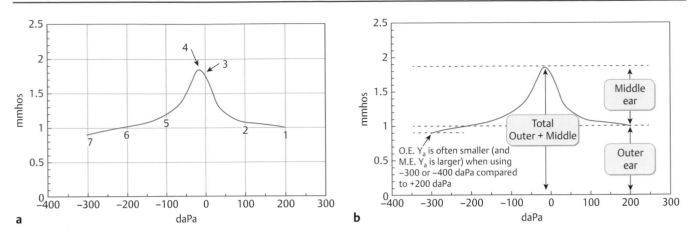

Fig. 7.4 **(a)** Example of an admittance (Y) tympanogram obtained at 226 Hz (or 220 Hz). Numbers refer to the text. **(b)** The same 226 Hz admittance tympanogram labeled to show total acoustic admittance, outer ear acoustic admittance, and middle ear (or peak-compensated static) acoustic admittance.

is now picking up more and more of the middle ear's admittance. The less the pressure, the less the tension on the eardrum, and the more the middle ear contributes. It is as though the eardrum has changed from being completely "opaque" to being progressively more "translucent." Because we know that 1.0 mmho is coming from the ear canal, we can deduce that the additional amounts of admittance (above 1.0 mmho) must be coming from the middle ear. Hence, the 1.75 mmhos of total admittance at 0 daPa represents 1.0 mmho from the ear canal and 0.75 mmho from the middle ear.

Returning to the tympanometry procedure, the pressure continues to be reduced below 0 daPa. Air is now being pumped out of the ear canal instead of into it, so that the pressure is becoming increasingly negative. We see that the admittance continues rising until it reaches a maximum of 1.85 mmhos when the pressure in the outer ear is −15 daPa (*point 4*). The total admittance then begins to fall again as the negative pressure increases. The maximum point is called the **peak** of the tympanogram. Using our visual analogy, this is where there is no longer any tension being imposed on the tympanic membrane, so that it becomes "transparent," allowing the probe tip to "see" all of the middle ear admittance. Because we know that the maximum (or peak) *total* admittance is 1.85 mmhos and that the *outer ear* admittance is 1.0 mmho, we can deduce that the *middle ear* admittance is 0.85 mmho. (The middle ear admittance is often referred to as the *static* admittance, or more accurately as *peak-compensated static* admittance, discussed below.)

By reducing the pressure below 0 daPa we are actually increasing the negative pressure. This causes the admittance to fall to 1.2 mmhos at −100 daPa (*point 5*), and to 1.0 mmho at −200 daPa (*point 6*). The falling admittance values indicate that the negative pressure is tensing the tympanic membrane, so that it again becomes progressively more opaque to sound. Continuing to increase the negative pressure causes the admittance to fall to only 0.9 mmho at −300 daPa (*point 7*), which is the lowest pressure used here. Thus, the admittance at −300 daPa is actually smaller than it was at +200 daPa. This means that the middle ear can be excluded from the measurement by applying either positive or negative pressure (i.e., at *point 1 or 7*; these two points are often called the positive and negative "tails").

Even though many audiologists use +200 daPa to estimate outer ear volume, the lowest point on the tympanogram is often obtained at −300 to −400 daPa. Compared with +200 daPa, it has been shown that −400 daPa more effectively removes the middle ear admittance and thus provides a more accurate measure of the outer ear volume (Shanks & Lilly 1981). It is suggested that (1) tympanograms should be obtained over a pressure range from +200 daPa down to −400 daPa (or at least −300 daPa); and that (2) the admittance of the middle ear should be based on (a) the tympanogram peak as the total admittance value and (b) the lower of the two "tails" as the outer ear admittance value.

Fig. 7.4a is redrawn in **Fig. 7.4b** to summarize the major components of the typical 226 Hz (or 220 Hz) tympanogram. Because the y-axis shows admittance in mmhos (or equivalent volume in ml), the overall height of the peak relative to 0 mmhos gives total admittance, and the overall height of the "tail" (at +200 daPa or −300 daPa) gives the outer ear volume. The height of the tympanogram's peak above its own baseline (i.e., one of the two tails) gives the middle ear admittance.

The peak of the tympanogram also provides us with an estimate of the pressure within the middle ear, which is −15 daPa in this example. Here is why: Recall that we exclude the middle ear by using air pressure to stress the eardrum. This stress occurs because there is more pressure on one side of the tympanic membrane than on the other (higher pressure in the outer ear than in the middle ear, or vice versa). The admittance will be highest (the peak) when the eardrum is not experiencing any stress due to a pressure difference. Thus, the positive or negative pressure used to obtain the peak pressure should be the same as the pressure that exists on the other side of the eardrum, that is, within the middle ear. This is so because having the same pressure on both sides of the eardrum will result in the least tension on the drum, and hence the highest total admittance value, so that the tympanogram peak provides us with an estimate of the pressure inside the middle ear.

Interpreting 226 Hz (Low-Frequency) Tympanograms

The major considerations that come into play when interpreting 226 Hz (or 220 Hz) tympanograms include static acoustic admittance, tympanometric gradient or width, ear volume, the pressure at which the tympanometric peak occurs, and the shape of the tympanogram. It is also possible to categorize tympanograms into a reasonably small number of types that summarize the majority of configurations found clinically. Several systems have been proposed for classifying 220 Hz (226 Hz) tympanograms (Lidén 1969; Jerger 1970; Lidén, Peterson, & Björkman 1970; Jerger, Anthony, Jerger, & Mauldin 1974; Lidén, Harford, & Hallén 1974; Feldman 1975; Paradise, Smith, & Bluestone 1976; Silman & Silverman 1991). The most widely utilized tympanogram classification system was originated by Jerger (1970). **Fig. 7.5** shows most of the tympanogram types in this system. These types were based on relative tympanograms obtained with an immittance bridge, and this format is retained in the figure. Notice that these tympanograms are expressed in arbitrary compliance units instead of absolute admittance in mmhos (static acoustic admittance and ear canal volume were measured separately).

Type A tympanograms had a distinctive peak in the vicinity of atmospheric pressure and were typical of normal patients, as well as those with otosclerosis. If the type A tympanogram had a very shallow peak, it was classified as type A_S, which was generally associated with otosclerosis but could also occur with otitis media. In contrast, very high (deep) type A tympanograms were designated as type A_D. These were found in otherwise normal ears that had scarred or flaccid eardrums, or in cases of ossicular interruptions. The type A_{DD} tympanogram was so deep that the peak was off-scale, and was found in ears with ossicular discontinuities.

Type B tympanograms were essentially flat across the pressure range, and were characteristic of patients with middle ear fluid and cholesteatoma. However, type B tympanograms can also be caused by entities such as eardrum perforations or impacted cerumen (or other obstructions) in the ear canal.

Type C tympanograms had negative pressure peaks beyond −100 daPa (mm H_2O), indicating negative middle ear pressure. They were associated with Eustachian tube disorders, and were also found in cases of middle ear fluid.

Not shown in the figure are tympanograms with notched peaks, which were classified as **type D** if the notch was narrow and **type E** if it was wide. These are rare occurrences when using 226 Hz (220 Hz) probe tones. Type D was associated with hypermobile or scarred (but otherwise normal) eardrums, whereas type E was found in cases of ossicular disruption.

Static Acoustic Immittance

Static acoustic immittance is the immittance of the middle ear at some "representative" air pressure. It was originally considered to be the middle ear impedance or admittance obtained under conditions of atmospheric pressure (Zwislocki & Feldman 1970; Feldman 1975, 1976). This point might seem confusing because we pressurized the ear to figure out the middle ear admittance. However, remember that the *total* admittance can be measured *without* applying any pressure, that is, at atmospheric pressure of 0 daPa. Pressure is used to stiffen the eardrum to obtain the outer ear component. This "pressurized" outer ear value is then *removed* from the total admittance at atmospheric pressure, leaving the middle ear admittance at the eardrum, which is also at atmospheric pressure. In any case, this is the situation that presumably exists in the patient's ear "under regular conditions" when the probe tip is not there. On the tympanogram, it is the value of Y_{ME} obtained at 0 daPa, which is 0.75 mmho in **Fig. 7.4a** (*point 3*). We will call this measurement "atmospheric static."

Fig. 7.5 Stylized examples of Jerger's (1970) classical 220 Hz (226 Hz) tympanogram types (shown in terms of the arbitrary compliance units used by relative immittance devices).

The alternative approach is to measure static admittance at whatever pressure corresponds to the peak of the tympanogram (Brooks 1969; Jerger 1970; Jerger, Jerger, & Mauldin 1972; Jerger, Anthony, et al 1974; Margolis & Popelka 1975). We will call this value "peak static." (More accurately, it is the *peak-compensated static* admittance.) It occurs at −15 daPa in **Fig. 7.4a**, where Y_{ME} is 0.85 mmho (*point 4*). The peak static method is preferred because it provides a more stable picture of middle ear admittance (Wiley, Oviatt, & Block 1987).

The static acoustic admittance measurements obtained from a patient are compared with the applicable normative admittance values. These norms are usually expressed as 90% normal ranges, which means that they include the admittance values that fall between the 5th and 95th percentiles for a large group of subjects with normal middle ears. **Table 7.1** shows representative normal ranges for the static acoustic admittance values with a 220/226 Hz probe tone in adults and children at least 6 months of age. Infants under 6 months are tested using higher-frequency probe tones, and are discussed later in this chapter.

Table 7.2 shows 90% normal ranges for static acoustic admittance values for older adults from two large-sample studies (Wiley, Nondahl, Cruickshanks, & Tweed 2005; Golding et al 2007). Notice that these ranges get wider with increasing age among older adults, and also that there are considerable differences between the two sets of results.

Two procedural variables warrant special mention. One of these is the effect of which "tail" is used for the ear canal value, as already discussed. The

other major procedural variable is pump speed, or how fast the pressure is changed while obtaining the tympanogram. As illustrated in **Table 7.3**, different pump speeds result in different normal ranges. This is an important variable to consider when interpreting tympanograms, especially when fast pump speeds are used, as is often the case during screening tests.

Table 7.1 Representative 90% normal ranges for peak static acoustic admittance (mmhos) using 220 and 226 Hz probe tones

Source	90% Normal range
Adults	
Wiley (1989)	0.37–1.66
Children	
Silman, Silverman, & Arick (1992)	0.35–1.25
Infants and Toddlers ≥ 6 months	
Roush et al (1995)	
6–12 months	0.20–0.50
12–18 months	0.20–0.60
18–24 months	0.20–0.70
6–12 months	0.20–0.50
Calandruccio, Fitzgerald, & Prieve (2006)	
6–12 months	0.16–0.60
2 years	0.21–1.03

Table 7.2 Ninety percent ranges for peak static acoustic admittance (mmhos) among older adults from two large-sample studies

Age (years)	Wiley et al (2005)[a]	Golding et al (2007)
48 (49)[b]–59	0.2–1.5	0.3–2.2
60–69	0.2–1.6	0.3–2.1
70–79	0.0–1.8	0.2–2.2
≥ 80	0.0–2.0	0.2–2.5

[a]Combined across right and left ears using baseline examination data.

[b]Range: 48–59 in Wiley et al (2005), and 49–59 in Golding et al (2007).

Table 7.3 Differences in 90% normal ranges for peak static acoustic admittance (mmhos) at slow and fast pump speeds[a]

Pumpspeed	Adults[b]	Children (3–5 years)[c]
Slow (≤ 50 daPa/s)	0.50–1.75	0.35–0.90
Fast (200 daPa/s)	0.57–2.0	0.40–1.03

[a]Modified from Van Camp et al (1986).
[b]Based on data from Wilson, Shanks, and Kaplan (1984a).
[c]Based on data from Koebsell and Margolis (1986).

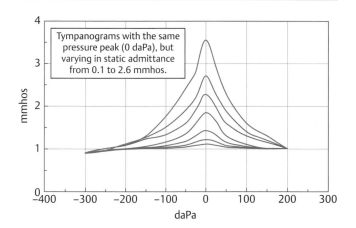

Fig. 7.6 Examples of tympanograms with static admittance values ranging from (top to bottom) 2.6, 1.7, 1.3, 0.9, 0.4, 0.2, to 0.1 mmho. These values are the distances in mmho between the height of the peaks and the ear canal value of 1.0 mmho at +200 daPa.

A given static admittance measurement is considered to be (1) within normal limits if it falls within the normal range, (2) abnormally low if it falls below the lower limit of the normal range, and (3) abnormally high if it is above the upper limit of the normal range. The seven tympanograms in **Fig. 7.6** show static admittance values ranging from 2.6 mmhos for the tympanogram with the highest peak down to only 0.1 mmho for the lowest one, which is close to being flat. Let us compare these to the normal range for adults in **Table 7.1**. The tallest tympanogram is abnormally high because its static admittance (2.6 mmhos) is well above the upper limit of 1.66 mmhos. The static value for the second tympanogram from the top is 1.7 mmhos, which is right on the upper limit (rounded to the nearest tenth of a mmho). We would probably consider it to be just within normal limits, especially if there is no air-bone-gap. (It is also within the upper limit of 1.75 mmhos in **Table 7.3**.) The third and fourth curves have static values of 1.3 and 0.9 mmhos and are clearly within normal limits. The next tympanogram (third from the bottom) shows a static admittance value of 0.4 mmho, which is just above the lower limit of 0.37. (Even though 0.4 mmho is below the 0.5 mmho lower limit in **Table 7.3**, most clinicians use lower limits closer to those in **Table 7.1**, and some use even lower criteria taken from other studies.)

The second tympanogram from the bottom in **Fig. 7.6** reveals static admittance of 0.2 mmho, and the static admittance shown on the lowest one is 0.1 mmho. Both of these are abnormally low compared with the normal range shown in **Table 7.1**.

Abnormally low static acoustic admittance corresponds to abnormally high impedance and is generally associated with disorders such as otitis media, cholesteatoma, and otosclerosis. On the other hand, abnormally high static admittance (and thus abnormally low impedance) is often associated with disorders such as ossicular discontinuity. Unfortunately,

the range of static admittance values found with the various types of disorders overlaps the normal range (Jerger 1970; Jerger, Anthony, et al 1974; Feldman 1976; Shahnaz & Polka 1997). There is even some degree of overlap between the ranges of static admittance values obtained from ears with otosclerosis and ossicular discontinuity (Silman & Silverman 1991).

If we apply the classical tympanogram types to the examples in **Fig. 7.6** we would categorize those having static admittance within the normal range as **type A**. The tympanogram with abnormally high admittance would be classified as either **type A_D** or **A_DD**. The two tympanograms with abnormally low admittance would be classified as **A_S**, although the lowest one might be considered "flat" enough to be categorized as **type B**. Notice that the tympanograms in this group have peaks at 0 daPa, so that the type A categories are straightforward. If these tympanograms had peak pressures of perhaps –165 daPa, then they would all have been classified as **type C**, and the differences in static admittance would have been obscured. (A possible exception is the lowest one, which might have been classified as type B.) This issue emphasizes the idea that details can be lost if one makes the mistake of considering tympanograms only by their letter designations.

Tympanometric Gradient and Width

We see in **Fig. 7.6** that the tympanogram peak becomes smaller as the static admittance becomes lower. If the admittance becomes low enough, then there will be no discernible peak, so that the tympanogram is described as *flat*. This is a common finding in ears with otitis media and cholesteatoma, where the static admittance may be as low as 0.06 or less (Jerger, Anthony, et al 1974). The flatness (versus peakedness) of a tympanogram can also be quantified by its **gradient**, which describes the relationship of its height and width. The gradient was originally calculated in terms of arbitrary units of compliance (Brooks 1969), as shown in **Fig. 7.7a**, and is determined as follows: (1) Draw a horizontal line where the width of the tympanogram is 100 mm H_2O (or daPa). (2) Measure the height of the peak above this line (hp), as well as the total height (ht) of the tympanogram from its peak to its baseline. In the figure hp is 3.6 compliance units and ht is 8 units. (3) Find the gradient by dividing hp/ht, which is 3.6/8 = 0.45 in the figure. The same procedure can be used to calculate the gradient of absolute tympanograms, except that the heights are measured in terms of mmhos or ml.

Tympanometric gradients less than 0.2 are considered to be abnormally low (Nozza, Bluestone, Kardatzke, & Bachman 1992) and are associated with the presence of middle ear fluid (Brooks 1969; Paradise, Smith, & Bluestone 1976; Fiellau-Nikolajsen 1983; Nozza et al 1992).

Another way to quantify the flatness of a tympanogram is to determine the **tympanometric width** (Koebsell & Margolis 1986; ASHA 1997), which is simply the width of the tympanogram in daPa measured at 50% of its static acoustic admittance value. The method for determining tympanometric width is illustrated by the example in **Fig. 7.7b**. The static admittance value is measured at the tympanogram peak and is found to be 0.85 mmho in this example. We measure down 0.425 mmho from the peak because this distance is half the static value, and draw a horizontal line intersecting both sides of the tympanogram. Next, we draw vertical lines from these intersection points down to the x-axis. The tympanogram width is the distance between these two lines. In the example the tympanogram width is 80 daPa because the vertical lines cross the x-axis at –40 daPa and +40 daPa (which are 80 daPa apart).

Tympanometric widths that are too wide are associated with middle ear effusion, and normative data may be used to help determine when this is the case (e.g., Koebsell & Margolis 1986; Margolis & Heller 1987; Nozza, Bluestone, Kardatzke, & Bachman 1992, 1994; Silman, Silverman, & Arick 1992; Roush, Bryant, Mundy, Zeisel, & Roberts 1995; AAA 1997; ASHA 1997; Shahnaz & Polka 1997; De Chicchis, Todd, & Nozza 2000). Representative upper cutoff values for tympanometric width are 235 daPa for infants and 200 daPa for 1-year-olds through school-age children (ASHA 1997). Typical 90% normal ranges for adults are 51 to 114 daPa (Margolis & Heller 1987) and 48 to 134 daPa (Shahnaz & Polka 1997).

Ear Volume

Tympanograms with extremely small or absent peaks are often referred to as essentially flat. These findings are usually attributed to extremely low middle ear admittance, and are typically associated with middle ear pathologies such as otitis media and cholesteatoma. However, we can reach this conclusion only if the volume (admittance at 226 Hz) measured at +200 daPa (or at –300 or –400 daPa) is attributable to the ear canal. If the volume is too large, then the

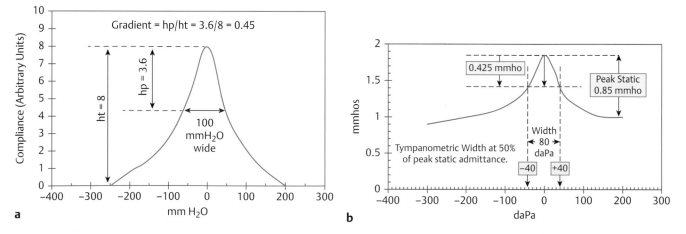

Fig. 7.7 Examples illustrating how to measure **(a)** tympanometric gradient (shown in terms of the arbitrary compliance units that were used by relative immittance bridges) and **(b)** tympanometric width.

flat tympanogram may be due to such causes as (1) a perforated tympanic membrane; (2) a patent myringotomy tube, if one is present; or (3) the absence of a hermetic seal. It is reasonable to consider the volume to be larger than normal when it exceeds 2.0 ml (mmhos) in children and 2.5 ml (mmhos) in adults (Van Camp et al 1986; Silman & Silverman 1991). On the other hand, the following causes are associated with volumes that are too small: (1) a clogged probe tip; (2) a probe tip that is pushed against the canal wall; (3) impacted cerumen or another obstruction in the ear canal; and (4) a clogged myringotomy tube if one is present. These cases are usually identified by volumes at or close to 0 ml (mmhos). **Fig. 7.8** demonstrates how the flat tympanograms associated with tympanic membrane perforation, otitis media with effusion, and a clogged probe tip are differentiated on the basis of their ear canal volumes. It is very important to keep this issue in mind when tympanograms are classified by type because the letter designation does not account for the ear volume. For example, we could not attribute the type B tympanogram in **Fig. 7.5** to middle ear effusion unless we also know the ear volume.

Tympanometric Peak Pressure

We know the pressure on the outer ear side of the eardrum because it is generated and measured using the air pump and manometer connected to the probe tip. In addition, we have learned that the tympanogram peak occurs when the same pressure exists on both sides of the tympanic membrane. Consequently, the ear canal pressure corresponding to the tympanogram peak is also an estimate of the pressure within the middle ear. **Fig. 7.9** shows otherwise identical tympanograms with peak pressures of 0, –50, –150, and –250 daPa. Notice how increasingly negative **tympanometric peak pressures** are shown moving to the left of 0 daPa. Even though "tympanometric peak pressure" and **"middle ear pressure"** are often used interchangeably, we distinguish between the two terms here to point out that they are not always the same, especially when the patient has a flaccid tympanic membrane (Elner, Ingelstedt, & Ivarsson 1971; Renvall & Lidén 1978, Margolis & Shanks 1985).

Abnormally negative tympanometric peak pressures are associated with Eustachian tube disorders, which can occur either with or without the presence of middle ear fluid. The amount of negative pressure needed to consider the tympanometric peak pressure *abnormally negative* is not clearly identifiable in the literature. Suggested cutoff values vary widely, including values such as –25 daPa (Holmquist & Miller 1972), –30 daPa (Feldman 1975), –50 daPa (Porter 1972), –l00 daPa (Jerger 1970; Jerger, Jerger, & Mauldin 1972; Jerger, Jerger, Mauldin, & Segal 1974; Fiellau-Nikolajsen 1983; Silman, Silverman, & Arick 1992), –150 daPa (Renvall & Lidén 1978; Davies, John, Jones, & Stephens 1988), –170 daPa (Brooks 1969), and –200 daPa (AAA 2012). In practice, –100 daPa appears to be a reasonable low cutoff value for tympanometric peak pressure. Lower pressures suggest the possibility of Eustachian tube dysfunction. Unfortunately, there does not seem to be a particular tympanometric peak pressure cutoff value that successfully distinguishes between the presence and absence of middle ear effusion. Several other tests of Eustachian tube function are described in the last section of this chapter.

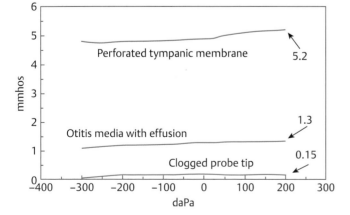

Fig. 7.8 Flat tympanograms from cases with tympanic membrane perforation (top), otitis media with effusion (middle), and a clogged probe tip (bottom). Ear canal volumes at +200 daPa are indicated for each.

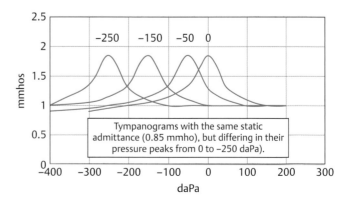

Fig. 7.9 Examples of tympanograms with tympanometric peak pressures of 0 daPa, –50 daPa, –150 daPa, and –250 daPa.

One can sometimes follow the course of recovery from a case of otitis media as tympanometric peak pressures that become progressively less negative over time (Feldman 1976). This course of events can be seen in stylized form by imagining that the series of tympanograms in **Fig. 7.9** follows a sequence going from –250 daPa toward 0 daPa over a period of several days.

Unlike the situation for negative middle ear pressure, the significance of abnormally high *positive* peak pressures (e.g., > 50 daPa) is not clear. In spite of the extensive literature on tympanometry and middle ear pathology, only a few papers have reported positive pressures in some cases of otitis media (Paradise et al 1976; Feldman 1976; Ostergard & Carter 1981). In addition, positive peak pressure has also been associated with nonpathologic causes such as rapid elevator rides, crying, or nose blowing (Harford 1980).

Tympanogram Shape

Low-frequency probe tones like 226 Hz are mainly sensitive to changes in stiffness (or compliance). The shapes of most 226 Hz (220 Hz) tympanograms do not provide much information because they are usually single-peaked or flat. The infrequent exception is the presence of a notch in the tympanogram peak. Notched tympanograms are produced when mass becomes a significant component of the ear's immittance, which occurs near and above its resonant frequency. For this reason notching is common with high-frequency probe tones, (e.g., 660 or 678 Hz) (Vanhuyse, Creten, & Van Camp 1975; Van Camp, Creten, van de Heyning, Decraemer, & Vanpeperstraete 1983; Van Camp et al 1986; Wiley, Oviatt, & Block 1987). Notching of the 226 Hz tympanogram is abnormal because it means that something is causing mass to play a greater than normal role in the ear. These changes can be produced by a scarred or flaccid tympanic membrane (even in an otherwise normal ear), as well as abnormalities such as ossicular discontinuities (which produce substantial hearing losses). Recall that these are the aberrations associated with type D and E tympanograms.

Vascular Pulsing

Although most tympanograms are smooth, they sometimes have regular ripples or undulations that are synchronized with the patient's pulse, which is their origin. Medical referral is indicated when vascular pulsing is present on the tympanogram because it tends to occur in patients with glomus jugulare tumors (Feldman 1976).

678 Hz (660 Hz) Tympanograms

"High-frequency" tympanograms are obtained with probe tones higher than the traditional "low-frequency" 226 Hz (or 220 Hz) probe tone. The "high-frequency" probe tone is usually 678 Hz (or 660 Hz). The combined use of 226 Hz and 678 Hz tympanograms is sometimes called **multiple frequency** (or **multifrequency**) **tympanometry**. However, this term is also used to describe various tympanometric methods that involve testing at many frequencies to arrive at the resonant frequency of the ear and other measures. Abnormally high resonant frequencies are associated with stiffening disorders, such as otosclerosis, whereas abnormally low resonant frequencies are associated with disorders that increase the mass component of the system, like ossicular discontinuity. The details of these and other advanced approaches are not covered here, but the interested student will find many readily available sources (e.g., Shanks, Lilly, Margolis, Wiley, & Wilson 1988; Shanks & Shelton 1991; Hunter & Margolis 1992; Margolis & Goycoolea 1993; Shahnaz & Polka 1997).

Separate tympanograms are obtained for susceptance (B) and conductance (G) when testing at 678 Hz (or 660 Hz) instead of a single admittance (Y) tympanogram. Depending on the instrumentation used, the B and G tympanograms may be obtained simultaneously (which is preferred), or they may be done one after the other. In either case, the interpretation is easier when they are plotted on the same tympanogram form.

Normal 678 (660) Hz Tympanograms

In contrast to 226 Hz tympanograms, 678Hz (660 Hz) B-G tympanograms are interpreted on the basis of their shapes and configurations (or morphology). There are four types of normal 678 Hz B-G tympanograms (Vanhuyse et al 1975; Van Camp et al 1983, 1986; Wiley et al 1987). They are named on the basis of the number of positive and negative peaks and must also meet a criterion for tympanogram width.

The first normal type of 678 Hz tympanogram is called **1B1G** because there is one peak for the B tympanogram and one peak for the G tympanogram **(Fig. 7.10a)**. The other three normal variations involve notches on one or both of the tympanograms. The second normal type has a notched peak on the B tympanogram and a single peak on the G tympanogram. Notice that the notch on the B tympanogram can be viewed as two positive peaks with a negative peak between them. The convention is to count these "peaks" or "extrema." Thus, this normal variation is called **3B1G** because B has three peaks and G has one

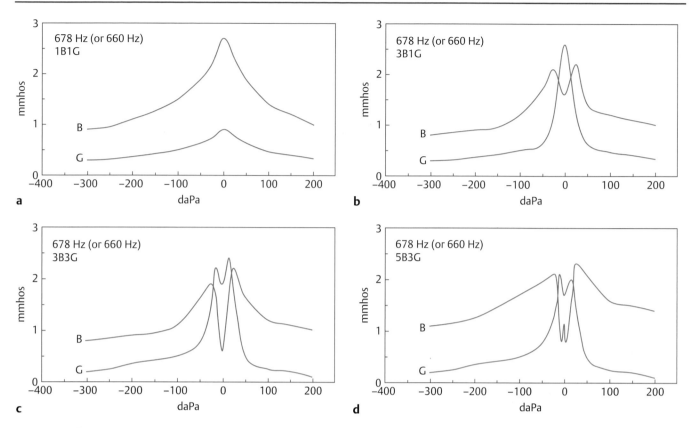

Fig. 7.10 Illustrative examples of normal B-G tympanograms obtained at 678 Hz (or 660 Hz): **(a)** 1B1G, **(b)** 3B1G, **(c)** 3B3G, and **(d)** 5B3G.

peak (**Fig. 7.10b**). The third normal variation is called **3B3G** because there are three peaks on both tympanograms (**Fig. 7.10c**). The last type of normal 678 Hz (or 660 Hz) configuration is called **5B3G** because it has five peaks on the B tympanogram and three peaks on the G tympanogram (**Fig. 7.10d**). In addition to having a maximum of five peaks for B and three peaks for G, the distance between the outermost peaks of normal 678 Hz B-G tympanograms should be (1) ≤ 75 daPa wide for 3B3G tympanograms and ≤ 100 daPa for 5B3G tympanograms, and (2) narrower for the G tympanogram than for the B tympanogram. **Table 7.4** shows the percentages of normal adults with each of the 678 Hz B-G tympanogram types.

Abnormal 678 (660) Hz Tympanograms

A 678 Hz (660 Hz) B-G tympanogram is considered abnormal if it fails to meet the criteria just outlined, that is, if it (1) has too many peaks and/or (2) is too wide. Abnormal 678 (660) Hz B-G tympanograms are principally associated with ossicular discontinuities, but they can also occur with tympanic membrane

Table 7.4 Percentages of normal 678 Hz (or 660 Hz) B-G tympanograms

	1B1G	3B1G	3B3G	5B3G
Van Camp et al (1983)	56.8	28.1	6.0	9.1
Wiley, Oviatt, & Block (1987)	75.8	17.4	5.5	1.2
Weighted average	69.4	21.0	5.7	3.9

abnormalities. We can often distinguish between them because ossicular discontinuities usually cause significant amounts of hearing loss and appreciably alter the acoustic reflex, which is generally not the case with eardrum abnormalities per se. In addition, many tympanic membrane abnormalities can be visualized otoscopically.

The 678 Hz (660 Hz) B-G tympanograms often help us to distinguish between ossicular discontinuities and other disorders, even when they are indistinguishable on the 226 Hz (220 Hz) tympanograms. **Fig. 7.11** shows 660 Hz B-G tympanograms from a case of ossicular discontinuity. This highly abnormal example is extremely wide and has an excessive number of peaks. In addition to being very abnormal this tympanogram is from a case that highlights the value of using 678 (660) Hz tympanometry. It is from a patient who previously had stapedectomy surgery in both ears for bilateral otosclerosis. He complained that the hearing in both ears worsened several years after the surgery, although he was not sure about the timing of the progression. His complaints were confirmed by much larger air-bone-gaps on his new audiogram. On the surface, this seemed to be a case of otosclerosis that progressed bilaterally after the surgery. No insights could be gleaned from the 220 Hz tympanograms. The 660 Hz tympanogram had not appreciably changed in his left ear, where the ossicular chain was again fixated by progression of the otosclerosis. However, the 660 Hz B-G tympanogram shown in the figure was a new finding in his right ear, revealing an ossicular discontinuity that occurred when the surgically installed prosthesis (Chapter 6) became dislodged.

Before leaving this topic, it is worth noting that it is possible for there to be a "stiffening" disorder like otosclerosis *medially* and a "loosening" anomaly such as a scarred or flaccid eardrum *laterally* in the same ear. Under these conditions the tympanogram will reflect characteristics of the more lateral eardrum problem (Feldman 1976).

■ Reflectance and Absorbance

We have been concentrating on *admittance* measurements using a *pure tone probe*, which is employed ubiquitously in regular audiological practice. However, the student should also be aware of another approach that measures power *reflectance* or *absorbance* across a wide range of frequencies using *wideband probe* signals like noises, chirps, and clicks. To understand reflectance, first imagine a sound going from the probe tip toward the eardrum. This is the *incident* sound. Some of the incident sound pressure might be *absorbed* into the middle ear system and some of it might be *reflected* back from the eardrum. *Pressure reflectance* is the ratio of the reflected pressure to the incident pressure, but using this measure is complicated because it also involves phase information. On the other hand, squaring the pressure reflectance yields power reflectance, which involves just a magnitude measurement without any phase information. So, in simplest terms, **power (or energy) reflectance** is the ratio of the sound reflected back

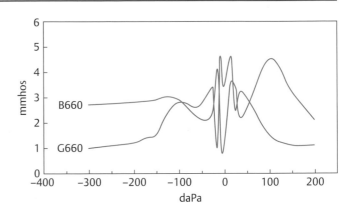

Fig. 7.11 The abnormal 660 Hz B-G tympanogram of a patient with ossicular discontinuity.

from the eardrum to the incident sound.[4] In other words, power reflectance is the proportion of the sound that is reflected from the eardrum, ranging from 0 when none of the sound is reflected to 1.0 when all of it is reflected. **Absorbance**, which is the proportion of the sound that flows into the middle ear, is simply *1 minus the reflectance*. More reflectance corresponds to less absorbance, and less reflectance corresponds to more absorbance. The term *wideband acoustic immittance* has been proposed to describe wideband reflectance and absorbance measurements, in contrast to *aural acoustic immittance*, which applies to the other measurements covered in this chapter (Feeney, Hunter, Kei, et al 2013).

Although wideband reflectance still is less common clinically than the other kinds of immittance measures we have been discussing, its use is definitely becoming more widespread. Thus, even the beginning student needs to be aware of some of its relevant features.

Reflectance and absorbance measurements are obtained clinically with instruments like the one shown in **Fig. 7.12a**, and are displayed graphically as a function of frequency between ~ 250 and 6000 Hz, as in **Fig. 7.12b**. The figure shows several idealized examples plotted in terms of power reflectance. The solid line in the figure shows the average power reflectance values at different frequencies for normal-hearing young adults, and the area shaded in gray

---

[4] For more precise definitions and rigorous explanations, see Rosowski, Stenfelt, and Lilly (2013) and Neely, Stenfelt, and Schairer (2013), as well as many of the other sources mentioned in this section.

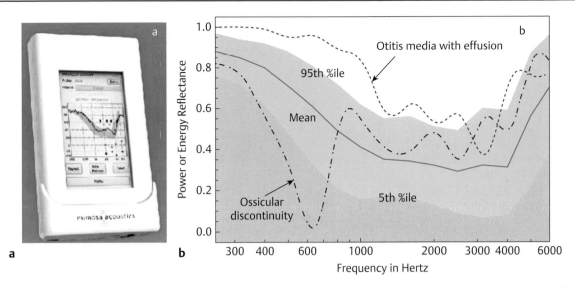

Fig. 7.12   **(a)** An example of a clinical power reflectance instrument. (Photograph courtesy of Mimosa Acoustics Inc.) **(b)** An example of mean power reflectance values as a function of frequency for young adults with normal hearing is shown by the thick solid line, and the corresponding 90% normal ranges are represented by the area shaded in gray between the 5th and 95th percentiles. The normative values shown are for Caucasian adults based on data by Shahnaz and Bork (2006) and Shaw (2009) as compiled by Shahnaz, Feeney, and Schairer (2013). Idealized examples of results from clinical cases of otitis media with effusion and ossicular discontinuity are shown by the broken lines.

shows the 90% normal range. Notice that reflectance is low between roughly 1000 and 4000 Hz, and then gets progressively higher as frequencies decrease below this range and when they increase above it.

The norms in **Fig. 7.12b** were obtained from normal-hearing Caucasian adults who were tested with a particular reflectance system. It is important to be aware that different norms must be used for Caucasian and Chinese populations (see, e.g., Shahnaz & Bork 2006; Beers, Shahnaz, Westerberg, & Kozak 2010; Shahnaz et al 2013); with children, especially newborns and infants for whom developmental changes in reflectance measures are large and clinically important (see, e.g., Keefe, Bulen, Arehart, & Burns 1993; Beers et al 2010; Werner, Levi, & Keefe 2010; Aithal, Kei, Driscoll, & Khan 2013; Kei, Sanford, Prieve, & Hunter 2013); and when using other reflectance instruments.

Reflectance can be measured clinically and provides useful information about a variety of conductive disorders in both children and adults, as well as having applications for newborn screening (e.g., Keefe et al 1993; Keefe & Simmons 2003; Jeng, Allen, Lapsley Miller, & Levitt 2008; Feeney, Grant, & Mills 2009; Shahnaz et al 2009; Beers et al 2010; Ellison et al 2012; Keefe, Sanford, Ellison, Fitzpatrick, & Gorga 2012; Hunter, Prieve, Kei, & Sanford 2013; Nakajima, Rosowski, Shahnaz, & Voss 2013; Prieve, Feeney, Stenfelt, & Shahnaz 2013). Contemporary

studies have found that similar reflectance outcomes are obtained when testing wideband reflectance at ambient air pressure and tympanometrically (e.g., Sanford, Keefe, Liu, et al 2009; Keefe et al 2012; Sanford, Hunter, Feeney, & Nakajima 2013). However, adjusting the outer ear pressure to counterbalance negative middle ear pressure (similar to measuring static immittance at TPP) has been recommended (Shaver & Sun 2013). In general, some of the key clinical findings have been that reflectance tends to be higher than normal when there is fluid in the middle ear and lower than normal when the ossicular chain is interrupted. Idealized examples of these situations are shown by the dotted lines labeled *otitis media with effusion* and *ossicular discontinuity* in **Fig. 7.12b**. Unfortunately, there is considerable overlapping of the reflectance results obtained from ears with otosclerosis and those with normal hearing.

■ The Acoustic Reflex

Presenting a sufficiently intense sound to either ear results in the contraction of the stapedius muscle in both ears; and is called the **acoustic** or **stapedius reflex**. This reflexive muscle contraction stiffens the conductive mechanism via the stapedius tendon, and therefore changes the ear's immittance. The acoustic reflex is easily measured because the immittance change is picked up by the probe tip and displayed on the immittance device meter.

Acoustic Reflex Arc

The acoustic reflex arc was described by Borg (1973), and its basic features are shown in **Fig. 7.13**. Let us follow this pathway assuming that the right ear was stimulated (highlighted by the shaded arrows in the figure). The afferent (sensory) part of the arc involves the auditory (eighth) nerve from the right ear, which goes to the right (ipsilateral) ventral cochlear nucleus. Neurons then go to the superior olivary complexes on both sides of the brainstem. The right and left superior olivary complexes send signals to the facial (seventh) nerve nuclei on their respective sides. Finally, the efferent (motor) legs of the acoustic reflex arc involve the right and left facial nerves, which direct the stapedius muscles to contract in both ears. Notice that the acoustic reflex involves the stapedius muscles. While the tensor tympani muscles do respond to extremely intense sounds, this is actually part of a startle reaction, and the accumulated evidence reveals that the acoustic reflex in humans is a stapedius reflex (Gelfand 2004). Certain kinds of nonacoustic stimulation also elicit contractions of the stapedius muscles (e.g., tactile stimulation of the external ear) or of both middle ear muscles (e.g., an air puff to the eye). These reflexes can be used in advanced diagnostic methods (Wiley & Block 1984).

Acoustic Reflex Tests

The basic acoustic reflex testing procedure involves presenting a sufficiently intense tone or noise to activate the reflex, and observing any resulting immittance change, which is usually seen as a decrease in the ear's admittance (i.e., an increase in its impedance). The immittance change caused by the contraction of the stapedius muscle is measured in the ear containing the probe tip, which is called the **probe ear**. The ear receiving the stimulus used to activate the reflex is called the **stimulus ear**. Either ear can be the stimulus ear because the stimulus can be delivered from the receiver in the probe tip (the fourth tube described earlier) or the earphone on the opposite ear. The **ipsilateral** or **uncrossed** acoustic reflex is being measured when the stimulus is presented to the probe ear, which is the same ear in which the immittance change is being monitored. In contrast, the **contralateral** or **crossed** acoustic reflex is being measured when the probe tip is in one ear and the stimulus goes to the opposite ear.

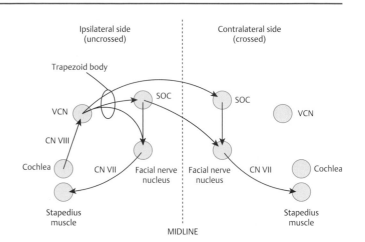

Fig. 7.13 Schematic diagram of the acoustic reflex pathways. The arrows highlight the ipsilateral (uncrossed) and contralateral (crossed) reflex arcs resulting from stimulation of one ear. Abbreviations: CN VII, seventh cranial (facial) nerve; CN VIII, eighth cranial (auditory) nerve; SOC, superior olivary complex; VCN, ventral cochlear nucleus.

It is easy to identify whether the right or left ear is being tested for the ipsilateral reflex because the reflex is activated and monitored in the same (probe) ear. However, there can be confusion about which ear is the "test ear" with contralateral reflexes because the stimulus and probe are in opposite ears. In fact, both ears (and the reflex pathway between them) are really being tested with the contralateral reflex. The convention is to identify a contralateral acoustic reflex according to the stimulated ear. Hence, a "right contralateral acoustic reflex" means that the stimulus is in the right ear (with the probe in the left ear), and a "left contralateral acoustic reflex" means that the stimulus is in the left ear (with the probe in the right ear). Another way to avoid confusion is to describe the test results as, for example, "stimulus right" or "probe left." The testing arrangements are shown schematically in **Fig. 7.14**. The usual reflex testing order is to do the left contralateral and right ipsilateral reflexes while the probe is in the right ear (**Fig. 7.14a**), and then to reverse the headset and do the right contralateral and left ipsilateral reflex test while the probe is in the left ear (**Fig. 7.14b**). To help the student sort out what goes where, **Fig. 7.15** summarizes the various reflex test arrangements in terms of both (a) the stimulus and the probe and (b) the right and left ears.

A variety of acoustic reflex tests are regularly used in clinical assessment. The two basic measurements are discussed here: the **acoustic reflex threshold**, which is the lowest stimulus level that produces a reflex response; and **acoustic reflex**

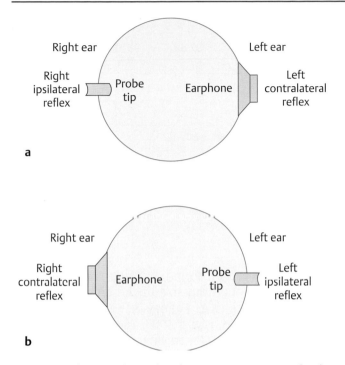

Fig. 7.14 The stimulus and probe are in opposite ears for the contralateral (crossed) acoustic reflex and in the same ear for the ipsilateral (uncrossed) acoustic reflex. Expressing the reflex according to the ear being stimulated, we measure the right ipsilateral and left contralateral reflexes when the probe is in the right ear **(a)**, and the left ipsilateral and right contralateral reflexes when the probe tip is in the left ear **(b)**.

a Arrangement in terms of stimulus and probe

TEST CONDITION	STIMULUS	PROBE
Right contralateral (crossed)	Right ear	Left ear
Left contralateral (crossed)	Left ear	Right ear
Right ipsilateral (uncrossed)	Right ear	Right ear
Left ipsilateral (uncrossed)	Left ear	Left ear

b Arrangement in terms of right ear and left ear

TEST CONDITION	RIGHT EAR	LEFT EAR
Right contralateral (crossed)	Stimulus	Probe
Left contralateral (crossed)	Probe	Stimulus
Right ipsilateral (uncrossed)	Stimulus & probe	
Left ipsilateral (uncrossed)		Stimulus & probe

Fig. 7.15 Summary of acoustic reflex testing arrangements and terminology in terms of the stimulus and probe **(a)** and the right ear and left ear **(b)**.

decay, which is a measure of how long the response lasts if the stimulus is kept on for a period of time. Some more advanced techniques include (1) **acoustic reflex magnitude and growth functions** (how the size of the response depends on stimulus level); (2) **acoustic reflex latency** (the time delay between the stimulus and the reflex response); and (3) **nonacoustic reflexes** (middle ear muscle reflexes that are stimulated tactually, electrically, or with air puffs instead of sound). The interested student will find these and related topics covered in many sources (Silman & Gelfand 1982; Bosatra, Russolo, & Silverman 1984; Silman 1984; Wiley & Block 1984; Silman & Silverman 1991; Wilson & Margolis 1991; Northern & Gabbard 1994; Gelfand 2009).

Acoustic Reflex Threshold

Acoustic reflex threshold (ART) testing involves finding the lowest level of a stimulus that causes a measurable change in acoustic immittance. **Fig. 7.16** shows the measurement of an ART under laboratory conditions and illustrates several characteristics of the reflex response. Notice that the immittance changes attributed to the reflex are associated in time with the stimulus presentations, and that the magnitude of the reflex response increases as the stimulus level is raised above the ART. Hence, we may also say that the ART is the smallest discernible immittance change that is associated in time with the presentation of a stimulus, and that responses should also be present (and generally larger) at higher stimulus levels. Clinical ARTs are usually obtained using pure tone stimuli at 500, 1000, and 2000 Hz. Even though some clinicians also use 4000 Hz, it is not recommended because even young, normal-hearing persons experience elevated ARTs at this frequency due to rapid adaptation (Gelfand 1984). Clinically, pure tone ARTs are obtained by changing the intensity of the stimulus in 5 dB steps while watching for admittance changes caused by the stimuli. These admittance changes are observed by watching for deflections on the admittance device meter, and the ART is considered to be the lowest intensity causing a deflection that can be distinguished from the background activity on the meter. This approach is often called "visual monitoring with 5 dB steps." It is sometimes necessary to test reflex thresholds using **broadband noise (BBN)** stimuli. Unlike pure tone ART testing, which can use visual monitoring with 5 dB steps, 1 or 2 dB steps and recorded responses are

Fig. 7.16 The acoustic reflex threshold is the lowest stimulus level resulting in an observable immittance change that is "time-locked" to a stimulus presentation. These data were obtained under laboratory conditions, using 1 dB stimulus steps and simultaneous recording of the stimulus presentations ("event marker") and reflex responses.

needed to accurately measure ARTs for *broadband noise* stimuli even for clinical purposes. This is due to the very small size of the reflex response at and just above the ART when broadband noise is used (Silman, Popelka, & Gelfand 1978; Gelfand 1984; Silman 1984; Silman, Gelfand, Piper, Silverman, & VanFrank 1984). These small reflex responses are often missed with visual monitoring, and the lowest level at which they occur is obscured with 5 dB steps. As a result, visual monitoring with 5 dB steps often causes the normal BBN ART to appear higher (poorer) than it really is, and also shrinks the size of the normal 20 dB noise-tone difference (Gelfand & Piper 1981; Gelfand 1984).

Normal ARTs with a 220 or 226 Hz probe tone occur between ~ 85 and 100 dB SPL for *pure tones* and ~ 20 dB lower when the stimulus is *broadband noise* (Gelfand 1984). Most clinical measurements involve pure tone ARTs. **Table 7.5** shows a representative set of contralateral and ipsilateral ARTs (in dB HL) for normal-hearing individuals. Acoustic reflex thresholds based on wideband reflectance measurements

generally have been found at lower (better) stimulus levels, although the size of the difference varies between studies (e.g., Feeney & Keefe 1999, 2001; Feeney, Keefe, & Marryott 2003; Feeney, Keefe, & Sanford 2004; Schairer, Ellison, Fitzpatrick & Keefe 2007). In addition, the difference between the ARTs for pure tones and broadband noise is the basis of many methods that attempt to identify or predict hearing loss from ARTs (Silman, Gelfand, Piper et al 1984; Silman, Gelfand, & Emmer 1987), as discussed below.

Acoustic Reflex Decay

In addition to the ART, it is also common practice to test for acoustic reflex decay (or adaptation), which is a measure of whether a reflex contraction is maintained or dies out during continuous stimulation (Anderson, Barr, & Wedenberg 1970; Jerger, Harford, Clemis, & Alford 1974; Wilson, Shanks, & Lilly 1984b). Reflex decay is tested at both 500 and 1000 Hz. Higher frequencies are not tested because even

Table 7.5 Acoustic reflex thresholds in dB HL for normal-hearing subjects, based on Wiley, Oviatt, and Block (1987)

		Pure tones (Hz)			Broadband noise
	500	1000	2000	4000	
Contralateral ART					
Mean	84.6	85.9	84.4	89.8	66.3
Standard deviation	6.3	5.2	5.7	8.9	8.8
Ipsilateral ART					
Mean	79.9	82.0	86.2	87.5	64.6
Standard deviation	5.0	5.2	5.9	3.5	6.9

normal people can have rapid reflex decay above 1000 Hz. The test involves presenting a stimulus tone continuously for 10 seconds at a level 10 dB above the reflex threshold. The magnitude of the reflex response will either stay the same or decrease over the course of the 10 second stimulus, as shown in **Fig. 7.17**. The central issue is whether the response decays to half of its original magnitude. If the magnitude of the reflex response does not decrease to 50% of its original size during the 10 second test period (**Fig. 7.17a,b**), then the outcome is considered negative. The test is considered positive if the magnitude of the reflex response does decay by 50% or more within this time period (**Fig. 7.17c**).

Conductive Hearing Loss

Conductive hearing losses cause acoustic reflexes to be either "elevated" or "absent." By "elevated" we mean that the ART is higher than normal, that is, it takes more intensity to reach the reflex threshold than would have been needed if there was no conductive loss. An "absent" reflex means that a reflex response cannot be obtained, even with the most intense stimulus available (which is usually 125 dB HL on most modern immittance devices). The effects of conductive loss can be summarized by two basic rules:

1. **Probe-ear rule** The presence of conductive pathology in the probe ear causes the acoustic reflex to be absent. Here, even though the stapedius muscle itself may actually be contracting, the presence of the pathology prevents us from being able to register any change in acoustic admittance that can be picked up by the probe tip. In fact, Jerger, Anthony, Jerger, and Mauldin (1974) found that the chances of having a measurable acoustic reflex fell to 50% when the air-bone-gap in the probe ear (averaged across frequencies) was only 5 dB.

2. **Stimulus-ear rule** A conductive loss in the stimulus ear causes the ART to be elevated by the amount of the conductive impairment. This occurs because the amount of the stimulus that actually reaches the cochlea will be reduced by the amount of the air-bone-gap. For example, suppose an otherwise normal patient develops otitis media with a 25 dB air-bone-gap. The 25-dB air-bone-gap causes the signal reaching her cochlea to be 25 dB weaker than the level presented from the earphone. If her ART would normally have been 85 dB HL (without the conductive loss), then the stimulus would now have to be raised by 25 dB to 110 dB HL to reach her cochlea at 85 dB HL. Hence, her ART would

Fig. 7.17 Acoustic reflex decay is considered negative if the reflex response does not decrease (tracing **a**) or if it decreases by less than half of its original magnitude (tracing **b**). Reflex decay is positive if the magnitude falls by 50% or more (tracing **c**).

now be elevated to 110 dB HL. In addition, if the air-bone-gap is large enough, then the ART will be elevated so much that the reflex will be absent. This occurs because the highest available stimulus level cannot overcome the size of the air-bone-gap and still deliver a large enough signal to the cochlea. Jerger, Anthony, et al (1974) found that the chances of having an absent acoustic reflex reached 50% when the conductive loss (averaged across frequencies) was 27 dB in the stimulus ear. This occurred because the (otherwise normal) average ART of ~ 85 dB HL plus an average air-bone-gap of 27 dB is more than 110 dB HL, which was the highest stimulus level available at that time. Modern immittance instruments allow testing up to 125 dB HL, so that the 50% point for absent reflexes is not reached until there is a 42 dB air-bone-gap in the stimulus ear (Gelfand 1984).

The following acoustic reflex configurations result from the two principles just described: For unilateral conductive losses, contralateral acoustic reflexes tend to be (1) absent when the probe is in the pathological ear, and (2) elevated or absent when the probe is in the normal ear. Contralateral acoustic reflexes tend to be absent in both ears when there is a bilateral conductive impairment. Ipsilateral acoustic reflexes are affected by both principles at the same time; that is, the air-bone-gap reduces the effective level of the stimulus that actually reaches the cochlea, and the conductive pathology prevents an immittance change from being monitored even if the reflex is activated. Consequently, ipsilateral acoustic reflexes tend to be absent when testing an ear with a conductive disorder, regardless of the condition of the opposite ear. These findings are illustrated in **Fig. 7.18** for a unilateral conductive loss and in **Fig. 7.19** for a bilateral conductive disorder.

Sensorineural Hearing Loss

Acoustic reflex thresholds depend on hearing sensitivity in a rather peculiar way (Popelka 1981; Silman & Gelfand 1981; Gelfand, Piper, & Silman 1983; Gelfand 1984; Gelfand & Piper 1984; Gelfand, Schwander, & Silman 1990). In this context "hearing sensitivity" represents a continuum going from normal hearing through various magnitudes of sensorineural hearing loss due to cochlear disorders. **Fig. 7.20**, **Fig. 7.21**, and **Fig. 7.22** show the 10th, 50th, and 90th percentiles of the ARTs at 500, 1000, and

2000 Hz for patients who have normal hearing or sensorineural losses associated with cochlear disorders. For example, **Fig. 7.20** provides the following information about patients who have thresholds of 5 dB HL at 500 Hz: 10% of them have ARTs up to 75 dB HL, 50% have ARTs up to 85 dB HL, and 90% have ARTs up to 95 dB HL. Similarly, **Fig. 7.21** shows that among patients who have thresholds of 60 dB HL at 1000 Hz, 10% have ARTs up to 85 dB HL, 50% have ARTs up to 95 dB HL, and 90% have ARTs up to 110 dB HL. Using the median (50th percentile) curves as a guide, we see that pure tone acoustic reflex thresholds (1) are about the same for people with normal hearing and sensorineural hearing losses of cochlear origin *up to roughly* 50 dB HL, and (2) become progressively higher as the amount of cochlear hearing loss increases *above about* 50 dB HL.

It is well established that patients with retrocochlear pathologies have acoustic reflexes that are elevated, often to the extent that the reflex is absent (Gelfand 1984). However, the decision about when an ART is "elevated" must account for the fact that the ARTs depend on the magnitude of the hearing loss in patients who do not have retrocochlear involvement. The 90th percentiles provide us with upper cutoff values for ARTs that meet this need. In fact, many prior inconsistencies about the diagnostic usefulness of the reflex were resolved by the introduction of 90th percentiles that account for the degree of hearing loss (Silman & Gelfand 1981; Gelfand 1984).

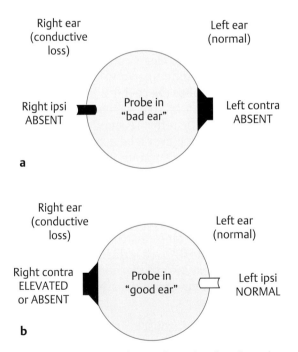

Fig. 7.18 Configuration of contralateral and ipsilateral acoustic reflexes in unilateral conductive hearing loss. The conductive loss affects the right ear in this example. Contralateral reflexes are absent with the probe in the abnormal ear ("probe ear rule," **a**), and are elevated (or absent) with the probe in the good ear and the contralateral stimulus going to the bad ear ("stimulus ear rule," **b**). The ipsilateral reflexes are absent when the probe is in the abnormal right ear **(a)**, and normal when the probe is in the normal left ear **(b)**.

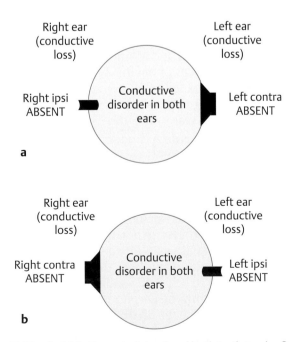

Fig. 7.19 **(a,b)** Both contralateral and both ipsilateral reflexes tend to be absent when there is a bilateral conductive disorder.

Fig. 7.20 Tenth, 50th, and 90th percentiles of acoustic reflex thresholds for a 500 Hz stimulus as a function of the hearing level at 500 Hz for people with normal hearing and sensorineural hearing losses of cochlear origin. (Adapted from Gelfand, Schwander, and Silman [1990], with permission of American Speech-Language-Hearing Association.)

Fig. 7.21 Tenth, 50th, and 90th percentiles of acoustic reflex thresholds for a 1000 Hz stimulus as a function of the hearing level at 1000 Hz for people with normal hearing and sensorineural hearing losses of cochlear origin. (Adapted from Gelfand, Schwander, and Silman [1990], with permission of American Speech-Language-Hearing Association.)

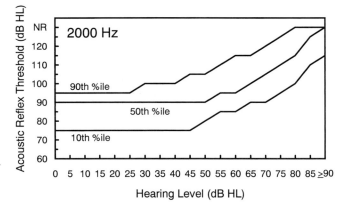

Fig. 7.22 Tenth, 50th, and 90th percentiles of acoustic reflex thresholds for a 2000 Hz stimulus as a function of the hearing level at 2000 Hz for people with normal hearing and sensorineural hearing losses of cochlear origin. (Adapted from Gelfand, Schwander, and Silman [1990], with permission of American Speech-Language-Hearing Association.)

Two sets of 90th percentile values are shown in **Table 7.6** (Silman & Gelfand 1981; Gelfand et al 1990) because both are in common use and distinguish between cochlear and retrocochlear ears with considerable success (Olsen, Bauch, & Harner 1983; Gelfand 1984; Sanders 1984; Gelfand et al 1990; Silman & Silverman 1991; Gelfand 2009).

In practice, the patient's ARTs are compared with the respective 90th percentiles that apply to his hearing thresholds for the frequencies tested. If an ART falls on or below the relevant 90th percentile, then it is considered to be essentially within the normal and/or cochlear distribution. However, ARTs

that fall above the applicable 90th percentiles are considered elevated because only a small proportion of normal and/or cochlear-impaired ears have ARTs that are so high. If the abnormally elevated or absent reflexes are not attributable to a conductive disorder, then the patient is considered to be at risk for eighth nerve pathology in the ear that receives the stimulus. In contrast, many patients with functional impairments (Chapter 14) have ARTs that are below the 10th percentiles (Gelfand 1994).

Abnormal reflex decay means that the response decreases rapidly, and is associated with retrocochlear disorders (Anderson et al 1970; Jerger, Harford, Clemis, & Alford 1974; Wilson et al 1984b). It is prudent to be suspicious of retrocochlear pathology in the stimulated ear if the reflex response decays by 50% or more within 10 seconds (as in **Fig. 7.17c**) at either 500 Hz and/or 1000 Hz. However, the student should be aware that there are differences in approach regarding whether abnormal decay should occur during the first 5 seconds versus any time during the 10 second test, as well as how to interpret reflex decay that occurs at one frequency and/or the other (Anderson et al 1970; Jerger, Harford, et al 1974; Hirsch & Anderson 1980; Olsen, Stach, & Kurdziel 1981; Wilson et al 1984b).

We have seen that acoustic reflex abnormalities such as elevated/absent reflexes and/or positive reflex decay are associated with retrocochlear pathologies in the ear receiving the stimulus tone. Testing both ARTs and reflex decay and considering a positive result on *either or both* tests as the criterion for suspecting retrocochlear pathology has

Table 7.6 Acoustic reflex threshold 90th percentile cutoff values as a function of hearing level at 500, 1000, and 2000 Hz

Hearing threshold (dB HL)	90th Percentile acoustic reflex threshold norms (dB HL)					
	Silman & Gelfand (1981)			Gelfand, Schwander, & Silman (1990)		
	500 Hz	1000 Hz	2000 Hz	500 Hz	1000 Hz	2000 Hz
0	95	100	95	95	95	95
5	95	100	95	95	95	95
10	95	100	100	95	95	95
15	95	100	100	95	95	95
20	95	100	100	95	95	95
25	95	100	100	95	95	95
30	100	100	105	95	95	100
35	100	100	105	95	95	100
40	100	105	105	95	95	100
45	100	105	105	95	95	105
50	105	105	110	100	100	105
55	105	105	110	105	105	110
60	105	110	115	105	110	115
65	105	110	115	110	110	115
70	115	115	125	115	115	120
75	115	115	125	120	120	125
80	125	125	125	120	125	NR[a]
85	125	125	125	NR	NR	NR
≥ 90	125	125	125	NR	NR	NR

[a]NR, no response at 125 dB HL.

been referred to as *acoustic reflexes combined (ARC)* (Turner, Frazer, & Shepard 1984; Turner, Shepard, & Frazer 1984). Acoustic reflex thresholds *and* decay should be routinely tested *because ARC with 90th percentiles* has a hit rate of ~ 85% for retrocochlear pathology and a false-positive rate of only 11% (Silman & Silverman 1991).

Acoustic Reflex Configurations

We have already seen that patients with conductive disorders typically have certain configurations of acoustic reflex findings (**Fig. 7.18** and **Fig. 7.19**). It

has also been pointed out that eighth nerve pathology (e.g., acoustic neuroma) is associated with reflex abnormalities affecting the stimulated ear, which is expected because the eighth nerve is the sensory leg of the acoustic reflex arc. A typical example is depicted in the **Fig. 7.23**. Notice that the right ear's ipsilateral (uncrossed) and contralateral (crossed) reflexes are both abnormal because they both stimulate the pathological auditory nerve, whereas both of the left ear reflexes are unaffected because they involve stimulating the normal eighth nerve. As one would expect, acoustic reflexes are typically absent in patients with auditory neuropathy spectrum disorder (e.g., Starr, Picton, Sininger, Hood, & Berlin 1996).

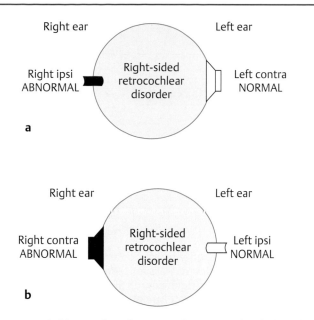

Fig. 7.23   (a,b) Typical configuration of acoustic reflex findings for an eighth-nerve (extra-axial retrocochlear) disorder in the right ear.

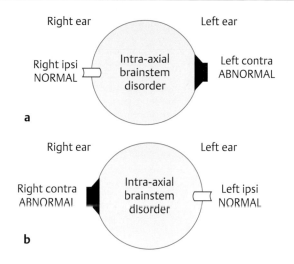

Fig. 7.24   (a,b) Typical configuration of acoustic reflex findings for intra-axial brainstem disorders.

In addition to retrocochlear lesions affecting the eighth nerve, acoustic reflex abnormalities are also associated with brainstem pathologies and facial nerve disorders, as well as demyelinating (e.g., multiple sclerosis) and neuromuscular (e.g., myasthenia gravis) diseases (Bosatra et al 1984; Gelfand 1984; Mangham 1984; Wiley & Block 1984; Wilson et al 1984b). Cortically involved patients have the same ARTs as normal and cochlear-impaired patients with similar hearing sensitivity (Gelfand & Silman 1982). Acoustic reflex configurations can help us distinguish among at least some of these categories of disorders, such as brainstem pathologies affecting the crossed reflex pathway and disorders of the facial nerve.

Pathologies *within* the brainstem are often called **intra-axial** to distinguish them from disorders such as acoustic tumors that are located outside the brainstem proper (which might be called **extra-axial**). Intra-axial brainstem pathologies often affect the reflex pathways going from one side to the other, while not impacting on the ipsilateral pathways (Jerger & Jerger 1977, 1983). This situation is shown in **Fig. 7.24**. Notice how the contralateral (crossed) reflexes are abnormal because they are affected by the intra-axial lesion, whereas the unaffected ipsilateral (uncrossed) reflexes are normal.

In contrast to eighth-nerve disorders that are associated with acoustic reflex abnormalities when the abnormal side is stimulated, *facial (seventh) nerve disorders* (e.g., Bell's palsy) are associated with abnormal reflexes when the probe tip is on the path-

ological side (Alford, Jerger, Coats, Peterson, & Weber 1973; Citron & Adour 1978; Wiley & Block 1984). This occurs because the facial nerve is the motor leg of the acoustic reflex arc that innervates the stapedius muscle. Hence, the abnormality is seen in the probe ear because this is where the effects of the muscle contraction are being monitored **(Fig. 7.25)**. Facial nerve disorders are generally discovered by observable signs of facial involvement and other neurological indicators besides stapedius reflex abnormalities. Thus, one of the major uses of acoustic reflexes has been to monitor the course of Bell's palsy through its recovery. However, it has been shown that seventh-nerve disorders can cause ipsilateral and contralateral acoustic reflex decay (with the probe tip on the abnormal side) even when there are no signs of facial palsy (Silman, Silverman, Gelfand, Lutolf, & Lynn 1988). Consequently, the possibility of seventh-nerve involvement should be kept in mind whenever acoustic reflexes are being interpreted.

Hearing Loss Identification and Prediction

Several approaches have been devised that attempt to identify the presence of hearing loss or to predict its extent from ARTs (Popelka 1981; Silman & Gelfand 1982; Silman, Gelfand, et al 1984; Silman, Gelfand, & Emmer 1987). As with other physiological methods, these acoustic reflex techniques were developed because we often have to evaluate the hearing of patients who cannot or will not respond reliably on routine behavioral tests. This might occur

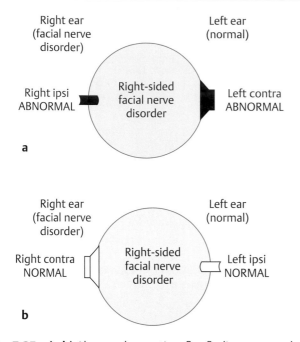

a

b

Fig. 7.25 **(a,b)** Abnormal acoustic reflex findings occur when the probe tip is located on the side of the facial nerve disorder. Thus, a right-sided facial nerve disorder will affect the right ipsilateral and left contralateral acoustic reflexes.

Fig. 7.26 Acoustic reflex thresholds are related to the degree of hearing loss in different ways for pure tone (left axis, dB HL) and broadband noise (right axis, dB SPL) stimuli. The relationships are shown as separate straight line functions for hearing losses below and above 50 dB HL to highlight the general concepts. (Based on data from Gelfand, Schwander, and Silman (1990) for pure tones and Popelka (1981) for broadband noise.

because the patient is too young for behavioral testing, or because the patient has one or more physical, cognitive, and/or emotional impairments that make behavioral testing difficult or impossible. Acoustic reflex-based methods for identifying or predicting hearing loss rely in various ways on the relationships of pure tone and broadband noise ARTs, and how these are affected by hearing loss. Recall that there is a 20 dB difference between the normal pure tone and broadband noise ARTs; and that tonal ARTs are independent of hearing thresholds for sensorineural losses up to roughly 50 to 60 dB HL, above which ARTs get higher as the amount of hearing loss increases. The opposite relationship exists for broadband noise ARTs, which become higher as hearing loss increases up to ~ 50 to 60 dB HL, and then remain more or less constant for greater amounts of hearing loss (Popelka 1981). These relationships are illustrated in **Fig. 7.26**.

The earliest hearing loss prediction methods attempted to predict the degree of hearing loss in decibels (Niemeyer & Sesterhenn 1974) or in categories (Jerger, Burney, Mauldin, & Crump 1974). The latter method, called **sensitivity prediction from the acoustic reflex (SPAR)**, was revised several times (Jerger, Hayes, Anthony, & Mauldin 1978). Unfortunately, these types of procedures were found to have large error rates in terms of false-positive and false-negative rates and the accuracy with which the severity of hearing loss was predicted (Silman, Gelfand, et al 1984). Another kind of approach tried to predict hearing loss from ARTs using formulas derived from statistical procedures called regression analyses (e.g., Baker & Lilly 1976; Rizzo & Greenberg 1979), although the predictive accuracy of these approaches was not very high (Hall & Koval 1982; Silman, Gelfand, et al 1984). The problems faced by methods that try to predict the degree of loss were due to several factors, such as (1) the peculiarities of the relationships shown in **Fig. 7.26** (e.g., the noise-tone difference gets smaller and then widens again as hearing loss increases); (2) regression formulas use the ART as the independent variable and hearing loss as the dependent variable, which is the opposite of the actual relationship; and (3) the range of ARTs is roughly 20 dB wide for any given amount of hearing loss (Popelka 1981; Gelfand 1984; Silman, Gelfand, et al 1984; Silman, Gelfand, & Emmer 1987).

A more successful approach involves the more conservative goal of simply identifying whether a significant hearing loss is present rather than trying to predict its magnitude. One approach of this type uses just the broadband noise ART because it is sensitive to even small amounts of hearing loss. Keith (1977) found that BBN ARTs were ≤ 85 dB SPL in 86.5% of normal-hearing individuals, and > 85 dB SPL in 96.9% of hearing-impaired patients. He therefore suggested using a broadband noise ART of 85 dB SPL as a cutoff value for distinguishing between normal and impaired hearing. However, Keith's sample did not include losses between 20 and 33 dB HL, and the age range of the subjects was unspecified. It has been confirmed that Keith's approach effectively separates those with normal hearing from those with substantial sensorineural hearing loss in young adults (Silman, Gelfand, et al 1984; Silman, Silverman, Showers, & Gelfand 1984), and it has also been found useful in patients who have cerebral palsy (Emmer & Silman 2003). However, patients with mild hearing losses and those with high-frequency hearing losses can have BBN ARTs falling on either side of the 85 dB SPL criterion (Silman, Gelfand, et al 1984; Silman, Silverman, et al 1984). Although these factors can limit the direct application of the 85 dB SPL cutoff value, especially with adults, they certainly do not detract from the value of the basic approach.

Another approach that has been widely used is the bivariate method, which uses both tonal and BBN ARTs (Popelka & Trumph 1976; Popelka 1981). It is called the **bivariate method** because the ART data are plotted on an x-y graph (**Fig. 7.27**). The x-axis shows the ratio of patient's BBN ARTs to tonal ARTs, and the y-axis shows the pure tone ARTs. A sample of reflex data from people with known hearing thresholds is then used to draw vertical and diagonal cutoff lines on the graph. In the original bivariate method (Popelka & Trumph 1976; Popelka 1981), these lines were placed so that at least 90% of normal-hearing

subjects had reflex data falling in a "normal area" to the left of the vertical line and under the diagonal. Young patients with significant hearing losses, defined as a pure tone average of 32 dB HL or more, were successfully identified by reflex data falling outside this normal area.

Correct identification rates with the bivariate method can be disappointing when trying to identify hearing losses in adults who may have mild and/or high-frequency as well as significant losses, especially when patients are ≥ 45 years old (Silman & Gelfand 1979; Silman, Gelfand, et al 1984; Silman, Silverman, Showers, & Gelfand 1984; Silverman, Silman, & Miller 1983). These problems are addressed by the **modified bivariate method** (Silman, Gelfand, et al 1984; Silman, Silverman, et al 1984), which differs from the original approach in terms of how the cutoff values are determined, and is used for patients who are under 45 years old. Using a reasonably large sample of patients with known thresholds, the cutoff lines of the modified bivariate plot are drawn to produce the best possible separation between normal and impaired ears, including the requirement that at least 90% of mild and sloping losses fall outside the normal area. Using the same group of 20- to 44-year-old adults, the original bivariate correctly identified 97% of normals but only 69% of hearing-impaired subjects, whereas the modified bivariate correctly identified 86% of normals and 96% with hearing losses (Silman, Gelfand, et al 1984; Silman, Silverman, et al 1984). Identifying hearing losses in adults who are ≥ 45 years old remains problematic; however, it was recommended that a hearing loss should be suspected for a patient in this population when the ART is > 95 dB SPL for broadband noise, or ≥ 105 dB SPL for 1000 or 2000 Hz (Silman, Gelfand, et al 1984; Silman, Silverman, et al 1984). Applying these criteria under clinical conditions correctly identified 93% of the patients whose hearing was within normal limits and 77% of those with hearing losses (Wallin, Mendez-Kurtz, & Silman 1986).

On High Stimulus Levels and the Acoustic Reflex

The student should be aware that the high stimulus levels involved in acoustic reflex testing do have rare but possible untoward effects. Several cases of threshold shifts and/or tinnitus attributable to the high stimulus levels used during acoustic reflex testing have been reported (Portmann 1980; Tanka, Ohhashi, & Tsuda 1981; Lenarz & Gulzow 1983; Miller, Hoffman, & Smallberg 1984; Arriaga & Luxford 1993; Hunter, Ries, Schlauch, Levine, & Ward 1999; Emanuel, Henson, & Knapp 2012). Noticeable

Fig. 7.27 Example of the bivariate plotting method. The original bivariate method places the cutoff lines where ≥90% of normal ears are in the normal area. The modified bivariate method places the cutoff lines where normal and impaired ears are maximally separated and ≥ 90% of ears with mild and sloping losses are outside of the normal area. Examples of typical normal and hearing loss cases are plotted.

minorities of audiologists surveyed by Emanuel et al (2012) reported some cases of patients with experiences such as discomfort and worsening of hearing loss and/or tinnitus associated with reflex testing. However, there was only *one* case of a patient who experienced *permanent* hearing loss and tinnitus among all 90 of the audiologists in the survey, and it was the only case ever encountered by a clinician who routinely employed reflex threshold and decay testing for over 20 years. Clearly, these instances are very uncommon, and they certainly must be weighed against the very valuable diagnostic potential of acoustic reflex tests.

Unfortunately, purely scientific and clinical considerations do not provide a resolution for this issue, let alone a neat one. One approach is to raise the stimulus level until a reflex response is obtained or the maximum level of 125 dB HL is reached. The opposite strategy is to limit testing to some presumably safe limit. Various limits have been suggested, such as 110 dB *SPL* (Wilson & Margolis 1999), 115 dB SPL (Hunter et al 1999), and 110 dB HL except when there is an air-bone-gap (Stach & Jerger 1991). Another possibility is to test up to a diagnostically relevant cutoff (above which the reflex would be considered elevated), such as the 90th percentile or perhaps 5 dB higher (Hunter et al 1999; Emanuel et al 2012). Regardless of philosophy, it is clear that one should be alert to complaints of hearing changes, dizziness, tinnitus, etc., during and after acoustic reflex testing.

■ Immittance Assessment in Infants

An important exception to the routine use of low-frequency probe tones occurs when the patient is an infant. Recall that normal tympanograms typically have a single peak at 220 or 226 Hz and are often multiple-peaked at 660 or 678 Hz. However, this relationship is reversed in neonates and infants below about 6 months of age (e.g., Sprague, Wiley, & Goldstein 1985; Mazlan, Kei, & Hickson 2009). As illustrated by the percentages in **Table 7.7** normal neonates usually have tympanograms with one peak when using high-frequency probes like 660/678 Hz and 1000 Hz, but that are multi-peaked or flat with low-frequency probes like 220/226 Hz. In addition, Baldwin (2006) found that the sensitivity of tympanograms for correctly identifying conductive disorders in 2- to 12-week-old babies was excellent (95–99%) with high-frequency probe tones (678 and 1000 Hz), but was extremely poor (2%) with a 226 Hz probe tone; this led her to conclude that low-frequency tympanometry is not valid with babies in this age range. It is thus not surprising that the use of high-frequency probe tones is standard practice for immittance tests in infants up to roughly 5 to 6 months of age (e.g., ASHA 2004; JCIH 2007; AAA 2012). Appropriate admittance norms using high-frequency probe tones are have been provided by several investigators (e.g., Kei, Allison-Levick, Dockray, et al 2003; Margolis, Bass-Ringdahl, Hanks, Holte, & Zapala 2003; Calandruccio, Fitzgerald, & Prieve 2006; Mazlan, Kei, Hickson, et al 2007; Swanepoel et al 2007; Mazlan, Kei, & Hickson 2009), and are illustrated in **Table 7.8**.

High-frequency probe tones are also used for acoustic reflex testing of neonates and infants up to ~ 5 to 6 months old. Their acoustic reflexes are often elevated or absent with a 220/226 Hz probe tone but are more likely to be present with ARTs more or less similar to those found in adults when using higher-frequency probe tones such as 660/678 and 1000 Hz (e.g., Bennett & Weatherby 1982; Gelfand 1984; Sprague, Wiley, & Goldstein 1985; Mazlan et al 2007, 2009; Swanepoel et al 2007). To illustrate this, **Table 7.9** compares the percentages of acoustic reflexes that are present in

Table 7.7 Percentages of single-peaked, multiple-peaked, and flat tympanograms obtained in normal neonates using low-frequency (220 Hz) versus high-frequency (660 and 1000 Hz) probe tones

Probe tone frequency	Tympanogram		
	Single peak	Multiple peaks	Flat
220 Hz[a]	17%	83%	0%
660 Hz[a]	99%	0%	1%
1000 Hz[b]	91.3%	0%	8.7%

[a]Based on data reported by Sprague, Wiley, and Goldstein (1985).
[b]Based on data reported by Mazlan, Kei, and Hickson (2009).

Table 7.8 Representative 90% normal ranges for peak compensated static acoustic admittance values (mmhos) using high-frequency probe tones

Source	Age	90% Normal range at	
		630/660/678 Hz	1000 Hz
Mazlan, Kei, Hickson, et al (2007)	At birth		0.38–1.18[a]
	6–7 weeks		0.49–1.53[a]
Kei, Allison-Levick, Dockray, et al (2003)	1–6 days		0.39–2.28[b]
Margolis, Bass-Ringdahl, Hanks, et al (2003)	0–20 weeks		0.60–4.30[c]
Calandruccio, Fitzgerald, & Prieve (2006)	4–10 weeks	0.08–1.28	0.20–2.26
	11–19 weeks	0.26–1.25	0.70–2.27
	20–26 weeks	0.44–1.16	0.62–2.18
	6–12 months	0.40–1.92	0.95–4.20
	2 years	0.69–4.54	1.12–4.07

[a]Ranges from one standard deviation below the mean to one standard deviation above the mean, rather than 90% normal ranges.
[b]Combined across both ears (the upper values [95th percentiles] were 2.28 mmhos for right ears and 1.95 mmhos for left ears).
[c]Based on the difference between the admittances at tympanometric peak pressure and at –400 daPa.

normal newborns when using 220, 660, and 1000 Hz probe tones. Notice that chances of obtaining measurable acoustic reflexes in neonates were lowest with the 220 Hz probe, higher with the 660 Hz probe, and even higher with the 1000 Hz probe tones. The corresponding mean ARTs are given in **Table 7.10**. Most contemporary immittance evaluations with these very young patients employ ipsilateral acoustic reflexes with a 1000 Hz probe tone; and several examples of 90% normal ranges are provided in **Table 7.11**.

■ Eustachian Tube Function Tests

We have already seen that Eustachian tube dysfunctions are inferred from the peak pressure of the tympanogram as a matter of routine. This section addresses several additional tests that are occasionally desirable when it is important to determine the adequacy of Eustachian tube functioning in a given patient. For example, adequate Eustachian tube functioning is often a factor when dealing with mat-

Table 7.9 Percentages of present acoustic reflexes in normal neonates using 220, 660, and 1000 Hz probe tones

Stimulus	Probe tone		
	220 Hz	660 Hz	1000 Hz
Ipsilateral acoustic reflex			
1000 Hz	43[a]	81[a]	86[b]
2000 Hz	—	—	91[c]
Broadband noise	51[a]	74[a]	91[c]
Contralateral acoustic reflex			
1000 Hz	34[a]	60[a]	—
Broadband noise	49[a]	83[a]	—

[a]Based on Sprague, Wiley, and Goldstein (1985).
[b]Based on Swanepoel, Werner, Hugo, et al (2007).
[c]Based on Mazlan, Kei, and Hickson (2009). The rate of present acoustic reflexes (91.3%) did not distinguish between the 2000 Hz and BBN stimuli.

Table 7.10 Mean acoustic reflex thresholds (dB HL) in normal neonates using 220, 660, and 1000 Hz probe tones

Stimulus	Probe tone		
	220 Hz	**660 Hz**	**1000 Hz**
Ipsilateral			
1000 Hz	82.6[a]	81.7[a]	93.0[b]
2000 Hz	—	—	76.2[c]
BBN	60.9[a]	54.6[a]	64.9[c]
Contralateral			
1000 Hz	92.2[a]	89.1[a]	—
BBN	70.0[a]	70.1[a]	—

[a]Based on Sprague, Wiley, and Goldstein (1985).
[b]Based on Swanepoel, Werner, Hugo, et al (2007).
[c]Based on Mazlan, Kei, and Hickson (2009).

ters such as inserting or removing a myringotomy tube, repairing a perforated tympanic membrane, adenoidectomy, and cleft palate surgery (e.g., Holmquist 1968; Bluestone, Paradise, Beery, & Wittel 1972; Hughes 1985; Hughes & Pensak 1997).

Before proceeding, it should be pointed out that the opposite problem occurs when the tube fails to close appropriately. This is called a **patulous Eustachian tube**. To test for patulous Eustachian tubes, McGrath and Michaelides (2011) recorded admittance while patients inhaled and exhaled over time. Ears with patulous Eustachian tubes were identified by > 0.07 ml immittance changes that were synchronized with the patients' breathing with ~ 84% sensitivity and ~ 95% specificity.

Eustachian tube functioning is usually assessed with an inflation test when the eardrum has a perforation or when a myringotomy tube is present (Bluestone 1975, 1980). This method involves using the immittance device to pump air into the ear through the probe tip while monitoring the increasing pressure on the manometer. A properly function-

ing Eustachian tube should be forced open by the increasing air pressure. Opening of the Eustachian tube releases the built-up air pressure, which is seen as a reasonably abrupt drop of the air pressure back down toward 0 daPa on the manometer. A second step is needed if the built-up air pressure does not open the tube. In this case the patient is instructed to swallow several times, which should cause the Eustachian tube to open, causing the pressure to fall back to 0 daPa on the manometer. A Eustachian tube dysfunction is considered to be present if the pressure cannot be completely vented by swallowing.

Several Eustachian tube function tests are used when the tympanic membrane is intact, including the Valsalva, Toynbee, and inflation and deflation tests (Bluestone 1975, 1980; Seifert, Seidemann, & Givens 1979; Riedel, Wiley, & Block 1987). Each of them involves determining (1) whether the pressure within the middle ear can be changed by a given activity, and (2) if swallowing will successfully ventilate the middle ear so that the pressure can return to its original value. The procedures outlined here are the ones proposed by Riedel, Wiley, and Block (1987).

■ Valsalva Test

To perform the Valsalva maneuver the patient is instructed to close her mouth and nose (by pinching her nostrils) and then to blow hard so that her cheeks puff up and air is forced into her ears, creating a sensation of fullness. The first step in the Valsalva test is to do a pretest tympanogram, which provides a baseline value for peak pressure. The patient is then instructed to perform the Valsalva maneuver. She is told not to swallow, and a second tympanogram is then obtained. It is expected that the peak pressure will increase in the positive direction compared with the baseline value, indicating that the maneuver successfully increased the middle ear pressure. The patient is then asked to swallow several times. This may be done while drinking water ("wet") or without

Table 7.11 Examples of 90% normal ranges for ipsilateral acoustic reflexes with a 1000 Hz probe tone in neonates

Source	Stimulus	90% Normal range (dB HL)
Swanepoel, Werner, Hugo, et al (2007)	1000 Hz	80–105
Mazlan, Kei, and Hickson (2009)	2000 Hz	65–90
	Broadband noise	55–80

drinking water ("dry"). These swallows are expected to open the Eustachian tube, so that the middle ear is ventilated and its pressure can return to normal (i.e., to the pretest baseline value). A third tympanogram is then done to determine whether the peak pressure returned to the baseline value as a result of the swallowing.

■ Toynbee Test

In the Toynbee maneuver the patient is instructed to swallow (dry) while holding his nose closed (by pinching his nostrils). The Toynbee maneuver is typically expected to make the middle ear pressure more negative, but it actually causes *either* a positive *or* negative shift in middle ear pressure (Riedel et al 1987). The Toynbee test follows the same procedures used for the Valsalva test, except that the Toynbee maneuver is used. (Although it is not an audiological technique, one should be aware that the **Politzer test** involves supplementing this maneuver by forcing air into one of the nostrils from a rubber bulb or other air pressure source.)

■ Inflation and Deflation Tests

The inflation and deflation tests are based on the notion that fairly large amounts of pressure in the outer ear will cause a slight change in middle ear pressure. The mechanism will become apparent as the test procedure is described. The first step in the inflation test is to measure the baseline peak pressure with a pretest tympanogram. Positive pressure of +400 daPa is then pumped into the ear canal. This is expected to push in on the tympanic membrane, making the middle ear volume slightly smaller. The patient is told to swallow (wet) several times while the positive pressure is being applied. This is expected to cause a small amount of negative pressure in the middle ear. A second tympanogram is now done, which is expected to show that the peak pressure is slightly more negative than the baseline. The pressure is then returned to 0 daPa and the patient is asked to swallow several times (wet or dry) in an attempt to ventilate the middle ear. A third tympanogram is then done, which is expected to show that the peak pressure has moved back to its baseline value. The inflation method appears to be the least useful of the various Eustachian tube tests because it produces the smallest amounts of pressure change.

The deflation test is procedurally identical to the inflation test, except that −400 daPa is used. The negative pressure in the outer ear is expected to pull back on the eardrum, so that the middle ear volume becomes slightly larger. The expected results are a slight increase in peak pressure during the second tympanogram, which returns to the baseline value on the third tympanogram.

There is no question that Eustachian tube tests should be performed when there is a specific need for the general information that they provide. However, it is noteworthy that Eustachian tube tests have not enjoyed general acceptance in spite of their longevity and the medical implications of Eustachian tube dysfunctions. This is at least partly due to the scarcity of criteria for normality and abnormality on these tests. Norms are not available for children. There are some adult norms for the sizes of the pressure shifts produced by each of the methods (Riedel et al 1987), but how well they can discriminate between normal and abnormal patients is not known. These points suggest that Eustachian tube function testing should be used and interpreted conservatively.

■ Study Questions

1. Describe how a tympanogram is obtained.
2. Define (a) total acoustic admittance, (b) peak-compensated static acoustic admittance, and (c) tympanometric peak pressure.
3. Define and contrast the classical types A, B, and C tympanograms.
4. What are 678 Hz (660 Hz) B-G tympanograms, and how can they help us distinguish between conductive disorders?
5. What is the acoustic reflex, and what are its principal characteristics?
6. Describe how the contralateral acoustic reflex is affected by a conductive disorder in the (a) probe ear and (b) stimulus ear.
7. How is the acoustic reflex threshold affected by cochlear hearing losses?
8. Describe how the contralateral acoustic reflex is affected by a retrocochlear disorder in the (a) probe ear and (b) stimulus ear.
9. What is acoustic reflex decay, and when is it expected to be abnormal?
10. Explain why an intra-axial brainstem lesion might result in abnormal contralateral acoustic reflexes but normal ipsilateral acoustic reflexes.

References

Aithal S, Kei J, Driscoll C, Khan A. Normative wideband reflectance measures in healthy neonates. Int J Pediatr Otorhinolaryngol 2013;77(1):29–35

Alford BR, Jerger JF, Coats AC, Peterson CR, Weber SC. Neurophysiology of facial nerve testing. Arch Otolaryngol 1973;97(2):214–219

American Academy of Audiology (AAA). 2012. Audiologic Guidelines for the Assessment of Hearing in Infants and Young Children. Available at: http://www.audiology.org/resources/documentlibrary/Pages/Pediatric-Diagnostics.aspx

American Academy of Audiology (AAA) Position Statement. Identification of hearing loss and middle-ear dysfunction in preschool and school-age children. Audiol Today 1997;9:21–23

American National Standards Institute (ANSI). 2012. American National Standard Specifications for Instruments to Measure Aural Acoustic Impedance and Admittance (Aural Acoustic Immittance). ANSI S3.39-(1987) (R2012). New York, NY: ANSI

American Speech-Language-Hearing Association (ASHA). 1997. Guidelines for Audiologic Screening. Rockville Pike, MD: ASHA

American Speech-Language-Hearing Association (ASHA). 2004. Guidelines for the Audiologic Assessment of Children from Birth to 5 Years of Age. Rockville Pike, MD: ASHA

Anderson H, Barr B, Wedenberg E. 1970. The early detection of acoustic tumors by the stapedial reflex test. In Wolstenholme GEW, Knight J, eds. Sensorineural Hearing Loss. London: Churchill; 275–289

Arriaga MA, Luxford WM. Impedance audiometry and iatrogenic hearing loss. Otolaryngol Head Neck Surg 1993;108(1):70–72

Baker S, Lilly DJ. 1976. Prediction of hearing level from acoustic reflex data. Paper presented at Convention of American Speech-Language-Hearing Association, Houston

Baldwin M. Choice of probe tone and classification of trace patterns in tympanometry undertaken in early infancy. Int J Audiol 2006;45(7):417–427

Beers AN, Shahnaz N, Westerberg BD, Kozak FK. Wideband reflectance in normal Caucasian and Chinese school-aged children and in children with otitis media with effusion. Ear Hear 2010;31(2):221–233

Bennett MJ, Weatherby LA. Newborn acoustic reflexes to noise and pure-tone signals. J Speech Hear Res 1982; 25(3):383–387

Bluestone CD, Paradise JL, Beery QC, Wittel R. Certain effects of cleft palate repair on eustachian tube function. Cleft Palate J 1972;9:183–193

Bluestone CD. 1975. Assessment of Eustachian tube function. In: Jerger J, ed. Handbook of Impedance Audiometry. Acton, MA: American Electromedics; 127–148

Bluestone CD. 1980. Assessment of Eustachian tube function. In: Jerger J, Northern J, eds. Clinical Impedance Audiometry. Acton, MA: American Electromedics; 83–108

Borg E. On the neuronal organization of the acoustic middle ear reflex. A physiological and anatomical study. Brain Res 1973;49(1):101–123

Bosatra A, Russolo M, Silverman CA. 1984. Acoustic-reflex latency: state of the art. In: Silman S, ed. The Acoustic Reflex: Basic Principles and Clinical Applications. Orlando, FL: Academic Press; 301–328

Brooks DN. The use of the electro-acoustic impedance bridge in the assessment of middle ear function. Int Audiol 1969;8:563–569

Calandruccio L, Fitzgerald TS, Prieve BA. Normative multifrequency tympanometry in infants and toddlers. J Am Acad Audiol 2006;17(7):470–480

Citron D III, Adour KK. Acoustic reflex and loudness discomfort in acute facial paralysis. Arch Otolaryngol 1978;104(6):303–306

Davies JE, John DG, Jones AH, Stephens SDG. Tympanometry as a screening test for treatable hearing loss in the elderly. Br J Audiol 1988;22(2):119–121

De Chicchis AR, Todd NW, Nozza RJ. Developmental changes in aural acoustic admittance measurements. J Am Acad Audiol 2000;11(2):97–102

Ellison JC, Gorga M, Cohn E, Fitzpatrick D, Sanford CA, Keefe DH. Wideband acoustic transfer functions predict middle-ear effusion. Laryngoscope 2012;122(4): 887–894

Elner A, Ingelstedt S, Ivarsson A. The elastic properties of the tympanic membrane system. Acta Otolaryngol 1971;72(6):397–403

Emanuel DC, Henson OEC, Knapp RR. Survey of audiological immittance practices. Am J Audiol 2012;21(1): 60–75

Emmer MB, Silman S. The prediction of hearing loss in persons with cerebral palsy using contralateral acoustic reflex threshold for broad-band noise. Am J Audiol 2003;12(2):91–95

Feeney MP, Grant IL, Mills DM. Wideband energy reflectance measurements of ossicular chain discontinuity and repair in human temporal bone. Ear Hear 2009; 30(4):391–400

Feeney MP, Hunter LL, Kei J, et al. Consensus statement: Eriksholm workshop on wideband absorbance measures of the middle ear. Ear Hear 2013;34(Suppl 1): 78S–79S

Feeney MP, Keefe DH. Acoustic reflex detection using wide-band acoustic reflectance, admittance, and power measurements. J Speech Lang Hear Res 1999; 42(5):1029–1041

Feeney MP, Keefe DH. Estimating the acoustic reflex threshold from wideband measures of reflectance, admittance, and power. Ear Hear 2001;22(4):316–332

Feeney MP, Keefe DH, Marryott LP. Contralateral acoustic reflex thresholds for tonal activators using wideband energy reflectance and admittance. J Speech Lang Hear Res 2003;46(1):128–136

Feeney MP, Keefe DH, Sanford CA. Wideband reflectance measures of the ipsilateral acoustic stapedius reflex threshold. Ear Hear 2004;25(5):421–430

Feldman AS. 1975. Acoustic impedance-admittance measurements. In: Bradford LJ, ed. Physiological Measures of the Audio-Vestibular System. New York, NY: Academic Press; 87–145

Feldman AS. 1976. Tympanometry—Procedures, interpretation and variables. In: Feldman AS & Wilber LA, eds. Acoustic Impedance and Admittance: The Measurement of Middle Ear Function. Baltimore, MD: Williams & Wilkins; 103–155

Fiellau-Nikolajsen M. Tympanometry and secretory otitis media: observations on diagnosis, epidemiology, treatment, and prevention in prospective cohort studies of three-year-old children. Acta Otolaryngol Suppl 1983;394(Suppl):1–73

Gelfand SA. 1984. The contralateral acoustic reflex threshold. In: Silman S, ed. The Acoustic Reflex: Basic Principles and Clinical Applications. Orlando, FL: Academic Press; 137–186

Gelfand SA. Acoustic reflex threshold tenth percentiles and functional hearing impairment. J Am Acad Audiol 1994;5(1):10–16

Gelfand SA. 2004. Hearing: An Introduction to Psychological and Physiological Acoustics, 4th ed. New York, NY: Marcel Dekker

Gelfand SA. 2009. The acoustic reflex. In: Katz J, Medwesty L, Burkard R, Hood L, eds. Handbook of Clinical Audiology, 6th ed. Baltimore, MD: Lippincott Williams & Wilkins; 189–221

Gelfand SA, Piper N. Acoustic reflex thresholds in young and elderly subjects with normal hearing. J Acoust Soc Am 1981;69(1):295–297

Gelfand SA, Piper N. Acoustic reflex thresholds: variability and distribution effects. Ear Hear 1984;5(4):228–234

Gelfand SA, Piper N, Silman S. Effects of hearing levels at the activator and other frequencies upon the expected levels of the acoustic reflex threshold. J Speech Hear Disord 1983;48(1):11–17

Gelfand SA, Schwander T, Silman S. Acoustic reflex thresholds in normal and cochlear-impaired ears: effects of no-response rates on 90th percentiles in a large sample. J Speech Hear Disord 1990;55(2):198–205

Gelfand SA, Silman S. Acoustic reflex thresholds in brain-damaged patients. Ear Hear 1982;3(2):93–95

Golding M, Doyle K, Sindhusake D, Mitchell P, Newall P, Hartley D. Tympanometric and acoustic stapedius reflex measures in older adults: the Blue Mountains Hearing Study. J Am Acad Audiol 2007;18(5):391–403

Hall JW III, Koval CB. Accuracy of hearing prediction by the acoustic reflex. Laryngoscope 1982;92(2):140–149

Harford ER. 1980. Assessment of Eustachian tube function. In: Jerger J, Northern J, eds. Clinical Impedance Audiometry. Acton, MA: American Electromedics; 40–64

Hirsch A, Anderson H. Audiologic test results in 96 patients with tumors affecting the eighth nerve. Acta Otolaryngol 1980;369(Suppl):1–26

Holmquist J. The role of the eustachian tube in myringoplasty. Acta Otolaryngol 1968;66(4):289–295

Holmquist J, Miller J. 1972. Eustachian tube evaluation using the impedance bridge. In: Rose D, Keating LW, eds. Mayo Foundation Impedance Symposium. Rochester, MN: Mayo Foundation; 297–307

Hughes GB, ed. 1985. Textbook of Clinical Otology. New York, NY: Thieme-Stratton

Hughes GB, Pensak ML, eds. 1997. Clinical Otology, 2nd ed. New York, NY: Thieme

Hunter LL, Margolis RH. Multifrequency tympanometry: current clinical application. Am J Audiol 1992;1:33–43

Hunter LL, Prieve BA, Kei J, Sanford CA. Pediatric applications of wideband acoustic immittance measures. Ear Hear 2013;34(Suppl 1):36S–42S

Hunter LL, Ries DT, Schlauch RS, Levine SC, Ward WD. Safety and clinical performance of acoustic reflex tests. Ear Hear 1999;20(6):506–514

Jeng PS, Allen JB, Lapsley Miller JA, Levitt H. Wideband power reflectance and power transmittance as tools for assessing middle-ear function. Perspectives on Hearing & Hearing Disorders in Childhood 2008;18(2):44–57

Jerger J. Clinical experience with impedance audiometry. Arch Otolaryngol 1970;92(4):311–324

Jerger J, Anthony L, Jerger S, Mauldin L. Studies in impedance audiometry. 3. Middle ear disorders. Arch Otolaryngol 1974;99(3):165–171

Jerger J, Burney P, Mauldin L, Crump B. Predicting hearing loss from the acoustic reflex. J Speech Hear Disord 1974;39(1):11–22

Jerger J, Harford E, Clemis J, Alford B. The acoustic reflex in eighth nerve disorders. Arch Otolaryngol 1974;99(6):409–413

Jerger J, Hayes D, Anthony L, Mauldin L. Factors influencing prediction of hearing level from the acoustic reflex. Maico Mongrs Contemp Audiol 1978;1:1–20

Jerger J, Jerger S, Mauldin L. Studies in impedance audiometry. I. Normal and sensorineural ears. Arch Otolaryngol 1972;96(6):513–523

Jerger S, Jerger J, Mauldin L, Segal P. Studies in impedance audiometry. II. Children less than 6 years old. Arch Otolaryngol 1974;99(1):1–9

Jerger S, Jerger J. Diagnostic value of crossed vs uncrossed acoustic reflexes: eighth nerve and brain stem disorders. Arch Otolaryngol 1977;103(8):445–453

Jerger S, Jerger J. Neuroaudiologic findings in patients with central auditory disorders. Semin Hear 1983;4:133–159

Joint Committee on Infant Hearing (JCIH), American Academy of Pediatrics. Year 2007 position statement: Principles and guidelines for early hearing detection and intervention programs. Pediatrics 2007;120(4):898–921

Keefe DH, Bulen JC, Arehart KH, Burns EM. Ear-canal impedance and reflection coefficient in human infants and adults. J Acoust Soc Am 1993;94(5):2617–2638

Keefe DH, Sanford CA, Ellison JC, Fitzpatrick DF, Gorga MP. Wideband aural acoustic absorbance predicts conductive hearing loss in children. Int J Audiol 2012;51(12):880–891

Keefe DH, Simmons JL. Energy transmittance predicts conductive hearing loss in older children and adults. J Acoust Soc Am 2003;114(6 Pt 1):3217–3238

Kei J, Allison-Levick J, Dockray J, et al. High-frequency (1000 Hz) tympanometry in normal neonates. J Am Acad Audiol 2003;14(1):20–28

Kei J, Sanford CA, Prieve BA, Hunter LL. Wideband acoustic immittance measures: developmental characteristics (0 to 12 months). Ear Hear 2013;34(Suppl 1):17S–26S

Keith RW. An evaluation of predicting hearing loss from the acoustic reflex. Arch Otolaryngol 1977;103(7):419–424

Koebsell KA, Margolis RH. Tympanometric gradient measured from normal preschool children. Audiology 1986;25(3):149–157

Lenarz T, Gülzow J. Akustisches Innenohrtrauma bei Impedanzmessung. Akutes Schalltrauma? [Acoustic inner ear trauma by impedance measurement. Acute acoustic trauma?]. Laryngol Rhinol Otol (Stuttg) 1983;62(2):58–61

Lidén G. The scope and application of current audiometric tests. J Laryngol Otol 1969;83(6):507–520

Lidén G, Harford E, Hallén O. Tympanometry for the diagnosis of ossicular disruption. Arch Otolaryngol 1974;99(1):23–29

Lidén G, Peterson JL, Björkman G. Tympanometry. Arch Otolaryngol 1970;92(3):248–257

Mangham CA. 1984. The effect of drugs and systemic disease on the acoustic reflex. In: Silman S, ed. The Acoustic Reflex: Basic Principles and Clinical Applications. Orlando, FL: Academic Press; 441–468

Margolis RH, Bass-Ringdahl S, Hanks WD, Holte L, Zapala DA. Tympanometry in newborn infants—1 kHz norms. J Am Acad Audiol 2003;14(7):383–392

Margolis RH, Goycoolea HG. Multifrequency tympanometry in normal adults. Ear Hear 1993;14(6):408–413

Margolis RH, Heller JW. Screening tympanometry: criteria for medical referral. Audiology 1987;26(4):197–208

Margolis RH, Popelka GR. Static and dynamic acoustic impedance measurements in infant ears. J Speech Hear Res 1975;18(3):435–443

Margolis RH, Shanks JE. 1985. Tympanometry. In: Katz J, ed. Handbook of Clinical Audiology, 3rd ed. Baltimore, MD: Williams & Wilkins; 438–475

Mazlan R, Kei J, Hickson L, et al. High frequency immittance findings: newborn versus six-week-old infants. Int J Audiol 2007;46(11):711–717

Mazlan R, Kei J, Hickson L. Test-retest reliability of the acoustic stapedial reflex test in healthy neonates. Ear Hear 2009;30(3):295–301

McGrath AP, Michaelides EM. Use of middle ear immittance testing in the evaluation of patulous Eustachian tube. J Am Acad Audiol 2011;22(4):201–207

Miller MH, Hoffman RA, Smallberg G. Stapedial reflex testing and partially reversible acoustic trauma. Hear Instr 1984;35:15–49

Nakajima HH, Rosowski JJ, Shahnaz N, Voss SE. Assessment of ear disorders using power reflectance. Ear Hear 2013;34(Suppl 1):48S–53S

Neely ST, Stenfelt S, Schairer KS. Alternative ear-canal measures related to absorbance. Ear Hear 2013;34(Suppl 1):72S–77S

Niemeyer W, Sesterhenn G. Calculating the hearing threshold from the stapedius reflex threshold for different sound stimuli. Audiology 1974;13(5):421–427

Northern JL, Gabbard SA. 1994. The acoustic reflex. In: Katz J, ed. Handbook of Clinical Audiology, 4th ed. Baltimore, MD: Williams & Wilkins; 300–316

Nozza RJ, Bluestone CD, Kardatzke D, Bachman R. Towards the validation of aural acoustic immittance measures for diagnosis of middle ear effusion in children. Ear Hear 1992;13(6):442–453

Nozza RJ, Bluestone CD, Kardatzke D, Bachman R. Identification of middle ear effusion by aural acoustic admittance and otoscopy. Ear Hear 1994;15(4):310–323

Olsen WO, Bauch CD, Harner SG. Application of Silman and Gelfand (1981) 90th percentile levels for acoustic reflex thresholds. J Speech Hear Disord 1983;48(3):330–332

Olsen WO, Stach BA, Kurdziel SA. Acoustic reflex decay in 10 seconds and in 5 seconds for Meniere's disease patients and for VIIIth nerve tumor patients. Ear Hear 1981;2(4):180–181

Ostergard CA, Carter DR. Positive middle ear pressure shown by tympanometry. Arch Otolaryngol 1981;107(6):353–356

Paradise JL, Smith CG, Bluestone CD. Tympanometric detection of middle ear effusion in infants and young children. Pediatrics 1976;58(2):198–210

Popelka GR. 1981. The acoustic reflex in normal and pathological ears. In: Popelka GR, ed. Hearing Assessment with the Acoustic Reflex. New York, NY: Grune & Stratton; 5–21

Popelka GR, Trumph A. 1976. Stapedial reflex thresholds for tonal and noise activating signals in relation to magnitude of hearing loss in multiple-handicapped children. Paper presented at Convention of American Speech-Language-Hearing Association, Houston

Porter T. Normal otoadmittance values for three populations. J Aud Res 1972;12:53–58

Portmann M. La mesure impédancemétrique n'est pas toujours sans risques. [Impedance audiometry is not always without risk]. Rev Laryngol Otol Rhinol (Bord) 1980;101(3-4):181–182

Prieve BA, Feeney MP, Stenfelt S, Shahnaz N. Prediction of conductive hearing loss using wideband acoustic immittance. Ear Hear 2013;34(Suppl 1):54S–59S

Renvall U, Liden G. 1978. Clinical significance of reduced middle ear pressure in school children. In: Harford ER, Bess FH, Bluestone CD, Klein JO, eds. Impedance Screening for Middle Ear Disease in Children. New York, NY: Grune & Stratton; 189–196

Riedel CL, Wiley TL, Block MG. Tympanometric measures of Eustachian tube function. J Speech Hear Res 1987;30(2):207–214

Rizzo S, Greenberg HJ. 1979. Predicting hearing loss from the acoustic reflex data. Paper presented at Convention of American Speech-Language-Hearing Association, Boston

Rosowski JJ, Stenfelt S, Lilly D. An overview of wideband immittance measurements techniques and terminology: you say absorbance, I say reflectance. Ear Hear 2013;34(Suppl 1):9S–16S

Roush J, Bryant K, Mundy M, Zeisel S, Roberts J. Developmental changes in static admittance and tympanometric width in infants and toddlers. J Am Acad Audiol 1995;6(4):334–338

Sanders JW. 1984. Evaluation of the 90th percentile levels for acoustic reflex thresholds. Paper presented at Convention of American Speech-Language-Hearing Association, San Francisco

Sanford CA, Hunter LL, Feeney MP, Nakajima HH. Wideband acoustic immittance: tympanometric measures. Ear Hear 2013;34(Suppl 1):65S–71S

Sanford CA, Keefe DH, Liu YW, et al. Sound-conduction effects on distortion-product otoacoustic emission screening outcomes in newborn infants: test performance of wideband acoustic transfer functions and 1-kHz tympanometry. Ear Hear 2009;30(6):635–652

Schairer KS, Ellison JC, Fitzpatrick D, Keefe DH. Wideband ipsilateral measurements of middle-ear muscle reflex thresholds in children and adults. J Acoust Soc Am 2007;121(6):3607–3616

Seifert MW, Seidemann MF, Givens GD. An examination of variables involved in tympanometric assessment of Eustachian tube function in adults. J Speech Hear Disord 1979;44(3):388–396

Shahnaz N, Bork K. Wideband reflectance norms for Caucasian and Chinese young adults. Ear Hear 2006;27(6):774–788

Shahnaz N, Bork K, Polka L, Longridge N, Bell D, Westerberg BD. Energy reflectance and tympanometry in normal and otosclerotic ears. Ear Hear 2009;30(2):219–233

Shahnaz N, Feeney MP, Schairer KS. Wideband acoustic immittance normative data: ethnicity, gender, aging, and instrumentation. Ear Hear 2013;34(Suppl 1):27S–35S

Shahnaz N, Polka L. Standard and multifrequency tympanometry in normal and otosclerotic ears. Ear Hear 1997;18(4):326–341

Shanks JE, Lilly DJ. An evaluation of tympanometric estimates of ear canal volume. J Speech Hear Res 1981;24(4):557–566

Shanks JE, Lilly DJ, Margolis RH, Wiley TL, Wilson RH; ASHA Working Group on Aural Acoustic-Immittance Measurements Committee on Audiologic Evaluation. Tympanometry. J Speech Hear Disord 1988;53(4):354–377

Shanks J, Shelton C. Basic principles and clinical applications of tympanometry. Otolaryngol Clin North Am 1991;24(2):299–328

Shaver MD, Sun X-M. Wideband energy reflectance measurements: effects of negative middle ear pressure and application of a pressure compensation procedure. J Acoust Soc Am 2013;134(1):332–341

Shaw J. 2009. Comparison of wideband energy reflectance and tympanometry measures obtained with Reflqin Interacoustics, Mimosa Acoustics and GSI Tympstar systems. Unpublished master's thesis. Vancouver: University of British Columbia. Available at: https://circle.

ubc.ca/bitstream/handle/2429/12715/ubc_2009_fall_shaw_jeffrey.pdf?sequence=1

Silman S. 1984. Magnitude and growth of the acoustic-reflex. In: Silman S, ed. The Acoustic Reflex: Basic Principles and Clinical Applications. Orlando, FL: Academic Press; 225–274

Silman S, Gelfand SA. Prediction of hearing levels from acoustic reflex thresholds in persons with high-frequency hearing losses. J Speech Hear Res 1979;22(4):697–707

Silman S, Gelfand SA. The relationship between magnitude of hearing loss and acoustic reflex threshold levels. J Speech Hear Disord 1981;46(3):312–316

Silman S, Gelfand SA. The acoustic reflex in diagnostic audiology—Part 2). Audiology (J Continuing Educ 1982;7:125–138)

Silman S, Gelfand SA, Emmer M. Acoustic reflex in hearing loss identification and prediction. Semin Hear 1987;8:379–390

Silman S, Gelfand SA, Piper N, Silverman CA, VanFrank L. 1984. Prediction of hearing loss from the acoustic-reflex threshold. In: Silman S, ed. The Acoustic Reflex: Basic Principles and Clinical Applications. Orlando, FL: Academic Press; 187–223

Silman S, Popelka GR, Gelfand SA. Effect of sensorineural hearing loss on acoustic stapedius reflex growth functions. J Acoust Soc Am 1978;64(5):1406–1411

Silman S, Silverman CA. 1991. Auditory Diagnosis: Principles and Applications. San Diego, CA: Academic Press

Silman S, Silverman CA, Arick DS. Acoustic-immittance screening for detection of middle-ear effusion in children. J Am Acad Audiol 1992;3(4):262–268

Silman S, Silverman CA, Gelfand SA, Lutolf J, Lynn DJ. Ipsilateral acoustic-reflex adaptation testing for detection of facial-nerve pathology: three case studies. J Speech Hear Disord 1988;53(4):378–382

Silman S, Silverman CA, Showers T, Gelfand SA. Effect of age on prediction of hearing loss with the bivariate-plotting procedure. J Speech Hear Res 1984;27(1):12–19

Silverman CA, Silman S, Miller MH. The acoustic reflex threshold in aging ears. J Acoust Soc Am 1983;73(1):248–255

Sprague BH, Wiley TL, Goldstein R. Tympanometric and acoustic-reflex studies in neonates. J Speech Hear Res 1985;28(2):265–272

Stach BA, Jerger JF. 1991. Immittance measures in auditory disorders. In: Jacobson JT, Northern JL, eds. Diagnostic Audiology. Austin, TX: Pro-Ed; 113–139

Starr A, Picton TW, Sininger Y, Hood LJ, Berlin CI. Auditory neuropathy. Brain 1996;119(Pt 3):741–753

Swanepoel W, Werner S, Hugo R, Louw B, Owen R, Swanepoel A. High frequency immittance for neonates: a normative study. Acta Otolaryngol 2007;127(1):49–56

Tanka K, Ohhashi K, Tsuda M. A case of unilateral acute sensorineural deafness after impedance audiometry. Clin Otol Jpn 1981;8:204–205

Turner RG, Frazer GJ, Shepard NT. Formulating and evaluating audiological test protocols. Ear Hear 1984;5(6):321–330

Turner RG, Shepard NT, Frazer GJ. Clinical performance of audiological and related diagnostic tests. Ear Hear 1984;5(4):187–194

Van Camp KJ, Creten WL, van de Heyning PH, Decraemer WF, Vanpeperstraete PM. A search for the most suitable immittance components and probe tone frequency in tympanometry. Scand Audiol 1983;12(1):27–34

Van Camp KJ, Margolis RH, Wilson, RH, Creten WL, Shanks JE. 1986. Principles of tympanometry. ASHA monographs no. 24

Vanhuyse VJ, Creten WL, Van Camp KJ. On the W-notching of tympanograms. Scand Audiol 1975;4:45–50

Wallin A, Mendez-Kurtz L, Silman S. Prediction of hearing loss from acoustic-reflex thresholds in the older adult population. Ear Hear 1986;7(6):400–404

Werner LA, Levi EC, Keefe DH. Ear-canal wideband acoustic transfer functions of adults and two- to nine-month-old infants. Ear Hear 2010;31(5):587–598

Wiley TL. Static acoustic-admittance measures in normal ears: a combined analysis for ears with and without notched tympanograms. J Speech Hear Res 1989; 32(3):688

Wiley TL, Block MG. 1984. Acoustic and nonacoustic reflex patterns in audiologic diagnosis. In: Silman S, ed. The Acoustic Reflex: Basic Principles and Clinical Applications. New York, NY: Academic Press; 387–411

Wiley TL, Nondahl DM, Cruickshanks KJ, Tweed TS. Five-year changes in middle ear function for older adults. J Am Acad Audiol 2005;16(3):129–139

Wiley TL, Oviatt DL, Block MG. Acoustic-immittance measures in normal ears. J Speech Hear Res 1987; 30(2):161–170

Wilson RH, Margolis RH. 1991. Acoustic-reflex measurements. In: Rintelmann WF, ed. Hearing Assessment, 2nd ed. Austin, TX: Pro-Ed; 247–319

Wilson RH, Margolis RH. 1999. Acoustic reflex measurements. In: Musiek FE, Rintelmann WF, eds. Contemporary Perspectives in Hearing Assessment. Boston, MA: Allyn & Bacon; 131–165

Wilson RH, Shanks JE, Kaplan SK. Tympanometric changes at 226 Hz and 678 Hz across 10 trials and for two directions of ear canal pressure change. J Speech Hear Res 1984a;27(2):257–266

Wilson RH, Shanks JE, Lilly DJ. 1984b. Acoustic-reflex adaptation. In: Silman S, ed. The Acoustic Reflex: Basic Principles and Clinical Applications. Orlando, FL: Academic Press; 329–386

Zwislocki J, Feldman AS. (1970). Acoustic impedance of pathological ears. ASHA monographs, no. 15

8 Speech Audiometry

As the principal avenue of human communication and interaction, it is clear that speech is the most important signal we hear. Consequently, the pure tone audiogram provides only a partial picture of the patient's auditory status because it does not give any direct information about his ability to hear and understand speech. To find out how a patient hears speech involves testing him with speech stimuli, and this process is called **speech audiometry**.

The instrument used for speech audiometry is the **speech audiometer**. Although devices designed specifically for speech audiometry were used in the past, this function is now incorporated into general-purpose clinical audiometers. The characteristics of audiometers, including those used for speech audiometry, are given in the *American National Standard Specifications for Audiometers* (ANSI S3.6-2010) and are described in Chapter 4. The **speech mode** (or the **speech channel**) of the clinical audiometer includes the following components: (1) various sources of recorded speech material, such as a tape deck, compact disk (CD) player, and a computer; (2) a microphone for live-voice testing; (3) an input selector to choose the desired source of the speech material; (4) an input level control, which is used with a VU meter to ensure that the speech signals are at the levels necessary for them to be properly calibrated; (4) an attenuator to control the level of speech being presented to the patient; (5) an output selector to direct the speech stimuli to the desired output transducer; and (6) output transducers (earphones, loudspeakers, bone vibrator). These components are illustrated in **Fig. 8.1**. In addition, there is a monitor earphone and/or loudspeaker (and level adjustment) to enable the audiologist to hear the speech signals that are being presented to the patient. Because speech audiometry is generally done in a two-room testing environment, there is also a patient (response) microphone that leads to an earphone and/or loudspeaker in the control room so that the audiologist can hear the patient's responses.

Recall that clinical audiometers have two channels because we sometimes need to present a signal to one ear and a masking noise to the opposite ear, or we might need to present different signals to the two ears on certain kinds of tests. The same thing applies to speech audiometry. Thus, a separate speech mode is provided for both channels of the audiometer. This allows us to send speech signals (not necessarily the same ones) to the two ears. Similarly, we might use one channel to present a speech test to one ear and use the second channel to present a masking noise to the opposite ear. Clinical masking is discussed in Chapter 9, and its appropriate use will be assumed throughout this chapter.

Calibrating the test signal(s) Calibration of the test materials is a necessary technical step in speech audiometry. Recorded materials always have a calibration signal, which is usually a 1000 Hz tone. The first steps are to select the appropriate input device (e.g., the tape deck) and set the interrupter switch to the constantly "on" position. The recorded calibration tone is then played while watching the level indicated on the VU meter. The input level dial is then turned up or down until the level of the calibration tone is at 0 dB on the VU meter. That's all there is to it. The input level control is kept in this position as long as this recording is being used. Now stop the calibration recording and proceed to administer the test materials on that recording. It will be necessary to recalibrate whenever you change recordings or move the input level dial. In practice it is desirable to calibrate the test material before each use. Throughout this chapter it will always be assumed that this simple calibration chore has already been completed for whatever tests are being used. Live-voice testing is trickier because the clinician must "balance" his vocal effort while talking into the microphone and setting the input level control to keep his speech "peaking" at 0 dB on the VU meter.

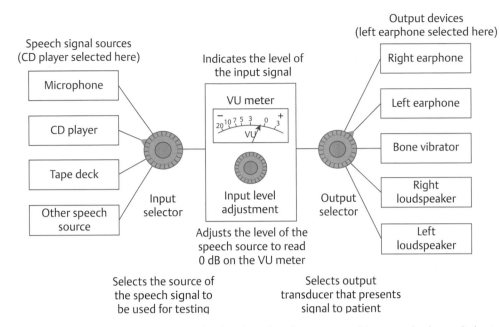

Fig. 8.1   Block diagram of the speech mode (channel) of a clinical audiometer. In this example the audiologist is using recorded speech from the CD player and is presenting that signal to the patient via the left earphone.

Thresholds for Speech

The threshold of a nonspeech signal such as a tone has a clear meaning: it is the level at which the presence of the sound is just audible. However, the threshold for speech can mean the lowest level at which speech is either just audible or just intelligible. The lowest level at which the presence of a speech signal can be heard 50% of the time is called the **speech detection threshold (SDT)** or the **speech awareness threshold (SAT)**. In contrast, the lowest level at which a speech signal is intelligible enough to be recognized or identified 50% of the time is the **speech recognition threshold** or **speech reception threshold (SRT)**. The SRT is usually obtained by asking the patient to repeat **spondee (or spondaic) words**, which are two-syllable words that have equal emphasis on both syllables, such as "baseball" or "railroad." Spondaic words lend themselves well to this use because a very small intensity increase causes the recognition of spondees to rise very rapidly from 0 to 100%. The SRT has also been called the **spondee threshold (ST)** when measured with spondaic words (ASHA 1979). All of these terms are readily understood in the field, but *speech detection threshold* and *speech recognition threshold* are the preferred usage (ASHA 1988).

Speech detection and recognition thresholds should be different because the SDT depends on audibility alone, whereas the SRT requires the stimuli to be heard and identified. This expectation has been borne out repeatedly by the finding that the average SDT tends to be roughly 7 to 9 dB lower (better) than the mean SRT (Thurlow, Silverman, Davis, & Walsh 1948; Chaiklin 1959; Beattie, Edgerton, & Svihovec 1975; Beattie, Svihovec, & Edgerton 1975; Cambron, Wilson, & Shanks 1991). Cambron, Wilson, and Shanks (1991) found the mean SDT-SRT difference to be 8 dB for a male talker and 8.2 dB for a female talker.

The speech reception threshold has several clinical functions: (1) to serve as a measure for corroborating pure tone thresholds, (2) to serve as a reference point for deciding on appropriate levels at which to administer suprathreshold speech recognition tests, (3) to determine hearing aid needs and performance, (4) to ascertain the need for aural (re)habilitation and progress in the management process, and (5) to determine hearing sensitivity for young children and others who are difficult to test. The speech detection threshold is generally used when an SRT is not obtainable.

Relation to the Pure tone Audiogram

Recall from Chapter 5 that the pure tone thresholds in the 500 to 2000 Hz range are associated with the SRT. We will see in Chapter 14 that a lack of reasonable consistency between the SRT and the pure tone thresholds is associated with functional hearing losses. In fact, as already mentioned, it is commonly accepted that one of the principal applications of the SRT is to corroborate the pure tone findings.

The SRT was originally compared with the pure tone average (PTA) of 500, 1000, and 2000 Hz (Fletcher 1929; Carhart 1946a), but it soon became apparent that this three-frequency PTA is not necessarily the combination of pure tone thresholds that comes closest to the SRT. This is especially true with sloping audiograms, where the pure tone thresholds may be quite different from one frequency to the other. Agreement between the SRT and PTA is improved under these conditions by using other combinations. Fletcher (1950) recommended using the average of the best two of these three frequencies, usually 500 and 1000 Hz. Carhart (1971) suggested that PTA-SAT agreement is maximized by a simple formula that involves subtracting 2 dB from the average of the 500 Hz and 1000 Hz thresholds. Single-frequency comparisons to the SRT are also sometimes appropriate. Carhart and Porter (1971) found that the single frequency with the highest correlation to the SRT is 1000 Hz, unless there is a sharply sloping hearing loss. When the audiogram slopes precipitously, it is often useful to compare the SRT to the one frequency that has the best threshold, which is often 500 Hz, and can even sometimes be 250 Hz (Gelfand & Silman 1985, 1993; Silman & Silverman 1991).

Materials for SRT Testing

As already indicated, most speech recognition thresholds are obtained using spondaic words, and we will concentrate on this method. Recorded 42-word spondee tests were originally developed at the Harvard Psychoacoustic Laboratory (PAL) by Hudgins, Hawkins, Karlin, and Stevens (1947). They tried to use phonetically dissimilar words from a familiar vocabulary that reasonably represented the sounds of English and were as homogeneous as possible with respect to their audibility. The PAL lists were provided in two recorded formats: all of the spondees were recorded at the same level in PAL Test No. 14, whereas they were attenuated by a fixed amount of 4 dB after every sixth word on PAL Test No. 9. Subsequently, Hirsh et al (1952) of the Central Institute for the Deaf (CID) improved upon the original spondaic materials by reducing the list to the 36 most familiar spondees and by recording the words in a way that made them homogeneous with respect to difficulty. This was done by adjusting the recording level by −2 dB

for the easiest spondees and by +2 dB for the hardest words. Six randomizations of the list were recorded with all of the spondees at the same level on the **CID W-1 Test**, and with an attenuation of 3 dB after every third word on the **CID W-2 Test**. In addition, each test word was preceded by the carrier phrase "Say the word . . . ," which was recorded at a level 10 dB higher than the test word itself. Contemporary studies using digital technology are addressing the issue of achieving homogeneous test materials in terms of the psychometric equivalence of recorded spondee words (e.g., Bilger, Matthies, Meyer, & Griffiths 1998; Wilson & Strouse 1999).

Numerous modifications and variations of the CID spondee materials have been introduced since the original lists and tests were distributed in the 1950s. A distinction is made between *lists* and *tests* because, for example, the CID W-1 Test refers to the specific recording just described. Presenting the same word list by live voice or from another recording actually constitutes a different test because of talker and recording differences. The spondaic word list recommended by ASHA (1988) is a revision of the CID W-1/W-2 list, emphasizing the criteria of dissimilarity among the words and homogeneous audibility. Recorded versions of the spondee tests (as well as many of the others discussed in this chapter) on cassette tapes and/or CDs are produced by Auditec of St. Louis, Virtual Corporation, and the Department of Veterans Affairs (VA). For example, the psychometrically equivalent spondee tests using a female talker developed by Wilson and Strouse (1999) are included in a CD produced by the Department of Veterans Affairs (1998). In addition, ASHA (1988) recommended a streamlined list of 15 highly homogeneous spondees based on research by Young, Dudley, and Gunter (1982), and a list of 20 spondees easily represented by pictures that are suitable for testing young children, based on findings by Frank (1980). Shortened lists like these are commonly used in clinical practice, but the student should be aware that shortening the word list lowers the SRT (Punch & Howard 1985; Meyer & Bilger 1997). Several examples of commonly used spondaic word lists may be found in Appendix B.

Although spondees are used in the overwhelming majority of routine clinical SRT measurements, they are not the only materials available for this purpose. Sentences are also used to obtain SRTs, principally against a background of noise or speech babble (the composite of several talkers all speaking at the same time). We will return to the use of these **sentence reception thresholds** later in this chapter.

Measuring the Speech Recognition Threshold

Instructions and Familiarization

The first part of the SRT testing process involves instructing the patient about the task and familiarizing him with the test words. As recommended by ASHA (1988), the instructions should indicate the nature of the task, that it involves speech material, how the patient is to respond, that he should continue responding even when the words are faint, and that guessing is encouraged. The following is an example of instructions that one might use:

> The next test is used to find the softest speech that you can hear and repeat back. I (*or a recorded voice*) will say two-syllable words like "baseball" or "railroad," and your job is to repeat each word. The words will start out being loud so that you can familiarize yourself with them. They will then get softer and softer. Your job is to keep repeating the words back to me, no matter how soft they become, even if you have to guess. Do you have any questions? (*Address these questions as necessary.*)

Notice that these instructions also refer to the familiarization process that precedes the actual testing. The purpose of familiarization is to ensure that the patient knows the test vocabulary and is able to recognize each word auditorily, and that the clinician can accurately interpret the patient's responses (ASHA 1988). The importance of the familiarization process is well established (Pollack, Rubenstein, & Decker 1959; Tillman & Jerger 1959; Conn, Dancer, & Ventry 1975). For example, Tillman and Jerger (1959) found that the average SRT is ~ 4 to 5 dB lower with familiarization than without it.

Recorded versus Monitored Live-Voice Testing

Spondaic words may be presented to the patient using readily available recorded materials or by **monitored live voice**, which means the words are spoken into a microphone by the audiologist, who monitors her voice level on the audiometer's VU meter. Recorded material is preferred for SRT testing, but presenting the stimuli by monitored live voice is also acceptable (ASHA 1988). Compared with monitored live-voice testing, recorded materials provide much better control over the level and quality of the speech signals being presented to the patient, as well as the obvious benefits of greater standardization. On the other hand, the flexibility afforded by monitored live-voice testing is often desirable or essential when testing patients who require any kind of modification

of the test procedure. Typical examples are elderly patients who might need more time to respond than is provided on the recording, children or others with restricted vocabularies, etc. The need for flexibility is not limited to patients who have special needs. For example, it is often desirable to test at a faster pace than is possible with recorded lists when testing some young, normal adults. In addition, the SRT is usually robust enough to withstand the limitations of live-voice testing, and has been found to be reliable under these conditions (Carhart 1946b; Creston, Gillespie, & Krohn 1966; Beattie, Forrester, & Ruby 1977). In fact, modified live voice is the most common way to present spondees for the SRT, and its use *for this purpose* is generally agreeable even to ardent proponents of recorded materials for most other kinds of speech recognition testing. However, the audiologic results should indicate that the SRT was obtained by monitored live voice when this is the case.

Carrier Phrase Use for SRT Testing

Whether the test word is introduced by a carrier phrase (e.g., "Say the word . . .") does not appear to have any substantive effect upon the resulting SRT (Silman & Silverman 1991). In fact, even though carrier phrases were included on the original Technisonics Studios phonograph recordings of W-1 and W-2, they are omitted from current commonly used spondee recordings such as those by Auditec of St. Louis and Virtual Corporation.

The Initial (Ballpark) SRT Estimate

It would unnecessarily fatigue the patient and waste time and effort to present many test words at levels well above or below the actual SRT. For this reason, SRT testing usually has an initial phase in which the level of the spondee words is changed in relatively large steps to make a quick, rough estimate of where the SRT is probably located. This ballpark estimate provides an efficiently placed starting level for the actual threshold search. Most SRT protocols specify the starting hearing level and technique for making this ballpark estimate, and this initial testing phase will be mentioned for each of the four SRT methods described below. However, one should be aware that many audiologists select the level to present the first word based on the patient's behavior or pure tone thresholds.

Testing Techniques

It is generally accepted that the SRT is the lowest hearing level at which a patient can repeat 50% of spondee words, but there are many ways to find this point and no single technique is universally accepted. Most SRT testing methods share several common features even though their specific characteristics can vary widely. The most common characteristic is that several spondee words are presented to the patient one at a time at the same hearing level. The **descending methods** begin presenting these blocks of test words *above* the estimated SRT so that the patient is initially able to repeat them, and then present subsequent blocks of spondee words at progressively lower hearing levels. This process is repeated until the patient misses a certain number of words, at which time the descending run is over. On the other hand, **ascending methods** start *below* the estimated threshold, where the patient cannot repeat the words, and then present subsequent blocks of test words at progressively higher hearing levels. This procedure is repeated until the patient correctly repeats a certain number of words, at which point the ascending run is terminated. What distinguishes the methods are features such as how many words are in a block, what are the criteria for starting and stopping an ascending or descending run, and how one defines the "50% correct" level.

One general group of SRT methods considers the SRT to be the lowest hearing level where half (or at least half) of a block of the words is correct. Three examples are illustrated in **Fig. 8.2**, although other techniques are also useful (e.g., Downs & Dickinson Minard 1996). The Chaiklin and Ventry (1964) method is a *descending technique* because it begins by presenting the spondee words at a level that is high enough for them to be heard and repeated easily, and

then searches for the SRT by presenting words at progressively lower hearing levels. The method involves presenting the spondees one at a time in blocks of up to six words per level. The intensity is decreased in 5 dB steps to find the lowest level where three words are repeated correctly. Two-decibel steps may also be used, but Chaiklin and Ventry (1964) found that 2 and 5 dB step sizes yield comparable results for clinical purposes. The initial testing phase begins 25 dB above the patient's two-frequency pure tone average, and involves presenting one word per level in decreasing 5 dB steps until one word is missed. The starting point for the main SRT search begins 10 dB above that level.

The Chaiklin-Ventry technique is illustrated in **Fig. 8.2a**. Suppose the first word was missed at 25 dB HL during the initial phase of testing, so that the starting level for our SRT search is 10 dB higher, at 35 dB HL. It is not necessary to present more than three words at the 35 dB starting level because they are all correct. The rationale is that three correct words out of a possible six indicates the performance is already at least 50%, so that nothing would be gained by presenting any more words at this level. This is why many of the blocks in the figure have fewer than six words even though the method is theoretically based on six words per level. In any case, because the patient repeated three words at 35 dB HL, we now know that the SRT must be 35 dB HL *or lower*. The level is thus reduced to 30 dB HL, where the same thing occurs, so we know the SRT is 30 dB HL or lower. When the level is reduced to 25 dB HL, the first two words are right but the third one is wrong. We

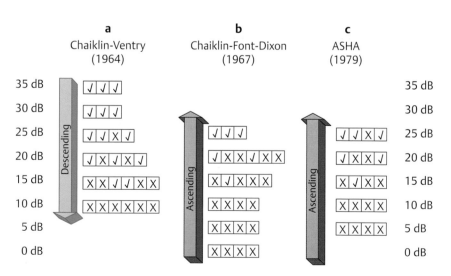

Fig. 8.2 Examples of measuring the SRT with **(a)** descending (Chaiklin & Ventry 1964), **(b)** ascending (Chaiklin, Font, & Dixon 1967), and **(c)** ascending (ASHA 1979) methods. The ASHA (1979) method includes a second ascending run beginning 10 dB below the first SRT measurement (*not shown*). The SRT is defined as the lowest hearing level where three out of a possible six spondee words are repeated correctly in **(a)** and **(b)**, and as the lowest level where at least three of the spondees are repeated correctly in **(c)**.

must now present another word because it is possible for the percentage of correct responses to be less than 50%. The fourth word is correct, bringing the tally to three right and one wrong at this level. Here, too, the score would be at least 50% if all six words were given, so there would be no benefit from presenting more words at this level. The SRT is now 25 dB HL or lower. Five words are needed at 20 dB HL. Let us see why. The first three words include an error, so a fourth is needed. The fourth word brings the tally to two right and two wrong. Based on a possible six words, the score could still be 33% (2 of 6), 50% (3 of 6), or even 67% (4 of 6). A fifth word is therefore presented, which is correct. This brings the tally to three correct out of a possible six, again meeting the criterion. The SRT is now 20 dB HL or lower. The intensity is reduced to 15 dB HL, where the following is found: one right out of three, two correct out of four, and two right out of five. Here a sixth word is needed to determine whether the score is 50% (3 of 6) or 33% (2 of 6). Word 6 is wrong, indicating that 15 dB is *below* the SRT. Thus, the SRT is *20 dB HL* in this example, because this is the lowest level where half of the spondee words are repeated correctly (out of a possible 6). The figure shows that 10 dB HL was also tested because the Chaiklin-Ventry method requires that we continue testing until all six words in a block are wrong, which occurs here at the next lower level.

Chaiklin, Font, and Dixon (1967) described an *ascending* SRT method that is otherwise very similar to the Chaiklin-Ventry technique in that it uses the same number of words per level, step size, and definition of the SRT. This method is illustrated in **Fig. 8.2b**. Because this is an ascending method, the starting level is now below the expected SRT. The initial testing phase with this approach begins at –10 dB HL, and involves presenting one word per level in ascending 10 dB steps until one word is repeated correctly. The main threshold search for SRT is then started 20 dB below that level. For example, if the first word was correctly repeated at 20 dB HL during the initial phase, then the starting level for the main test would be 20 dB lower, or 0 dB HL, which is shown in the figure. In the ascending method, we are working upward until the patient finally repeats correctly three out of a theoretical six words per level. The reasoning for how many words to use per level is analogous to the Chaiklin-Ventry method, except that we must be mindful of the direction. At least four words must be presented and missed before raising the test level because this is the smallest number of misses that can tell us that we are still *below* the SRT. In other words, the patient must miss four out of a possible six words before we really know that he cannot possibly repeat three of them. This explains why four errors are shown at each ascending level from

the starting level of 0 dB HL through 20 dB. Only four words are needed if the patient misses all of them (e.g., at 0, 5, and 10 dB HL), but five words must be used if one is correct (e.g., at 15 dB HL), and six words are needed if two are right (e.g., at 20 dB HL). The SRT in this example is *25 dB HL* because this is the first level where three words are repeated correctly. It is not necessary to go above this point because the SRT is defined as the lowest level where the patient correctly repeats three of a possible six spondees. Incidentally, just because the patient got all three words correct in a row in our example does not mean this is always the case. Any combination of three correct spondees in a block of up to six words at the same hearing level will do (e.g., "x✓x✓✓" or "x✓x✓x✓" or "xxx✓✓✓").

The *ascending* SRT method recommended by ASHA (1979) is illustrated in **Fig. 8.2c**. Its initial testing phase is similar to the Chaiklin, Font, and Dixon (1967) approach, except that the starting level for the main test is 15 dB below the level where the first word is correctly repeated. This is why the two methods have different starting levels in the figure. The ASHA (1979) method has the following characteristics: Four spondee words are presented at each hearing level. The hearing level is increased by 5 dB until *at least three* of the words are correctly repeated at the same level (which is 25 dB HL in the figure). The intensity is then reduced by 10 dB, and a second ascending series of presentations is administered using the same technique (not shown in the figure). The SRT is defined as the lowest level at which at least three words are correctly repeated, based on at least two ascending runs.

The methods just described are similar in that the SRT is the hearing level of the block of words that meets some criterion (such as 3 of 6 or 3 of 4 words correct). Another general group of SRT methods involves interpolating the 50% correct level using the responses obtained from several blocks of words (Hudgins et al 1947; Tillman & Olsen 1973; Wilson, Morgan, & Dirks 1973; ASHA 1988), and is based on well-established statistical principles (Spearman 1908). This technique is often called the **Tillman-Olsen method** and is incorporated into the ASHA (1988) guidelines for SRT testing.

The initial phase of the ASHA (1988) method is a ballpark estimate. It begins by presenting one spondee word at 30 dB or 40 dB HL. If the original intensity is too low for the patient to repeat the first word, then it is increased in large, 20 dB steps (giving one word per step) to quickly find where she can repeat a word. Regardless of whether the first word is repeated at 30 dB HL or at 70 dB HL, then one word per level is presented in decreasing 10 dB steps until the patient misses a word, at which point a second word is presented. This descending strategy continues until she misses two consecutive words at the same level. The *starting level* for the main SRT determination will be 10 dB higher than the level where the two words were missed. Thus, if the patient misses two consecutive words at 40 dB HL, the starting level would be 50 dB HL.

Having arrived at a starting level, we are now ready to find the SRT using the ASHA (1988) procedure. The testing itself is similar to the other methods, except five words are given at every level and we keep track of whether each word is right or wrong on a tally sheet such as the one shown in **Fig. 8.3**. First, five spondee words are presented one at a time at the starting level, where the patient usually repeats all of them correctly. We then decrease the hearing level by 5 dB and present another five words, tallying the results for each word. This *descending* procedure continues until the patient misses all five words at the same level. This "stopping level" is 35 dB HL in the example. Notice that the patient's performance goes from 100% correct at the starting level down to 0% correct at the stopping level. The SRT is interpolated from this range by, in effect, giving 1 dB of credit for each correctly repeated word. The calculation is done by following these steps:

1. Record the starting level (50 dB in the example).
2. Count all the correct words, including the starting level (10 words in the example).
3. Subtract the number of correct words from the starting level (50 – 10 = 40).
4. Add a 2 dB correction factor to the difference found in step 3 (40 + 2 = 42).

The result in step 4 is the SRT, expressed in dB HL (SRT = 42 dB HL). The ASHA (1988) method can also be done with 2 dB steps (**Fig. 8.4**). Here, we present two words per level and stop testing when the patient misses five out of six words. The calculation is also the same, except that the correction factor is 1 dB.

In general, the differences between SRTs obtained with the various test methods tend to be either not statistically significant or too small to be of any major clinical relevance. For example, SRTs are ~ 2.7 to 3.7 dB better (lower) with the ASHA (1988) method compared with the ASHA (1979) procedure, but the 1979 method has a slight edge with respect to agreement between the SRT and pure tone averages (Huff & Nerbonne 1982; Wall, Davis, & Myers 1984; Jahner, Schlauch, & Doyle 1994). The 1988 method took less time to administer than the 1979 technique in two studies (Huff & Nerbonne 1982; Wall et al 1984), but Jahner et al (1994) found that the 1988 method took 4 seconds longer plus 11 seconds for the SRT calculation. It is hard to demonstrate a singularly "best" method, although the ASHA (1988) approach appears to be the most appealing one on conceptual grounds.

Testing by Bone-Conduction

Bone-conduction speech audiometry most often involves obtaining an SRT. This approach has been used to (1) help indicate whether a conductive loss is present (by comparison to the air-conduction SRT) in children and other patients when reliable pure tone results are lacking, (2) provide insight about

Speech level	Word number					
(dB HL)	1	2	3	4	5	
50	√	√	√	√	√	Starting level
45	√	√	X	√	√	
40	X	√	X	X	X	
35	X	X	X	X	X	Stop: 5 missed on same level

Count correct words from startng level to stopping level (10 in this example)

Calculation of SRT (in dB HL):

Record the starting level: 50
Subtract number of correct words: – 10
Subtotal: 40
Add the 2-dB correction factor: + 2
Seech recognition threshold (SRT) = 42

Fig. 8.3 Tally sheet and calculation of the SRT with 5 dB steps according to the ASHA (1988) method.

Speech level (dB HL)	Word no. 1	Word no. 2	
50	√	√	Starting level
48	√	√	
46	X	√	Count correct words from starting level to stopping level (9 in this example)
44	√	X	
42	√	X	
40	X	√	
38	√	X	
36	X	X	
34	X	X	Stop: 5 of 6 words missed

Calculation of SRT (in dB HL):

Record the starting level:	50
Subtract number of correct words:	− 9
Subtotal:	41
Add the 1-dB correction factor:	+ 1
Speech recognition threshold (SRT) =	42

Fig. 8.4 Tally sheet and calculation of the SRT with 2 dB steps according to the ASHA (1988) method.

the status of the cochlea before and after middle ear surgery, and (3) corroborate bone-conduction pure tone thresholds (Bess 1983; Olsen & Matkin 1991). Although reference values are provided for presenting speech stimuli by bone-conduction (see Chapter 4), it is a wise choice to calibrate on an empirical basis for the presentation of speech by bone-conduction.

Comfortable and Uncomfortable Loudness Levels for Speech

The **most comfortable loudness level (MCL)** for speech is the hearing level at which the patient experiences speech material to be most comfortable, that is, where she prefers to listen to speech material. In contrast, the **uncomfortable loudness level (UCL)** for speech is the hearing level at which the patient considers speech material to be uncomfortably loud. The uncomfortable loudness level is also known as the **loudness discomfort level (LDL)**.

The types of speech material typically used for obtaining the MCL and UCL include continuous discourse, spondee words, and sentences. "Continuous discourse" (or "cold running speech") is usually a recorded selection of some prose material. Relatively uninteresting selections are used so that the patient can focus on the loudness of the material without being distracted by its content.

Both the MCL and UCL are affected by the testing method used and the instructions given to the

patient, although generally accepted, standardized methods for their measurement are lacking (Punch, Joseph, & Rakerd 2004a). The basic approach involves adjusting the speech level up or down until the patient indicates that it is comfortably loud for the MCL and uncomfortably loud for the UCL. Another approach employs category rating methods like the **Contour Test** (Cox, Alexander, Taylor, & Gray 1997). Originally designed for use with tonal stimuli, the Contour Test was successfully used to measure MCLs and UCLs for spondee words by Punch, Rakerd, & Joseph (2004b). In this test, the patient listens to spondee words presented one at a time at different levels, and rates the loudness of each of them based on a choice of descriptive categories. An example would be a seven-point scale, where **1** is "very soft," **2** is "soft," **3** is "comfortable, but slightly soft," **4** is "comfortable," **5** is "comfortable, but slightly loud," **6** is "loud, but OK," and **7** is "uncomfortably loud."

As they try to find *the* MCL, new clinicians learn rather quickly that many patients report comfortable loudness at several hearing levels. This experience reveals that the MCL is actually a *range of levels* instead of *a level* (Dirks & Morgan 1983; Punch et al 2004a). Because ascending tests produce low estimates of the MCL and descending tests produce high estimates, it has been suggested that these two measurements might be used to identify the lower and upper ends of the MCL range, in which case the midpoint between them might be used when a single value is desired (Dirks & Kamm 1976; Punch et al 2004b).

Why are descending MCLs higher than ascending MCLs? The stimuli start at high levels (from which they are lowered) in a descending test, whereas they start at low levels (from which they are raised) in an ascending test. Thus, the patient's MCL judgment is affected by the point of reference provided by the preceding sounds, which are much louder when a descending test is done and much softer when an ascending test is done (Punch et al 2004a). Consistent with this, Punch et al (2004b) showed that MCLs were influenced by whether they were tested before or after UCLs. Specifically, MCLs were significantly elevated when they followed a UCL measurement. (However, UCLs were not appreciably affected by test order.) The clinical implications are that (1) ascending MCL estimates should be done before descending MCL estimates when both are being used to establish the MCL range, and (2) MCL testing should be completed before UCL testing (Punch et al 2004b)

When testing for the UCL, it is important for the patient to understand that he should indicate when the experience of *loudness* becomes uncomfortable (Dirks & Morgan 1983). For example, the instructions for the Contour Test tell the patient to "Keep in mind that an uncomfortably loud sound is louder than you would ever choose on your radio no matter what mood you are in" (Cox et al 1997, p. 390). This is an important point because we are interested in when the sound becomes uncomfortably loud rather than the patient's capacity to endure pain. In other words, we are concerned with sound levels that begin to produce an uncomfortable *auditory* experience, as opposed to the *tactile* sensations (e.g., tickle, feeling, pain) associated with the highest tolerable sound intensities. For this reason, *uncomfortable loudness level* is often preferred over other terms that include words like *discomfort* and *tolerance*, such as *loudness discomfort level, tolerance level,* or *threshold of discomfort.*

The range in decibels between the patient's SRT and UCL is called the **dynamic range**. It is, in effect, the patient's usable listening range. For example, if a patient has an SRT of 15 dB HL and a UCL of 100 dB HL, then her dynamic range would be 100 – 15 = 85 dB wide. This means that the patient's hearing can accommodate a range of sound intensities that is 85 dB wide. One of the major problems faced by many patients with sensorineural hearing losses is that their thresholds are elevated but their UCLs remain essentially unchanged, which results in a constricted dynamic range. For example, a patient's SRT might be elevated to 65 dB HL, but her UCL might still be 100 dB HL, so that her dynamic range would be 100 – 65 = 35 dB wide. Notice the difference between this situation and the prior example. There would be no problem "fitting" the wide range of intensities in the real world into a usable (dynamic) listening range that is 85 dB wide. However, the patient in the second example has a usable listening range that is only 35 dB wide, which is too narrow to accommodate the range of intensities found in the real world of sound. Imagine the implications of a restricted dynamic range for hearing aid use: Amplifying sound levels so they become audible (which is desirable) will also cause many sounds to exceed the patient's UCL (which is undesirable). Consequently, in addition to amplifying them, we must also try to "squeeze" the wide range of real-world sounds into the patient's narrower dynamic range.

■ Assessing Speech Recognition

There is a readily understandable distinction between the threshold for speech and the ability to understand the speech that is heard. Consider the following complaints expressed by a variety of hearing-impaired patients: "I can hear speech but I can't understand it"; "Words aren't clear"; "Speech sounds muffled [or distorted]"; or "I mistake one word for another." The common theme here is that the speech heard by the patient is lacking in intelligibility. This problem is experienced in terms of inaccurately received messages and/or reduced clarity. Speech recognition measures have been used in every phase of audiology, such as (1) to describe the extent of hearing impairment in terms of how it affects speech understanding, (2) in the differential diagnosis of auditory disorders, (3) for determining the needs for amplification and other forms of audiologic rehabilitation, (4) for making comparisons between various hearing aids and amplification approaches, (5) for verifying the benefits of hearing aid use and other forms of audiologic rehabilitation, and (6) for monitoring patient performance over time for either diagnostic or rehabilitative purposes.

Speech intelligibility can be tested clinically in a straightforward manner. The most common approach is to present the patient with a list of test words. The percentage of test words correctly repeated by the patient is called the **speech recognition score**, the **word recognition score**, or the **speech discrimination score**. *Speech recognition score* is the preferred term because it describes the task in terms of the patient's response, which involves recognizing or identifying the test items. It is often called the "suprathreshold speech recognition score" because these tests are typically performed at levels above the threshold for speech. *Word recognition score* is an equally acceptable term provided the test items are words, which is usually the case. Even though it is a popular term, *speech discrimination score* is less desirable because it refers to a different kind of test than that usually performed. Specifically, a speech *discrimination* test involves comparing two (or more) items and judging whether they are the same or different. Speech recognition scores are sometimes called "PB scores" for reasons that will become clear, although this term is technically correct only when "PB" materials are used. One sometimes sees references to "articulation testing" and "articulation scores," particularly in the older literature. Even though this term is rarely used anymore, it was actually quite appropriate because it alludes to the degree of correspondence between the stimulus and the response.

The student has probably noticed that *speech recognition score* looks and sounds a lot like *speech recognition threshold*. The possible confusion of these terms is one reason that many audiologists continue to use the terms *speech reception threshold* and *speech discrimination score* even though the preferred nomenclature is more descriptive and precise.

Traditional Test Materials

Speech recognition tests were originally devised to assess the effectiveness of telephone and radio communication systems, and various different kinds of speech material were used for this purpose. The most commonly used materials for clinical speech recognition testing are monosyllabic words that are presented in an open-set format. An **open-set** format means the patient must respond without any prior knowledge of what the possible alternatives might be, whereas a **closed-set** format means the patient is provided with a choice of several possible response alternatives. In other words, an open-set item is much like a fill-in question and a closed-set item is much the same as a multiple-choice question.

This section outlines the development of the W-22 and NU-6 lists, which are the most widely used speech recognition tests in general clinical practice. We can then discuss the fundamental aspects and implications of speech recognition testing without being overwhelmed by the details of alternative kinds of tests. Other speech recognition materials will be discussed later in the chapter.

The common features of the W-22 and NU-6 speech recognition tests include an open-set format; 50-word lists composed of reasonably familiar monosyllabic words, each of which is preceded by a carrier phrase (such as "You will say . . ." or "Say the word . . ."); and phonetic or phonemic balance within each list. Several recorded versions of these tests are commercially available. The CID W-22 and NU-6 test lists may be found in Appendices C and D.

The first monosyllabic word materials to enjoy wide clinical use were the Harvard **PAL PB-50 test** (Egan 1948). The PB-50 test is the precursor of the W-22 and NU-6 materials, which have supplanted it in day-to-day speech recognition testing. Each of the 20 PB-50 lists included 50 words that were phonetically balanced (hence the name "PB-50"). **Phonetic balance** means that the relative frequencies of the phonemes on the test list are as close as possible to the distribution of speech sounds used in English, which was in turn based on Dewey's (1923) analysis of 100,000 words in newsprint. To improve word familiarity and phonetic balance, Hirsh et al (1952) included 120 of the 1000 PB-50 words in the **CID W-22 test** lists. The W-22 test includes 200 words arranged in four 50-word lists (1–4), each of which was recorded using six randomizations. Phonetic balance on the W-22 lists is based on an analysis of spoken English (business telephone conversations) by French, Carter, and Koenig (1930), as well as the Dewey word counts, where 95% of the words on the W-22 lists are among the 4000 most common words found by Thorndike (1932).

Northwestern University Auditory Test No. 6, or the **NU-6 test**, is composed of four lists of 50 phonemically balanced **consonant-vowel nucleus-consonant**, or **CNC**, words (Tillman & Carhart 1966). Just as the W-22 test was derived from the PB-50 materials, the NU-6 lists were based on the earlier work of Lehiste and Peterson (1959; Peterson & Lehiste 1962). Lehiste and Peterson (1959) modified the concept of phonetic balance to one of **phonemic balance** in recognition of the fact that speech recognition is accomplished on a phonemic rather than a phonetic basis. This is a real distinction because **phonemes** are actually groups of speech sounds (each of which is a **phonetic element**) that are classified as being the same by native speakers of the language. Thus, all phonetic differences are not phonemically relevant. For example, phonetically different variants of the phoneme /p/ (**allophones** of /p/) are identified as /p/ even though they vary in terms of their articulatory and acoustic (i.e., phonetic) characteristics in different speech sound contexts (e.g., /p/ as in /pat/ versus /pit/, or initially versus finally as in /pɛp/) and from production to production. To achieve a reasonable degree of phonemic balance, Lehiste and Peterson developed test lists from 1263 monosyllabic words. These were all CNC words drawn from the Thorndike and Lorge (1944) word counts. The original CNC lists were subsequently modified to replace the least familiar words (Peterson & Lehiste 1962), so that all but 21 of the words on the final version of the CNC lists have a frequency of ≥ 5/million. Tillman, Carhart, and Wilber (1963) used 95 of Lehiste and Peterson's CNC words and 5 others to construct two 50-word lists known as the NU-4 test, which may be viewed as an intermediate step in the development of the NU-6 test. The 100 CNCs on the NU-4 lists were increased to 200 words (185 of which are from the Lehiste and Peterson materials) to develop the four 50-word lists that compose the NU-6 test (Tillman & Carhart 1966).

Speech Recognition Testing

The speech recognition testing process is extremely simple. We will assume that the test is being done with either recorded W-22 or NU-6 materials, but the fundamentals are largely the same regardless of which test is used. The patient is instructed to listen to the test recording and to repeat each test word, guessing if necessary. The attenuator is then set to the desired presentation level, and the speech materials are presented to the patient through the desired output transducer (e.g., one of the earphones). The clinician keeps a tally of right and wrong responses during the test and then calculates a percent correct score. Each word is worth 2% on a 50-word test. For example, the speech recognition score would be 92% if four words are missed or repeated incorrectly, 86% if seven words are wrong, etc. Foreign language speakers and those who cannot give a verbal response can often be tested effectively by having them respond by pointing to the response word from a choice of alternative words or pictures (Spitzer 1980; Wilson & Antablin 1980; Comstock & Martin 1984; McCullough, Cunningham, & Wilson 1992; McCullough, Wilson, Birck, & Anderson 1994; Aleksandrovsky, McCullough, & Wilson 1998).

Speech recognition scores are generally expected to be ~ 90 to 100% in normal-hearing individuals. The range of speech recognition scores is typically between 80 and 100% with most conductive losses (e.g., otitis media, otosclerosis), but has been found to be as low as 60% in cases of glomus tumor; and the range for sensorineural losses is anywhere from 0 to 100%, depending on etiology and degree of loss (Bess 1983). In general, speech recognition scores that are "abnormally low" are associated with retrocochlear lesions; however, there is no clear cutoff value for this decision (e.g., Johnson 1977; Olsen, Noffsinger, & Kurdziel 1975; Bess 1983). As we shall see in the next section, a lower than expected speech recognition score can also occur if the test level is not high enough. Thus, an atypically low speech recognition score often means the clinician must retest at a higher hearing level.

When is a speech recognition score "too low" with respect to the patient's audiogram? There is a rough relationship in which speech recognition scores tend to become lower as sensorineural hearing loss worsens, but it is hardly predictive and is complicated because the notion of "better" and "worse" on an audiogram often involves considering both the amount and configuration of the loss. Some guidance was provided by 98% lower cutoff values for PB-50 test scores associated with various amounts of cochlear hearing loss among patients younger than 56 years of age (Yellin, Jerger, & Fifer 1989). However, those cutoff values based on PB-50 test scores do not seem applicable to scores obtained with more commonly used tests such as CID W-22 (Gates, Cooper, Kannel, & Miller 1990). Dubno, Lee, Klein, Matthews, and Lam (1995) reported 95% lower cutoff values for the NU-6 test (Auditec version) as a function of the patient's three-frequency PTA. These lower cutoff values are shown for both 50- and 25-word lists in **Fig. 8.5**.

Performance-Level Functions

The percentage of words that are repeated correctly depends on more than just the patient's speech recognition ability. It also depends on the conditions of the test, such as the level at which the words are presented. The graph in **Fig. 8.5** is called a **performance-level (PL) function** because it shows how the patient's speech recognition *performance* (in percent correct on the y-axis) depends on the *level* of the test materials (along the x-axis). The more traditional term, **performance-intensity (PI) function**, is often used as well. The PL function is a type of **psychometric function**, which shows performance (in this case speech recognition) as a function of some stimulus parameter (in this case the speech level). It is often called a **PL-PB** or **PI-PB function** when phonetically or phonemically balanced (PB) words are used.

The PL function in **Fig. 8.6** is from a normal-hearing individual. Notice how his speech recognition scores are low when the words are presented at very soft levels, and that the scores improve as the intensity increases. In this case, a maximum score of 100% is eventually achieved when the intensity reaches a level of 30 dB HL. The maximum score on the PI-PB function is traditionally called PB_{max}. Notice that the PL function flattens (or becomes asymptotic) as the intensity is raised above the level where PB_{max} is found. This plateau establishes the fact that PB_{max} has been reached, because it shows that the score does not improve any more when the intensity continues to be raised. (This is a moot point when 100% is reached, but it is a real issue when PB_{max} is lower than 100%.) This maximum score is used to express a patient's speech recognition performance. It is assumed that a patient's "speech recognition score" refers to PB_{max} unless otherwise indicated. Thus, we must be confident that PB_{max} has been obtained (or at least approximated).

Fig. 8.5 Lower 95% confidence limits for PB_{max} when obtained using the NU-6 test (Auditec) as a function of the degree of hearing loss. (Based on data by Dubno, Lee, Klein, Matthews, and Lam 1995.)

Fig. 8.6 The performance-level function of a normal-hearing individual whose maximum speech recognition score *(PB_{max})* is 100%.

Fig. 8.7 Several representative examples of various kinds of performance-intensity functions. **(a)** The same normal performance-level (PL) function from **Fig. 8.6**. **(b)** The same normal PL function displaced rightward by 30 dB HL due to a conductive loss. **(c)** The PL function of a patient with sensorineural loss whose scores reach PB_{max} of 80% at 70 dB HL and remain essentially the same at higher levels. **(d)** The PL function of a patient with sensorineural loss with PB_{max} of 76% at 70 dB HL, which rolls over slightly at higher intensities. **(e)** A PL function with PB_{max} of 64% and pathologic rollover in a patient with retrocochlear pathology.

Fig. 8.7 shows some representative examples of PL functions. The normal PL function from **Fig. 8.6** is shown as curve **a** for comparison with the others. Curve **b** shows what might happen if this normal patient were to develop a conductive hearing loss. Notice that this PL function is displaced to the right by 30 dB HL due to a conductive loss, but is otherwise the same as curve **a**. In other words, all the speech recognition scores would be the same as long as the intensity of the words is increased sufficiently to overcome the effects of the air-bone-gap. Performance-intensity function **c** is from a typical patient with a sensorineural hearing loss of cochlear origin. This patient's maximum speech recognition score is 80% and her PL function is essentially asymptotic above the level where PB_{max} is first obtained, as in curves **a** and **b**. Curve **d** is from another patient with a cochlear impairment, for whom PB_{max} is 76%. In this case raising the intensity above the level where PB_{max} was obtained results in speech recognition scores that fall somewhat below PB_{max}.

The PL function shown in curve **e** is from a patient with retrocochlear pathology. The maximum speech recognition score here is only 64%, which we will assume is atypically low for his audiogram. Atypically low speech recognition scores are considered a risk factor for retrocochlear pathology. In addition, notice that the speech recognition scores drop substantially as the intensity is raised above the level where PB_{max} was obtained. This is an example of how the PL function provides diagnostic information in addition to the maximum speech recognition

score, that is, by revealing the presence of abnormal PI rollover. **Rollover of the PL function** (often called **PL** or **PI rollover**) is defined as a reduction of speech recognition scores that occurs at intensities above the level where PB_{max} is obtained. Mild rollover as depicted in curve **d** is not considered abnormal; however, significant amounts of rollover as in curve **e** are pathologic and are associated with retrocochlear disorders (Jerger & Jerger 1971; Dirks, Kamm, Bower, & Betsworth 1977).

Curve **e** from **Fig. 8.7** is replotted in **Fig. 8.8** to show how to determine when rollover is clinically significant. In addition to PB_{max}, a second point is now highlighted on the PL function, labeled **PB_{min}**. This is the lowest speech recognition score obtained at intensity levels higher than where PB_{max} was obtained. These two scores are used to calculate a number called the **rollover index (RI)** (Jerger & Jerger 1971), as follows:

$$RI = \frac{\left(PB_{max} - PB_{min}\right)}{PB_{max}}$$

Retrocochlear pathology is suggested when the rollover index is greater than 0.45 when using PAL

PB-50 materials (Jerger & Jerger 1971; Dirks et al 1977). When the NU-6 test is used, the cutoff value has been reported to be from 0.25 (Bess, Josey, & Humes 1979) to 0.35 (Meyer & Mishler 1985). Abnormal rollover exists for the case in **Fig. 8.8** because the rollover index is 0.41, which is significant for the NU-6 materials. Abnormal rollover also occurs in some elderly patients (Gang 1976; Dirks et al 1977; Shirinian & Arnst 1980). These findings have been associated with neural presbycusis (Jerger & Jerger 1976; Dirks et al 1977; Shirinian & Arnst 1980), and exemplify the concept that audiological tests reflect the site of the disorder (e.g., retrocochlear) rather than its etiology (e.g., acoustic tumor) (Jerger & Jerger 1976).

Speech Recognition Testing Considerations

There are several considerations that must be addressed when choosing and administering speech recognition tests. Deciding which test to use for speech recognition assessment involves choosing the most efficient test for the purpose at hand. For most routine audiological evaluations this will be one of the widely accepted, open-set tests such as CID W-22 and NU-6. Other tests that might be used, as well as special-purpose tests, are outlined later in this chapter and elsewhere in the text with respect to specific assessment issues. When and how to use masking is handled in Chapter 9. Here we will address several issues that pertain to word recognition testing per se,

such as lexical considerations, test forms and form equivalency, phonetic/phonemic balance, carrier phrases, choosing an initial testing level, whole-word versus phonemic scoring, foreign language considerations, recorded versus monitored live-voice testing, and test size. The last two issues are controversial. About 82% of audiologists use **monitored live voice** instead of **recorded** speech recognition tests; and 56% use **shortened test lists** (typically 25-word "**half-lists**") instead of **full lists**, while 30% stop testing after 25 words unless the patient makes errors (Martin, Champlin, & Chambers 1998).[1] These practices might maximize convenience and minimize testing time, but, as we shall see, the most cogent evidence supports the use of recorded materials and a larger test size. Wiley, Stoppenbach, Feldhake, Moss, and Thordardottir (1995) present an insightful discussion dealing with issues such as these that should be read by even the beginning audiology student.

Lexical Considerations

Speech recognition performance is affected by more than just how accurately the sounds of speech are heard. **Lexical considerations** come into play when the test materials are words, which is almost always the case in clinical speech recognition testing. **Word familiarity** has a substantial effect upon speech recognition performance (e.g., Owens 1961), and was addressed above in the discussion of how the traditional speech recognition tests were developed. Word familiarity must also be considered when deciding which test to use, especially when dealing with children.

Word familiarity is not the only lexical consideration involved in word recognition. There is a well-established effect of **word frequency**, with a significant bias favoring the recognition of words with a higher frequency of occurrence compared with lower-frequency words (see, e.g., Luce & Pisoni 1998). The ability to correctly repeat a test word is also affected by whether it has many or few similar-sounding alternatives, that is, other possible words that could be confused with the test word if one of the phonemes is misheard. These similar-sounding alternatives compose the **lexical neighborhood** of the test word. Test words with many similar-sounding alternatives (*dense lexical neighborhoods*) are more difficult than words with a smaller number of

Fig. 8.8 This is the same PL function with abnormal rollover from **Fig. 8.7**, now indicating PB$_{max}$, PB$_{min}$, and how to calculate the rollover index.

---

[1] By commenting that only 4% of audiologists attend to the relationship between sample size and measurement error, the survey implied that only 4% of clinicians use standard 50-word lists.

similar-sounding alternatives (*sparse lexical neighborhoods*). The manner in which these effects are involved in speech recognition is described by the **neighborhood activation model**[2] (Luce 1990; Luce & Pisoni 1998).

Test Forms and Equivalency

The clinician must know about the alternative **test forms** that are available for each test she uses. More than one form of the same test is usually provided because more than one administration is almost always necessary. For example, we routinely test the speech recognition of each ear separately, and often have to do this at more than one hearing level. Different test forms are desirable for each of these administrations. The audiologist must also be aware of **test form equivalency**, which refers to how well various alternative forms of the same test agree with one another. The various forms of a given test tend to produce comparable results, but some forms are easier or harder than others for a given test, and the audiologist must be aware of these differences for the tests that she uses.

Not all speech recognition tests use a fixed set of alternative test forms. For example, the Tri-Word Test or CASRA (Gelfand 1993, 1998; Gelfand & Gelfand 2012), described below, produces one-time-use test forms that are balanced for difficulty by assigning equal numbers of high-, middle-, and low-difficulty words to each test list. These "difficulty ratings" are based on empirically obtained error rates, which in effect accounts for all factors affecting the recognition of the words in the pool. The unique test forms are used in the same order in which they were generated, so that any patient must hear all 450 words in the pool before any test word is repeated.

Phonetic/Phonemic Balance

The concept of **phonetic/phonemic balance** played a major role in the development of many speech recognition tests. However, phonetic/phonemic balance

has been found to have little practical impact on the outcome of speech recognition tests, and its clinical relevance is at best questionable (Tobias 1964; Carhart 1970; Aspinall 1973; Bess 1983; Martin, Champlin, & Perez 2000). In fact, attempts to achieve phonetic/ phonemic balance have largely been abandoned over the course of time in the development of many speech recognition tests.

Carrier Phrases

Carrier phrase use also appears to be a minor issue during speech recognition testing. Some studies found statistically significant advantages for speech recognition scores obtained with a carrier phrase (Gladstone & Siegenthaler 1971; Gelfand 1975), but others found no significant differences (Martin, Hawkins, & Bailey 1962; McLennan & Knox 1975). Some patients are able to perform better with the carrier phrases, perhaps because they serve as alerting signals, whereas other patients are annoyed or even distracted by them. Thus, regardless of whether the audiologist uses carrier phrases as a matter of routine, she should be alert to the patient's responsiveness and be prepared to add, change, or omit carrier phrases as conditions warrant.

Testing Level

Routine speech recognition testing is often done at one hearing level for each ear. Some audiologists add a second measurement at high levels to screen for the possibility of rollover, and the testing of speech recognition at more than one level is strongly encouraged (e.g., Boothroyd 2008a). In any case, it is necessary to choose a speech level that will most likely result in the highest speech recognition score for the ear being tested.

Some audiologists perform routine speech recognition testing at MCL, but this is not desirable because the MCL is actually a range rather than a level, and the highest speech recognition score is often obtained at levels above the MCL (Clemis & Carver 1967; Ullrich & Grimm 1976; Posner & Ventry 1977; Dirks & Morgan 1983; Beattie & Zipp 1990; Guthrie & Mackersie 2009).

Many audiologists do routine speech recognition testing at 30, 35, or 40 dB above the patient's SRT (dB SL re: SRT). The information in **Fig. 8.9** reveals why 40 dB SL seems to be the optimal choice among them by showing how scores change with testing level in dB SL re: SRT. The upper curve shows that the average scores for normal-hearing subjects began to flatten at ~ 30 dB SL and were maximized by 40 dB SL. On the other hand, the hearing-impaired patients'

---

[2] The neighborhood activation model of spoken language recognition is outside the scope of this text. In oversimplified terms, the sound patterns of a stimulus word are compared with acoustic-phonetic representations in the listener's memory. On a probability basis, these representations are activated depending on how similar they are to the stimulus—the greater the similarity, the greater the degree of activation. This is followed by a lexical selection process among all words in memory that are potential matches to the stimulus, which is biased by word frequency. See, e.g., Luce and Pisoni (1998) for a comprehensive discussion, and Kirk et al (1995, 1999) for informative summaries.

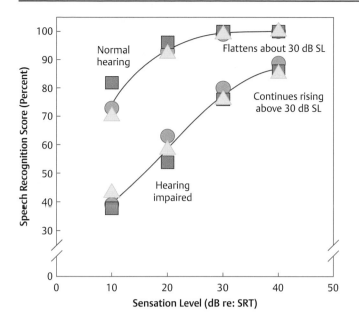

Fig. 8.9 Speech recognition scores tend to improve up to ~ 30 dB SL for normals and 40 dB SL for patients with sensorineural losses. Data points are means for NU-6 (*circles*), Pascoe high-frequency (*triangles*), and California Consonant (*squares*) tests based on Maroonroge and Diefendorf (1984); best-fit curves are shown to highlight the general relationships. Notice that the same pattern of results was found for all three of the tests used.

scores continued improving up to at least 40 dB SL, which was the highest level tested. Clearly, the hearing-impaired patients' speech recognition would have been understated by a single test done below 40 dB SL.

However, routine speech recognition testing at 40 dB SL re: SRT is by no means always the best choice, for at least two reasons. First, many patients with sensorineural hearing losses have sloping audiograms, often with pure tone thresholds that are much better for the lower frequencies and much worse for the higher frequencies. Recall here that the SRT is often similar to the better pure tone thresholds for the lows. Thus, testing this patient at 40 dB above the SRT will often mean that she cannot hear many of the higher-frequency cues that are important for accurate speech recognition. For example, consider a patient with an SRT of 25 dB HL whose pure tone thresholds are ~ 20 or 25 dB HL up to 1000 Hz, and then slope sharply to 60 dB HL or more at 2000 Hz and higher. Testing speech recognition at 40 dB SL would mean that the speech would be presented at 25 + 40 = 65 dB HL, which means that the speech would be barely or not at all audible in the high frequencies. The second limitation is that 40 dB

SL re: SRT has been found to be uncomfortably loud for a majority of patients with sensorineural hearing losses greater than 50 dB HL (Kamm, Dirks, & Mickey 1978) or even ≥ 35 dB HL (Guthrie & Mackersie 2009).

Comparisons of various presentation level methods led Guthrie and Mackersie (2009) to conclude that the highest scores tend to be obtained when the speech is presented 5 dB below the patient's UCL for speech (UCL – 5 dB) for hearing losses ranging from *mild through severe*. They also found that the same results can be achieved for patients with *mild to moderate sloping losses* by presenting the speech at certain levels relative to the 2000 Hz threshold (dB re: 2000 Hz), as shown in **Table 8.1**.

All things considered, it appears that the presentation levels in **Table 8.1** are reasonable choices for use in routine speech recognition testing. Overall, the table suggests using 40 dB SL re: SRT for patients with normal hearing through mild losses with only slight slopes, and using Guthrie and Mackersie's recommendations in most other cases.

Whole-Word versus Phonemic Scoring

Speech recognition tests that use words are usually scored on a whole-word basis. Whole-word scoring reflects the patient's correct reception of the intended word, but also misrepresents how well the patient is able to make use of the acoustical cues of speech. For example, a CNC word such as "cat" is correct only when the patient repeats "cat"; but whole-word scoring considers the response to be *equally* wrong regardless of whether the patient incorrectly repeats one, two, or all three of its phonemes (e.g., "pat," "pot," "pack," "tack," or "seed") or cannot repeat any part of the word at all.

An alternative approach is to score word recognition on a phoneme-by-phoneme basis, which has been done successfully for quite some time (Groen & Helleman 1960; Boothroyd 1968a,b, 1970, 1984, 2006, 2008a, 2008b; Markides 1978; Duffy 1983; Boothroyd & Nittrouer 1988; Gelfand 1993, 1998; Olsen, Van Tasell, & Speaks 1997; Mackersie, Boothroyd, & Minniear 2001; Guthrie & Mackersie 2009; Gelfand & Gelfand 2012). Compared with whole-word scoring, the use of phonemic scoring (1) provides a more precise and more valid measure of the correct reception of the acoustic cues of speech; (2) improves reliability by maximizing the number of scorable items; (3) makes it possible to obtain meaningful scores from patients whose whole-word scores would have been zero; (4) gives a better idea of which speech sounds are misperceived; and (5) minimizes the effects of nonacoustic factors such as word familiarity, word-level predictability, con-

Table 8.1 Recommended levels for presenting the speech materials for routine speech recognition testing

Hearing range	Present the speech recognition test at a level of	If the 2000 Hz threshold is
Normal through mild hearing loss (only slight slopes)	40 dB SL re: SRT or Speech UCL – 5 dB	
Mild through moderate sloping hearing loss[a]	Speech UCL – 5 dB or 25 dB SL re: 2000 Hz[b]	≤ 45 dB HL
	20 dB SL re: 2000 Hz	50–55 dB HL
	15 dB SL re: 2000 Hz	60–65 dB HL
	10 dB SL re: 2000 Hz	70–75 dB HL
Moderately severe through severe hearing loss [a]	Speech UCL – 5 dB	

[a] Based on Guthrie and Mackersie (2009).
[b] The levels in dB SL re: 2000 Hz refer to the *dial reading* at which the attenuator is set when presenting the speech and the dial reading of the attenuator for the 2000 Hz threshold.

text, and differences between word lists. Moreover, comparing word scores and phoneme scores makes it possible to estimate the benefit to speech recognition provided by taking advantage of lexical information (e.g., Boothroyd & Nittrouer 1988; Nittrouer & Boothroyd 1990; Olsen et al 1997).

The benefits of phonemic scoring are optimized by instructing the patient to repeat whatever he hears because partial credit is given for any part of a word or any individual sounds that are correct, even if the word itself is unintelligible (Markides 1978). Also, the examiner should be able to see the patient's face and should ask for clarification of equivocal replies to minimize the chances of misperceiving the patient's intended response. Because of partial credit for any correct part of a "mix-heard" word, the phoneme score obtained on a test will be higher than the word score for the same test. (Exceptions occur when the score is 0 or 100%, and when all phonemes are wrong for every word that is wrong.) For this reason, one should state when phonemic scoring has been used.

Recorded versus Monitored Live-Voice Testing

The distinction between lists of test words and recorded tests is particularly relevant when testing speech recognition because the intelligibility of the same words is affected by speech differences among talkers, and even the same person does not produce

a given word the same way each time it is spoken. In effect, one could propose that the same word list spoken by two different talkers constitutes two different tests (Kreul, Bell, & Nixon 1969).[3] Significantly different speech recognition results are often obtained for the same test materials when they are administered by different talkers (Penrod 1979; Gengel & Kupperman 1980; Hood & Poole 1980; Bess 1983), and even when using different recordings made over time by the same speaker (Brandy 1966). Clinicians also differ with regard to how they say test words, some using a conversational manner and others attempting to speak clearly. In fact, clinicians can inadvertently adjust their speech production depending on the nature of the patient's responses. This can be a significant factor because intelligibility is affected by the use of *conversational* versus *clear speech* (Picheny, Durlach, & Braida 1985). These points provide a forceful argument for the use of recorded speech recognition materials whenever possible. Of course, monitored live-voice testing is often appropriate when the special needs of the patient call for a flexible approach and when a recorded version of the speech recognition test being used is not available.

---

[3] In this context, one should also be aware that norms have been published for contemporary recordings of the various speech recognition tests (e.g., Heckendorf, Wiley, & Wilson, 1997; Wilson & Oyler, 1997; Stoppenbach, Craig, Wiley, & Wilson, 1999).

Test Size

Even though most standard speech recognition tests include 50 monosyllabic words, many attempts have been made to reduce the test size to 25 or even fewer words (for a review, see Bess 1983). After determining the relative difficulty of the words on the W-22 lists, Runge and Hosford-Dunn (1985) suggested a speech recognition testing strategy that involves presenting the most difficult words first. They recommended presenting the 10 *most difficult words first*, and stopping if these are all correct. If any of the first 10 words are missed, then the next 15 words would be given, for a total of 25 words. Testing would then be terminated if there are no more than four errors based on the first 25 words. Otherwise, the entire 50-word list would be used. About 30% of audiologists stop testing after 25 words if the patient makes no errors (Martin, Champlin, & Chambers 1998), suggesting that some aspects of this strategy have been adopted by many audiologists.

The problem with reducing test size is that reliability depends on the size of the test. Shortening a test also makes it less reliable. Let us see why. The variability of speech recognition scores is largely defined by the binomial distribution (Boothroyd 1968a; Hagerman 1976; Thornton & Raffin 1978; Raffin & Schafer 1980; Raffin & Thornton 1980; Gelfand 1993, 1998, 2003; Carney & Schlauch 2007). Specifically, the variability of a test score can be described in terms of its standard deviation, which depends on the percent correct *and* the number of scorable items in the test. For the math-minded, this relationship may be written as

$$SD = 100\sqrt{\left[(p)(1-p)/n\right]}$$

where SD is the standard deviation (in percent), p represents the test score (as a proportion from 0.0 to 1.0), and n is the number of scorable items.

This relationship is shown graphically in **Fig. 8.10**. The y-axis shows the standard deviation of the test score in percent. A larger standard deviation means the score is more variable, or less reliable. The x-axis shows the test score in percent correct. The various curves show what happens when the test has 10 items, 25, 50, etc., up to 450 items. This figure depicts several principles. (1) Reliability improves as the number of test items increases and gets worse as the number of items gets smaller. Egan (1948) made this point in the original description of the PAL PB-50 test. (2) Speech recognition scores become more variable (less reliable) as they go from either extreme (100% or 0%) toward 50% correct. (3) The improvement in reliability that comes with adding more test

Fig. 8.10 Test scores become more variable (less reliable) (1) as the number of tested items becomes smaller, and (2) when the percent correct approaches 50%. Notice how reducing the size of the test has a bigger effect when the test size is relatively small (e.g., going from 50 items to 25 or 10) compared with when it is relatively large (e.g., going from 450 items to 400 or 350).

items is greatest when the test has fewer items and gets progressively smaller as the test size increases, as shown by the convergence of the curves. The third curve from the top applies to the standard 50-item test list and the second curve from the top applies to a 25-word half-list. Notice how the test gets much more variable (less reliable) moving from the 50-word list to a 25-word half-list.

What does all this mean clinically? Consider the following. All tests have some degree of variability. Suppose we have two different tests for the same phenomenon. If the phenomenon is weight, the two different tests might be two different scales. The variability of scale A is ±2 pounds and the variability of scale B is ±4 pounds. Because scale A can vary by 2 pounds either way, a weight of 130 pounds really means 130 ± 2 pounds. On the other hand, 130 pounds on scale B really means 130 ± 4 pounds. If a dieter weighed 130 pounds 2 weeks ago, continued to follow the diet, and now weighs 127 pounds, can she really say that she lost weight? The answer is "yes" using scale A because the 3-pound change from 130 to 127 is larger than what could have been due to the variability of the scale (i.e., the test). However, the answer must be "no" (or, at least, "we can't confidently say yes") using the more variable scale B. The reason is that the 3-pound change could also have been due to the random fluctuations in the readings provided by the scale (i.e., the variability of the test).

Let us now extend this line of reasoning to speech recognition testing. The variability of a speech recognition test refers to the chance fluctuations of the scores obtained with that test. To be considered different, two scores must differ by an amount larger than what could have occurred by chance. Before we can confidently say that two speech recognition scores are different from each other, the difference must be wider than the size of the fluctuations associated with the test itself. In turn, the size of this variability depends on the size of the test: for any given score, variability is wider for a test with fewer items and narrower for tests with more items. Cutoff values that may be used to determine whether two word recognition scores are significantly different from one another take the form of **95% confidence limits** (Thornton & Raffin 1978; Raffin & Schafer 1980; Raffin & Thornton 1980). **Table 8.2** shows the cutoff values that should be used when comparing scores obtained using 50-, 25-, 10-, and 100-word test lists, respectively. This table is based on values derived from Carney and Schlauch (2007) using modern computer simulation methods along with slightly different ones from the seminal work of Thornton and Raffin (1978). The classical Thornton-Raffin values were in regular use between ~ 1978 and 2007, and are provided for reference purposes because many clinical records from that period will continue to remain active for quite some time.

To be considered a true difference the spread between two speech recognition scores must be *wider* than the applicable confidence limits shown in **Table 8.3**, **Table 8.4**, **Table 8.5**, and **Table 8.6**. If the difference between two test scores is *within* the applicable confidence limits, then it cannot be considered to reflect an actual performance difference because the same disparity could have occurred by chance (due just to the inherent variability of the test). For example, to be considered significantly different from a score of 80%, a second score must fall outside of the (a) 68 to 89% range on a 100-item test, (b) 64 to 92% range on a standard 50-word test, (c) 56 to 96% range on 25-word (half-list) test, and (d) 50 to 100% if only 10 words are used. Notice how a larger test size makes it possible to make finer distinctions between two test results.

Foreign Language Influences and Implications

It is often necessary to test a patient whose native language is not English or who may not speak English at all. This can be a problematic clinical issue because speech audiometry involves material that is inherently linguistic in nature, so the results may be influenced by such factors as differences in phonology and morphologic rules between languages, and are exacerbated by word familiarity effects. Hence, nonnative speakers of the language often obtain lower scores on English speech recognition tests than do native speakers of the language (e.g., Gat & Keith 1978), and speakers of Spanish score lower on a nonsense syllable test using English phonemes than do English or bilingual speakers (Danhauer, Crawford, & Edgerton 1984). Audiologists everywhere face the same problem; only the local language changes.

Bilingual patients can usually be tested in English, but we must be mindful of linguistic influences when interpreting the results, especially if they are lower than expected. Fortunately, this issue is receiving increasing attention (e.g., Bradlow & Pisoni 1999; Bradlow & Alexander 2007; Cutler, Garcia Lecumberri, & Cooke 2008; Smiljanic & Bradlow 2011; Calandruccio & Smiljanic 2012a), and a sentence test has been developed for use with those who speak English as a second language (Calandruccio & Smiljanic 2012a,b).

But what about a patient who does not speak the language? The perfect solution is for every patient to be tested in his native language by an audiologist who is also a native speaker or at least a fluent speaker of that language. This may be possible, but it is far from the norm. The opposite approach is simply to test foreign language patients using standard English language tests, which is the worst alternative because it confounds the results with the largest number of linguistic problems. A commonsense solution is for the English-speaking audiologist to use test materials that are available in the patient's own language (e.g., Weisleder & Hodgson 1989; Harris et al 2007; Soli & Wong 2008). In the United States, this often involves lists of Spanish bisyllabic words, which tend to yield results analogous to those found with English monosyllabic word lists (Weisleder & Hodgson 1989). Several examples of Spanish lists are shown in Appendix E. Recordings should be used whenever possible so that the phonology of the language is actually embodied in the test items.

Linguistic limitations on the part of the clinician are a concern when English-speaking audiologists score verbal responses in a foreign language. However, Cokely and Yager (1993) found that English-speaking audiologists can competently score verbal responses in Spanish. It is hard to generalize their findings to other languages. However, Cakiroglu and Danhauer (1992) found that different linguistic backgrounds do not seem to have a major impact on the results when English words are being used. They had talkers of Turkish, East Indian, and American origin record W-22 word lists, and then administered these tests to groups of listeners from each of these

Table 8.2 Examples of 95% confidence limits for speech recognition scores obtained with 50-word test lists[a]

Original test score	95% Confidence limits		Original test score	95% Confidence limits	
	Carney-Schlauch	Thornton-Raffin		Carney-Schlauch	Thornton-Raffin
0	0–6	0–4	52	34–70	34–70
2	0–10	0–10	54	36–72	36–72
4	0–14	0–14	56	38–74	38–74
6	0–18	2–18	58	40–76	40–76
8	2–20	2–22	60	42–76	42–78
10	2–24	2–24	62	44–78	44–78
12	4–26	4–26	64	46–80	46–80
14	4–28	4–30	66	48–82	48–82
16	6–32	6–32	68	50–84	50–84
18	6–34	6–34	70	52–84	52–86
20	8–36	8–36	72	54–86	54–86
22	10–38	8–40	74	56–88	56–88
24	10–42	10–42	76	58–90	58–90
26	12–44	12–44	78	62–90	60–92
28	14–46	14–46	80	64–92	64–92
30	16–48	14–48	82	66–94	66–94
32	16–50	16–50	84	68–94	68–94
34	18–52	18–52	86	72–96	70–96
36	20–54	20–54	88	74–96	74–96
38	22–56	22–56	90	76–98	76–98
40	24–58	22–58	92	80–98	78–98
42	24–60	24–60	94	82–100	82–98
44	26–62	26–62	96	86–100	86–100
46	28–64	28–64	98	90–100	90–100
48	30–66	30–66	100	94–100	96–100

[a]Based on data by Carney and Schlauch (2007) and Thornton and Raffin (1978). All values are in percent. Scores within the confidence limits ranges are not significantly different from the original scores ($p > 0.05$).

backgrounds. The only significant influence of talker background occurred for the Turkish subjects who heard the list recorded by the Indian talker. Overall, however, the linguistic backgrounds of the talkers and listeners did not pose a problem for clinical evaluation purposes.

The use of closed-set tests is a less biased approach to performing speech audiometry across languages. In this way, recorded test items can be presented in the patient's language and her responses can be scored without being influenced by the perceptions of the clinician. Several tests have been devel-

Table 8.3 Examples of 95% confidence limits for speech recognition scores obtained with 25-word test lists[a]

Original test score	95% Confidence limits		Original test score	95% Confidence limits	
	Carney-Schlauch	Thornton-Raffin		Carney-Schlauch	Thornton-Raffin
0	0–12	0–8	52	28–76	28–76
4	0–20	0–20	56	32–80	32–80
8	0–28	0–28	60	36–84	36–84
12	0–32	4–32	64	40–84	40–84
16	4–40	4–40	68	44–88	44–88
20	4–44	4–44	72	48–92	48–92
24	8–48	8–48	76	52–92	52–92
28	8–52	8–52	80	56–96	56–96
32	12–56	12–56	84	60–96	60–96
36	16–60	16–60	88	68–100	68–96
40	16–64	16–64	92	72–100	72–100
44	20–68	20–68	96	80–100	80–100
48	24–72	24–72	100	88–100	92–100

[a]Based on data by Carney and Schlauch (2007) and Thornton and Raffin (1978). All values are in percent. Scores within the confidence limits ranges are not significantly different from the original scores (p > 0.05).

oped in which the patient points to one of a choice of pictures corresponding to the test word, which was presented in a foreign language, such as Spanish or Russian. The pictures may be presented on paper (Spitzer 1980; Comstock & Martin 1984) or a computer screen (McCullough et al 1994; Aleksandrovsky, McCullough, & Wilson 1998).

Types of Speech Recognition Tests

The remainder of this chapter provides the student with a sample of the types of speech recognition tests that are available in addition to the traditional ones already described. Keep in mind that this is by no means an exhaustive listing—many fine tests and testing approaches are not included. Examples of tests intended principally for use with children are discussed in Chapter 12.

Many different kinds of speech recognition tests exist, which may be categorized in a variety of ways. Here we will distinguish between tests that use real words and those that use nonsense syllables, and between open- and closed-set formats.

Open-Set Tests

Open-set monosyllabic word tests are the most popular method for clinically assessing speech recognition, and the majority of practicing clinicians use the NU-6 and W-22 tests in day-to-day practice. Other tests involve different approaches to open-set word recognition testing, some of which are outlined in this section.

High-frequency word lists include a preponderance of words with high-frequency consonants because these are often missed by patients with sensorineural hearing losses, and were originally designed to help find performance differences between hearing aids. Pascoe's (1975) list included 50 monosyllabic words in which 63% of the consonants are voiceless. Gardner (1971, 1987) originally proposed two 25-word lists including the consonants /p, t, k, s, f, θ, h/ with the vowel /I/, and were expanded to an alphabetical listing of 200 monosyllabic words with a variety of vowels. An interesting variation of this approach are the **low-mid-high word lists** (Koike, Brown, Hobbs, & Asp 1989; Koike 1993). These 30-word lists have an equal num-

Table 8.4 Examples of 95% confidence limits for speech recognition scores obtained with 10-word test lists[a]

Original test score	95% Confidence limits	
	Carney-Schlauch	Thornton-Raffin
0	0–20	0–20
10	0–40	0–50
20	0–50	0–60
30	10–70	10–70
40	10–70	10–80
50	20–80	10–90
60	30–90	20–90
70	30–90	30–90
80	50–100	40–100
90	60–100	50–100
100	80–100	80–100

[a]Based on data by Carney and Schlauch (2007) and Thornton and Raffin (1978). All values are in percent. Scores within the confidence limits ranges are not significantly different from the original scores (p > 0.05).

ber of words emphasizing relatively low-frequency ("move"), mid-frequency ("tag"), and high-frequency ("teeth") speech sounds.

The **AB isophonemic word lists** were developed by Boothroyd (1968a, 1984; Boothroyd & Nittrouer 1988). The isophonemic word lists include CNC words drawn from a pool of 30 consonants. Each list includes 10 words that are presented in an open-set format and are scored phonemically, so that the resulting speech recognition score is based on 30 items. The original British English version of the test (Boothroyd 1968a) included 15 lists, which were revised slightly for use in the United States at the Clark School for the Deaf (Boothroyd 1984). The current version includes five additional lists and is shown in Appendix F. It is used in the **Computer-Assisted Speech Perception Assessment (CASPA) Test** (Boothroyd 2006, 2008a,b), which also includes 20 Spanish lists developed by Haro (2005). Sixteen of the 20 isophonemic lists have been shown to be equivalent, but lists 3, 6, 7, and 16 were found to be easier than the others (Mackersie et al 2001).

The **Tri-Word Test (TWT)**, originally called the **Computer-Assisted Speech Recognition Assessment (CASRA) test** (Gelfand 1993, 1998; Gelfand & Gelfand 2012), was developed (1) to minimize test variability by maximizing the number of scorable items, and (2) to enhance sensitivity for misperceived speech sounds by using phonemic scoring, while at the same time (3) retaining the major characteristics of a traditional word recognition test. These traditional test characteristics include the use of monosyllabic words, an open-set format, verbal responses, right/wrong scoring, and no more than 50 test presentations. A test size of 450 was chosen because the benefits of additional test items reach diminishing returns with ~ 450 scorable items, which is shown by the converging curves in **Fig. 8.10**. This seemingly paradoxical combination of test characteristics is made possible by using an interactive computer program to administer 150 digitized CNC words in 50 three-word presentations, without a carrier phrase. The words are repeated by the patient and scored by the audiologist on a phoneme-by-phoneme basis. The result is a test size of 450 scorable items (50 presentations × 3 words × 3 phonemes). The computer selects and presents the words, and is used to keep track of all the bookkeeping details. A test form generation program distributes a 450-word pool into three 150-word lists at a time, which are balanced for word difficulty. This program also minimizes semantic and syntactic cues within each three-word group. An added benefit of using digitized words and a computer in place of a tape recorder is that the intervals between word presentations automatically adjust to how long it takes the patient to respond.

The Tri-Word Test optimizes reliability because the advantage of adding items becomes negligible by the time the test size reaches ~ 450. However, optimized reliability is not always needed clinically, providing the variability of the test is consistent with what the audiologist is trying to do with it. Thus, the size of the TWT can be reduced to what the clinician considers acceptable for the intended purpose (Gelfand 2003). For example, shortening the TWT to 25 presentation sets provides a score based on 25 sets × 3 words × 3 phonemes = 225 scorable test items; 20 presentations yield 20 × 3 × 3 = 180 items; and 10 presentations provide 10 × 3 × 3 = 90 items. Gelfand (2003) found that performance on both the 20- and 25-set versions of the TWT accounted for ~ 97% of the variance on the full (50-set) test. Thus, the 20-set version is probably the best compromise when trying to shorten the test without appreciably losing reliability. However, the 10-set version still accounted for 88% of full-test variance, and its 90 scorable items makes it more reliable than a traditional test using 75 words. Thus, the 10-set version of the TWT

Table 8.5 Examples of 95% confidence limits for speech recognition scores obtained with 100-word test lists[a]

Original test score	95% Confidence limits Carney-Schlauch	Original test score	95% Confidence limits Carney-Schlauch	Thornton-Raffin
0	0–3	50	37–63	37–63
1	0–6	51	38–64	38–64
2	0–7	52	39–65	39–65
3	0–9	53	40–66	40–66
4	1–11	54	41–67	41–67
5	1–12	55	42–68	42–68
6	1–14	56	43–69	43–69
7	2–15	57	44–70	44–70
8	3–17	58	45–71	45–71
9	3–18	59	46–72	46–72
10	4–19	60	47–72	47–73
11	4–21	61	48–73	48–74
12	5–22	62	49–74	49–74
13	6–23	63	50–75	50–75
14	6–24	64	51–76	51–76
15	7–26	65	52–77	52–77
16	8–27	66	53–78	53–78
17	8–28	67	54–79	54–79
18	9–29	68	55–80	55–80
19	10–30	69	56–80	56–81
20	11–32	70	57–81	57–81
21	11–31	71	58–82	58–82
22	12–34	72	59–83	59–83
23	13–35	73	61–84	60–84
24	14–36	74	62–85	61–85
25	15–37	75	63–85	63–86
26	15–38	76	64–86	64–86
27	16–39	77	65–87	65–87
28	17–41	78	66–88	66–88
29	18–42	79	69–89	67–89

30	19–43	80	68–89	68–89
31	20–44	81	70–90	69–90
32	20–45	82	71–91	71–91
33	23–46	83	72–92	72–92
34	22–47	84	73–92	73–92
35	23–48	85	74–93	74–93
36	24–49	86	76–94	75–94
37	25–50	87	77–94	77–94
38	26–51	88	78–95	78–95
39	27–52	89	79–96	79–96
40	28–53	90	81–96	81–96
41	28–54	91	82–97	82–97
42	29–55	92	83–97	83–98
43	30–56	93	85–98	85–98
44	31–57	94	86–99	86–99
45	32–58	95	88–99	88–99
46	33–59	96	89–99	89–99
47	34–60	97	91–100	91–100
48	35–61	98	93–100	92–100
49	36–62	99	94–100	94–100
50	37–63	100	97–100	97–100

[a]Based on data by Carney and Schlauch (2007) and Thornton and Raffin (1978). All values are in percent. Scores within the confidence limits ranges are not significantly different from the original scores (p > 0.05).

method represents a very practical approach that may be employed in many clinical speech recognition assessments.

Closed-Set Tests

Closed-set speech recognition tests have several advantages over the open-set approach. Closed-set testing reduces (1) the effects of word frequency in the language, (2) the effects of a patient's familiarity with the test words and alternative choices, and (3) learning effects. An added advantage of closed-set tests is that they can focus on particular aspects of speech recognition by carefully arranging the choices for each stimulus, so the clinician can analyze the patient's errors and confusions in some detail.

Perhaps the best-known closed-set word recognition tests are the Modified Rhyme Test and the California Consonant Test. There are certainly many other closed-set word tests, although the fundamental features are illustrated by these two. The **Modified Rhyme Test (MRT)** (House, Williams, Heker, & Kryter 1965; Kreul et al 1968) presents the patient with six alternatives for each stimulus word. Twenty-five of the 50 test words have choices that differ by their initial consonants, such as

bent went sent tent dent rent

The other 25 test items involve final consonant distinctions, such as

mass mad mat map man math

Several variations of the MRT are also available, such as the *Rhyming Minimal Contrasts Test* (Griffiths 1967) and the *Distinctive Feature Discrimination Test* (McPherson & Pang-Ching 1979). The **California Consonant Test (CCT)** (Owens & Schubert 1977) has two 100-item test forms. Four closed-set choices are provided for each of the 36 initial consonant test items, such as

pin kin tin thin

and for each of the 64 final consonant items, for example,

path patch pack pat

The student should also be aware of the **University of Oklahoma Closed Response Speech Test (UOCRST)** (Pederson & Studebaker 1972), which adds a medial vowel subtest to the initial and final consonant subtests, and also uses several replications of each test item. These two characteristics can be very useful, and are atypical of most other real-word tests.

The **Speech Pattern Contrast (SPAC) test** (Boothroyd 1984, 1988) provides information about the patient's ability to perceive phonologically relevant distinctions, that is, those that affect the meaning of what is being said. This kind of information has many uses in aural rehabilitation, and when assessing needs and progress with various sensory aids (such as hearing aids, cochlear implants, and tactile devices). The SPAC test uses a closed-set format in which the patient is presented with a test word (or phrase), which must then be identified from choices that are written or that appear on a computer screen. The alternatives are contrasting in terms of particular characteristics of speech. Eight segmental contrasts and two suprasegmental contrasts are examined on the SPAC test: vowel height ("fall"-"fool"), vowel place ("feel"-"fool"), initial consonant voicing ("tip"-"dip"), initial consonant continuance ("tip"-"sip"), final consonant voicing ("do"-"too"), final consonant continuance ("fate"-"face"), initial consonant place ("big"-"dig"), final consonant place ("bid"-"big"), stress ("THESE new clocks"-"these NEW clocks"), and pitch rise/fall ("That's yours."-"That's yours?"). Separate subtests allow two segmental contrasts to be tested at a time by giving four alternatives for each item. For example, the four choices for "tip" are

zip sip dip tip

If the response is "sip," then an error would be counted for *continuance* because /t/ and /s/ dif-

fer for this characteristic; however, *voicing* would be counted as correct because both /t/ and /s/ are unvoiced. The suprasegmental contrast subtests give two choices for each item. Two subtests that do not involve phonologically significant contrasts are also available. These assess the ability to distinguish between male and female voices (talker sex) and natural versus monotonous speech (pitch range).

Nonsense-Syllable Tests

Nonsense-syllable tests use meaningless syllables rather than real words to evaluate a patient's ability to accurately perceive speech sounds. They are probably the most sensitive approach for examining the details of a patient's speech recognition difficulties, but they are also the most abstract and are not as generally accepted as real-word tests in routine clinical practice. The **City University of New York Nonsense Syllable Test (CUNY-NST)** (Resnick, Dubno, Hoffnung, & Levitt 1976; Levitt & Resnick 1978) and the **Nonsense Syllable Test (NST)** (Edgerton & Danhauer 1979) are two carefully developed and widely known tests of this type. The CUNY-NST is a closed-set test made up of seven subtests that include between seven and nine consonant-vowel (CV) or vowel-consonant (VC) nonsense syllables, as shown in **Table 8.6** (as well as some optional subtests). All of the syllables on a given subtest are offered as choices for each other. Each subtest of the CUNY-NST is composed of the consonants most likely to be confused by hearing-impaired patients. A **Modified CUNY Nonsense Syllable Test (MNST)** (Gelfand, Schwander, Levitt, Weiss, & Silman 1992) can be used in situations where it is necessary to test for all possible confusions among 16 CV syllables and 21 VC syllables. In contrast to the CUNY-NST, the **Edgerton-Danhauer Nonsense Syllable Test (NST)** is an open-set test in which the patient must identify 25 nonsense bisyllables, that is, meaningless consonant-vowel-consonant-vowel (CVCV) items such as /ʃeθɑ/ or /sɛfɛ/.

Sentence Tests

Speech recognition testing can also be accomplished by presenting the test material in the form of sentences, which makes it possible to look at the patient's speech recognition ability in a variety of ways. Performance on these tests is usually expressed as the percentage of correctly recognized words in each of the sentences. This percentage might be based on scoring all of the words in the sentence or only certain **key words**. The **CID Everyday Sentences** test

Table 8.6   The CUNY nonsense syllable test

Subtest	Stimuli and response alternatives								
1	ɑf	ɑʃ	ɑt	ɑk	ɑs	ɑp	aθ		
2	uθ	up	us	uk	ut	uf	uʃ		
3	iʃ	if	it	ik	is	iθ	ip		
4	ab	ɑð	ɑd	ɑm	ɑz	ɑg	ɑn	ɑŋ	ɑv
5	fɑ	tɑ	pɑ	hɑ	θɑ	tʃɑ	sɑ	ʃɑ	kɑ
6	lɑ	bɑ	dɑ	gɑ	rɑ	jɑ	dʒɑ	wɑ	
7	nɑ	vɑ	mɑ	zɑ	gɑ	bɑ	ðɑ	dɑ	

Modified from Levitt and Resnick (1978) with permission of *Scandinavian Audiology*.

(Silverman & Hirsh 1955; Davis & Silverman 1978) and the **IEEE** (or **Harvard**) **Sentences** test (IEEE 1969) are the classic tests in this category. There are 10 test lists in CID Everyday Sentences and 72 in the IEEE Sentences. Both tests contain 10 sentences per list, composed of various numbers of words per sentence, and a total of 50 key words. These tests are still used from time to time, but are being replaced by more contemporary tests, such as the ones that follow.

The **Connected Speech Test (CST)** (Cox, Alexander, & Gilmore 1987; Cox, Alexander, Gilmore, & Pusakulich 1988, 1989) is a carefully constructed and standardized approach that includes a total of 48 passages dealing with a variety of familiar topics. Each passage is composed of 10 test sentences that contain 25 scorable key words. In addition, the CST is available in both audio and audiovisual formats.

The **AzBio Sentence Lists** (Spahr & Dorman 2004; Spahr, Dorman, Litvak, et al 2012) include sentences recorded by four different talkers (two males and two females) instead of a single talker for the whole list. Each test list contains 20 sentences varying in length from 3 to 12 words, and between 133 and 159 key words depending on the list. An example is shown in Appendix G. The test score is simply the percentage of the correctly repeated words based on the total number of words in the whole list. For example, the list in the table has a total of 143 words, so correctly repeating 112 of them would yield a score of (122/143) × 100 = 85%. There are 15 lists in the standard clinical version of the AzBio test (Spahr et al 2012; Auditory Potential n.d.), and another 8 lists in a test battery for adults with cochlear implants (MSTB 2011; Spahr et al 2012). Ten of the 15 lists appear to produce scores that are similar enough to

be considered equivalent forms of the test (Schafer, Pogue & Milrany 2012).[4] Based on binomial confidence limits like those described for word tests earlier in this chapter, Spahr et al (2012) suggested that a patient's performance on two test administrations (e.g., before versus after intervention) may be considered significantly different if the AzBio scores are at least 15% apart, or 11% apart when double lists are used.

The **Perceptually Robust English Sentence Test Open-set (PRESTO)** (Gilbert, Tamati, & Pisoni 2013) uses lists composed of 18 sentences spoken by a variety of different talkers from several different parts of the United States. Each 18-sentence list contains 76 key words, and the score itself is based on how many of the key words are repeated correctly. As a result, performance on PRESTO involves the listener's ability to quickly accommodate to the different talkers and dialects among the test sentences. When the PRESTO was presented against a multi-talker babble, those with very high versus very low PRESTO scores also performed differently on measures of vocabulary size, and short-term and working memory, discriminating talker gender, and categorizing regional dialects (Tamati, Gilbert & Pisoni 2013).

The **Basic English Lexicon (BEL) Sentences** test (Calandruccio & Smiljanic 2012a,b) is unique because it was designed to be appropriate for testing people who are second-language speakers of English,

---

[4] Specifically, lists 2, 3, 4, 5, 8, 9, 10, 11, 13, and 15 produced similar scores and were thus recommended for regular use by Schafer et al (2012).

as well as native speakers of the language. This was done by deriving the test words from the short conversations of 100 people with diverse backgrounds who were second-language speakers of English, and using sentences with simple and consistent structures. Each list is composed of 25 sentences with four key words per sentence, so that the test scores are based on 100 key words. Two of the test's lists are shown in Appendix H. Twenty BEL lists are available, which is a very useful feature because it allows the test to be presented to the same person several times without having to repeat sentences. In addition, the test CD (Calandruccio & Smiljanic 2012b) includes three recordings for each list (by two female talkers and one male).

The **Speech Perception in Noise (SPIN) test** (Kalikow, Stevens, & Elliott 1977; Bilger 1984; Bilger, Nuetzel, Rabinowitz, & Rzeczkowski 1984) is based on scoring the last word in each test sentence. Thus, the SPIN actually assesses monosyllabic word recognition in a sentence context, in contrast to the nature of the other sentence tests described in this section. Two kinds of sentences are used in the SPIN test. The test word at the end of a **probability-high (PH-SPIN)** sentence is somewhat predictable from the information provided by the body of the sentence, such as

We shipped the furniture by TRUCK.

On the other hand, the test word at the end of a **probability-low (PL-SPIN)** sentence cannot be predicted from the sentence, as in

Mary could not discuss the TACK.

Comparing a patient's performance on the Pl-SPIN and PH-SPIN allows us to assess the patient's ability to make use of contextual cues. The revised SPIN test (Bilger 1984) includes eight lists of 50 sentences each. Each list contains 25 PL-SPIN sentences and 25 PH-SPIN sentences. As its name suggests, the SPIN can be presented in quiet or against a background noise (a 12-talker babble), which is provided on a second channel of the test.

The **Synthetic Sentence Identification (SSI) test** (Speaks & Jerger 1965; Jerger, Speaks, & Trammell 1968) uses a very different approach to speech recognition assessment with sentences, and has been used in a variety of clinical applications. The SSI uses sentences that are third-order approximations to English, which means they are composed of words selected at random except that every three-word sequence must be syntactically correct. This idea can be understood by analyzing each three-word sequence in a typical SSI test sentence, *Women view men with green paper should:*

Women view men
    view men with
        men with green
            with green paper
                green paper should.

Notice how the sentence is grammatically correct even though its meaning is irrational.

The SSI test is administered in a closed-set format. Before the test starts, the patient is provided with a written list of 10 numbered SSI sentences. After each sentence is presented, the patient responds by indicating its number on the list. The SSI recordings are provided with the test sentences on one channel of the recording and a story being read by the same talker on the other channel. The story is used as a competing message. In actual use, the SSI sentences are presented while the competing message is simultaneously being directed into the opposite ear (SSI with contralateral competing message, **SSI-CCM**) or into the same ear (SSI with ipsilateral competing message, **SSI-ICM**).

Speech Recognition Performance as Signal-to-Noise (Babble) Ratio

So far, we have been addressing speech recognition performance in terms of percent-correct scores. Another approach is to present the speech test against a background of noise or speech babble, and to find the signal-to-noise ratio (SNR) or signal-to-babble ratio (SBR) needed for the patient to achieve 50% intelligibility. Assessing speech perception in noise is important and revealing because it represents one of the major complaints of people with sensorineural hearing loss, and cannot simply be inferred from the patient's audiogram. In fact, those with sensorineural impairments often face problems with both **audibility,** typically expressed as the hearing loss itself, and **distortion**, usually expressed in terms of a SNR (e.g., Plomp 1968; Soli & Wong 2008; Vermiglio, Soli, Freed, & Fisher 2012).

Speech perception in noise is usually tested by obtaining a **sentence recognition** (or **reception**) **threshold** (SRT[5]) in the presence of noise or speech babble using any of a variety of sentence tests (Plomp & Mimpen 1979; Hagerman 1982; Gelfand, Ross, & Miller 1988; Smoorenburg 1992; Killion & Villchur 1993; Nilsson, Soli, & Sullivan 1994; Versfeld, Daalder, Festen, & Houtgast 2000; Cox, Gray,

---

[5] One can usually tell from the context whether "SRT" means the traditional speech recognition threshold for spondee words, discussed earlier, or the sentence recognition threshold, as used here.

& Alexander 2001; Killion, Niquette, Gudmundsen, & Banerjee 2004; Wilson, McArdle, & Smith 2007; Dawson, Hersbach, & Swanson 2013). A variety of variables are involved in the measurement of SRTs in noise (see, e.g., Theunissen, Swanepoel, & Hanekom 2009), but the basic approach is quite simple. For example, we might present the noise at a fixed level of 60 dB HL, and then raise and lower the level of the sentences until we find the speech level where the patient correctly repeats 50% of the items. If the SRT in the presence of the noise is 66 dB HL, then the SNR is +6 dB. Alternatively, we could also keep the speech at a fixed level and vary the level of the noise, again resulting in the SNR for 50% intelligibility.

A lower SNR indicates better speech perception in noise and a higher SNR means poorer speech perception in noise. This is so because +6 dB SNR means that the speech has to be 6 dB stronger than the noise for the patient to get 50% of the items right, and +14 dB SNR means that the patient needs the speech to be 14 dB stronger than the noise. Thus, the SNR approach gives us a straightforward way of assessing the patient's speech recognition ability in noise. In fact, we can express a patient's **signal-to-noise ratio loss (SNR loss)** as the difference between his SNR and an average value obtained by normal-hearing listeners.

The **Hearing in Noise Test** (**HINT**; Nilsson et al 1994) includes 25 lists of 10 sentences each that are presented according to a set of rules that allows the clinician to find the patient's SRT in noise. A convenient and useful feature of the HINT is that it is available with normative data in several languages other than English (Soli & Wong 2008). In addition to the standard method of administration, the HINT sentences can also be scored on a percent-correct basis, although the resulting scores are susceptible to ceiling effects when the materials are presented in quiet (e.g., Gifford, Shallop, & Peterson 2008).

The **Quick Speech-in-Noise (QuickSIN)** test (Killion et al 2004) is a highly efficient instrument for clinical use, in which one test sentence is presented against a speech babble of each of six SNRs from +25 dB to 0 dB. The patient's task is to repeat the sentences, each of which contains five scorable key words, and the SRT in noise is found using a technique analogous to the Tillman-Olsen method described earlier in this chapter. This test and its precursor, the **Speech-in-Noise (SIN)** test (Killion & Villchur 1993), were derived from the IEEE sentences and use 5 dB increments.

The **Bench-Koval-Bamford Speech-in-Noise (BKB-SIN)** test (Niquette, Arcaroli, Revit, et al 2003; Etymotic Research 2005) is a new version of the SIN test approach derived from an Americanized version of the Bench-Koval-Bamford (BKB) sentences

test (Bench, Koval, & Bamford 1979; see Chapter 12), and uses three key words in but one sentence per list (which has four SNRs between –6 and +21 dB in 3 dB steps. The **Australian Sentence Test in Noise (AuSTIN)** (Dawson et al 2013) is another sentence test using BKB-like sentences. In addition to including a very a large number of test lists, AuSTIN innovatively increases or decreases the SNR based on whether ≥ 50% of the morphemes are correct in each sentence and calculates the SRT by fitting the results to a psychometric function.

The **Words-in-Noise** (**WIN**; Wilson 2003; Wilson, Abrams, & Pillion 2003; Wilson et al 2007) test is a similar kind of measure that uses monosyllabic words instead of sentences. In this test, the patient is asked to repeat 10 CNC words against a background of speech babble at each of seven SNRs from +24 dB to 0 dB. The original 70-word WIN was split into two 35-word tests composed of 5 words per level for more rapid testing (Wilson & Burks 2005), and a third list was added that can be used for familiarization and practice[6] (Wilson & Watts 2012).

People with sensorineural losses require higher SNRs than normal-hearing people to reach SRTs in noise. However, average SNRs vary between studies from roughly –2.5 to 5 dB for normal-hearing adults and ~ 5 to 14 dB for those with hearing loss, depending on which test was used, methodological details, and other factors (e.g., Nilssen et al 1994; Wilson 2003; Wilson et al 2003; Killion et al 2004; Etymotic Research 2005; Duncan & Aarts 2006; McArdle, Wilson, & Burks 2005; Tadros et al 2005; Wilson et al 2007). The study by Wilson et al (2007) is particularly informative because it provided SNRs obtained with selected lists from four different speech-in-noise tests (BKB-SIN, HINT, QuickSIN, and WIN) for both normal-hearing and hearing-impaired individuals. As illustrated in **Fig. 8.11**, hearing-impaired listeners had similar average SNRs of 3.3 to 4.3 dB for the HINT, QuickSIN, and WIN, and just 0.8 dB for the BKB-SIN. On the other hand, normal-hearing listeners had average SNRs that were more disparate among the tests, ranging from 5 dB on the BKB-SIN to 14 dB on the WIN. We might use the difference between the SNRs of the two groups to illustrate the SNR deficit experienced by hearing-impaired patients compared with those with normal hearing (shown by the arrows in the figure). These differences averaged 4.2 dB on the BKB-SIN, 5.6 dB on the HINT, 7.9 dB on the QuickSIN, and 10.1 dB on the WIN. Overall, the Quick-

---

[6] Lists 1 and 2 are essentially parallel forms; however, list 3 performance is poorer and should not be compared with lists 1 and 2 (Wilson & Watts, 2012).

Fig. 8.11 Mean signal-to-noise ratios in decibels needed to achieve the speech recognition threshold (50% recognition) in noise for four tests for persons with normal hearing (*gray bars*) and sensorineural hearing loss (*black bars*). The *double-headed arrows* highlight the difference between the two groups in dB SNR. The SNRs are based on data for two representative lists from each test (HINT, lists 1 and 8; BKB-SIN, lists 1A and 2A; QuickSIN, lists 1 and 8; WIN, lists 1 and 2). (Based on data reported by Wilson et al [2007], used with permission of Dr. Richard H. Wilson.)

SIN and WIN were more challenging tasks and more effectively distinguished between the normal and impaired speech-in-noise performance, compared with the BKB-SIN and HINT. Based on these findings, Wilson et al (2007) insightfully recommended that the QuickSIN or WIN be included in routine clinical assessments, and that the easier BKB-SIN and/or HINT be used when there is considerable severe impairment (e.g., cochlear implant assessments) and when testing younger children.

■ Study Questions

1. What is the speech recognition threshold (SRT) and how is it typically measured?
2. Explain the expected relationship between the SRT and the pure tone audiogram.
3. What are speech recognition scores and how are they typically measured?
4. Explain the differences between whole-word and phonemic scoring.
5. Define most comfortable level (MCL) and uncomfortable listening level (UCL), and describe how they may be measured.
6. Define and explain the characteristics of performance-intensity (PI) functions for monosyllabic word recognition.
7. Explain why speech recognition scores are less reliable when they are measured with shorter word lists compared with longer lists.
8. How can we determine if the difference between two speech recognition scores is significant for a particular patient?
9. Define signal-to-noise ratio loss (SNR loss).
10. Describe the various factors that come into play in the measurement and interpretation of speech recognition performance.

References

Aleksandrovsky IV, McCullough JK, Wilson RH. Development of suprathreshold word recognition test for Russian-speaking patients. J Am Acad Audiol 1998;9(6):417–425

American National Standards Institute (ANSI). 2010. American National Standard Specifications for Audiometers. ANSI S3.6-2010. New York, NY: ANSI

American Speech-Language-Hearing Association (ASHA). Guidelines for determining the threshold level for speech. ASHA 1979;20:297–301

American Speech-Language-Hearing Association (ASHA). Guidelines for determining threshold level for speech. ASHA 1988;30(3):85–89

Aspinall KB. 1973. The effect of phonetic balance on discrimination for speech in subjects with sensorineural hearing loss. Unpublished doctoral dissertation. Boulder: University of Colorado

Auditory Potential, LLC. N.d. The AzBio Sentence Lists. Available at http://www.auditorypotential.com/

Beattie RC, Edgerton BJ, Svihovec DV. An investigation of the Auditec of St. Louis recordings of the Central Institute for the Deaf spondees. J Am Audiol Soc 1975;1(3):97–101

Beattie RC, Forrester PW, Ruby BK. Reliability of the Tillman-Olsen procedure for determination of spondee threshold using recorded and live voice presentations. J Am Audiol Soc 1977;2(4):159–162

Beattie RC, Svihovec DV, Edgerton BJ. Relative intelligibility of the CID spondees as presented via monitored live voice. J Speech Hear Disord 1975;40(1):84–91

Beattie RC, Zipp JA. Range of intensities yielding PB Max and the threshold for monosyllabic words for hearing-impaired subjects. J Speech Hear Disord 1990;55(3):417–426

Bench J, Kowal A, Bamford J. The BKB (Bamford-Kowal-Bench) sentence lists for partially-hearing children. Br J Audiol 1979;13(3):108–112

Bess FH. 1983. Clinical assessment of speech recognition. In: Konkle DF, Rintelmann WF, eds. Principles of Speech Audiometry. Baltimore, MD: University Park Press; 127–201

Bess FH, Josey AF, Humes LE. Performance intensity functions in cochlear and eighth nerve disorders. Am J Otol 1979;1(1):27–31

Bilger RC. 1984. Speech recognition test development. In: Elkins E, ed. Speech Recognition by the Hearing Impaired. ASHA Reports 14; 2–15

Bilger RC, Matthies ML, Meyer TA, Griffiths SK. Psychometric equivalence of recorded spondaic words as test items. J Speech Lang Hear Res 1998;41(3):516–526

Bilger RC, Nuetzel JM, Rabinowitz WM, Rzeczkowski C. Standardization of a test of speech perception in noise. J Speech Hear Res 1984;27(1):32–48

Boothroyd A. Developments in speech audiometry. Sound 1968a;2:3–10

Boothroyd A. Statistical theory of the speech discrimination score. J Acoust Soc Am 1968b;43(2):362–367

Boothroyd A. Developmental factors in speech recognition. Int Audiol 1970;9:30–38

Boothroyd A. Auditory perception of speech contrasts by subjects with sensorineural hearing loss. J Speech Hear Res 1984;27(1):134–144

Boothroyd A. Perception of speech pattern contrasts from auditory presentation of voice fundamental frequency. Ear Hear 1988;9(6):313–321

Boothroyd A. 2006. Computer-Assisted Speech Perception Assessment CASPA 5.0 Software. San Diego, CA: A Boothroyd

Boothroyd A. The performance/intensity function: an underused resource. Ear Hear 2008a;29(4):479–491

Boothroyd A. 2008b. Computer-Assisted Speech Perception Assessment CASPA 5.0 Manual. San Diego, CA: A Boothroyd

Boothroyd A, Nittrouer S. Mathematical treatment of context effects in phoneme and word recognition. J Acoust Soc Am 1988;84(1):101–114

Bradlow AR, Alexander JA. Semantic and phonetic enhancements for speech-in-noise recognition by native and non-native listeners. J Acoust Soc Am 2007;121(4):2339–2349

Bradlow AR, Pisoni DB. Recognition of spoken words by native and non-native listeners: talker-, listener-, and item-related factors. J Acoust Soc Am 1999;106(4 Pt 1): 2074–2085

Brandy WT. Reliability of voice tests in speech discrimination. J Speech Hear Res 1966;9:461–465

Cakiroglu S, Danhauer JL. Effects of listeners' and talkers' linguistic backgrounds on W-22 test performance. J Am Acad Audiol 1992;3(3):186–192

Calandruccio L, Smiljanic R. New sentence recognition materials developed using a basic non-native English lexicon. J Speech Lang Hear Res 2012a;55(5):1342–1355

Calandruccio L, Smiljanic R. 2012b. Basic English Lexicon (BEL) Sentences. Compact disk. Chapel Hill, NC: Lauren Calandruccio

Cambron NK, Wilson RH, Shanks JE. Spondaic word detection and recognition functions for female and male speakers. Ear Hear 1991;12(1):64–70

Carhart R. Speech reception in relation to pattern of pure tone loss. J Speech Disord 1946a;11:97–108

Carhart R. Monitored live voice as a test of auditory acuity. J Acoust Soc Am 1946b;17:339–349

Carhart R. 1970. Discussion, questions, answers, comments. In: Rojskjer C, ed. Speech Audiometry. Denmark: Second Danavox Symposium; 229

Carhart R. Observations on relations between thresholds for pure tones and for speech. J Speech Hear Disord 1971;36(4):476–483

Carhart R, Porter LS. Audiometric configuration and prediction of threshold for spondees. J Speech Hear Res 1971;14(3):486–495

Carney E, Schlauch RS. Critical difference table for word recognition testing derived using computer simulation. J Speech Lang Hear Res 2007;50(5):1203–1209

Chaiklin JB. The relation among three selected auditory speech thresholds. J Speech Hear Res 1959;2:237–243

Chaiklin JB, Font J, Dixon RF. Spondaic thresholds measured in ascending 5 dB steps. J Speech Hear Res 1967;10:141–145

Chaiklin JB, Ventry IM. Spondee threshold measurement: a comparison of 2- and 5-dB steps. J Speech Hear Disord 1964;29:47–59

Clemis JD, Carver WF. Discrimination scores for speech in Ménière's disease. Arch Otolaryngol 1967;86(6): 614–618

Cokely JA, Yager CR. Scoring Spanish word-recognition measures. Ear Hear 1993;14(6):395–400

Comstock CL, Martin FN. A children's Spanish word discrimination test for non-Spanish-speaking clinicians. Ear Hear 1984;5(3):166–170

Conn M, Dancer J, Ventry IM. A spondee list for determining speech reception threshold without prior familiarization. J Speech Hear Disord 1975;40(3):388–396

Cox RM, Alexander GC, Gilmore C. Development of the Connected Speech Test (CST). Ear Hear 1987;8(5, Suppl):119S–126S

Cox RM, Alexander GC, Gilmore C, Pusakulich KM. Use of the Connected Speech Test (CST) with hearing-impaired listeners. Ear Hear 1988;9(4):198–207

Cox RM, Alexander GC, Gilmore C, Pusakulich KM. The Connected Speech Test version 3: audiovisual administration. Ear Hear 1989;10(1):29–32

Cox RM, Alexander GC, Taylor IM, Gray GA. The contour test of loudness perception. Ear Hear 1997;18(5): 388–400

Cox RM, Gray GA, Alexander GC. Evaluation of a revised speech in noise (RSIN) test. J Am Acad Audiol 2001; 12(8):423–432

Creston JE, Gillespie M, Krohn C. Speech audiometry: taped vs live voice. Arch Otolaryngol 1966;83(1):14–17

Cutler A, Garcia Lecumberri ML, Cooke M. Consonant identification in noise by native and non-native listeners: effects of local context. J Acoust Soc Am 2008;124(2):1264–1268

Danhauer JL, Crawford S, Edgerton BJ. English, Spanish, and bilingual speakers' performance on a nonsense syllable test (NST) of speech sound discrimination. J Speech Hear Disord 1984;49(2):164–168

Davis H, Silverman SR. 1978. Hearing and Deafness, 4th ed. New York, NY: Holt, Rinehart & Winston

Dawson PW, Hersbach AA, Swanson BA. An adaptive Australian Sentence Test in Noise (AuSTIN). Ear Hear 2013;34(5):592–600

Department of Veterans Affairs. 1998. Speech Recognition and Identification Materials (disc 2.0). Mountain Home, TN: VA Medical Center

Dewey G. 1923. Relative Frequency of English Speech Sounds. Cambridge, MA: Harvard University Press

Dirks DD, Kamm C. Psychometric functions for loudness discomfort and most comfortable loudness levels. J Speech Hear Res 1976;19(4):613–627

Dirks DD, Kamm C, Bower D, Betsworth A. Use of performance-intensity functions for diagnosis. J Speech Hear Disord 1977;42(3):408–415

Dirks DD, Morgan DE. 1983. Measures of discomfort and most comfortable loudness. In: Konkle DF, Rintelmann WF, eds. Principles of Speech Audiometry. Baltimore, MD: University Park Press; 203–229

Downs D, Dickinson Minard P. A fast valid method to measure speech-recognition threshold. Hear J 1996;49(8):39–44

Dubno JR, Lee F-S, Klein AJ, Matthews LJ, Lam CF. Confidence limits for maximum word-recognition scores. J Speech Hear Res 1995;38(2):490–502

Duffy JK. The role of phoneme-recognition audiometry in aural rehabilitation. Hear J 1983;37:24–28

Duncan KR, Aarts NL. A comparison of the HINT and Quick SIN Tests. J Speech Lang Pathol Audiol 2006;30:86–94

Edgerton BJ, Danhauer JL. 1979. Clinical Implications of Speech Discrimination Testing Using Nonsense Stimuli. Baltimore, MD: University Park Press

Egan JP. Articulation testing methods. Laryngoscope 1948;58(9):955–991

Etymotic Research. 2005. Bamford-Kowal-Bench Speech-in-Noise Test (v. 1.03). Compact disk. Elk Grove Village, IL: Etymotic Research

Fletcher H. 1929. Speech and Hearing in Communication. Princeton: Van Nostrand Reinhold

Fletcher H. A method of calculating hearing loss for speech from an audiogram. Acta Otolaryngol Suppl 1950;90:26–37

Frank T. Clinical significance of the relative intelligibility of pictorially represented spondee words. Ear Hear 1980;1(1):46–49

French NR, Carter CW Jr, Koenig W Jr. The words and sounds of telephone conversations. Bell Syst Tech J 1930;9:290–324

Gang RP. The effects of age on the diagnostic utility of the rollover phenomenon. J Speech Hear Disord 1976;41(1):63–69

Gardner HJ. Application of a high-frequency consonant discrimination word list in hearing-aid evaluation. J Speech Hear Disord 1971;36(3):354–355

Gardner HJ. High frequency consonant word lists. Hear Instr 1987;38:28–29

Gat IB, Keith RW. An effect of linguistic experience. Auditory word discrimination by native and non-native speakers of English. Audiology 1978;17(4):339–345

Gates GA, Cooper JC Jr, Kannel WB, Miller NJ. Hearing in the elderly: the Framingham cohort, 1983–1985. Part I. Basic audiometric test results. Ear Hear 1990;11(4):247–256

Gelfand SA. Use of the carrier phrase in live voice speech discrimination testing. J Aud Res 1975;15:107–110

Gelfand SA. 1993. A clinical speech recognition method to optimize reliability and efficiency. Paper presented at Convention of American Academy of Audiology, Phoenix

Gelfand SA. Optimizing the reliability of speech recognition scores. J Speech Lang Hear Res 1998;41(5):1088–1102

Gelfand SA. Tri-word presentations with phonemic scoring for practical high-reliability speech recognition assessment. J Speech Lang Hear Res 2003;46(2):405–412

Gelfand SA, Gelfand JT. Psychometric functions for shortened administrations of a speech recognition approach using tri-word presentations and phonemic scoring. J Speech Lang Hear Res 2012;55(3):879–891

Gelfand SA, Ross L, Miller S. Sentence reception in noise from one versus two sources: effects of aging and hearing loss. J Acoust Soc Am 1988;83(1):248–256

Gelfand SA, Schwander T, Levitt H, Weiss M, Silman S. Speech recognition performance on a modified nonsense syllable test. J Rehabil Res Dev 1992;29(1):53–60

Gelfand SA, Silman S. Functional hearing loss and its relationship to resolved hearing levels. Ear Hear 1985;6(3):151–158

Gelfand SA, Silman S. Functional components and resolved thresholds in patients with unilateral nonorganic hearing loss. Br J Audiol 1993;27(1):29–34

Gengel RW, Kupperman GL. Word discrimination in noise: effect of different speakers. Ear Hear 1980;1(3):156–160

Gifford RH, Shallop JK, Peterson AM. Speech recognition materials and ceiling effects: considerations for cochlear implant programs. Audiol Neurotol. 2008;13(3):193–205

Gilbert JL, Tamati TN, Pisoni DB. Development, reliability, and validity of PRESTO: a new high-variability sentence recognition test. J Am Acad Audiol 2013;24(1):26–36

Gladstone VS, Siegenthaler BM. Carrier phrase and speech intelligibility score. J Aud Res 1971;11:101–103

Griffiths JD. Rhyming minimal contrasts: a simplified diagnostic articulation test. J Acoust Soc Am 1967;42(1):236–241

Groen JJ, Hellema AC. Binaural speech audiometry. Acta Otolaryngol 1960;52:397–414

Guthrie LA, Mackersie CL. A comparison of presentation levels to maximize word recognition scores. J Am Acad Audiol 2009;20(6):381–390

Hagerman B. Reliability in the determination of speech discrimination. Scand Audiol 1976;5:219–228

Hagerman B. Sentences for testing speech intelligibility in noise. Scand Audiol 1982;11(2):79–87

Haro N. (2005). Spanish word lists for speech audiometry (unpublished report). San Diego: San Diego State University. [Cited by Boothroyd (2006).]

Harris RW, Nissen SL, Pola MG, McPherson DL, Tavartkiladze GA, Eggett DL. Psychometrically equivalent

Russian speech audiometry materials by male and female talkers. Int J Audiol 2007;46(1):47–66

Heckendorf AL, Wiley TL, Wilson RH. Performance norms for the VA compact disc versions of CID W-22 (Hirsh) and PB-50 (Rush Hughes) word lists. J Am Acad Audiol 1997;8(3):163–172

Hirsh IJ, Davis H, Silverman SR, Reynolds EG, Eldert E, Benson RW. Development of materials for speech audiometry. J Speech Hear Disord 1952;17(3):321–337

Hood JD, Poole JP. Influence of the speaker and other factors affecting speech intelligibility. Audiology 1980;19(5):434–455

House AS, Williams CE, Heker MH, Kryter KD. Articulation-testing methods: consonantal differentiation with a closed-response set. J Acoust Soc Am 1965;37:158–166

Hudgins CV, Hawkins JE Jr, Karlin JE, Stevens SS. The development of recorded auditory tests for measuring hearing loss for speech. Laryngoscope 1947;57(1):57–89

Huff SJ, Nerbonne MA. Comparison of the American Speech-Language-Hearing Association and revised Tillman-Olsen methods for speech threshold measurement. Ear Hear 1982;3(6):335–339

Institute of Electrical and Electronic Engineers (IEEE). IEEE Recommended Practice for Speech Quality Measures. IEEE Trans Audio Electroacoust 1969;17(3):225–246

Jahner JA, Schlauch RA, Doyle T. A comparison of American Speech-Language Hearing Association guidelines for obtaining speech-recognition thresholds. Ear Hear 1994;15(4):324–329

Jerger J, Jerger S. Diagnostic significance of PB word functions. Arch Otolaryngol 1971;93(6):573–580

Jerger J, Jerger S. Comment on "The effects of age on the diagnostic utility of the rollover phenomenon." J Speech Hear Disord 1976;41(4):556–557

Jerger J, Speaks C, Trammell JL. A new approach to speech audiometry. J Speech Hear Disord 1968;33(4):318–328

Johnson EW. Auditory test results in 500 cases of acoustic neuroma. Arch Otolaryngol 1977;103(3):152–158

Kalikow DN, Stevens KN, Elliott LL. Development of a test of speech intelligibility in noise using sentence materials with controlled word predictability. J Acoust Soc Am 1977;61(5):1337–1351

Kamm C, Dirks DD, Mickey MR. Effect of sensorineural hearing loss on loudness discomfort level and most comfortable loudness judgments. J Speech Hear Res 1978;21(4):668–681

Killion MC, Niquette PA, Gudmundsen GI, Revit LJ, Banerjee S. Development of a quick speech-in-noise test for measuring signal-to-noise ratio loss in normal-hearing and hearing-impaired listeners. J Acoust Soc Am 2004;116(4 Pt 1):2395–2405

Killion MC, Villchur E. Kessler was right—partly: but SIN test shows some aids improve hearing in noise. Hear J 1993;4 6(9):31–35

Kirk KI, Eisenberg LS, Martinez AS, Hay-McCutcheon M. Lexical Neighborhood Test: test-retest reliability and interlist equivalency. J Am Acad Audiol 1999;10:113–123

Kirk KI, Pisoni DB, Osberger MJ. Lexical effects on spoken word recognition by pediatric cochlear implant users. Ear Hear 1995;16(5):470–481

Koike KJM. Verifying speech amplification with low-mid-high frequency words. Hear Instr 1993;44:11–13

Koike KJM, Brown B, Hobbs H, Asp C. 1989. New generation speech discrimination test: Tennessee Tonality Test. Proc 6th Conf Rehab Eng 11, 324–326

Kreul EJ, Bell DW, Nixon JC. Factors affecting speech discrimination test difficulty. J Speech Hear Res 1969;12(2):281–287

Kreul EJ, Nixon JC, Kryter KD, Bell DW, Lang JS, Schubert ED. A proposed clinical test of speech discrimination. J Speech Hear Res 1968;11:536–552

Lehiste I, Peterson GE. Linguistic considerations in the study of speech intelligibility. J Acoust Soc Am 1959;31:280–286

Levitt H, Resnick SB. Speech reception by the hearing-impaired: methods of testing and the development of new tests. Scand Audiol Suppl 1978;(6):107–130

Luce PA. 1990. Neighborhoods of Words in the Mental Lexicon. (Research on Speech Perception Technical Report 6). Bloomington, IN: Indiana University

Luce PA, Pisoni DB. Recognizing spoken words: the neighborhood activation model. Ear Hear 1998;19(1):1–36

Mackersie CL, Boothroyd A, Minniear D. Evaluation of the Computer-Assisted Speech Perception Assessment Test (CASPA). J Am Acad Audiol 2001;12(8):390–396

Markides A. Whole-word scoring versus phoneme scoring in speech audiometry. Br J Audiol 1978;12(2):40–46

Maroonroge S, Diefendorf AO. Comparing normal hearing and hearing-impaired subject's performance on the Northwestern Auditory Test Number 6, California Consonant Test, and Pascoe's High-Frequency Word Test. Ear Hear 1984;5(6):356–360

Martin FN, Champlin CA, Chambers JA. Seventh survey of audiometric practices in the United States. J Am Acad Audiol 1998;9(2):95–104

Martin FN, Champlin CA, Perez DD. The question of phonetic balance in word recognition testing. J Am Acad Audiol 2000;11(9):489–493, quiz 522

Martin FN, Hawkins RR, Bailey HA. The non-essentiality of the carrier phrase in phonetically balanced (PB) word testing. J Aud Res 1962;2:319–322

McArdle RA, Wilson RH, Burks CA. Speech recognition in multitalker babble using digits, words, and sentences. J Am Acad Audiol 2005;16(9):726–739, quiz 763–764

McCullough JA, Cunningham LA, Wilson RH. Auditory-visual word identification test materials: computer application with children. J Am Acad Audiol 1992;3(3):208–214

McCullough JA, Wilson RH, Birck JD, Anderson LG. A multimedia approach for estimating speech recognition of multilingual clients. Am J Audiol 1994;3:19–22

McLennan RO Jr, Knox AW. Patient-controlled delivery of monosyllabic words in a test of auditory discrimination. J Speech Hear Disord 1975;40(4):538–543

McPherson DF, Pang-Ching GK. Development of a distinctive feature discrimination test. J Aud Res 1979; 19(4):235–246

Meyer TA, Bilger RC. Effect of set size and method on speech reception thresholds in noise. Ear Hear 1997; 18(3):202–209

Meyer DH, Mishler ET. Rollover measurements with Auditec NU-6 word lists. J Speech Hear Disord 1985; 50(4):356–360

Minimum Speech Test Battery for Adult Cochlear Implant Users (MSTB) Manual. 2011. Available at http://www.auditorypotential.com/MSTBfiles/MSTBManual2011-06-20%20.pdf

Nilsson M, Soli SD, Sullivan JA. Development of the Hearing in Noise Test for the measurement of speech reception thresholds in quiet and in noise. J Acoust Soc Am 1994;95(2):1085–1099

Niquette P, Arcaroli J, Revit L, et al. 2003. Development of the BKB-SIN Test. Paper presented at meeting of American Auditory Society, Scottsdale, AZ

Nittrouer S, Boothroyd A. Context effects in phoneme and word recognition by young children and older adults. J Acoust Soc Am 1990;87(6):2705–2715

Olsen WO, Matkin ND. 1991. Speech audiometry. In: Rintelmann WF, ed. Hearing Assessment, 2nd ed. Austin, TX: Pro-Ed; 39–140

Olsen WO, Noffsinger D, Kurdziel S. Speech discrimination in quiet and in white noise by patients with peripheral and central lesions. Acta Otolaryngol 1975;80(5-6):375–382

Olsen WO, Van Tasell DJ, Speaks CE. The Carhart Memorial Lecture, American Auditory Society, Salt Lake City, Utah 1996. Phoneme and word recognition for words in isolation and in sentences. Ear Hear 1997;18(3):175–188

Owens E. Intelligibility of words varying in familiarity. J Speech Hear Res 1961;4:113–129

Owens E, Schubert ED. Development of the California Consonant Test. J Speech Hear Res 1977;20(3):463–474

Pascoe DP. Frequency responses of hearing aids and their effects on the speech perception of hearing-impaired subjects. Ann Otol Rhinol Laryngol 1975;84(5 pt 2, Suppl 23):1–40

Pederson OT, Studebaker GA. A new minimal-contrasts closed-response-set speech test. J Aud Res 1972; 12:187–195

Penrod JP. Talker effects on word-discrimination scores of adults with sensorineural hearing impairment. J Speech Hear Disord 1979;44(3):340–349

Peterson GE, Lehiste I. Revised CNC lists for auditory tests. J Speech Hear Disord 1962;27:62–70

Picheny MA, Durlach NI, Braida LD. Speaking clearly for the hard of hearing I: Intelligibility differences between clear and conversational speech. J Speech Hear Res 1985;28(1):96–103

Plomp R. A signal-to-noise ratio model for the speech-reception threshold of the hearing impaired. J Speech Hear Res 1986;29(2):146–154

Plomp R, Mimpen AM. Improving the reliability of testing the speech reception threshold for sentences. Audiology 1979;18(1):43–52

Pollack I, Rubenstein H, Decker L. Intelligibility of known and unknown message sets. J Acoust Soc Am 1959;31:273–279

Posner J, Ventry IM. Relationships between comfortable loudness levels for speech and speech discrimination in sensorineural hearing loss. J Speech Hear Disord 1977;42(3):370–375

Punch JL, Howard MT. Spondee recognition threshold as a function of set size. J Speech Hear Disord 1985;50(2):120–125

Punch J, Joseph A, Rakerd B. Most comfortable and uncomfortable loudness levels: six decades of research. Am J Audiol 2004a;13(2):144–157

Punch J, Rakerd B, Joseph A. Effects of test order on most comfortable and uncomfortable loudness levels for speech. Am J Audiol 2004b;13(2):158–163

Raffin MJM, Schafer D. Application of a probability model based on the binomial distribution to speech-discrimination scores. J Speech Hear Res 1980;23(3):570–575

Raffin MJM, Thornton AR. Confidence levels for differences between speech-discrimination scores. A research note. J Speech Hear Res 1980;23(1):5–18

Resnick SB, Dubno JR, Hoffnung S, Levitt H. Phoneme errors on a nonsense syllable test. J Acoust Soc Am 1976;58(Suppl 1):114

Runge CA, Hosford-Dunn H. Word recognition performance with modified CID W-22 word lists. J Speech Hear Res 1985;28(3):355–362

Schafer EC, Pogue J, Milrany T. List equivalency of the AzBio sentence test in noise for listeners with normal-hearing sensitivity or cochlear implants. J Am Acad Audiol 2012;23(7):501–509

Shirinian MJ, Arnst DJ. PI-PB rollover in a group of aged listeners. Ear Hear 1980;1(1):50–53

Silman S, Silverman CA. 1991. Auditory Diagnosis: Principles and Applications. San Diego, CA: Academic Press

Silverman SR, Hirsh IJ. Problems related to the use of speech in clinical audiometry. Ann Otol Rhinol Laryngol 1955;64(4):1234–1244

Smiljanić R, Bradlow AR. Bidirectional clear speech perception benefit for native and high-proficiency non-native talkers and listeners: intelligibility and accentedness. J Acoust Soc Am 2011;130(6):4020–4031

Smoorenburg GF. Speech reception in quiet and in noisy conditions by individuals with noise-induced hearing loss in relation to their tone audiogram. J Acoust Soc Am 1992;91(1):421–437

Soli SD, Wong LLN. Assessment of speech intelligibility in noise with the Hearing in Noise Test. Int J Audiol 2008;47(6):356–361

Spahr AJ, Dorman MF. Performance of subjects fit with the Advanced Bionics CII and Nucleus 3G cochlear implant devices. Arch Otolaryngol Head Neck Surg 2004;130(5):624–628

Spahr AJ, Dorman MF, Litvak LM, et al. Development and validation of the AzBio sentence lists. Ear Hear 2012;33(1):112–117

Speaks C, Jerger J. Method for measurement of speech identification. J Speech Hear Res 1965;8:185–194

Spearman C. The method of "right and wrong cases" ("constant stimuli") without Guass's formulae. Br J Psychol 1908;2:227–242

Spitzer JB. The development of a picture speech reception threshold test in Spanish for use with urban U.S. residents of Hispanic background. J Commun Disord 1980;13(2):147–151

Stoppenbach DT, Craig JM, Wiley TL, Wilson RH. Word recognition performance for Northwestern University Auditory Test No. 6 word lists in quiet and in competing message. J Am Acad Audiol 1999;10(8):429–435

Tadros SF, Frisina ST, Mapes F, Kim S, Frisina DR, Frisina RD. Loss of peripheral right-ear advantage in age-related hearing loss. Audiol Neurootol 2005;10(1):44–52

Tamati TN, Gilbert JL, Pisoni DB. Some factors underlying individual differences in speech recognition on PRESTO: a first report. J Am Acad Audiol 2013;24(7):616–634

Theunissen M, Swanepoel W, Hanekom J. Sentence recognition in noise: variables in compilation and interpretation of tests. Int J Audiol 2009;48(11):743–757

Thorndike DL. 1932. A Teacher's Word Book of Twenty Thousand Words Found Most Frequently and Widely in General Reading for Children and Young People. New York, NY: Columbia University Press

Thorndike DL, Lorge I. 1944. The Teacher's Word Book of 30,000 Words. New York, NY: Columbia University Press

Thornton AR, Raffin MJM. Speech-discrimination scores modeled as a binomial variable. J Speech Hear Res 1978;21(3):507–518

Thurlow WR, Silverman SR, Davis H, Walsh TE. A statistical study of auditory tests in relation to the fenestration operation. Laryngoscope 1948;58(1):43–66

Tillman TW, Carhart R. 1966. An Expanded Test for Speech Discrimination Utilizing CNC Monosyllabic Words. Northwestern University Auditory Test No. 6. Tech Report SAM-TR-66–55.Brooks AFB, TX: USAF School of Aerospace Medicine

Tillman TW, Carhart R, Wilber L. 1963. A test for speech discrimination composed of CNC monosyllabic words. Northwestern Univ. Auditory Test No. 4. Brooks AFB, TX: USAF School of Aerospace Med. Tech. Report SAM-TDR-62–135

Tillman TW, Jerger JF. Some factors affecting the spondee threshold in normal-hearing subjects. J Speech Hear Res 1959;2(2):141–146

Tillman TW, Olsen WO. 1973. Speech audiometry. In: Jerger J, ed. Modern Developments in Audiology, 2nd ed. New York, NY: Academic Press; 37–74

Tobias JV. On phonemic analysis of speech discrimination tests. J Speech Hear Res 1964;7:98–100

Ullrich K, Grimm D. Most comfortable listening level presentation versus maximum discrimination for word discrimination material. Audiology 1976;15(4):338–347

Vermiglio AJ, Soli SD, Freed DJ, Fisher LM. The relationship between high-frequency pure-tone hearing loss, hearing in noise test (HINT) thresholds, and the articulation index. J Am Acad Audiol 2012;23(10):779–788

Versfeld NJ, Daalder L, Festen JM, Houtgast T. Method for the selection of sentence materials for efficient measurement of the speech reception threshold. J Acoust Soc Am 2000;107(3):1671–1684

Wall LG, Davis LA, Myers DK. Four spondee threshold procedures: a comparison. Ear Hear 1984;5(3):171–174

Weisleder P, Hodgson WR. Evaluation of four Spanish word-recognition-ability lists. Ear Hear 1989;10(6):387–392

Wiley TL, Stoppenbach DT, Feldhake LJ, Moss KA, Thordardottir ET. Audiologic practices: what is popular versus what is supported by evidence. Am J Audiol 1995;4:26–34

Wilson RH. Development of a speech-in-multitalker-babble paradigm to assess word-recognition performance. J Am Acad Audiol 2003;14(9):453–470

Wilson RH, Antablin JK. A picture identification task as an estimate of the word-recognition performance of nonverbal adults. J Speech Hear Disord 1980;45(2):223–238

Wilson RH, Abrams HB, Pillion AL. A word-recognition task in multitalker babble using a descending presentation mode from 24 dB to 0 dB signal to babble. J Rehabil Res Dev 2003;40(4):321–327

Wilson RH, Burks CA. Use of 35 words for evaluation of hearing loss in signal-to-babble ratio: a clinic protocol. J Rehabil Res Dev 2005;42(6):839–852

Wilson RH, McArdle RA, Smith SL. An evaluation of the BKB-SIN, HINT, QuickSIN, and WIN materials on listeners with normal hearing and listeners with hearing loss. J Speech Lang Hear Res 2007;50(4):844–856

Wilson RH, Morgan DE, Dirks DD. A proposed SRT procedure and its statistical precedent. J Speech Hear Disord 1973;38(2):184–191

Wilson RH, Oyler AL. Psychometric functions for the CID W-22 and NU Auditory Test No. 6. Materials spoken by the same speaker. Ear Hear 1997;18(5):430–433

Wilson RH, Strouse A. Psychometrically equivalent spondaic words spoken by a female speaker. J Speech Lang Hear Res 1999;42(6):1336–1346

Wilson RH, Watts KL. The Words-in-Noise Test (WIN), list 3: a practice list. J Am Acad Audiol 2012;23(2):92–96

Yellin MW, Jerger J, Fifer RC. Norms for disproportionate loss in speech intelligibility. Ear Hear 1989;10(4):231–234

Young LL Jr, Dudley B, Gunter MB. Thresholds and psychometric functions of the individual spondaic words. J Speech Hear Res 1982;25(4):586–593

It seems reasonable to assume that sounds presented to the right ear are heard by the right ear, and that sounds presented to the left ear are heard by the left ear. However, this is not necessarily true. In fact, it is common to find that the sound being presented to one ear is actually being heard by the opposite ear. This phenomenon is called **cross-hearing** or **shadow hearing**. To avoid confusion it is customary to call the ear currently being tested the **test ear (TE)** and to call the opposite ear, which is the one not being tested, the **nontest ear (NTE)**. Cross-hearing results in a false picture of the patient's hearing. Even the possibility that the sounds being presented to the TE are really being heard by the NTE causes the outcome of a test to be suspect, at best. This chapter explains why this situation occurs, how it is recognized, and the manner in which the NTE is removed from the test.

■ Cross-Hearing and Interaural Attenuation

Suppose we know for a fact that a patient's right ear is essentially normal and that his left ear is completely deaf. We would expect the audiogram to show air- and bone-conduction thresholds of perhaps 0 dB HL to 10 dB HL for the right ear and "no response" symbols for both air-conduction and bone-conduction at the maximum testable levels for the left ear, as in **Fig. 9.1a**. However, this does not occur. Instead, the actual audiogram will be more like the one shown in **Fig. 9.1b**. Here the thresholds for the right ear are just as expected. On the other hand, the left air-conduction thresholds are in the 55 to 60 dB HL range, and the left bone-conduction thresholds are the same as for the right ear. How can this be if the left ear is deaf?

Cross-Hearing for Air-Conduction

Let us first address this question for the air-conduction signals. Since the patient cannot hear anything in the left ear, the level of an air-conduction test tone presented to that ear will be raised higher and higher. Eventually, the tone presented to the deaf ear will be raised so high that it can actually be heard in the opposite ear, at which point the patient will finally respond. The patient's response to the signal directed to his deaf ear (the TE) is the result of hearing that signal in the other ear (the NTE). Thus, the left ear's threshold curve in **Fig. 9.1b** is due to cross-hearing, and is often called a **shadow curve**.

In order for the tone to be heard in the NTE it must be possible for a signal presented to one ear to be transmitted across the head to the other ear. This phenomenon is called **signal crossover**. The intensity of the sound reaching the NTE is less than what was originally presented to the TE because it takes a certain amount of energy to transmit the signal across the head. The number of dB that are "lost" in the process of signal crossover is called **interaural attenuation (IA)** (Chaiklin 1967).

In **Fig. 9.1b**, the patient's right air-conduction threshold at 1000 Hz is 10 dB HL. Even though his *left* ear is completely deaf, he also responded to a 1000 Hz tone presented from the *left* earphone at 60 dB HL. This means that the 60 dB HL tone presented to the left ear must have reached a level of 10 dB HL in the *right* ear. Consequently, IA at 1000 Hz in this case must be 50 dB (60 dB – 10 dB = 50 dB). Similarly, the amount of IA at 4000 Hz in this case is 55 dB (60 dB – 5 dB = 55 dB)

Crossover occurs when the signal is *physically present* in the opposite ear, whereas cross-hearing occurs only when it is *audible*. The distinction is clarified using the following example based on our hypothetical patient: The level of the 1000 Hz tone

Fig. 9.1 **(a)** Imagined (incorrect) audiogram without cross-hearing for a patient who is deaf in the left ear, showing "no response" for air-conduction or bone-conduction signals. **(b)** Actual audiogram for such a patient, reflecting the fact that the signals presented to the left side were heard in the right ear by cross-hearing. **(c)** Audiogram obtained when the left thresholds are retested with masking noise in the right ear.

reaching this person's right (nontest) ear will always be 50 dB less than the amount presented from the left earphone due to IA. Consider these three cases:

dB HL at left earphone	− IA	= dB HL present at right cochlea
(a) 60 dB	− 50 dB	= 10 dB (at threshold)
(b) 80 dB	− 50 dB	= 30 dB (20 dB SL)
(c) 55 dB	− 50 dB	= 5 dB (5 dB below threshold)

These three examples are shown graphically in **Fig. 9.2**. In (a) the tone reaches the right ear at 10 dB HL, and is heard because this is the right ear's threshold. In (b) the tone reaches the right ear at 30 dB HL and is heard because this level is 20 dB above the right ear's threshold (20 dB SL). In both of these cases signal crossover resulted in cross-hearing. However, the tone in (c) reaches the right ear at only 5 dB HL, which is 5 dB *below* threshold and is thus inaudible.

Here, there is crossover because the signal is present in the NTE but there is no cross-hearing because it is below threshold.

Assuming the bone-conduction threshold remained at 10 dB HL, how would cross-hearing be affected if the IA was changed from 50 dB to another value, such as 40 dB or 60 dB? Some time with paper and pencil will reveal that the cross-hearing situation would change considerably.

Cross-Hearing for Bone-Conduction

The right and left bone-conduction thresholds are the same in **Fig. 9.1b** even though the right ear is normal and the left one is deaf. The implication is that the bone-conduction signal presented to the left side of the head is being received by the right ear. This should come as no surprise, since we found in Chapter 5 that a bone-conduction vibrator stimulates

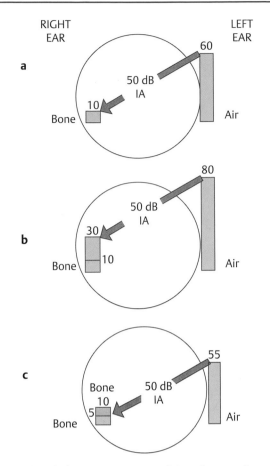

RIGHT EAR   LEFT EAR

a

50 dB IA

Bone   10   60   Air

b

50 dB IA

30
Bone   10   80   Air

c

Bone
50 dB IA
10
5
Bone   55   Air

Fig. 9.2 **(a–c)** Three crossover conditions (see text).

both cochleae about equally. From the cross-hearing standpoint, we may say that there is no interaural attenuation (IA = 0 dB) for bone-conduction. Thus, the right and left bone-conduction signals result in the same thresholds because they are both stimulating the same (right) ear.

Overcoming Cross-Hearing with Masking Noise

The above example demonstrates that there are times when the NTE is (or at least may be) responding to the signals intended for the TE. How can we stop the NTE from hearing the tones being presented to the TE? First, consider an analogy from vision testing. Looking at an eye chart with two eyes is akin to the cross-hearing issue. We all know from common experience that to test one eye at a time the optometrist simply blindfolds the nontest eye. In other words, one eye is tested while the other eye is **masked**. In effect, we do the same thing in audiology,

except that the auditory "blindfold" is a noise that is directed into the NTE. The noise in the NTE stops it from hearing the sounds being presented to the TE. Just as the nontest eye is masked by the blindfold, so is the nontest ear masked by the noise.

Returning to our example, **Fig. 9.1c** shows the results obtained when the air- and bone-conduction thresholds of the left (test) ear are retested with appropriate masking noise in the right (nontest) ear. The thresholds here are shown by different symbols than the ones in frames (a) and (b), to distinguish them as *masked* results. Because the left ear in this example is completely deaf, the masked thresholds have downward-pointing arrows indicating no response at the maximum limits of the audiometer. Notice that the **masked results** in frame (c) are at the same hearing levels as the ones in frame (a). The important difference is that the **unmasked thresholds** in frame (a) could never have actually occurred because of cross-hearing. Note the dramatic difference between the unmasked results in frame (b) and the patient's real hearing status, revealed by the masked thresholds in frame (c).

We see that when cross-hearing occurs it is necessary to retest the TE while directing a masking noise into the NTE. The purpose of the masking noise is to prevent the NTE from hearing the tone (or other signal) intended for the TE. Thus, the issue of whether cross-hearing might be occurring is tantamount to the question, is masking (of the NTE) necessary?

Principal Mechanism of Crossover

Signal crossover (and therefore cross-hearing) for bone-conduction signals obviously occurs via a bone-conduction route, as depicted in **Fig. 9.3a**. It occurs because a bone-conduction signal is transmitted to both cochleae.

Because crossover for air-conduction requires a reasonably substantial signal to be produced by the earphone (recall that interaural attenuation was ~ 50 dB in the prior example), common sense seems to suggest that air-conduction signals might reach the opposite ear by an air-conduction route. This might occur by sound escaping through the earphone cushion on the test side, traveling around the head, and then penetrating the earphone cushion on the nontest side. Alternatively, earphone vibration on the test side might be transmitted via the headset to the earphone on the nontest side. In either of these two scenarios, the signal from the test side would enter the ear canal of the NTE, that is, as an air-conduction signal. As compelling as these explanations may seem, they are not correct. It has been shown repeatedly that the actual crossover route for air-conduc-

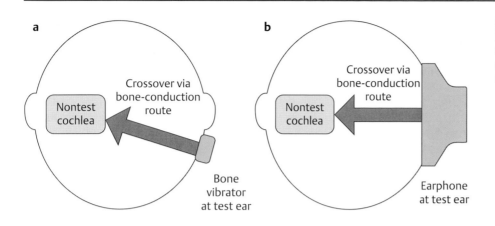

Fig. 9.3 Signal crossover and cross-hearing occur via the bone-conduction route to the opposite cochlea, as indicated by the arrows for both **(a)** bone-conduction and **(b)** air-conduction.

tion signals occurs principally by *bone-conduction* to the cochlea of the opposite ear (Sparrevohn 1946; Zwislocki 1953; Studebaker 1962), as depicted in **Fig. 9.3b**.

Interaural Attenuation for Air-Conduction

Cross-hearing of a test signal renders a test invalid. We must therefore identify cross-hearing whenever it occurs so that we can mask the NTE. The cost of failing to do so is so great that we want to employ masking every time that cross-hearing is even possible. Once we have obtained the unmasked audiogram, we are left with the following question: Is the air-conduction signal being presented to the TE great enough to cross the head and reach the bone-conduction threshold of the NTE? In other words, is this difference greater than the value of interaural attenuation? The corollary problem is to determine the IA value.

Interaural attenuation for air-conduction using supra-aural earphones typical of the type used in audiological practice has been studied using a variety of approaches (Littler, Knight, & Strange 1952; Zwislocki 1953; Liden 1954; Liden, Nilsson, & Anderson 1959a; Chaiklin 1967; Coles & Priede 1970; Snyder 1973; Smith & Markides 1981; Sklare & Denenberg 1987). **Fig. 9.4** shows the mean IA values found in four of these studies, as well as the maximum and minimum amounts of IA obtained across all four studies. Average IA values are ~ 50 to 65 dB, and there is a general tendency for IA to become larger with frequency. The range of IA values is very wide, and the means are much larger than the minimum IA values. Consequently, we cannot rely on average IA values as a red flag for cross-hearing in clinical practice because many cases of cross-hearing would be missed in many patients on the lower side of the IA range. For this reason it is common practice to use *minimum* IA values to identify possible cross-hearing, that is, to decide when masking may be needed. As anticipated from the figure, the minimum IA value typically suggested to rule out crossover for clinical purposes is **40 dB** (Studebaker 1967; Martin 1974, 1980).

Interaural Attenuation for Insert Earphones

The IA values just described are obtained using typical supra-aural audiometric earphones, such as Telephonics TDH-49 and related receivers. In contrast, insert earphones such as Etymotic ER-3A and EARtone 3A receivers provide much greater amounts of IA (Killion, Wilber, & Gudmundsen 1985; Sklare & Denenberg 1987). This occurs because the amount of IA is inversely related to the contact area between the earphone and the head (Zwislocki 1953), and the contact area between the head and earphone is much less for insert receivers than it is for supra-aural earphones. **Fig. 9.5** shows some of the results obtained by Sklare and Denenberg (1987), who compared the IA produced by TDH-49 (supra-aural) and ER-3A (insert) earphones on the same subjects. They found that mean IA values were from 81 to 94+ dB up to 1000 Hz and 71 to 77 dB at higher frequencies, for insert receivers.

As already explained, we are most interested in the minimum IA values, which are shown by the bottoms of the error lines in the graph. Sklare and Denenberg found that insert receivers produced minimum IA values of 75 to 85 dB at frequencies up to 1000 Hz, and 50 to 65 dB above 1000 Hz. This is substantially greater than the minimum IA values found for the TDH-49 earphone, which ranged from 45 to 60 dB.

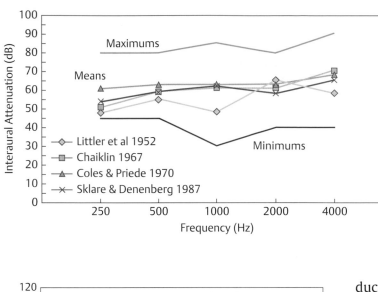

Fig. 9.4 Interaural attenuation values for supra-aural earphones from four representative studies. Lines with symbols are means for each study. The "minimum" and "maximum" lines show the smallest and largest IA values across all four studies.

Fig. 9.5 Interaural attenuation for TDH-49 (supra-aural) versus ER-3A (insert) earphones. Bars show means and error lines show ranges. Some actual values were higher than shown. (This occurred because some individual IA values were higher than the limits of the equipment.) (Based on the data of Sklare and Denenberg [1987]).

It should be noted that the IA values just described were obtained using insert receivers that were inserted to the proper depth into the ear canal. Insert receivers produce much less IA when their insertion into the ear canal is shallow compared with deep (Killion et al 1985).

Interaural Attenuation for Bone-Conduction

It is commonly held that interaural attenuation is 0 dB for all bone-conduction signals, but this concept requires qualification. There is essentially no IA for bone-conduction signals presented by a bone-conduction vibrator using *frontal placement* (Studebaker 1967). However, IA for the more commonly used *mastoid placement* of the bone-conduction oscillator depends on the frequency being tested, and is also variable among patients (Studebaker 1964, 1967). Interaural attenuation values for bone-conduction signals presented at the mastoid are ~ 0 dB at 250 Hz and rise to ~ 15 dB at 4000 Hz (Studebaker 1967). The author's experience agrees with others' clinical observations that IA for bone-conduction varies among patients from roughly 0 to 15 dB at 2000 and 4000 Hz (Silman & Silverman 1991).

■ Clinical Masking

Recall that masking per se means to render a tone (or other signal) inaudible due to the presence of a noise in the same ear as the tone. Thus, masking the right ear means that a noise is put into the right ear, so that a tone cannot be heard in the right ear. *Clinical masking* is an application of the masking phenomenon used to alleviate cross-hearing. In clinical masking we put noise into the nontest ear because we want to assess the hearing of the test ear. In other words, the masking noise goes into the NTE, and the test signal goes into the TE. Also, the noise is delivered to the NTE by *air-conduction*, regardless of whether the TE is being tested by air- or bone-conduction. These rules apply in all but the most unusual circumstances. The kinds of masking noises used with various test signals are covered in a later section. In the meantime, it is assumed that the appropriate masking noise is always being used.

The meaning is clear when an audiologist says that she will "retest the left bone-conduction threshold with masking noise in the right ear." However, masking terminology is usually more telegraphic. As such, it suffers from ambiguity and can be confusing to the uninitiated. It is therefore worthwhile to familiar-ize oneself with typical masking phrases and what these really mean. *Unmasked air-conduction* (or just *unmasked air*) refers to an air-conduction threshold that was obtained without any masking noise. Simi-larly, *unmasked bone-conduction* (or *unmasked bone*) means a bone-conduction threshold obtained without any masking noise. For example, *unmasked right bone* means the bone-conduction threshold of the right ear that was obtained without any masking noise.

Masked air-conduction (or *masked air*) refers to an air-conduction threshold (in the TE) that was obtained with masking noise in the opposite ear. *Masked bone-conduction* (*masked bone*) denotes a bone-conduction threshold obtained with masking noise in the NTE. Thus, *masked right air* is referring to the air-conduction threshold of the right ear that was obtained while masking noise was being pre-sented to the left (nontest) ear. By the same token, *masked left bone* means the bone-conduction thresh-old of the left ear that was obtained with masking noise in the right ear.

The process of *masking for air-conduction* (*mask-ing for air*) means to put masking noise into the NTE while testing the TE by air-conduction. Likewise, the operation of *masking for bone-conduction* (*masking for bone*) means to put masking noise into the NTE while testing the TE by bone-conduction.

Instructions for Testing with Masking

The first step in clinical masking is to explain to the patient what is about to happen and what she is sup-posed to do. The very idea of being tested with "noise in your ears" can be confusing to some patients, especially when they are being evaluated for the first time. The author has found that most patients readily accept the situation when they are told that putting masking noise in the opposite ear is the same as an optometrist covering one eye while testing the other.

Noises Used for Clinical Masking

What kind of noise should be used to mask the non-test ear? The answer to this question depends on the signal being masked. If the signal being masked has a wide spectrum, such as speech or clicks, then the masker must also have a wide spectrum. (The student might wish to refer back to Chapter 1 to review the relevant physical concepts.) For example, masking for speech tests commonly uses white noise (actually broadband noise), pink noise, speech-shaped noise, or multitalker babble. Speech-shaped noise has a spectrum that approximates that of the long-term spectrum of speech. Multitalker babble is made by

recording the voices of many people who are talking simultaneously, resulting in an unintelligible babble.

Complex noises (e.g., sawtooth noise) composed of a low fundamental frequency along with many harmonics were also used in the past. These noises were poor and unreliable maskers, but one should be aware of them if only for historical perspective.

Pure tones can also be masked by wide-band noises, but this is not desirable. Recall from Chapter 3 that if we are trying to mask a given pure tone, only a rather limited band of frequencies in a wide-band noise actually contributes to masking that tone. This is the critical band (ratio). The parts of a wide-band noise that are higher and lower than the critical band do not help mask the tone, but they do make the noise sound louder. Thus, wide-band noise is a poor choice for masking pure tones because it is both inef-ficient and unnecessarily loud.

It would therefore seem that the optimal masking noises for pure tones would be critical bands. In prac-tice, however, audiometers actually provide masking noise bandwidths that are wider than critical bands. This type of masking noise is called **narrow-band noise (NBN)**. Audiometric NBNs may approximate bandwidths that are one-third octaves, one-half octaves, or other widths, and also vary widely in how sharply intensity falls outside the pass band (i.e., the rejection rate or steepness of the filter skirts). If an NBN is centered around 1000 Hz, then we can call this a 1000 Hz NBN; if it is centered around 2000 Hz, then it is a 2000 Hz NBN, and so forth. **Table 9.1** summarizes the bandwidths for narrow-band mask-ing noises specified by the ANSI S3.6-2010 standard.

When to Mask for Bone-Conduction

It might seem odd to discuss the bone-conduction masking rule before the one for air-conduction (AC) because this is the reverse of the order used to obtain unmasked thresholds. However, masked thresholds are tested in the opposite order, bone-conduction (BC) before AC. This is done because the rule for determining when masking is needed for air-con-duction depends upon knowing the true bone-con-duction thresholds. This means that if masking is needed for BC, it must be done first.

Bone-conduction testing presents us with a pecu-liar dilemma if we take it for granted that we always need to know which ear is actually responding to a signal. This is so because there is little if any IA for BC, so we rarely know for sure which cochlea is actually responding to a signal, no matter where the vibrator is placed. (Although mastoid placement is assumed throughout this book unless specifically indicated, it should be noted that the bone oscillator and both

Table 9.1 Allowable lower and upper cut-off frequencies for narrow-band masking noises[a]

	Frequency (Hz)										
	125	250	500	750	1000	1500	2000	3000	4000	6000	8000
Lower cutoff frequency (Hz)											
Minimum	105	210	420	631	841	1260	1680	2520	3360	5050	6730
Maximum	111	223	445	668	891	1340	1780	2670	3560	5350	7130
Upper cutoff frequency (Hz)											
Minimum	140	281	561	842	1120	1680	2240	3370	4490	6730	8980
Maximum	149	297	595	892	1190	1780	2380	3570	4760	7140	9510

[a]Based on ANSI S3.6-2010.

earphones are usually in place from the outset when forehead placement is used.)

This situation might seem to imply that masking should always be used whenever bone-conduction is tested. This approach was recommended by ANSI (2004) on the grounds that bone-conduction calibration is based on data that were obtained with masking the opposite ear.

However, this approach is not encouraged because it has several serious problems in addition to being unnecessarily conservative at the cost of wasted effort (Studebaker 1964, 1967). When bone-conduction thresholds are *always* tested with masking, the opposite ear will always be occluded with an earphone (both ears would probably be occluded with forehead placement). Thus, one cannot know when or where an occlusion effect occurs, or how large it is. But you need to know the size of the occlusion effect in the first place to calculate how much noise is needed for bone-conduction masking. In addition, always having the headset in place denies the clinician the ability to cross-check for bone-conduction oscillator placement errors, which cause falsely elevated bone-conduction thresholds. Also, placement problems can be clouded by an occlusion effect and/ or by unwittingly attributing a higher threshold to the masking. The headset itself only exacerbates vibrator placement problems.

Another questionable technique relies on the Weber test to determine which ear is hearing a bone-conduction signal. These results are not sufficiently accurate or reliable for this purpose. Even its proponents admit that it is best to disregard unlikely Weber results (Studebaker 1967).

Because a given unmasked bone-conduction threshold could as likely be coming from either ear, a practical approach to deciding when to mask for bone-conduction is based on whether knowing which

cochlea is actually responding affects how the audiogram is interpreted. In other words, when does it make a difference whether a given bone-conduction threshold is coming from one cochlea or the other?

A bone-conduction threshold should be retested with masking in the NTE whenever there is an air-bone-gap (ABG) within the test ear that is greater than 10 dB, that is, 15 dB or more, which may be written as:

ABG > 10 dB .

Because testing is done in 5 dB steps, this rule also can be stated this way: *A bone-conduction threshold should be retested with masking in the NTE whenever the air-bone-gap (ABG) within the test ear is 15 dB or more*, or

ABG ≥ 15 dB

This principle is shown schematically in **Fig. 9.6a**. This rule is consistent with the one recommended by Yacullo (1996, 2009), but differs from a stricter approach that calls for masking whenever the ABG is ≥ 10 dB (Studebaker 1964; ASHA 2005).[1] The underlying concept for suggesting the less stringent masking criterion is as follows: The variability of a clinical threshold is usually taken to be ± 5 dB. Applying this principle to both the air- and bone- conduction thresholds for the same frequency allows them to be as much as 10 dB apart. Thus, for practical purposes, an ABG ≤ 10 dB is too small to be clinically relevant.

---

[1] The > 10 dB (≥ 15) rule encouraged here was included in the first two editions of this text. It was changed to the Studebaker (1964) recommendation in the third edition because the ≥ 10 dB rule continued to be endorsed in the ASHA (2005) guidelines. However, the current edition is returning to the > 10 dB (≥ 15) rule because it is considered to be the more compelling approach.

With this in mind, consider the unmasked thresholds in the following example:

Right air conduction	50 dB HL
Left air conduction	70 dB HL
Bone conduction	45 dB HL

We do not know which ear is really responsible for the bone-conduction threshold of 45 dB. First consider the situation from the standpoint of the *right* ear. If we assume that the unmasked bone-conduction threshold was heard in the right cochlea, then it would have a 5 dB ABG (50 – 45 = 5). It is therefore not necessary to retest the bone-conduction of the right ear with masking noise in the left ear, because our rule says we should mask when the ABG > 10 dB. But one may say that we still do not know if the bone-conduction threshold is really from the right ear; how can this be acceptable? There are only two options:

1. If the tone was heard by the *right* cochlea, then the ABG is only 5 dB. This is too small to be clinically relevant and the 50 dB loss in the right ear would be interpreted as essentially sensorineural.

2. What if the bone-conduction threshold of 45 dB is really coming from the *left* ear? This option would mean the left cochlea must be more sensitive than the right one. This means the right ear's real bone-conduction threshold would be 50 dB. If so, then the right ear is *still* sensorineural (because the air-conduction threshold is 50 dB HL). Thus, there is no reason to mask the opposite (left) ear in this case because the clinical outcome for the right ear is the same regardless of which cochlea really heard the tone.

The situation is different for the *left* ear, which has an air-conduction threshold of 70 dB. If we assume that the 45 dB bone-conduction threshold is from the *left* ear, then its ABG would be 70 – 45 = 25 dB. It would then be necessary to retest the left ear's bone-conduction threshold with masking in the opposite (right) because an ABG of 25 dB meets our > 10 dB masking criterion. Consider some of the alternatives: Suppose we put the appropriate masking into the opposite (right) ear and find that the left ear's bone-conduction threshold really is 45 dB. This would mean that there really is a 25 dB ABG in the left ear, indicating the presence of a conductive component. In fact, with masking in the right ear, we might find that the real bone-conduction threshold of the left ear is anywhere between 45 and 70 dB. This would mean that the left ABG could be anywhere from 25

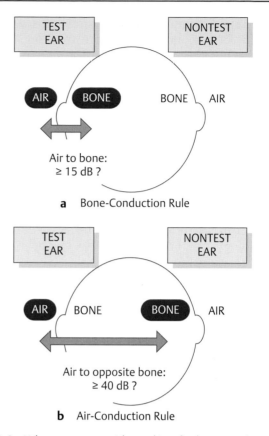

Fig. 9.6 When to retest with masking for bone- and air-conduction when using standard audiometric (supra-aural) earphones. **(a)** The bone-conduction masking rule asks whether the air-bone-gap is ≥ 15 dB (i.e., > l0 dB) within the test ear. **(b)** The air-conduction masking rule asks whether there is a difference of ≥ 40 dB between the air-conduction threshold on the test side and the bone-conduction thresholds on the nontest side.

dB (a mixed loss) down to 0 dB (a sensorineural loss). Here, we *do* need to know which cochlea is really hearing the bone-conduction signal.

When to Mask for Air-Conduction

Recall that we must use masking whenever cross-hearing might occur. Cross-hearing for an air-conduction signal occurs via the bone-conduction route, and depends on three parameters: (1) the sound level in dB HL presented to the TE; (2) the amount of IA in dB, which determines how much of the signal crosses over; and (3) the *true bone-conduction threshold* in dB HL of the NTE, which determines whether this signal is audible in the NTE.

Consequently, one must mask for air-conduction whenever the sound (in dB HL) being presented to the TE is able to reach the bone-conduction threshold (in dB HL) of the NTE. Because we need to know the NTE's real bone-conduction thresholds, we must mask for bone-conduction before masking for air-conduction. This also means that the unmasked air- and bone-conduction thresholds should be obtained before any masking is accomplished.

The rule for when to mask for air-conduction is shown in **Fig. 9.6b** and may be stated in several ways. Using the minimum IA value of 40 dB as our criterion, *masking for AC is needed whenever the test ear's air-conduction threshold (AC_T) and the nontest ear's bone-conduction threshold (BC_N) differ by 40 dB or more.* Some audiologists call the spread between AC_T and BC_N an **air-opposite-bone-gap (AOBG)** or an **air-contralateral-bone-gap (ACBG)**. Using this terminology, masking is necessary whenever the following relationship applies:

$$AOBG \geq 40 \text{ dB}.$$

For the mathematically minded, it is necessary to retest an air-conduction threshold with masking whenever:

$$\left(AC_T - BC_N\right) \geq 40 \text{ dB}$$

Of course, this comparison is done individually for each test frequency (usually between 250 and 4000 Hz), and one compares the two ears at the same frequency. (One should remember that the 40 dB figure being used here and elsewhere assumes that standard, supra-aural audiometric earphones are being used. It should be replaced with the appropriate minimum IA value (**Fig. 9.5**) when testing with insert earphones.)

The rule just described is really simpler than it might seem. Suppose the *right air-conduction* threshold is 50 dB HL and the *left bone-conduction* threshold is 5 dB HL (at the same frequency, of course). Are they at least 40 dB apart? The answer is yes (50 – 5 = 45, and 45 dB is certainly ≥ 40 dB). Therefore, the right air-conduction threshold must be retested with masking noise in the left ear. In a second example, the *right air-conduction* threshold is 50 dB HL and the *left bone-conduction* threshold is 15 dB HL. Are they at least 40 dB apart? The answer is no (50 – 15 = 35, and 35 dB is less than the 40 dB criterion). Therefore, the right ear's air-conduction threshold does *not* need to be retested with masking noise in the left ear. In other words, the right ear's original air-conduction threshold of 50 dB HL is considered to be its true threshold. Consider one more example, in which the right ear's air-conduction threshold is 75 dB HL and the left ear's bone-conduction threshold is 35 dB HL. The right ear needs to be retested with masking because the AOBG is 40 dB, which meets the ≥ 40 dB

criterion. It must be emphasized that the comparison made in the air-conduction masking decision is always between *air-conduction* on the *test* side and *bone-conduction* on the *nontest* side, because this is the crossover route. It cannot validly be based on a comparison between the air-conduction thresholds of the two ears. A logical exception occurs when the air-conduction threshold of the NTE is better than its bone-conduction threshold at the same frequency— for example, when the air-conduction threshold is 10 dB HL and the bone-conduction threshold is 20 dB HL. Here, one uses the *better* air-conduction threshold (10 dB HL in this example).

Central Masking

As a scientific phenomenon, masking means a threshold shift for a signal that occurs when the noise and signal are presented to the *same* ear. Very technically, this is called "direct, ipsilateral masking," and it occurs because the noise and signal are present within the same cochlea. In *clinical* masking we are trying to cause direct, ipsilateral masking of the *nontest* ear so that we can be sure that only the test ear is actually hearing the test signal.

Central masking can occur when the signal and noise are presented to different ears. Suppose that the right ear gets the tone and the left ear gets the noise. Let us also assume that we know for a fact that there is no crossover for either the signal or the noise. (We know this because both the tone and the noise levels being used are well below interaural attenuation.) Clearly, direct ipsilateral masking cannot occur because the signal is in one cochlea and the noise is in the other cochlea. We find that the right ear's threshold is consistently shifted (from, say, 5 dB HL to 10 dB HL) whenever there is noise in the left ear. The reason a noise in one ear can cause a threshold shift (masking) in the other ear is as follows. Even though the peripheral ears are physically separate, the neural signals that come from the two cochleae are combined in the central auditory nervous system (CANS). The noise in one ear can interfere with the ability to hear a tone in the other ear because they interact in the CANS.

Although central masking is a real phenomenon, it is not the effect of interest during clinical masking. In fact, central masking actually complicates matters in clinical masking. For this reason, the amount of central masking that occurs is of some importance when clinical masking is being done. Clinicians generally consider the central masking effect to be ~ 5 dB; however, threshold shifts as large as 15 dB have been reported (Liden, Nilsson, & Anderson 1959b), and the effect increases with the magnitude of the masking noise (Studebaker 1962; Dirks 1964; Dirks & Malmquist 1964). More information about the nature and parameters of central masking may be found in Gelfand (2010). We will follow the conservative practice of allowing for 5 dB of central masking during clinical masking procedures.

Effective Masking Calibration

If the audiometer is set up to produce a 1000 Hz pure tone, then an attenuator dial reading of 50 means that a 1000 Hz tone will be presented to the patient at 50 dB HL. If the patient can hear this, then we know her 1000 Hz tonal threshold is 50 dB HL or less. If we change the input selector from "tone" to "NBN," then many audiometers will produce a 1000 Hz NBN at 50 dB HL. This means a narrow band of noise is centered around 1000 Hz, which has an overall level equal to that of a 1000 Hz tone at 50 dB HL. If the patient can hear this, then we know her 1000 Hz NBN threshold is 50 dB HL or less.

However, what if we want to use the noise to mask a 50 dB HL 1000 Hz tone? To meet this goal, the level of a NBN noise would have to be increased. The ANSI audiometer standard (ANSI S3.6-2010) provides corrections to be built in to the audiometer's masking channel, so that the masking level dial is calibrated in **decibels of effective masking (dB EM)**. These corrections are shown in **Table 9.2**. However, it is up to the clinician to verify that these dial readings actually provide effective masking on her own equipment, and if necessary to determine the proper masking noise settings. Specifically, she must determine the difference in decibels between the level of a given tone and the level of the noise that just masks that tone. This difference is often called the **effective masking level (EML)**, but is more readily understood if it is called the **minimum effective masking correction (MEMC)** because it is the correction that must be added to the tone's level to arrive at a *minimum noise level* that will *effectively mask* that tone. For example, suppose it takes 55 dB HL of NBN to just mask a 50 dB HL tone. This means that to mask a tone, the noise has to be 5 dB higher than the tone; that is, the MEMC in this case is 55 dB – 50 dB = 5 dB.

The clinician arrives at a set of MEMCs for each audiometer by performing a simple biological (psychoacoustic) calibration study using normal-hearing subjects. There are various approaches, but the one about to be outlined is probably the simplest. The audiometer must have two channels. One channel will produce the tone, and the second channel will produce the masking noise. The output selector is set up so that both channels are directed into the same earphone, that is, both the tone and the noise are directed into the same ear because we want to find out how much noise is needed to mask the tone. Most audiometers automatically set the tone and the NBN to the same frequency. If the audiometer has separate frequency controls for the two channels, then they should both be set to the same frequency (after all, we do not want to use a 4000 Hz NBN to mask a 1000 Hz tone).

We will go through the basic sequence at 1000 Hz. The noise attenuator is turned to a comfortable level, such as 40 dB HL, and the noise is set to the constantly on position. We now have a continuous 1000 Hz narrow-band noise at 40 dB HL. Next, we find the tone's threshold against the background of the continuously on noise. Many clinicians use a pulsing tone for this purpose because it makes the listening task somewhat easier. Having found the threshold for the tone (where it is *just audible* over the noise), the tone is then decreased in 5 dB steps until it is just *inaudible*. This is where the tone is *just masked* by the noise. Suppose we find that the tone's level is 35 dB HL at this point. We can now say that a 1000 Hz NBN at 40 dB will just mask a 35 dB 1000 Hz tone, or that a 35 dB tone is just masked by a 40 dB noise at 1000 Hz. Either way, the noise has to be 5 dB higher than the tone to just mask it in this example.

Table 9.2 Amounts in decibels (dB) to be added to the reference equivalent threshold sound pressure level (RETSPL) to achieve effective masking (dB EM) for one-third and one-half octave-band masking noises[a]

	Frequency (Hz)										
	125	250	500	750	1000	1500	2000	3000	4000	6000	8000
For one-third octave-band noise	4	4	4	5	6	6	6	6	5	5	5
For one-half octave-band noise	4	4	6	7	7	8	8	7	7	7	6

[a]Based on ANSI S3.6-2010.

This strategy is repeated several times to arrive at an average value, which represents that subject's MEMC at 1000 Hz. The procedure is then repeated at the remaining frequencies.

After testing at least 10 subjects, the clinician calculates a mean MEMC at each frequency. For example, the average correction at 500 Hz might be 8.5 dB, rounded to an MEMC of 10 dB; the mean at 1000 Hz MEMC might be 4.6 dB, rounded to 5 dB, etc. These MEMC values are then employed during clinical masking. For purposes of illustration, we will always assume that the MEMC is 5 dB.

This type of procedure can also be used to arrive at minimal effective masking levels on an individual patient basis (Veniar 1965). Veniar's method involves presenting the tone at a constant level and increasing the noise (in the same earphone) until the patient no longer hears the tone. The student should also be aware that physical masking noise calibration methods based on electroacoustic measurements and/or calculations are also available (e.g., Sanders 1972; Townsend & Schwartz 1976), although most clinicians are probably best served by the psychoacoustic approach.

Some audiometers, such as portable instruments and those mainly intended for screening purposes, do not allow one to direct the tone and noise into the same channel. In this case, a simple mixing circuit must be built to properly combine the noise and tone in the same earphone (see Studebaker 1967, p. 362). Fortunately, this is rarely necessary in modern practice.

The Initial Masking Level

Once we have decided to retest the TE with masking noise in the NTE, we must decide how much masking noise to use. The recommended approach is the initial masking level method described by Martin (1967, 1974, 1980). Other formulas have also been proposed (Liden, Nilsson, & Anderson 1959b; Studebaker 1964). However, they are more complex and have been shown to yield similar masking levels to the recommended approach (Martin 1974). Obviously, we must start with enough noise to render the test tone inaudible in the NTE. It is important to remember at this juncture that we already have an unmasked threshold; we are just not sure about which ear is hearing it. If the threshold is really coming from the NTE, then we must start with enough noise to mask the NTE at threshold.

Initial Masking Level for Air-Conduction

We will assume that we have previously determined the average minimum effective masking correction for our audiometer to be 5 dB higher than the hearing level of the test tone at every frequency. In other words, the masking noise level must be 5 dB higher than the tone level. For example, the noise level would have to be set to 15 dB HL to mask a 10 dB HL tone, or 60 dB HL to mask a 55 dB HL tone. We must also add a 10 dB **safety factor** because the MEMC is an *average*. Adding a 10 dB safety factor means that our starting masking level will have an attenuator (dB HL) dial reading that is 15 dB higher than the unmasked threshold in the NTE. For example, if the NTE's air-conduction threshold is 20 dB HL, then the initial masking level will be:

	20 dB HL	(AC threshold of the tone we want to mask)
+	5 dB	(MEM correction)
=	25 dB HL	(Average MEM level for a 20 dB HL tone)
+	10 dB	(Safety factor)
=	35 dB HL	(Initial Masking Level)

In other words, if the air-conduction threshold of the NTE is 20 dB HL, we will use 35 dB HL of masking noise as the starting masking level. This value is the **initial masking level (IML)**. For the mathematically oriented, the initial masking level (in dB HL) directed into the NTE may be reduced to the formula

$$IML = HL_N + MEMC + SF$$

where HL_N is the air-conduction threshold hearing level of the NTE, MEMC is the minimum effective masking correction, and SF is the safety factor.

Initial Masking Level for Bone-Conduction and the Occlusion Effect

The IML for bone-conduction testing is similar to the one used for air-conduction with the important addition of a factor to account for the **occlusion effect (OE)**. This is done because the earphone covering the NTE can introduce an occlusion effect, which is an increase in the level of a bone-conduction signal due to occluding the ear canal.

A simple example will show how the OE affects a masked bone-conduction threshold. Suppose an unmasked bone-conduction threshold is 35 dB HL, and the test ear needs to be retested with masking. (To keep things simple, the NTE has a 35 dB HL sensorineural loss.) The 35 dB HL bone-conduction threshold was obtained without any earphones covering the ear canals, and is thus an *unoccluded* bone-conduction threshold. Here the NTE receives the tone at 35 dB HL (at the cochlea). When we retest this bone-conduction with masking, the NTE is covered with the earphone used to deliver the masking noise. In so doing, we change the bone-conduction test from *unoccluded* to *occluded*, which may cause an occlusion effect to occur. Let us assume that the OE is 15 dB. This means that a 35 dB HL bone-conduction signal from the audiometer will be boosted by 15 dB to 50 dB HL at the cochlea of the NTE. Consider what this means from the standpoint of the IML. If we use the above IML formula intended for air-conduction testing, we would be unsuccessfully trying to mask what is really a 50 dB HL signal with a noise that can only mask a tone as high as 35 dB HL. In other words, since occluding the NTE effectively boosted the tone level by 15 dB, we would also need to increase the amount of masking noise by 15 dB in order to account for the occlusion effect, as follows:

	35 dB HL	(AC threshold of the tone we want to mask)
+	5 dB	(MEM correction)
=	40 dB HL	(Average MEM level for a 35 dB HL tone)
+	10 dB	(Safety factor)
=	50 dB HL	(IML, unoccluded)
+	15 dB	(Correction for the OE)
=	65 dB HL	(Initial masking level accounting for the OE)

The initial masking level formula for bone-conduction testing accounts for the OE, and may be written as

$$IML = HL_N + MEMC + SF + OE$$

Determining the Occlusion Effect

We need to know the size of the OE to determine the IML. One approach is to use fixed OE values (e.g., Studebaker 1979; Goldstein & Newman 1985;

Yacullo 2009), such as the ones shown in **Table 9.3**. The alternative approach, which is recommended here, is that clinicians should determine the presence and magnitude of the OE on an individual patient basis. The reason is that we cannot assume any predetermined value because the occlusion effect (1) differs with frequency, (2) is highly variable among people, and (3) is absent when there is a conductive pathology. Consequently, we must first perform an easy but important test to determine the presence and size of the OE before determining IMLs for bone-conduction.

The recommended procedure employs the **audiometric Bing test** (Martin, Butler, & Burns 1974), and is as follows: Having already obtained the unmasked bone-conduction thresholds, the audiologist places the earphone over the NTE and retests the bone-conduction *without any noise*. An OE is considered to be present if the occluded threshold is better (lower) than the unoccluded one; the size of the OE is simply the difference between them. In the case of the above example, the unoccluded bone-conduction threshold would be 35 dB and the occluded bone-conduction threshold would be 20 dB HL, revealing that the OE is 35 – 20 = 15 dB. The resulting OE value is then used in the calculation of the IML. The bone-conduction IML formula is the same as the air-conduction formula when the OE is zero. This is done for each frequency up to and including 1000 Hz, which is the region where OEs are expected to occur.

This procedure works because the OE increases the level of signal reaching the cochlea, so the dial reading of the threshold is lowered by the amount of the OE (which was 15 dB in our example).

There are at least two supplemental benefits of the audiometric Bing test. First, it provides supportive diagnostic information because the OE tends to be present in ears that are normal or have sensorineural impairments, and tends to be absent in ears with conductive or mixed losses. Second, the

Table 9.3 Occlusion effect values recommended by Yacullo (2009) for use when calculating initial masking levels for bone-conduction testing

	Apparent status of the nontest ear		Air-bone-gap ≤ 20 dB
	No conductive component		
Frequency	TDH-39/49/50 supra-aural earphones	EARTone 3A insert earphones	
250 Hz	30 dB	10 dB	0 dB
500 Hz	20 dB	10 dB	
1000 Hz	10 dB	0 dB	

clinician can be alerted to the inadvertent displacement of the bone-conduction vibration by occluded thresholds that are poorer (higher) than the unoccluded thresholds.

Using the Initial Masking Level

Once we have determined that masking is necessary, the first step is to retest the threshold in question while masking noise is being presented to the NTE at the IML.

After instructing the patient and setting up the equipment for masked testing (see below), the masking noise is turned on. With the IML in the NTE, we now retest the threshold for the TE. As previously mentioned, we will allow for 5 dB of central masking during clinical masking procedures. If the patient responds within 5 dB of the same level obtained previously without masking, then we consider the original threshold to be confirmed as being derived from the test ear. This is so because the patient can still hear the tone even though the NTE is being masked; if the NTE is not hearing the tone, then it must have been heard in the TE. For example, suppose that the right ear's unmasked threshold was 40 dB HL. This threshold is considered to be true if it stays at 40 dB HL (or shifts only 5 dB to 45 dB HL) with the initial masking level in the left (nontest) ear. The 40 dB HL is now called a masked threshold, and the masking procedure is finished for this tone.

The alternative outcome is that the IML causes the threshold to shift by more than 5 dB from its original, unmasked value. For example, the right ear's unmasked threshold of 40 dB HL might shift to 50 dB HL with the IML in the left ear. In this case, even though the tone was directed into the right ear, the original (unmasked) threshold must have come from the left (nontest) ear. Why? Because if the tone was really heard in the right ear, then putting noise into the left would not have changed anything—it would still be heard in the right ear. If appropriate masking noise in the left ear stops the patient from hearing a tone from the right earphone, then the original threshold must have been originally picked up in the left ear via cross-hearing. Under these circumstances we must now move to the next phase of the masking procedure, which involves finding the actual threshold of the test ear using the **threshold shift** or **plateau method**.

We may summarize the use of the initial masking level as follows: (1) The original threshold is confirmed if it stays the same (within 5 dB) at the initial masking level. (2) An unmasked threshold was probably heard in the non-test ear if the initial masking level causes it to shift more than 5 dB.

The Plateau Method

The plateau method is a widely accepted strategy for finding the true masked threshold of the TE and was described by Hood (1960). (A more efficient approach that can be used if the unmasked air-conduction thresholds differ by ≥ 25 dB between the ears is described later in the chapter.) Sometimes called the threshold shift method, the logic of the plateau strategy can be understood in terms of **Fig. 9.7**, which shows the results of a hypothetical test. The ordinate represents the threshold of the tone in the test ear when it is presented alone (unmasked) and when various levels of masking noise are being presented to the NTE. The abscissa shows the level of the masking noise in the NTE, as well as the unmasked (unm) situation. In this example, the apparent threshold of the test tone is 50 dB HL, indicated by the symbol for the unmasked (unm) situation. This is not the actual threshold of the TE because the lowest masking level used (20 dB) caused it to shift to 60 dB HL. Notice that the rest of the graph breaks down into three distinct ranges, labeled *undermasking, plateau,* and *overmasking.*

Undermasking

When a tone is really being heard by the nontest ear via cross-hearing, then raising the level of the masking noise will cause the masked threshold to increase. This occurs because the noise and tone are both in the same (nontest) ear. For example, **Fig. 9.7** shows that raising the masking noise from 20 to 35 dB HL caused the apparent tonal threshold to rise from 60 to 75 dB HL. The one-for-one elevation occurs because masking increases linearly with masker level, as we learned in Chapter 3. This linear increase of apparent threshold with masking noise

Fig. 9.7 The masking plateau (see text). Abbreviation: unm, unmasked. In this example, the unmasked threshold of the test tone is 50 dB HL, and its masked threshold is 75 dB HL.

level indicates that the tone is still being picked up by the NTE. We call this undermasking because the amount of noise is not sufficient to exclude the NTE from the test. Thus, undermasking occurs when there is not enough masking noise, so that the tone is being heard by the nontest ear, as in **Fig. 9.8a**.

The Plateau

The plateau occurs when the NTE is effectively masked by the noise so that the tone is heard by the test ear. Here the tone is picked up only by the test ear and the noise is picked up only by the nontest ear. When the tone is really being heard in the test ear, then raising the masking noise level will not cause the threshold to change. This is seen in the middle part of **Fig. 9.7** and conceptually in **Fig. 9.8b**, where the threshold for the tone stays the same at 75 dB HL even though the masking noise is raised from 35 to 65 dB. This plateau reveals the test ear's true masked threshold for the tone. The width of the plateau is sometimes called the range of **effective masking**.

The plateau occurs because the noise is effectively masking the nontest ear so that the test ear can hear the tone. Raising the noise in the NTE continues to keep it effectively masked; thus the test ear remains free to respond to the tone at its own threshold. A visual analogy will make this clearer. Let us say that you can read the 20-20 vision line of an eye chart with both eyes. However, you can only read down to the 20-30 line if you cover (mask) your right eye with a small piece of paper. The left eye must have 20-30 vision because your right eye is covered. Now, what would happen if you were to cover the right eye with a larger piece of paper, then a bigger piece, and then an even larger one? You would find that the size of the paper would not make a difference as long as it covers just the right eye. The size of the paper used to mask the nontest eye is analogous to the level of the noise used to mask the nontest ear: once the noise is effectively masking the nontest ear, you can add more noise without affecting the threshold because the amount of noise "covering" the NTE has nothing to do with the TE—at least within limits.

Overmasking

Overmasking occurs when so much noise is presented to the NTE that it crosses over and masks the test ear. Let us return to the vision example. If you keep increasing the size of the paper covering the right eye, it will eventually get big enough to cover the left eye as well, and this will have an obvious outcome. This is analogous to what would happen if we continue increasing the level of the masking noise.

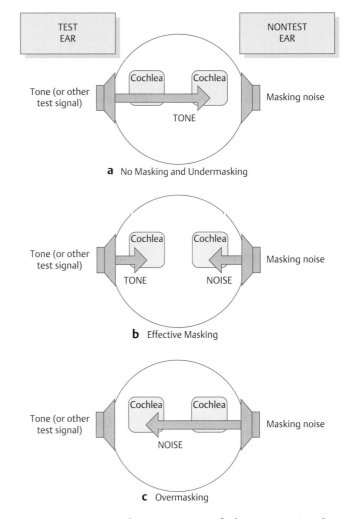

Fig. 9.8 Conceptual representation of what is occurring during **(a)** undermasking, **(b)** effective masking along the plateau, and **(c)** overmasking. No arrow is shown for the noise in **a** because it is not preventing the NTE from hearing the tone (the same picture also describes cross-hearing without masking). No arrow is shown for the tone in **c** because the noise is preventing the TE from hearing it.

Eventually, the noise will become sufficiently intense to cross over to the test ear. Once this occurs, the threshold for the tone will start to rise again as the masking level is increased. This range on the plateau graph is aptly called **overmasking**, and is illustrated by the diagonal line on the right side of **Fig. 9.7** and also in **Fig. 9.8c**. Overmasking will be covered further in a subsequent section.

Plateau Width

Masking plateaus become narrow when there is a conductive loss in the nontest (masked) ear: the wider the air-bone-gap, the smaller the plateau. The situation becomes exacerbated when both ears have air-bone-gaps, as will be described below.

The width of the plateau is important for at least two reasons. First, the wider the plateau the more confidence you can have in the validity of the masked threshold. Audiologists typically require a plateau to be at least 15 to 20 dB wide before accepting a masked threshold as valid. Second, a very narrow plateau can be missed altogether during testing, in which case a masked threshold cannot be obtained. In fact, sometimes there is no plateau between the undermasking and overmasking ranges so that a usable masked threshold cannot be obtained. One must then indicate that obtaining a masked threshold was at least attempted, often with a phrase such as "no plateau" or "could not mask."

Factors that increase the likelihood of overmasking have the effect of making the masking plateau narrower. Everything else being equal, the plateau becomes smaller as (1) interaural attenuation values get smaller, (2) the test ear's bone-conduction threshold gets lower, (3) the masked ear's air-conduction threshold gets higher, and (4) the occlusion effect gets larger (when masking for bone-conduction). The first two factors increase the chances that a given amount of masking noise will reach and cause masking in the test ear's cochlea. The second pair makes it necessary for a higher masking noise level to be used.

Overmasking and the Maximum Masking Level

Overmasking occurs when too much noise is presented to the NTE, so that the noise crosses the head and actually masks the tone in the TE. This is represented by the large arrow in **Fig. 9.9**. In other words, the noise that was intended to prevent cross-hearing in the NTE is also stopping the test ear from hearing the signal. Since the patient can no longer hear the tone, the clinician will increase the tone level until the patient can hear it over the noise. The resulting threshold shift (represented by the small arrow in **Fig. 9.9**) is a false estimate of the threshold. Thus, a valid measurement cannot be obtained starting with the lowest noise level that causes overmasking, and for all higher noise levels. Clearly, the clinician must be constantly alert to the possibility of overmasking whenever masking is used.

Overmasking depends on the same cross-hearing effect that occurs when a tone is received by the NTE, except in the opposite direction. Because crossover occurs via the bone-conduction route, we must now think about how many decibels of the noise being delivered to the nontest ear reach the cochlea of the

test ear. This means that the noise level being presented to the NTE exceeds IA by an amount that reaches the bone-conduction threshold of the TE. For this reason it has been proposed (Martin 1991) that overmasking occurs when the level of the noise in the nontest ear (MN_N) is equal to or more than IA plus the bone-conduction threshold of the test ear (BC_T), or when

$$MN_N \geq \left(IA + BC_T \right)$$

For example, suppose that we present masking noise to the NTE of a patient whose TE has a bone-conduction threshold of 30 dB HL at 2000 Hz, and that her IA at this frequency is 50 dB. When will overmasking occur? To answer this important clinical question, we simply substitute these values into the formula:

$$MN_N \geq \left(IA + BC_T \right)$$

$$MN_N \geq \left(50 \text{ dB} + 30 \text{ dB HL} \right)$$

$$MN_N \geq 80 \text{ dB HL}$$

In other words, overmasking should occur in this case when the masking noise is 80 dB HL or more.

This commonly employed rule is actually too strict when the masking noise level just equals IA + BC_T. At this level what actually occurs is cross-hearing of the noise by the TE. The noise is at threshold

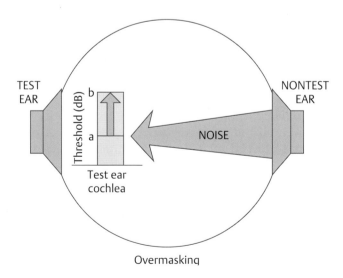

Fig. 9.9 Overmasking occurs when the masking noise (large arrow) crosses to and masks the test ear. This causes a threshold shift in the test ear (small arrow), causing a false elevation of its threshold (from **a** to **b**).

(is just audible) in the TE, but this does not mean it can also cause masking in the TE. In terms of the example, the 80 dB HL noise presented to the NTE arrives at the TE's cochlea at 30 dB HL, which is the bone-conduction threshold. Hence, the noise is audible in the TE at 30 dB HL. However, it does not mean this 30 dB noise is capable of masking a 30 dB tone in that ear. This should not be surprising. Recall that we calibrated the MEML of our masking noise on a group of normal listeners, and found that the HL of a masking noise has to be an average of 5 dB higher than the HL of the tone it can mask (i.e., on average, it took 45 dB HL of noise to mask a 40 dB HL tone). For this reason, the 30 dB HL noise that reaches the test ear at threshold can be heard, but it will take an additional 5 dB (the minimum effective masking correction, MEMC) to actually mask the TE. For this reason, we can say that over-masking occurs when

$$MN_N \geq \left(IA + BC_T + MEMC\right)$$

Thus, overmasking in our example actually occurs when the noise presented to the NTE reaches 85 dB HL:

$$MN_N \geq \left(IA + BC_T + MEMC\right)$$

$$MN_N \geq \left(50\ dB + 30\ dB\ HL + 5\ dB\right)$$

$$MN_N \geq 85\ dB\ HL$$

Overmasking becomes problematic as early in the masking process as when one is deciding on the initial masking level. Once the IML is determined, the clinician must ask herself whether overmasking is already occurring at this starting level. This problem is particularly noticeable when the air-conduction threshold of the NTE is poorer than that of the TE. Consider the following example, where the thresholds (at some frequency) are:

Right AC:	50 dB HL (masked)
Right BC:	50 dB HL (masked)
Left AC:	25 dB HL (unmasked, masking not needed)
Left BC:	10 dB HL (*unmasked, masking needed*)

(To simplify the illustration, let's ignore any other considerations that might arise, and also assume that the right air- and bone-conduction thresholds have just been obtained with masking in the left ear even though this implies a test order somewhat different from what was suggested earlier.)

The left bone-conduction threshold still needs to be retested with masking. This involves putting the appropriate IML into the right ear, which in this case is:

	50 dB HL	(Threshold of the tone we want to mask)
+	5 dB	(Our MEM correction)
=	55 dB HL	(MEML for 50 dB HL)
+	10 dB	(Safety factor)
=	65 dB HL	(Initial masking level)

Assuming that IA = 40 dB, then the 65 dB starting noise level presented to the right ear will reach the left cochlea at 65 dB HL – 40 dB = 25 dB HL. Logically, overmasking occurs because 25 dB HL of noise in the left cochlea is more than sufficient to cause masking of its 10 dB bone-conduction threshold. This is confirmed with the overmasking formula, which shows that the 65 dB IML exceeds 55 dB, which is the level where overmasking begins in this case:

$$MN_N \geq \left(IA + BC_T + MEMC\right)$$

$$65\ dB \geq \left(40 + 10 + 5\right)$$

$$65\ dB \geq 55\ dB$$

The chances of overmasking become even greater when bone-conduction is being tested with masking. This can occur because covering the NTE with the earphone can result in an occlusion effect, which would increase the level of the bone-conduction signal in the nontest ear. Suppose a 15 dB occlusion effect results when the right ear is covered with the earphone used to deliver the masking noise. If this occurs, then the IML must be increased to overcome the enhanced bone-conduction signal reaching the nontest cochlea at 65 + 15 = 80 dB HL. Under these conditions, overmasking could occur even if IA was as high as 65 dB! This is so because 85 dB ≥ (65 + 10 + 5).

The maximum masking level (MML) is the highest masking noise level that can be used without causing overmasking to occur. Recall that the typical increment for an audiometric signal is 5 dB. It should thus make sense that the MML is simply 5 dB below the lowest noise level that causes overmasking. For example, if we determine that the lowest level for overmasking is 80 dB HL, then the MML is simply 80 – 5 = 75 dB HL.

For the math-minded, overmasking occurs whenever

$$MN_N \geq \left(IA + BC_T + MEMC\right)$$

Thus, the lowest level at which overmasking occurs is

$$MN_N = \left(IA + BC_T + MEMC\right)$$

Maximum masking occurs one attenuator step (5 dB) below this minimum overmasking value, or when

$$MN_N = \left(IA + BC_T + MEMC\right) - 5$$

It is important to note that while one must always be on the alert for overmasking, one should not be too quick to write "could not mask" or "masking dilemma" on the audiogram without bothering to at least try to obtain a masked threshold. If the previously unmasked threshold is not shifted with the IML, then it has been confirmed as a masked threshold. If the unmasked threshold is shifted by the IML, then one should try to obtain a plateau beginning with lower masking levels. (This is actually what was called for in Hood's original description of the plateau.) At least sometimes an acceptable plateau (and therefore a masked threshold) is obtained. Of course, one's suspicions about overmasking will have been confirmed if no plateau is obtained. In that case, one can indicate "no plateau" on the audiogram, and know that this comment is *empirically* based.

The Masking Dilemma

A special case in which overmasking occurs at the initial masking level is aptly called the **masking dilemma** (Naunton 1960). This problem occurs when the unmasked audiogram reveals large air-bone-gaps in both ears. **Fig. 9.10** shows a typical example of the masking dilemma in which the ABGs are ~ 55 dB wide. This situation is a dilemma because we must retest both ears with masking even though overmasking would occur at the initial masking levels. For example, the IML of a noise needed to mask the right ear at 1000 Hz would be 55 + 5 + 10 = 70 dB HL, but the unmasked bone-conduction threshold is 0 dB HL. Overmasking occurs because presenting the IML to the right ear would cause masking at the left cochlea, which would shift the left ear's air- and bone-conduction thresholds. In such a case, we do not really know whether the left ear's threshold shifted because of (1) effective masking or (2) overmasking.

Optimized Masking Method for Asymmetrical Audiograms

Turner (2004a,b) described an **optimized masking method** that can be used when testing the *poorer* ear (with masking noise in the better ear) *if* the unmasked air-conduction thresholds at the test frequency *differ by ≥ 25 dB* between the ears. This approach is

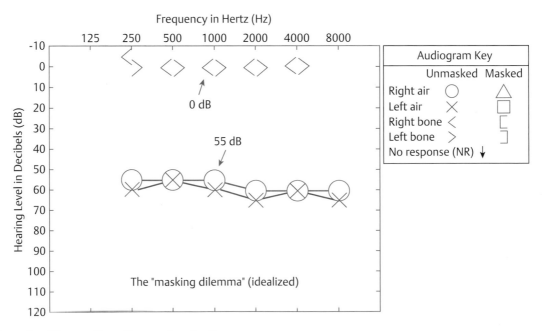

Fig. 9.10 Example of the masking dilemma (see text).

more efficient than the traditional plateau method because it identifies the threshold of the test ear in fewer steps. Let's examine the optimized method in terms of the example in **Fig. 9.11**, which involves the same example that was used to illustrate the plateau method in **Fig. 9.7**.

As before, the apparent (unmasked) air-conduction threshold is 50 dB HL (point *a* in the figure). The first step is to retest with some initial level of masking noise in the NTE. Unlike the traditional technique, the initial masking level used in the optimized method is set to the air-conduction threshold of the *test* ear minus 10 dB, or

$$IML = HL_T - 10$$

Since the apparent threshold of the test ear is 50 dB in our example, the IML presented to the NTE is 50 – 10 = 40 dB. If the IML does not change the threshold of the test ear (or if it shifts by a small amount attributable to central masking), then the original threshold of 50 dB HL would be confirmed as the true one. However, we find that the IML raised the threshold of the test ear to 75 dB HL (point *b* in the figure). As in the plateau method, the next step is to retest with a higher level of masking noise in the NTE. However, unlike the plateau method, the optimized method increases the masker level by the size of the threshold shift caused by the IML. In our example, the IML caused a 25 dB threshold shift from 50 to 75 dB HL. Thus, the next masking level will be 25 dB above the IML, or 40 + 25 = 65 dB. As shown by point *c* in the figure, the 75 dB HL threshold stayed the same with this masking level, confirming that it is the true masked threshold of the test ear. Notice that the optimized method identified the masking plateau with fewer retests than would have been required by the traditional technique.

If the 65 dB masker had caused the threshold to shift again, then we would have repeated the last step by retesting with the masking level raised by the amount of that threshold shift. For example, if the 65 dB noise caused the threshold to shift by 15 dB to 90 dB HL, then we would have retested with a masking level of 65 + 15 = 80 dB in the NTE. This strategy is repeated until the plateau is identified or maximum levels are reached.

The optimized method is the same for bone-conduction testing except for the initial masking level. When masking for bone-conduction, the IML is set to either (a) the unmasked bone-conduction threshold plus 30 dB (IML = BC + 30) or (b) the level used by the clinician's masking protocol, whichever is higher. This IML accounts for occlusion effects as great as 20 dB (Turner 2004b).

Fig. 9.11 Identifying the masking plateau (true threshold of the test ear) with the optimized masking method (see text).

■ Some Considerations for Bone-Conduction Masking

As already pointed out, masking is completed first for bone-conduction thresholds because these are needed to make air-conduction masking decisions. Unlike masking for AC, where the earphones are worn in the regular way, masking for bone-conduction involves a special arrangement of the bone vibrator and earphones. The transducer setup for masked bone-conduction testing is shown in **Fig. 9.12**. The bone-conduction oscillator is placed on the test ear's mastoid process, and the nontest ear is covered with the earphone being used to deliver the masking noise. The test ear is left *uncovered*, and its earphone is placed on the side of the head between the test ear and eye as shown in the figure. It is very important to make sure that the bone vibrator and NTE earphone are properly placed. This is an important step because the earphone headset can easily interfere with the bone vibrator's headband. It is also important to tell the patient (1) that this peculiar arrangement is being done on purpose; (2) to keep as still as comfortably possible to avoid jostling the equipment on her head; and (3) to let you know immediately if anything slips out of place. This setup is reversed when it is time to test for the other ear's masked bone-conduction thresholds.

The *unmasked* bone-conduction thresholds should be rechecked with the earphone headset in place before testing is done with masking noise. This is done for two purposes. One reason is to determine whether covering the NTE results in an occlusion effect, which constitutes administering the audiometric Bing test (Martin et al 1974). The size of the occlusion effect is noted for each frequency where it occurs (typically up to 1000 Hz) because this value must be added to the IML used for BC, as already described.

Fig. 9.12 Typical arrangement of **(a)** the bone vibrator and **(b)** earphones during masking for bone-conduction.

Another reason for rechecking the unmasked bone-conduction thresholds with the earphone in place is to assure that the bone-conduction vibrator placement has not been compromised by the addition of the headset. This is done by making sure that the bone-conduction thresholds with the earphone headset in place are not worse than they were originally. Here one should use a frequency of at least 1000 Hz, preferably higher. The reason for using a higher frequency is that the occlusion effect can cloud the ability to detect a placement problem at frequencies up to ~ 1000 Hz. For example, suppose we retest at 500 Hz and find that the bone-conduction is unchanged by the addition of the headset. This could mean that the vibrator placement is fine and there is also no occlusion effect; but it can also mean that the bone-conduction threshold is 15 dB poorer because the vibrator moved, but that this was counteracted by a 15 dB occlusion effect. Needless to say, the vibrator and earphone headset should be adjusted and rechecked if a placement problem is found.

Insert Earphones

Insert earphones such as the EARtone 3A and ER-3A receivers are readily available for audiological use. Their use provides two significant advantages over standard supra-aural audiometric earphones as far as masking is concerned. These advantages occur because properly used insert receivers (1) increase interaural attenuation (Zwislocki 1953) and (2) alleviate the occlusion effect.

The interaural attenuation values provided by insert earphones have been reported by several studies (Killion et al 1985; Sklare & Denenberg 1987; Van Campen, Sammeth, & Peek 1990). For example, **Fig. 9.5** shows the IA values obtained for both supra-aural and insert earphones by Sklare and Denenberg (1987). Recall that interaural attenuation is pivotal to the decision about when masking must be used. In fact, the rule to mask for air-conduction when the AOBG is ≥ 40 dB is based on the premise that IA is often as small as 40 dB when using standard supra-aural earphones. Using insert receivers makes the need for air-conduction masking quite rare by increasing the amount of IA to the values shown in that figure, which are, on average, over 70 dB. Moreover, using insert receivers to present the masking noise reduces the amount of noise reaching the test ear, thereby making overmasking less of a problem.

Sensorineural Acuity Level (SAL) Test

An indirect technique for estimating the sensorineural component (i.e., the bone-conduction thresholds) of a hearing loss was originated by Rainville (1955) and modified for more efficient clinical use as the **Sensorineural Acuity Level (SAL)** Test by Jerger and Tillman (1960). The SAL test is no longer used routinely, but it can be helpful when one needs to know about a patient's hearing sensitivity at the cochlea, and standard bone-conduction thresholds are equivocal, such as when there is a masking dilemma.

In the SAL test, each of the patient's air-conduction thresholds is tested twice. The first threshold is measured as always (in quiet), but the second threshold is measured while a masking noise is being presented at its maximum level from a bone vibrator at the forehead (in noise). This noise is thus transmitted by bone-conduction to the cochlea, where it will mask the air-conduction test tone. Raising the level of the air-conduction tone will enable the patient to hear it over the noise. The SAL test involves measuring the size of this threshold shift for a given patient and comparing it to the threshold shifts of normal listeners. The original method used a white noise masker and supra-aural earphones to present the test tones, but the contemporary approaches often use narrow band masking noises and insert earphones (Hall 2005).

Before using the SAL test on patients, we must find out how much masking is produced by the noise being used. This is done by testing a group of normal persons. For example, suppose we find that the bone-conduction noise causes the 1000-Hz air-conduction thresholds of normal people to *shift* from 0 dB HL to 55 dB HL. This is illustrated for the case labeled "normal" in **Fig. 9.13**. Clinically, we would expect the same amount of threshold shift if the patient's hearing is normal *at the cochlea* and less of a threshold shift (or none at all) if there is a hearing loss *at the cochlea.*

Because the cochlea is normal when there is a conductive loss, all of the masking noise from the bone vibrator will be just as effective as it is in a person with normal hearing. Therefore, the bone-conduction noise will cause the threshold for the test tone to *shift* by the same amount (55 dB with our noise) in a conductive loss as it does in normal people. For example, a 50 dB HL threshold would shift by 55 dB to 105 dB HL, as for the case labeled "conductive" in **Fig. 9.13**. On the other hand, the masking noise will cause a smaller amount of threshold shift in cases of sensorineural loss because less (or even none) of the masking noise will be heard by the disordered cochlea. For example, the masking noise in our example would be only slightly audible at the cochlea of somebody with a 50 dB HL sensorineural loss. As shown for the case labeled "sensorineural" in

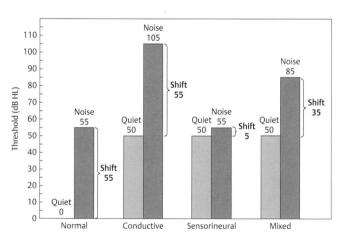

Fig. 9.13 Examples of SAL test outcomes for listeners with normal hearing and those with 50 dB HL conductive, sensorineural, and mixed hearing losses. For each pair, the left bar represents the air-conduction threshold in quiet and the right bar is the air-conduction threshold with masking noise being presented from a bone-conduction vibrator on the forehead.

Fig. 9.13, the original 50 dB HL threshold would shift by only 5 dB to 55 dB HL while the noise is present.

The last case in **Fig. 9.13** shows what might happen in the case of a 50 dB HL mixed hearing loss. Here, the noise shifts the threshold by 35 dB to 85 dB HL. The shift is now smaller than 55 dB because the effectiveness of the bone-conducted noise is *weakened by the sensorineural part* of the mixed loss. Since the bone-conduction noise is 20 dB less effective than what it normally is, then the bone-conduction threshold in this case must be 20 dB HL.

Notice from these examples that the SAL test can be used to find a bone-conduction threshold by subtracting the actual shift caused by the noise from expected shift (55 dB here). For our three cases with 50-dB HL air-conduction thresholds, the SAL test shows that the bone-conduction thresholds are (a) 55 (expected shift) – 55 (actual shift) = 0 dB HL when the loss is conductive, (b) 55 – 5 = 50 dB HL when the loss is sensorineural, and (c) 55 – 35 = 20 dB HL when the loss is mixed.

Masking for Suprathreshold Tonal Tests

The discussion of clinical masking so far has focused on pure tone thresholds. Let us now address masking for tests that use pure tones presented at levels above threshold, for example, tone decay, SISI, etc. (see Chapter 10). It is readily apparent that if masking was required to obtain the threshold for a tone, then it will also be needed for tests performed above threshold. For example, suppose 35 dB of masking noise in the left ear was needed to obtain a 50 dB HL threshold in the right ear. We now want to assess the right ear with the Olsen-Noffsinger tone decay test (TDT), which begins at 20 dB SL (Chapter 10). Clearly, if masking was needed to make sure that only the test ear was receiving a tone at 50 dB HL, then masking will also be needed if that same tone is presented at 70 dB HL. Moreover, the masking noise must be raised to account for the higher level of the tone now being presented to the test ear. In other words, even though the 35 dB HL noise (in the NTE) was fine when 50 dB HL was being presented to the test ear, it will not suffice when the test tone is raised to 70 dB HL. The noise needs to be 20 dB higher because the tone is now 20 dB higher.

Finally, since most special auditory tests are presented at *supra*threshold levels, they will often have to be administered with masking in the NTE even though masking was not needed when the threshold was obtained at the same frequency. This is so because cross-hearing will occur whenever the amount of the test signal that exceeds IA can reach the NTE's bone-conduction threshold. For example, suppose the air-conduction threshold of the right ear (TE) is 40 dB HL and the bone-conduction threshold of the left ear (NTE) is 10 dB HL. The right air-conduction threshold does not have to be retested with masking because the AOBG is 40 – 10 = 30 dB, which is less than the 40 dB AOBG criterion. Now consider what happens with a suprathreshold test such as the Olsen-Noffsinger TDT. This test begins at 20 dB above the 40 dB HL threshold, which means the test tone will be presented to the TE at 60 dB HL. If we properly extend the definition of the "A" ("air") in AOBG to mean the *level at which the test tone is presented* to the TE (instead of just its threshold), then the AOBG in our example becomes 60 – 10 = 50 dB. The 50 dB AOBG exceeds the 40 dB AOBG criterion, indicating that cross-hearing is possible and therefore masking is indicated.

Thus, the rule for when masking is needed for any tonal suprathreshold test is simply a generalization of the already familiar concept, which is to mask whenever the AOBG is ≥ 40 dB *except* that "A" ("air") now means the *presentation level* of the test tone (in dB HL). The 40 dB criterion can be replaced with the individual's actual IA value if it is known (see below). As before, this comparison is made separately at each test frequency where a suprathreshold tonal test is being considered.

Recall that the 40 dB criterion is used as a conservative rule of thumb because we usually do not know an individual's own IA for a given signal. In practice, we sometimes do know this value, especially after the threshold has been established. Here is how: Suppose a patient's thresholds at 1000 Hz are (1) 5 dB HL for both air- and bone-conduction in the right ear, and (2) 60 dB HL in the left ear. This patient's IA cannot be 40 dB because if it were, she would have responded at 45 dB HL in the left ear. Because she did not respond to the tone in the left ear until it reached 60 dB HL, then her actual minimum IA at this frequency must be 60 – 5 = 55 dB. In cases such as this we are able to replace the 40 dB value with the individually determined amount.

The amount of masking noise needed during suprathreshold tonal tests requires some calculations, which must account for several factors: (1) How much of the test signal reaches the nontest cochlea? This involves (a) the presentation level of the signal at the TE, (b) the bone-conduction threshold of the NTE, and (c) interaural attenuation. (2) How much of the masking noise presented to the NTE actually reaches its cochlea? This means that we must account for any air-bone-gap in the nontest ear. (3) Finally, we must remember to account for the effective masking ability of the noise, which involves the MEMC and the safety factor. Thus, the amount of noise that must be presented to the NTE when masking for a suprathreshold tonal test is determined as follows:

	Presentation level at the TE in dB HL (P_T)
–	Interaural attenuation (IA, 40 dB if unknown)
=	Level crossing over to NTE cochlea
+	Air-bone-gap of the NTE (ABG_N)
+	Minimum effective masking correction (MEMC)
+	10 dB safety factor (SF)
=	Masking noise level in NTE IN dB HL (MNN)

This calculation can also be written as a formula:

$$MNN = P_T - IA + ABG_N + MEMC + SF$$

Just because one is able to calculate the correct masking level does not mean that it can be used blindly. One must first estimate whether overmasking is possible or likely, as described earlier. This is especially important when using masking with suprathreshold tests, which require the use of higher noise levels than those used for threshold measures.

A peculiar problem is encountered when masking is used during sweep-frequency Bekesy audiometry (see Chapter 10) because the frequency keeps changing over the course of the test instead of staying the same. For this reason, some audiometers that support Bekesy audiometry provide NBN maskers that change in frequency in synchrony with the changing test frequency, and some clinicians use broadband noise maskers. The problem does not stop here. Optimum masking noise levels (however one goes about determining what they should be) must also change "on the fly" as the test sweeps across the audiogram because the amount of hearing loss is rarely the same at every frequency. In fact, the author has never come across a truly adequate masking approach for sweep frequency Bekesy audiometry.

Effects of Masking on Test Results

The fact that central masking has already been considered highlights the fact that the noise in the NTE can have an impact on the test results. Even the beginning student should be aware of some of the effects that a contralateral masking noise can have on test outcomes, if only generally.

The presence of masking in the NTE can result in tone decay among subjects without threshold adaptation in the absence of the noise (Shimizu 1969; Priede & Coles 1975), and affects the results of the short increment sensitivity index (SISI) (Blegvad & Terkildsen 1967; Blegvad 1969; Shimizu 1969;

Swisher, Dudley, & Doehring 1969). Even though effects vary widely among the subjects in these studies, SISI scores were typically higher with noise in the NTE compared with the scores obtained without masking. In fact, it was not uncommon for masking noise to cause SISI scores to change from one diagnostic category to another (e.g., a negative score might become questionable or positive).

Several studies have also revealed that the outcome of Bekesy audiometry is affected by masking in the NTE (Dirks & Norris 1966; Blegvad 1967, 1968; Grimes & Feldman 1969). Compared with unmasked results, the presence of masking noise in the NTE caused thresholds to become poorer (more so for continuous than for pulsed tracings), narrowing of excursion widths, and widening of the separation between the pulsed and continuous tracings. In light of these specific effects, it is not surprising that masking caused the diagnostic classifications of Bekesy audiograms to change from Type I to Type II or IV, and from Type II to Type IV.

■ Masking for Speech Audiometry

The basic concepts already learned about masking for tonal tests can be applied to masking for speech audiometry (Chapter 8) with a few modifications.

Effective Masking Calibration for Speech

Minimum effective masking corrections can be determined for speech materials in a similar way to that described earlier for tones. Briefly, the masking noise and speech material are directed into the same earphone, with the noise turned on at a reasonably comfortable level (such as 40 dB HL or 50 dB HL) throughout the procedure. Beginning at a higher level than the noise, the subject is presented with a predetermined number of test words (e.g., six or eight), which are to be repeated. This procedure is continued in decreasing steps of 5 dB until a speech level is found where all of the words are missed by the listener. The difference between this speech level and that of the noise is the MEMC for that listener. The procedure is repeated using at least 10 normal-hearing subjects, and the clinician then calculates an average. As we have already done for NBN masking, this average value is then used as the MEMC along with a safety factor for clinical masking.

The procedure just described actually applies to the kind of noise and speech materials used—for example, speech noise and spondee words. Additional MEMC values can be arrived at in the same way for other materials and/or masking noises—for example, monosyllabic words, white noise, etc.

When to Mask During Speech Audiometry

We already know that the "when to mask" question involves three factors. The first factor is the level of the signal being presented to the TE. In speech audiometry this will typically be spondee words when obtaining the speech reception threshold (SRT) and monosyllabic words for speech recognition testing. Interaural attenuation is the second factor. Individual IA values for speech using standard audiometric earphones range from 48 to 68 dB across studies (Liden 1954; Liden, Nilsson, & Anderson 1959a; Snyder 1973; Smith & Markides 1981; Sklare & Denenberg 1987). The 48 dB minimum supports the use of 45 dB as the IA criterion for deciding when to mask for speech (assuming 5 dB test steps), as suggested by Konkle and Berry (1983) and Goldstein and Newman (1985). However, the author prefers using the more conservative value of 40 dB, at least under typical conditions. This concurs with others (e.g., Martin 1991). Using insert receivers increases IA for speech up to the 68 to 84 dB range (Sklare & Denenberg 1987).

The third factor to be considered is the bone-conduction threshold of the NTE. However, bone-conduction thresholds are rarely obtained for speech. It is therefore necessary to use one or more of the *pure tone* bone-conduction thresholds of the NTE. ASHA (1988) guidelines suggest considering the frequencies between 500 and 4000 Hz with the most sensitive (lowest or best) bone-conduction threshold being used for this purpose. However, the author's experience suggests that 250 Hz might also be considered, especially when thresholds are decidedly better at low frequencies compared with higher ones.

Thus, masking should be employed during speech audiometry when the speech level in the test ear (S_T) minus interaural attenuation equals or exceeds the "best" pure tone bone-conduction threshold of the NTE (BC_N). For those who like formulas, masking for speech audiometry is indicated when

$$S_T - IA \geq BC_N$$

Here, IA may be 40 or 45 dB, although 40 dB provides a more conservative margin of safety.

Masking for the Speech Reception Threshold

The masking procedure for SRT testing is analogous to the one used for pure tone thresholds. To begin with, the initial masking level is equal to the SRT of the nontest ear plus the MEMC and a safety factor, or

$$IML_{SRT} = SRT_N + MEMC + SF$$

The original SRT is considered to be confirmed if the SRT stays the same with the IML in the NTE, or if it shifts by only 5 dB, attributable to central masking (Martin, Bailey, & Pappas 1965; Martin 1966; Frank & Karlovich 1975). If the IML causes the SRT to shift by ≥ 10 dB, then the SRT must be found using the plateau (threshold shift) method. The masking strategy is the same as that described for tonal testing, except one uses the test technique appropriate for obtaining an SRT rather than a pure tone threshold (see Chapter 8).

Masking for Speech Recognition and Other Suprathreshold Speech Tests

A calculation is needed to determine the correct amount of masking noise to be used during speech recognition and other suprathreshold speech tests. This calculation is actually the same as the one described above for suprathreshold tonal tests, except the presentation level now refers to that of the speech material. By now the student already knows that one must be ever vigilant about the possibility of overmasking, especially when performing any suprathreshold test.

A nifty rule-of-thumb that often works to arrive at the needed amount of noise for masking during speech audiometry is to use a masking noise level (in the NTE) that is 20 dB less than the level of the speech material being presented to the test ear (Jerger & Jerger 1971; Hannley 1986; Yacullo 1996, 1999, 2009). When properly used, this approach causes the masking noise in the NTE to be at least 20 dB greater than any speech signal that might cross over to it from the test ear. The author has found that this maneuver works especially well for symmetrical sensorineural hearing losses, and when masking the better ear while testing the poorer ear with asymmetrical sensorineural losses. However, after estimating how much masking noise to use with this technique, you *must* remember to consider whether either under- or overmasking might occur. Problems will arise if there is a conductive loss in the nontest ear.

Maximum Masking and Overmasking During Speech Audiometry

The maximum masking and overmasking rules for speech audiometry are similar to the ones already discussed, except that one attends to the *best* bone-conduction threshold of the test ear.

Masking for Speech Tests by Bone-Conduction

Speech testing by bone-conduction is relatively uncommon, but one must still be prepared to mask during these conditions should they arise. Here, the "when to mask" question follows the one used for tones, except that the comparison is made between the speech level and the best bone-conduction threshold. The issue of how much masking to use for bone-conduction speech stimuli must account for the occlusion effect. Even though the average occlusion effect for speech is ~ 6 dB when the vibrator is at the mastoid (or 9 dB when stimulating from the forehead), individual values can be as large as 20 dB (Klodd & Edgerton 1977). Because of this variability, it is recommended that the size of the occlusion effect for speech be determined on an individual patient basis using the same approach already described for tonal signals.

■ Study Questions

1. Define cross-hearing and explain its implications in hearing assessment.
2. Define interaural attenuation and explain its characteristics for air-conduction and bone-conduction.
3. What is clinical masking and why is it used?
4. Describe and explain the criteria for deciding when masking is needed during (a) air-conduction testing, and (b) bone-conduction testing.
5. Explain the use of the initial masking level.
6. Define central masking and describe its implications in clinical masking.
7. Define the occlusion effect and describe its implications in clinical masking.
8. Describe the plateau method, and explain why the plateau reveals the actual threshold of the test ear.
9. What is overmasking and why does it occur?
10. What are the benefits of insert earphones in the context of cross-hearing and clinical masking?

References

American National Standards Institute (ANSI). 2010. American National Standard Specifications for Audiometers. ANSI S3.6-2010. New York, NY: ANSI

American National Standards Institute (ANSI). 2004. Methods for Manual Pure-Tone Threshold Audiometry. ANSI S3.21-2004. New York, NY: ANSI

American Speech-Language-Hearing Association (ASHA). Guidelines for determining threshold level for speech. ASHA 1988;30(3):85–89

American Speech-Language-Hearing Association (ASHA). 2005. Guidelines for Manual Pure-Tone Threshold Audiometry. Rockville, MD: ASHA

Blegvad B. Contralateral masking and Békésy audiometry in normal listeners. Acta Otolaryngol 1967;64(2):157–165

Blegvad B. Békésy audiometry and clinical masking. Acta Otolaryngol 1968;66(3):229–240

Blegvad B. Differential intensity sensitivity and clinical masking. Acta Otolaryngol 1969;67(4):428–434

Blegvad B, Terkildsen K. Contralateral masking and the SISI-test in normal listeners. Acta Otolaryngol 1967;63(6):557–563

Chaiklin JB. Interaural attenuation and cross-hearing in air-conduction audiometry. J Aud Res 1967;7:413–424

Coles RRA, Priede VM. On the misdiagnoses resulting from incorrect use of masking. J Laryngol Otol 1970;84(1):41–63

Dirks D. Factors relating to bone-conduction reliability. Arch Otolaryngol 1964;79:551–558

Dirks D, Malmquist C. Changes in bone-conduction thresholds produced by masking in the non-test ear. J Speech Hear Res 1964;7:271–278

Dirks DD, Norris JC. Shifts in auditory thresholds produced by ipsilateral and contralateral maskers at low-intensity levels. J Acoust Soc Am 1966;40(1):12–19

Frank T, Karlovich RS. Effect of contralateral noise on speech detection and speech reception thresholds. Audiology 1975;14(1):34–43

Gelfand SA. 2010. Hearing: An Introduction to Psychological and Physiological Acoustics, 5th ed. London: Informa

Goldstein BA, Newman CW. 1985. Clinical masking: A decision making process. In: Katz J, ed. Handbook of Clinical Audiology, 3rd ed. Baltimore, MD: Williams & Wilkins; 170–201

Grimes CT, Feldman AS. Comparative Bekesy typing with broad and modulated narrow-band noise. J Speech Hear Res 1969;12(4):840–846

Hall JW. The clinical challenges of bone-conduction measurement. Hear J. 2005;58(3):10–15

Hannley M. 1986. Basic Principles of Auditory Assessment. Boston, MA: College-Hill

Hood JD. The principles and practice of bone conduction audiometry: a review of the present position. Laryngoscope 1960;70:1211–1228

Jerger J, Jerger S. Diagnostic significance of PB word functions. Arch Otolaryngol 1971;93(6):573–580

Jerger J, Tillman T. A new method for clinical determination of sensorineural acuity level (SAL). Arch Otolaryngol 1960;71:948–953

Killion MC, Wilber LA, Gudmundsen GI. Insert earphones for more interaural attenuation. Hear Instr 1985;36:34–36

Klodd DA, Edgerton BJ. Occlusion effect: bone conduction speech audiometry using forehead and mastoid placement. Audiology 1977;16(6):522–529

Konkle DF, Berry GA. 1983. Masking in speech audiometry. In: Konkle DF, Rintelmann WF, eds. Principles of Speech Audiometry. Baltimore, MD: University Park Press; 285–319

Liden G. Speech audiometry; an experimental and clinical study with Swedish language material. Acta Otolaryngol Suppl 1954;114:1–145

Liden G, Nilsson G, Anderson H. Narrow-band masking with white noise. Acta Otolaryngol 1959a;50(2):116–124

Liden G, Nilsson G, Anderson H. Masking in clinical audiometry. Acta Otolaryngol 1959b;50(2):125–136

Littler TS, Knight JJ, Strange PH. Hearing by bone conduction and the use of bone-conduction hearing aids. Proc R Soc Med 1952;45(11):783–790

Martin FN. Speech audiometry and clinical masking. J Aud Res 1966;6:199–203

Martin FN. A simplified method for clinical masking. J Aud Res 1967;7:59–62

Martin FN. Minimum effective masking levels in threshold audiometry. J Speech Hear Disord 1974;39(3):280–285

Martin FN. The masking plateau revisited. Ear Hear 1980;1(2):112–116

Martin FN. 1991. Introduction to Audiology, 4th ed. Englewood Cliffs, NJ: Prentice-Hall

Martin FN, Bailey H, Pappas J. The effect of central masking on thresholds for speech. J Aud Res 1965;5:293–296

Martin FN, Butler EC, Burns P. Audiometric Bing test for determination of minimum masking levels for bone-conduction tests. J Speech Hear Disord 1974;39(2):148–152

Naunton RF. A masking dilemma in bilateral conductive deafness. Arch Otolaryngol 1960;72:753–757

Priede VM, Coles RRA. Masking of the non-test ear in tone decay, Békésy audiometry, and SISI tests. J Laryngol Otol 1975;89(3):227–236

Rainville MJ. Nouvelle méthode d'assourdissement pour le releve des courbe de conduction osseuse. J. Francais Oto-laryngologie 1955;72:752–757

Sanders JW. 1972. Masking. In: Katz J, ed. Handbook of Clinical Audiology, 1st ed. Baltimore, MD: Williams & Wilkins; 111–142

Shimizu H. Influence of contralateral noise stimulation on tone decay and SISI tests. Laryngoscope 1969;79(12):2155–2164

Silman S, Silverman CA. 1991. Auditory Diagnosis: Principles and Applications. San Diego, CA: Academic Press

Sklare DA, Denenberg LJ. Interaural attenuation for tubephone insert earphones. Ear Hear 1987;8(5):298–300

Smith BL, Markides A. Interaural attenuation for pure tones and speech. Br J Audiol 1981;15(1):49–54

Snyder JM. Interaural attenuation characteristics in audiometry. Laryngoscope 1973;83(11):1847–1855

Sparrevohn UR. Some audiometric investigations of monaurally deaf persons. Acta Otolaryngol 1946;34:1–10

Studebaker GA. On masking in bone-conduction testing. J Speech Hear Res 1962;5:215–227

Studebaker GA. Clinical masking of air- and bone-conducted stimuli. J Speech Hear Disord 1964;29:23–35

Studebaker GA. Clinical masking of the nontest ear. J Speech Hear Disord 1967;32(4):360–371

Studebaker GA. 1979. Clinical masking. In: Rintelmann WF, ed. Hearing Assessment. Baltimore, MD: University Park Press; 51–100

Swisher LP, Dudley JG, Doehring DG. Influence of contralateral noise on auditory intensity discrimination. J Acoust Soc Am 1969;45(6):1532–1536

Townsend TH, Schwartz DM. Calculation of effective masking using one octave and one-third octave analysis. Audiol Hear Ed 1976;2:27–34

Turner RG. Masking redux. I: An optimized masking method. J Am Acad Audiol 2004a;15(1):17–28

Turner RG. Masking redux. II: A recommended masking protocol. J Am Acad Audiol 2004b;15(1):29–46

Van Campen LE, Sammeth CA, Peek BF. Interaural attenuation using etymotic ER-3A insert earphones in auditory brain stem response testing. Ear Hear 1990;11(1):66–69

Veniar FA. Individual masking levels in pure tone audiometry. Arch Otolaryngol 1965;82(5):518–521

Yacullo WS. 1996. Clinical Masking Procedures. Boston, MA: Allyn & Bacon

Yacullo WS. Clinical masking in speech audiometry: a simplified approach. Am J Audiol 1999;8(2):106–116

Yacullo WS. 2009. Clinical masking. In: Katz J, Medwetsky L, Burkard R, Hood L, eds. Handbook of Clinical Audiology, 6th ed. Baltimore, MD: Lippincott Williams & Wilkins; 80–115

Zwislocki J. Acoustic attenuation between the ears. J Acoust Soc Am 1953;25:752–759

10 Behavioral Tests for Audiological Diagnosis

This chapter deals to a large extent with behavioral tests used for identifying the anatomical location ("site") of the abnormality ("lesion") causing the patient's problems—those traditionally referred to as **site-of-lesion tests**. At this juncture it is wise to distinguish between medical and audiological diagnosis. Medical diagnosis involves determining the location of the abnormality and also its etiology, which involves the nature and cause of the pathology, and how it pertains to the patient's health. In this sense, audiological tests contribute to medical diagnosis in at least two ways, depending on who sees the patient first. When the patient sees the audiologist first, they can act as screening tests to identify the possibility of conditions that indicate the need for referral to a physician. If the patient has been referred to the audiologist by a physician, then these tests provide information that assist in arriving at a medical diagnosis. In contrast, audiological diagnosis deals with ascertaining the nature and scope of the patient's auditory problems and their ramifications for dealing with the world of sound in general and communication in particular.

Diagnostic audiological assessment was traditionally viewed in terms of certain site-of-lesion tests specifically intended for this purpose. However, solving the diagnostic puzzle really starts with the initial interview and case history. After all, this is when we begin to compare the patient's complaints and behaviors with the characteristics of the various clinical entities that might cause them. Moreover, *direct* site-of-lesion assessment is already under way with the pure tone audiogram and routine speech audiometric tests. For example, we compare the pure tone air- and bone-conduction thresholds to determine whether the hearing loss is conductive, sensorineural, or mixed. This is the same question as asking whether the problem is located in the conductive mechanism (the outer and/or middle ear), the sensorineural mechanism (the cochlea or eighth nerve), or a combination of the two. In addition, the acoustic immittance tests that are part of almost every routine evaluation constitute a powerful audiological diagnostic battery in and of themselves.

In this chapter, we will briefly consider whether asymmetries between the right and left ears on the pure tone audiogram help us to identify retrocochlear disorders; after which we will consider the classical site-of-lesion tests. As discussed in Chapter 6, terms like *acoustic neuroma* or *tumor, vestibular schwannoma,* and *eighth* nerve tumor will be used interchangeably. Following the traditional tests, we will cover the behavioral measures used to identify cochlear dead regions and some aspects of the assessment of central auditory processing disorders.

■ Asymmetries between the Ears

Recall from Chapters 5 and 6 that cochlear and eighth nerve lesions cannot be distinguished from one another based on the pure tone audiogram. In fact, any degree and configuration of hearing loss can be encountered in patients with retrocochlear pathology (e.g., Johnson 1977; Gimsing 2010; Suzuki, Hashimoto, Kano, & Okitsu 2010). In spite of this, a significant difference between the ears is a very common finding in patients with acoustic tumors (e.g., Matthies & Samii 1997), so that the index of suspicion is raised when an asymmetry is found. Although we will be focusing here on asymmetries in the pure tone audiogram, it is important to stress that other asymmetries also raise the flag for ruling out retrocochlear pathology. Unilateral tinnitus (e.g., Sheppard, Milford & Anslow 1996; Dawes & Jeannon 1998; Obholzer, Rea, & Harcourt 2004; Gimsing 2010) and differences in speech recognition scores between the ears (e.g., Welling, Glasscock, Woods, & Jackson 1990; Ruckenstein, Cueva, Morrison, & Press 1996; Robinette, Bauch, Olsen & Cevette 2000) are among the other examples of asymmetries that become apparent early in the evaluation process.

However, many patients without retrocochlear pathology often have some degree of difference between their ears, as well; and there can be disagreement about whether a hearing loss is symmetrical or asymmetrical even among expert clinicians (Margolis & Saly 2008). It is therefore desirable to have criteria for identifying when a sensorineural hearing loss involves a clinically significant asymmetry. Thus, it is not surprising that various criteria have been suggested for identifying asymmetries in the pure tone audiogram that are clinically significant. Many of these criteria are summarized in **Table 10.1**, although other kinds of approaches using mathematical and statistical techniques have also been developed (e.g., Nouraei, Huys, Chatrath, Powles, & Harcourt 2007; Zapala et al 2012).

Some of the methods in **Table 10.1** use an inter-ear difference of ≥ 15 dB as the criterion for a clinically significant asymmetry, while others use require ≥ 20 dB. They also differ with respect to which frequencies are considered, how many of them are involved, and how the differences are calculated. The first two methods in the figure consider a difference between the ears to be clinically significant even if it occurs at just one frequency between 500 and 4000 Hz; and each of the next two considers only one specific frequency. The third set of methods require an asymmetry to be present for at least two frequencies in a range, but differ in terms of whether they can be any two frequencies or only ones that are adjacent to one another. Finally, the last group of methods compare an average of the thresholds for a certain range of frequencies. Also notice that a few methods use different criteria based on gender, on whether the hearing loss is unilateral versus bilateral but asymmetrical, and even on whether the next step in the process would be magnetic resonance imaging (MRI) or auditory brainstem responses (ABR). So, with all these differences, which criteria should be used?

At least part of the answer to this question is provided in the last two columns of the table, which are based on the findings by Zapala et al (2012) for patients with hearing losses that were known to be either medically benign or associated with vestibular schwannomas. The **sensitivity** (also known as the **hit rate**) column shows the percentage of patients who had vestibular schwannomas who were correctly identified by the criteria. In contrast, the **specificity** column shows the percentage of patients who did not have tumors and who were correctly identified by the criteria. For example, the criteria by Welling et al (1990) had 49.5% sensitivity and 89.4% specificity. This means that their method correctly identified 49.5% of the patients with tumors and 89.4% of those without tumors. This also means that 100 − 49.5 = 50.5% of the patients with tumors were missed by the method (**false negatives**), and that it also incorrectly flagged 100 − 89.4 = 10.6% of those who did not have tumors (**false positives**). Overall, we see that these provide up to ~ 50% specificity and roughly 14% specificity. Somewhat better performance can be achieved with a statistical approach that allows the clinician to estimate the sensitivity and false positive rate for a given patient (Zapala et al 2012). This method uses the average difference between the ears at 250 to 4000 Hz (including 3000 Hz) and includes adjustments for the patient's age, gender, and noise exposure history.

Which method is "best"? The answer to this question depends on how the comparison is made, and provides a convenient opportunity to introduce some useful concepts.

One way to identify the optimal method is to find the one that has the highest sensitivity and the highest specificity. In these terms, the overall top-performing criteria in the table were *≥ 15 dB for ≥ 2 frequencies between 250 and 8000 Hz* (Ruckenstein et al 1996; Cueva 2004) with 49.9% sensitivity and 89.8% specificity, and *≥ 15 dB for 1 frequency between 500 and 4000 Hz* (Welling et al 1990) with 48.5% sensitivity and 89.4% specificity.[1]

Another way to compare the methods is to graph the hit rate against the false alarm rate.[2] (We will bypass the details, but interested students will want to know that this approach comes from the **theory of signal detection**, and the plot is called a **receiver operating characteristic** or **ROC curve** [see, e.g., Gelfand 2010].) With this approach, Zapala et al (2012) found that their statistical method was the most effective method for distinguishing vestibular schwannomas from medically benign cases, followed by a close tie between *≥ 15 dB for the 250 to 8000 Hz average* (Sheppard et al 1996) and *≥ 15 dB* for the *500 to 3000 Hz average (*Robinette et al 2000).

The picture that emerges is that a significantly asymmetrical hearing loss provides up to ~ 50% sensitivity along with good specificity, and that the criteria just highlighted seem to be reasonable choices for use. Considering the limited sensitivity and high specificity of the criteria, a referral to rule out retrocochlear pathology is certainly warranted when a significant asymmetry is identified.

---

[1] A noticeable exception occurred for women with a history of noise exposure, for whom sensitivity was 40% with the Welling et al (1990) method compared with 30% for the Ruckenstein et al (1996) criteria (Zapala et al 2012).

[2] Because of the high level used, a 90 dB SPL broadband masking noise is presented to the opposite ear.

Table 10.1 Examples of various criteria for clinically significant asymmetries between the two ears on the pure tone audiogram

Asymmetry criteria					Tumor vs. nontumor[b]	
Size (dB)	Based on	Frequencies (Hz)	Comments	Source	Sensitivity (%)	Specificity (%)
≥ 15	1 frequency	500–4000		Welling et al (1990)	48.5	89.4
≥ 20	1 frequency	500–4000		Suzuki et al (2010)	—	—
≥ 15	1 frequency	3000		Saliba et al (2009)	45.7	86.4
≥ 20	1 frequency	4000	Females	Schlauch et al (1995)	35.6[c] 20.0[d]	95.2[c] 94.1[d]
≥ 15	≥ 2 frequencies	250–8000		Ruckenstein et al (1996); Cueva (2004)	49.9	89.8
≥ 15 ≥ 20	≥ 2 neighboring frequencies	250–8000	Unilateral Asymmetric	Obholzer et al (2004)	39.3	95.9
≥ 20	≥ 2 neighboring frequencies	Any		Gimsing (2010)	41.4	93.6
≥ 15	≥ 2 frequencies	2000–8000			45.9	90.7
≥ 20	≥ 2 neighboring frequencies	250–8000		Dawes & Jeannon (1998)	39.3	95.9
≥ 15	Average	500–3000		Robinette et al (2000)	38.1	97.3
≥ 15	Average	1000–8000		Hunter et al (1999)	40.9	96.7
≥ 15	Average	250–8000		Sheppard et al (1996)	34.6	98.6
≥ 20	Average	1000–8000	For MRI[a]	Mangham (1991)	32.5	98.4
≥ 20	Average	1000–4000	Males	Schlauch et al (1995)	39.2[c] 28.7[d]	98.7[c] 98.9[d]

[a]Mangham (1991) suggested asymmetry criteria of ≥ 20 dB to refer for MRI and 5–15 dB to refer for ABR. The 5–15 dB criterion is excluded from the table because its 72.5% sensitivity came at the cost of a 39.2% false-positive rate (or 70.8% specificity).
[b]All values are based on the findings reported by Zapala et al (2012), and unless otherwise noted show the *overall* correct identification of cases with tumors (sensitivity) and without tumors (specificity), combined for males and females and for those with and without noise exposure.
[c]For individuals *without* noise exposure.
[d]For individuals *with* noise exposure.

Classical Behavioral Tests

A common thread among many of the traditional behavioral tests for distinguishing cochlear and retrocochlear disorders is the perception of intensity and how it is affected by pathology. We shall see, however, that the ability of these kinds of tests to confidently separate cochlear and retrocochlear disorders has actually been rather disappointing, and their use has decreased over the years (Martin, Champlin, & Chambers 1998). In spite of this, we will cover these tests in some detail not just because one will find the need to use them from time to time, but also because this knowledge provides the future clinician with (a) insight into the nature of hearing impairment, (b) familiarity with various approaches used to assess auditory skills, and (c) the all-important foundation needed for understanding the literature in the field.

Threshold Tone Decay Tests

A continuous tone sounds less loud after it has been on for some time compared with when it was first turned on, or it may fade away altogether. The decrease in the tone's loudness over time is usually called **loudness adaptation**, and the situation in which it dies out completely is called **threshold adaptation** or **tone decay**. Adaptation is due to the reduction of the neural response to continuous stimulation over time, and is common to all sensory systems (Marks 1974). Adaptation per se is a normal phenomenon, but excessive amounts of adaptation reflect the possibility of certain pathologies. It is for this reason that adaptation tests are often used as clinical site-of-lesion tests.

Most clinical adaptation procedures are **threshold tone decay tests**, which measure adaptation in terms of whether a continuous tone fades away completely within a certain amount of time, usually 60 seconds. The patient's task is easily understood in terms of these typical instructions: "You will hear a continuous tone for a period of time, which might be a few seconds or a few minutes. Raise your finger (or hand) as soon as the tone starts and keep it up as long as the tone is audible. Put your finger down whenever the tone fades away. Pick it up again if the tone comes back, and hold it up as long as you can still hear it. It is very important that you do not say anything or make any sounds during this test because that would interrupt the tone. Remember, don't make any sounds, keep your finger raised whenever you hear the tone, and down whenever you don't hear it." Because the patient may be holding his hand or finger up for some time, it is a good idea to have him support his elbow on the arm of his chair. Many audiologists have the patient press and release a response signal button instead of holding up and lowering his finger or hand.

Carhart (1957) suggested that tone decay tests (TDTs) be administered to each ear at 500, 1000, 2000, and 4000 Hz, but most audiologists select the frequencies to be tested on a patient-by-patient basis. Both ears should be tested at each frequency selected because this permits the clinician to compare the two ears as well as to determine whether abnormal tone decay is present bilaterally. Of course, each ear is tested separately.

Carhart Tone Decay Test

In the **Carhart threshold tone decay test** (1957), a test tone is presented to the patient at threshold (0 dB SL) for 60 seconds. If the patient hears the tone for a full minute at the initial level, then the test is over. However, if the patient lowers his finger, indicating that the tone faded away before 60 seconds have passed, then the audiologist (1) increases the level by 5 dB without interrupting the tone, and (2) begins timing a new 60-second period as soon as the patient raises his hand. If the tone is heard for a full minute

at 5 dB SL, then the test is over. However, if the tone fades away before 60 seconds are up, then the level is again raised 5 dB and a new minute is begun. This procedure continues until the patient is able to hear the tone for 60 seconds, or until the maximum limits of the audiometer are reached.

Tone decay test results are expressed as the *amount of tone decay*, which is simply the sensation level at which the tone was heard for 60 seconds. For example, if the tone was heard for 1 minute at threshold, then there would be 0 dB of tone decay; and if the tone was heard for 60 seconds at 5 dB SL, then there was 5 dB of tone decay. Similarly, if the tone could not be heard for a full minute until the level was raised to 45 dB SL, then there would be 45 dB of tone decay.

Normal individuals and those with conductive abnormalities are expected to have little or no threshold adaptation. Cochlear losses may come with varying degrees of tone decay, which may range up to perhaps 30 dB, but excessive tone decay of *35 dB or more* is associated with retrocochlear pathologies (Carhart 1957; Tillman 1969; Morales-Garcia & Hood 1972; Olsen & Noffsinger 1974; Sanders, Josey, & Glasscock 1974; Olsen & Kurdziel 1976). Thus, if the TDT is viewed as a test for retrocochlear involvement, then ≤ 30 dB of tone decay is usually interpreted as "negative," and > 30 dB of tone decay is "positive."

Tone decay test outcomes should be documented separately for each ear in terms of the number of decibels of tone decay at each frequency tested, to which one might add an interpretation (such as "positive" or "negative"). One should never record "positive" or "negative" without the actual results. You can always figure out whether a result was positive or negative from the amount of tone decay, but you could never go back and deduce the actual amount of tone decay from a record that says only "positive" or "negative." These points apply to all diagnostic procedures.

Olsen-Noffsinger Tone Decay Test

The **Olsen-Noffsinger tone decay test** (1974) is identical to the Carhart TDT except that the test tone is initially presented at 20 dB SL instead of at threshold. Beginning at 20 dB SL is desirable for several reasons. It makes the test simpler for the patient to take because a 20 dB SL test tone is much easier to detect than one given at threshold. It is also easier to distinguish it from any tinnitus that the patient may have. In addition, starting the test at 20 dB SL can shorten the test time by as much as 4 minutes for every frequency tested. Reducing the test time makes the experience less fatiguing for the patient and saves clinician time, which is always at a premium. The Olsen-Noffsinger modification relies on the premise that amounts of tone decay up to 20 dB on the Carhart TDT are interpreted as negative. Thus, omitting the test trials that would have been given at 0 to +15 dB SL should not change any diagnostic decisions. It has been found that the Carhart and Olsen-Noffsinger procedures yield similar results in terms of when the results are positive versus negative (Olsen & Noffsinger 1974; Olsen & Kurdziel 1976).

The outcome of the Olsen-Noffsinger TDT is recorded as follows: If the patient hears the initial (20 dB SL) test tone for a full minute, then one records the results as "≤ 20 dB tone decay." Greater amounts of tone decay are recorded in the same way as for the Carhart TDT.

The Olsen-Noffsinger TDT is sometimes misconstrued as a tone decay "screening" test because most patients are able to hear the initial test tone for the full 60 seconds. It should be stressed that the reason why many patients do not have to be tested beyond the 20 dB SL starting level is simply that they do not have more than 20 dB of tone decay. One should remember that the Olsen-Noffsinger is a full-fledged TDT that yields the actual amount of significant tone decay > 20 dB, just like the Carhart procedure.

Other Modifications of the Carhart Tone Decay Test

There are several other modifications of the Carhart TDT of which the student should be aware. The **Yantis** (1959) **modification** begins testing at 5 dB SL instead of at threshold. This modification is so commonly used that it is not distinguished from the Carhart by most clinicians. **Sorensen's** (1960, 1962) **modification** requires the patient to hear the test tone for 90 seconds instead of 60 seconds, and is performed only at 2000 Hz. This procedure is rarely used.

The **Rosenberg** (1958, 1969) **modified tone decay test** begins like the Carhart test but lasts only 60 seconds from start to finish. If the patient hears the tone for 60 seconds at threshold, then the test is over and there is 0 dB of tone decay. If the tone fades away before the end of one minute, then the clinician does the following: As with the Carhart TDT, she increases the intensity in 5 dB steps without interrupting the tone until the patient raises his hand. Every time the patient lowers his hand, the audiologist again raises the tone in 5 dB steps until the patient hears the tone again, and so on. However, unlike the Carhart TDT, she does *not* begin timing a new minute with every level increment. Instead, the clock keeps running until a total of 60 seconds has elapsed since the tone was originally turned on. The amount of tone decay is the sensation level reached at the end of 60 sec-

onds. For example, if the threshold was 35 dB HL, the tone starts at this level and one begins timing for 60 seconds. If the attenuator has been raised by a total of 25 dB to 60 dB HL at the end of one minute, then there has been 25 dB of tone decay. Notice that the Rosenberg test ignores how long the tone was actually heard at any given level.

Green's (1963) **modified tone decay test** involves administering the Rosenberg 1-minute test with a significant change in the instructions. The patient is told to lower his hand completely if the tone fades away and to lower his hand partially if the tone *loses its tonal quality* (even though it might still be audible). The modified instructions are based on the observation that some patients with retrocochlear pathologies hear a change in the character of the tone in which it loses it tonal quality, becoming noise-like, before its audibility is completely lost (Pestalozza & Cioce 1962; Sorensen 1962; Green 1963). This phenomenon is called **atonality** or **tone perversion** (Parker & Decker 1971).

Owens Tone Decay Test

Owens (1964a) introduced a modification of a tone decay procedure originated by Hood (1955). Unlike the Carhart test and its modifications, which concentrate on the amount of adaptation, the **Owens tone decay test** focuses upon the *pattern* of tone decay. The test begins by presenting a continuous test tone at 5 dB SL. As with the Carhart TDT, the Owens test ends if the patient hears the tone for 60 seconds at this initial level. However, if the tone fades away before 60 seconds, the tone is turned off for a 20-second rest (recovery) period. After the 20-second rest, the tone is reintroduced at 10 dB SL (i.e., 5 dB higher), and a new 60-second period begins. If the tone is heard for a full minute at 10 dB SL, then the test is over. However, if the tone fades away before a full minute, then the tone is turned off for another 20-second rest period, after which it is given again at 15 dB SL. The same procedure is followed for the 15 dB SL tone. If necessary, the tone is presented for another 1-minute period at 20 dB SL, but this is the last level tested regardless of whether the tone is heard for 60 seconds or less. The audiologist records how many seconds the tone was heard at each of the levels presented, and the test is interpreted in terms of the pattern of how many seconds the tone was heard at each of the four test levels.

Fig. 10.1 shows the various patterns (types) of tone decay described by Owens (1964a). The type I pattern involves being able to hear the initial (5 dB SL) tone for a full minute, and is associated with normal ears and those with cochlear impairments.

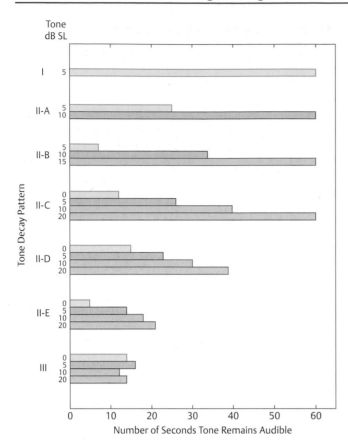

Fig. 10.1   Tone decay patterns on the Owens tone decay test. (Based on data by Owens [1964a].)

There are five type II patterns, called II-A through II-E. The type II patterns share two characteristics: (1) the tone fades away before 60 seconds for at least the lowest sensation level, and (2) the tone is heard progressively longer at increasingly higher sensation levels. The tone is finally heard for a full minute at 10 dB SL in type II-A, at 15 dB in type II-B, and at 20 dB SL in type II-C. In the type II-D pattern, the tone fades away in less than a minute at all four sensation levels, but it does remain audible for appreciably longer periods of time with each successively higher sensation level. Cochlear impairments are most commonly associated with types II-A through II-D.

In the type II-E pattern each 5 dB rise in sensation level produces only a small increase in how long the tone is heard (averaging 4 to 7 seconds per 5 dB level). This pattern is found in either cochlear or retrocochlear abnormalities.

The type III pattern is principally associated with retrocochlear disorders. Here, increasing the sensation level does not cause the tone to be heard for longer periods of time.

Rate of Tone Decay

Wiley and Lilly (1980) proposed a modification of the Owens TDT in which (1) the rest period between tones is reduced to 10 seconds, and (2) the test level continues to be raised until the tone remains audible for a full minute (or the audiometer's maximum level is reached). This modification allowed them to distinguish between the rates of tone decay in the two ears of a patient who had a cochlear disorder in one ear and an acoustic tumor in the other ear. The importance of looking at the rate of tone decay was also shown by Silman, Gelfand, Lutolf, and Chun (1981) in a patient whose hearing loss was so severe that the Owens TDT was the only usable tone decay method.

Overall Assessment of Threshold Tone Decay Tests

Tone decay appears to be the only classical site-of-lesion technique that is still routinely used by a majority of audiologists (Martin et al 1998). Several studies have compared the accuracy of threshold adaptation tests as indicators of retrocochlear pathology (e.g., Parker & Decker 1971; Olsen & Noffsinger 1974; Sanders, Josey, & Glasscock 1974). Overall, they have shown the Carhart-type TDTs are most sensitive procedures. This appears to hold true whether the test begins at threshold, 5 dB SL (Yantis 1959), or 20 dB SL (Olsen & Noffsinger 1974). This kind of TDT is thus the one of choice, with the Olsen-Noffsinger modification being the most efficient. The Owens TDT is particularly valuable when the severity of a hearing loss makes it impossible to determine the amount of tone decay using the Carhart or similar procedures (Silman et al 1981). In contrast, the Rosenberg 1-minute TDT is not as effective at identifying retrocochlear lesions as the Carhart, Olsen-Noffsinger, or Owens procedure (Parker & Decker 1971; Olsen & Noffsinger 1974) and is not recommended.

Green's modification of the Rosenberg TDT has not been compared with other tests that do not use the atonality criterion. It is not clear whether atonality per se should be used as a criterion for tone decay testing because little if any research actually addresses this issue. More tone decay can be obtained when the patient responds to either atonality or inaudibility compared with inaudibility alone. However, the experience of the author and his colleagues (e.g., Silman & Silverman 1991) has been that using the atonality criterion increases the number of false-positive TDT results, and this is especially problematic when testing elderly patients. Even though several earlier papers suggested accounting for the loss of tonal quality (e.g., Sorenson 1962; Pestalozza & Cioce 1962;

Flottorp 1964; Johnson 1966; Sung, Goetzinger, & Knox 1969; Olsen & Noffsinger 1974), it appears that only ~ 10% of audiologists use the atonality criterion (Martin, Woodrick Armstrong, & Champlin 1994).

As a group, threshold TDTs correctly identify retrocochlear lesions among anywhere from 64 to 95% of the cases, and correctly classify non-retrocochlear disorders ~ 77 to 96% of the time (Owens 1964a; Gjaevenes & Söhoel 1969; Tillman 1969; Olsen & Noffsinger 1974; Sanders et al 1974; Olsen & Kurdziel 1976; Antonelli, Bellotto, & Grandori 1987; Josey 1987). Part of this variability comes from differences in which tone decay tests were used and how they were administered and interpreted, and also from differences in the patient populations. Turner, Shepard, and Frazer (1984) have shown that TDT results are correct in an average of 70% of retrocochlear cases and 87% for ears that do not have retrocochlear lesions, across studies.

■ Suprathreshold Adaptation Test

Jerger and Jerger (1975a) suggested a tone decay test performed at high levels instead of beginning at threshold, called the **suprathreshold adaptation test (STAT)**. Here, a *continuous* test tone lasting a total of 60 seconds is presented at 110 dB SPL.[2] (This corresponds to ~ 105 dB HL when the test is done at 1000 Hz, and to 100 dB HL when testing at 500 Hz or 2000 Hz.) As with threshold tone decay tests, the patient is told to keep her hand raised as long as she hears the tone, and to lower her hand if it fades away completely. If the high-intensity tone is heard for the full minute, then the test is over and the result is negative. If the tone fades away before 60 seconds are up, then the patient is retested with a *pulsing* tone for confirmatory purposes. If the patient keeps her hand up for the full 60 seconds in response to the pulsing tone, then her failure to keep responding to the continuous tone is attributed to abnormal adaptation. The test is thus confirmed to be positive, suggesting a retrocochlear disorder. However, if she fails to respond to the pulsing tone for 1 minute, then the test result is not considered to be valid because tone decay should not occur with a pulsed tone. The correct identification rates for cochlear and retrocochlear cases, respectively, are 100% and 45% when the STAT is done at 500 and 1000 Hz, 95% and 54% at 500 to 2000 Hz, and 13% and 70% at 500 to 4000 Hz (Jerger & Jerger 1975a; Turner et al 1984).

---

[2] Because of the high level used, a 90 dB SPL broadband masking noise is presented to the opposite ear.

■ Loudness Recruitment and Loudness Balance Testing

Loudness Recruitment

We all have had the experience of being told to "speak up" by a hearing-impaired relative. Upon complying with this request, we are then told to "stop shouting." This common experience reveals an important facet of many cochlear impairments: Even though more intensity (i.e., a higher than normal HL) is needed for a sound to be heard, once the sound is raised above this elevated threshold, the now higher-intensity sound is as loud to the patient as it would be to a normal-hearing person. Consider a normal person whose threshold for a tone is 0 dB HL and a patient whose threshold is 50 dB HL for the same tone. If the tone is raised to 80 dB HL, it will now be 80 dB above the normal person's threshold but only 30 dB above the patient's threshold. Yet the tone will sound *as loud* to the patient (at 30 dB SL) as it does to the normal individual (at 80 dB SL). For this patient, the 30 dB level increase was perceived as an *increase in loudness* by an amount that took an 80 dB level increase for the normal person. In other words, the patient has experienced an abnormally rapid growth of loudness. This is called **loudness recruitment**.

When there is a sensorineural hearing loss, loudness recruitment is associated with a cochlear site of lesion, whereas the absence of loudness recruitment is associated with retrocochlear pathologies (Dix, Hallpike, & Hood 1948; Hallpike & Hood 1951, 1959; Jerger 1961; Hallpike 1965; Davis & Goodman 1966; Hood 1969; Priede & Coles 1974; Coles & Priede 1976).

Alternate Binaural Loudness Balance (ABLB) Test

The nature of the **alternate binaural loudness balance (ABLB) test** (Fowler 1936) is described by its name. A tone is presented *alternately* between the two ears (*binaurally*). The level of the tone stays the same in one ear (the "fixed" ear), but is varied up and/or down in the other ear (the "variable" ear), as shown schematically in **Fig. 10.2**. The patient reports when the tone sounds louder in the right ear, when it is louder in the left ear, and when it sounds equally loud in both ears. We say that a *loudness balance* has been obtained when the tones sound equally loud in both ears. The tester then records the two levels (in dB HL) where the loudness balance occurred.

Let us see what happens when the ABLB is given to a *normal*-hearing person who has the same thresholds in both ears. The results of a series of loudness

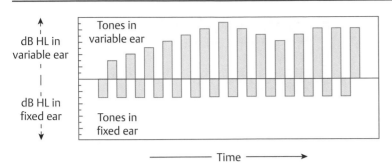

Fig. 10.2 Schematic representation of the alternate binaural loudness balance (ABLB) test, showing a tone being presented alternately between the two ears. Its level is fixed in one ear and is variable in the other ear.

balances at the same frequency in 20 dB intervals are shown in the left panel of **Fig. 10.3**. We assume that 0 dB HL in the right ear and 0 dB HL in the left ear are equally loud because they are both at threshold. Moving on to the loudness balances themselves, notice that 20 dB HL in the right ear sounded as loud as 20 dB HL in the left ear, 40 dB HL in the right ear was just as loud as 40 dB HL in the left ear, etc. Although ABLB results can be recorded numerically, it is more convenient to show them diagrammatically. The diagram in the middle panel of **Fig. 10.3** is called a **laddergram** for obvious reasons. Hearing level is shown going down the y-axis just as on an audiogram. For each loudness balance, we draw a circle at the hearing level in the right ear and an X at the hearing level for the left ear, and then join the two symbols with a line to show they are equally loud. The horizontal lines ("rungs") indicate that equal loudness occurs at the same intensity for both ears. We can also show the results on a **Steinberg-Gardner plot** like the one in the right panel of the figure. Here, each point shows the coordinates of the levels in the two ears

that sound equally loud. In this example, all of the points fall along a diagonal line because there was a one-to-one relationship between the equally loud levels in the two ears. Whenever the points fall along this 45° line, it means that equal intensities sound equally loud.

Clinical Use of the ABLB

The ABLB is used clinically to determine whether loudness recruitment is present in the abnormal ear of a patient who has a unilateral hearing loss. Loudness balances are made between the patient's abnormal ear and his normal ear. Normal thresholds are needed in the better ear because the ABLB works by comparing loudnesses between the two ears. After all, if we are trying to find out whether loudness is growing at a faster than normal rate in the abnormal ear by comparing it to the other ear, then we must know that loudness is growing at a normal rate in the other ear. Thus, the thresholds must be normal

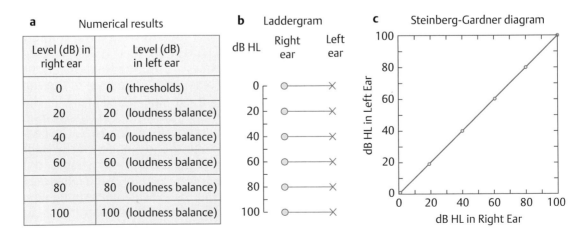

Fig. 10.3 Loudness balance results for a normal-hearing person shown **(a)** numerically, **(b)** on a laddergram, and **(c)** on a Steinberg-Gardner plot. When equal sound levels are equally loud, points are joined by horizontal lines on the laddergram and fall along the 45° line on the Steinberg-Gardner diagram.

in the opposite ear for the frequencies being tested. Further, the threshold of the abnormal ear should be at least 35 dB HL at each frequency tested.

Types of Recruitment

Suppose a patient has a threshold of 0 dB HL in his normal right ear and 45 dB HL in his abnormal, left ear at the frequency we are testing. Since we assume that loudnesses are equal at threshold, this means that 0 dB HL in the right ear sounds as loud as 45 dB HL in the left ear. For simplicity, this will be the starting point in all of our examples. The abnormal, left ear will be used as the fixed ear and the normal right ear will be the variable ear, and we will do loudness balances in 20 dB increments. In other words, we will adjust the level of the tone in the right ear until it balances in loudness with a 65 dB HL tone in the left ear, after which we will repeat the procedure at 85 dB HL in the fixed ear, and finally at 105 dB in the fixed ear.

Complete recruitment occurs when the loudness balances at higher levels occur at the same intensities in both ears, that is, when equal intensities sound equally loud. This is what occurred in the earlier example, where the thresholds were 0 dB HL

in the good ear and 50 dB HL in the bad ear, and yet 80 dB HL sounded equally loud in both ears.

Complete recruitment is shown in **Fig. 10.4a**. Here, even though the thresholds are 0 dB HL and 45 dB HL, equal loudness is eventually obtained when both ears receive 105 dB HL. In practice, recruitment is generally considered complete if equal loudness occurs at equal hearing levels (dB HL) ± 10 dB (Jerger 1962). This is shown by the flattening of the rungs on the laddergram. In this example, a 60 dB rise (from 45 to 105 dB HL) in the abnormal ear sounds like a 105 dB rise (from 0 to 105 dB HL) in the normal ear. In terms of sensation level, 60 dB SL in the bad ear is experienced as being just as loud as 105 dB SL in the good ear (**Fig. 10.5a**).

Complete recruitment is easily seen on the Steinberg-Gardner plot (**Fig. 10.4a**), which plots the level in the abnormal ear on the x-axis and the equally loud level in the good ear on the y-axis. The normal one-to-one loudness-growth relationship is shown by a 45° line for comparison purposes. Any points that fall on this diagonal indicate that equal intensities sound equally loud. The plot of the test results begins 45 dB to the right (i.e., x = 45, y = 0) because the thresholds are 45 dB in the abnormal ear and

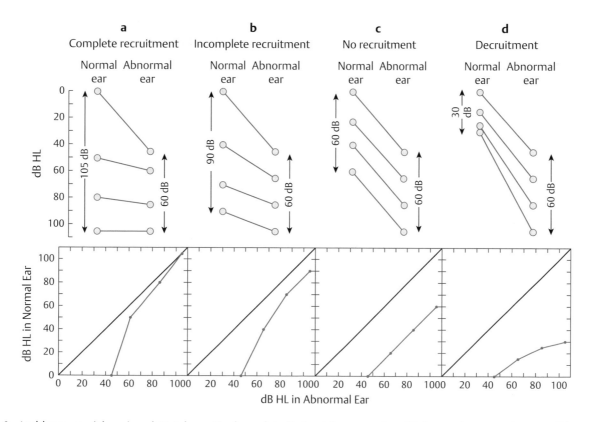

Fig. 10.4 Laddergrams (above) and Steinberg-Gardner plots (below) for examples of **(a)** complete recruitment, **(b)** incomplete (partial) recruitment, **(c)** no recruitment, and **(d)** decruitment.

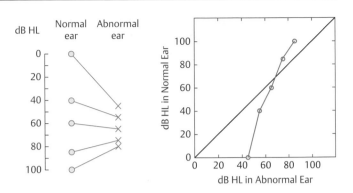

Fig. 10.6   An example of hyper-recruitment (over-recruitment).

Fig. 10.5   Loudness balance test results in terms of sensation levels.

0 dB in the normal ear, but it rises at a sharp angle and eventually meets the 45° line at the point corresponding to 105 dB HL in both ears. The steeply rising line on the Steinberg-Gardner diagram gives a clear picture of what we mean when we say that recruitment is an abnormally rapid growth of loudness. As already pointed out, complete recruitment suggests a cochlear site of lesion.

Some patients with Meniere's disease may exhibit a special case of recruitment in which the loudness in the abnormal ear not only catches up with the normal ear, but actually overtakes it (Dix et al 1948; Hallpike & Hood 1959; Hood 1977). This finding is called **hyper-recruitment** (or **over-recruitment**), and is shown in **Fig. 10.6**. Hyper-recruitment is revealed on the laddergram by rungs that first flatten and then reverse direction. In this example, 85 dB HL in the abnormal ear actually sounds as loud as 100 dB HL in the normal ear. This is shown on the Steinberg-Gardner diagram when the line that shows the patient's equal loudness judgments crosses above the diagonal line. One should note that hyper-recruitment is something of a controversial issue, and the likelihood of finding it seems to be affected by how the ABLB test is performed (Hood 1969, 1977; Coles & Priede 1976).

Incomplete (or **partial**) **recruitment** occurs when the results fall between complete recruitment and no recruitment (discussed below). This is shown as a partial flattening of the laddergram or by a line that rises toward but does not quite reach the diagonal on the Steinberg-Gardner plot. An example is shown in **Fig. 10.4b** and **Fig. 10.5b**. Audiologists are inconsistent about how they interpret incomplete recruitment, and it is not surprising that its diagnostic value has been questioned (Priede & Coles 1974).

No recruitment occurs when the relationship between the levels at the two ears is the same for the loudness balances as it is at threshold. An example is shown in **Fig. 10.4c** and **Fig. 10.5c**. Here, the same 45 dB spread that exists between the left and right thresholds is also found for each of the loudness balances. This is seen as parallel lines on the laddergram. The situation is even clearer on the Steinberg-Gardner plot. In spite of the threshold difference between the ears, the line showing equally loud levels rises at a 45° angle just like the normal line. This shows that the spread between the two ears is maintained at high levels. It also means that a 20 dB increase in the abnormal ear sounds just as loud as a 20 dB increase in the normal ear; that is, loudness is growing at the same rate with increasing intensity in both ears. Consequently, loudness must be growing at the normal rate in the abnormal ear. As a practical guideline, one might say that there is no recruitment if equal loudness occurs at equal sensation levels (dB SL) ± l0 dB (Jerger 1962).

No recruitment is the expected result when the loss in the abnormal ear is conductive. In fact, Fowler (1936) originally conceived of the ABLB as a test to distinguish between otosclerosis (a conductive disorder) and sensorineural hearing losses. However, the ABLB is not used with conductive losses because its actual purpose is to help to distinguish between cochlear and retrocochlear disorders. Thus, finding no recruitment in a case of unilateral sensorineural loss is the same as failing to argue in favor of a cochlear disorder. By inference, this would lead us to suspect retrocochlear pathology.

In some cases, loudness grows at a slower than normal rate as intensity increases in the abnormal ear. This is called **decruitment** (Davis & Goodman 1966) or **loudness reversal** (Priede & Coles 1974) and is associated with retrocochlear pathology. In the example in **Fig. 10.4d**, 105 dB HL in the bad ear sounds only as loud as 30 dB HL in the good ear. In other words, 60 dB SL in the abnormal ear sounds like only 30 dB SL in the normal ear (**Fig. 10.5d**). In effect, loudness is lost rather than gained as intensity is raised.

ABLB Testing Approaches

Different procedures have been suggested for administering the ABLB. In Jerger's (1962) protocol, the tone alternates between the ears automatically every 500 milliseconds (as in **Fig. 10.2**), with the fixed level in the abnormal ear and the variable signal in the normal ear. The patient changes the intensity of the tone in the variable ear using the method of adjustment (see Chapter 3) until it sounds equal in loudness to the tone in the fixed ear. Loudness balances are made at 20 dB intervals above the bad ear's threshold, and are plotted on a laddergram.

One should note that because the tone alternates between the two ears every 500 milliseconds, it will be off for 500 milliseconds in each ear. This off-time ensures that the test tones will not be subject to adaptation. This requirement is met if the tone is off for at least a certain **critical off-time**, which is ~ 200 to 250 milliseconds (Dallos & Tillman 1966; Jerger & Jerger 1966; Tillman 1966).

Hood (1969, 1977) suggested manual control over the presentation of the tones according to the method of limits (see Chapter 3), using the good ear as the fixed-level ear, and plotting the results on a Steinberg-Gardner diagram. Others have suggested presenting the fixed-level tone to the bad ear and testing according to Hood's method (Priede & Coles 1974; Coles & Priede 1976), or randomizing the use of the good and bad ears as the fixed-level ear under computer control (Fritze 1978).

Actual ABLB techniques vary widely among audiologists, many of whom use hybrid methods. For example, one might use automatically alternating tones with the fixed level in the bad ear, employ a modified method of limits or bracketing, and have the patient respond with hand signals, or by saying "right," "left," or "equal."

An interesting ABLB modification by Miskolczy-Fodor (1964) uses the Bekesy tracking method (see below) to keep the level in the variable ear equally loud as the one in the reference ear, and the results are automatically plotted on paper. **Fig. 10.7** shows an example. Two sets of results must be combined for accurate loudness balances with this method, one using the good ear as the reference and one using the bad ear (Carver 1970; Gelfand 1976). Otherwise, it over- or underestimates the loudness balance points. Other variations have also been reported (Sung & Sung 1976).

Fig. 10.7 In Miskolczy-Fodor's modification of the ABLB, the level in the reference ("target") ear steadily rises instead of remaining fixed. The level in the variable ear is kept equally loud with the reference ear using a Bekesy tracking technique. Loudness balance tracings are shown here when the good ear is the reference, and when the poor ear is the reference. (From Gelfand [1976] with permission.)

Simultaneous versus Alternate Loudness Balance

The ABLB involves presenting the test tones alternately between the ears. This must be distinguished from presenting the tones to the two ears at the same time, which is called the **simultaneous binaural loudness balance test**. Jerger and Harford (1960) showed that the results of the alternate and simultaneous balance tests disagree in terms of which intensities are "equally loud" at the two ears. This happens because the two methods are testing two different things. The alternate balance test yields the levels that sound equally loud at the two ears. In contrast, the simultaneous test is really a lateralization task. In other words, presenting simultaneous tones to the two ears causes the patient to hear a single, fused image somewhere in the head between the left and right ears. Rather than showing the levels that cause the two sounds to be equally loud, the simultaneous test really shows the levels that cause the fused image to be lateralized in the middle of the head (which is called a "median-plane localization"). Consequently, one should not use simultaneous balances to measure equal loudness between the ears.

Alternate Monaural Loudness Balance Test

The ABLB often cannot be done because (1) it requires a normal ear (or at least an ear with normal hearing at the frequency being tested), and (2) most people with sensorineural losses have bilateral impairments. This dilemma was addressed with the **alternate monaural loudness balance (AMLB) test** (Reger 1935). The AMLB is similar to the ABLB except that the loudness balance is done for *two different tones within the same ear*. Consider a patient with a bilateral loss that slopes sharply above 1000 Hz. The thresholds in one of her ears might be 0 dB HL at 500 Hz and 50 dB at 2000 Hz. In such a case, 500 Hz and 2000 Hz tones might be alternately presented to the same ear. The level would remain fixed at one frequency, and the level at the other frequency would be varied up and down until the two tones sound equally loud. The results are interpreted in the same general way as for the ABLB, but a correction is needed to account for loudness level differences (Chapter 3) between frequencies (Denes & Naunton 1950). Moreover, the interfrequency loudness balance task tends to be difficult for many patients. The AMLB is rarely used because of these problems.

Diagnostic Accuracy of the ABLB

We can consider the ABLB from the standpoint of how well it distinguishes between cochlear disorders (where there should be recruitment) and retrocochlear pathologies (where there should be no recruitment or decruitment). The ABLB has been found to identify the correct site of lesion in ~ 90% of cases for cochlear disorders and only ~ 59% for retrocochlear pathologies across studies (Turner et al 1984). These figures show that many acoustic tumor cases are misclassified as cochlear on the basis of having positive recruitment. It is possible that some retrocochlear cases might have recruitment or other characteristics of cochlear disorders (e.g., high SISI scores; see below) because of *secondary damage* to the cochlea (Dix & Hallpike 1958; Benitez, Lopez-Rios, & Novon 1967; Perez de Moura 1967; Buus, Florentine, & Redden 1982a). The basic concept involves these two steps: (1) the tumor damages the cochlea by putting pressure on its blood supply and/or adversely altering the chemistry of the cochlear fluids; and (2) the resulting cochlear disorder then produces positive recruitment. Also, there may well be a coexisting cochlear disorder having nothing to do with retrocochlear pathology. For example, a patient with an acoustic tumor may well have a noise-induced cochlear impairment. These points apply to the results of other site-of-lesion tests as well.

■ Intensity Difference Limen Tests

Recall from Chapter 3 that the smallest difference in intensity that can be perceived is called the **difference limen for intensity (DLI)**. The DLI is smaller than normal in patients who have loudness recruitment, and thus several DLI tests have found their way into and out of clinical use over the years. The DLI tests assess one ear at a time, so they can be used with either bilateral or unilateral hearing losses.

In the **Lüscher-Zwislocki test** (1949) the patient heard an *amplitude-modulated (AM) tone* at 40 dB SL. An AM tone is one that undulates in level at a regular rate such as twice per second (**Fig. 10.8a**). The patient was asked to listen to this tone and to indicate whether it sounded continuous or if it seemed to undulate in level. This boils down to whether she can discern the intensity difference between the peaks and troughs of the undulating tone, which is called the *amount of amplitude modulation*. The smallest amount of AM that could be detected was thus the patient's difference limen for intensity. The DLIs were smaller for patients who had recruitment than for those without recruitment. This test was originally done at 40 dB SL, but modifications have been done at ≥ 80 dB HL (Lüscher 1951) and at 15 dB SL (Jerger 1952).

Another approach was used in the **Denes-Naunton test** (1950). Here, the patient was presented with a pair of tones, one after the other, and had to decide whether they were equal or if one was louder than the other (**Fig. 10.8b**). Many pairs of tones were presented to the patient. To find the DLI, the first tone was always kept at the same level, but the second tone would be changed in level (or vice versa). The procedure continued until the tester found the smallest level difference that the patient could detect. This was done for tone pairs presented at 4 dB SL and at 44 dB SL. The test was interpreted by comparing the *relative* sizes of the DLIs obtained at these two SLs. Intensity DLs were found to stay the same or get larger going from 4 dB SL to 44 dB SL in ears with recruitment. On the other hand, the DLIs were smaller at the higher SL in ears without recruitment. A modification by Jerger (1953) combined testing at two levels (10 and 40 dB SL) with the simpler-to-do AM procedure.

The use of these DLI tests almost came to an abrupt halt after Hirsh, Palva, and Goodman (1954) reported similar DLIs in recruiting, nonrecruiting, and normal ears. The discrepancies between their findings and those described above may partly be due to different methods of measuring the DLI, resulting in dissimilar results. [The interested student might see the discus-

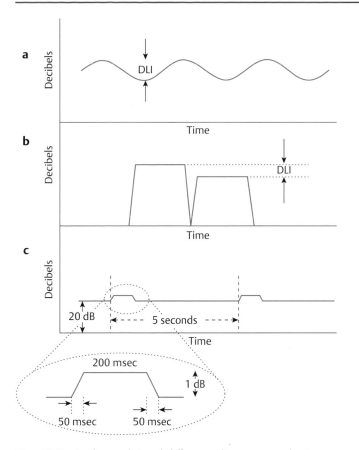

Fig. 10.8 In the traditional difference limen tests, the intensity difference limen (DLI) was determined by finding the smallest perceptible difference between **(a)** the peaks and troughs of an amplitude-modulated (AM) tone, or **(b)** the levels of two tones presented one after the other. **(c)** In the short increment sensitivity (SISI) test, the patient has to detect 1 dB increments that are superimposed on a carrier tone.

sions in Buus, Florentine, and Redden (1982a,b) or Gelfand (2010) in this regard.] There is also support for the distinction between the DLI and loudness recruitment (Lamoré & Rodenburg 1980). However, the DLI-recruitment controversy diverted the focus of the diagnostic issue, which has more to do with distinguishing between cochlear and retrocochlear sites of lesion than with whether abnormally small DLIs are akin to loudness recruitment.

■ Short Increment Sensitivity Index

The DLI issue was refocused by Jerger, Shedd, and Harford (1959), who pointed out that the ability to detect small intensity differences is useful in the dif-

ferential diagnosis no matter what the DLI-recruitment relation may or may not be. They also modified the nature of the intensity discrimination test, making the task easier for the patient to take, and easier for the clinician to administer and interpret. Instead of directly measuring the size of the DLI, their **short increment sensitivity index (SISI)** presents the patient with increments having a predetermined size of (usually) 1 dB, and simply asks her to indicate when she hears them.

The basic structure of the SISI is depicted in **Fig. 10.8c**, which shows that the stimulus in the SISI has two aspects. The first component is an ongoing tone that stays on for the entire duration of the test. This *carrier tone* is presented at 20 dB SL. The second element is a 200-millisecond increment of 1 dB that is superimposed on top of the carrier tone. Twenty 1 dB pulses are superimposed on the carrier tone, spaced at 5-second intervals; and the patient simply listens to the carrier tone and indicates whenever these brief pulses are heard.

Several 5 dB pulses, which are easily detected by almost everybody, are used at the start of the test to demonstrate the stimulus and to ensure that the patient knows how to respond appropriately. A familiarization/training strategy may be used, which begins with a 5 dB pulse, and then the sizes of the pips are reduced 1 dB at a time until reaching the 1 dB test increments (Harford 1967). A few other 5 dB pulses are scattered among the 1 dB increments to make sure the patient continues to respond properly. This is especially important when a patient is missing many or all of the 1 dB increments. In addition, several "catch trials" are distributed among the 1 dB pips over the course of the test. A catch trial is the *absence* of a pulse that occurs at a 5-second interval where a 1 dB pulse would have been presented. This helps to ensure that the patient is responding to the increments and not to just the expectation of a pulse every 5 seconds. These "nonpulses" are especially important when the patient is responding to many or all of the 1 dB increments. The 5 dB and empty trials are important for the proper administration of the SISI test because they provide the clinician with guidance about the validity of the results, and often indicate when it is necessary to reinstruct the patient or to make some other change. However, only the 20 one-decibel pulses are used to score the test.

The SISI test is scored by simply counting how many of the 1 dB increments out of the 20 were heard, and expressing the result in percent. For example, a SISI score of 100% means that all 20 pulses were heard, and a score of 40% means that only 8 of them were detected.

The fundamental principle of the SISI test is that many of the pulses should be heard if the ear being tested has a cochlear disorder. On the other hand, fewer increments should be detected if the test ear has a retrocochlear disorder, a conductive loss, or normal hearing. Presuming the test is done when there is a sensorineural hearing loss, this boils down to a distinction between cochlear and retrocochlear sites of lesion. Scores ≥ 70% are usually considered "positive" or "high," and suggest a cochlear disorder. Scores that are ≤ 30% are "negative" or "low," and suggest retrocochlear involvement if there is a sensorineural hearing loss. Results falling between these ranges are generally considered to be "questionable." However, the student should be aware that other cutoff values have been proposed over the years.

Jerger et al (1959) found that the SISI scores of eight patients with Meniere's disease were 70 to 100% at 1000 Hz and 95 to 100% at 4000 Hz, but were 0% at both frequencies for three retrocochlear cases. Also, SISI scores were only 0 to 15% for conductive losses. Patients with high-frequency sensorineural losses due to noise exposure had low scores (0 to 40%) at 1000 Hz where their thresholds were normal, and high scores (95 to 100%) at 4000 Hz where their thresholds were elevated. In their case, the low scores at 1000 Hz were the correct outcomes associated with normal sensitivity and not a false indication of retrocochlear impairment. Presbycusic patients, whose thresholds ranged between 0 and 65 dB HL at 1000 Hz and between 30 and 75 dB HL at 4000 Hz, had SISI scores anywhere from 0 to 100% at both frequencies. The wide range of scores for these patients with age-related hearing loss probably reflects the effects of both their widely disparate thresholds and the variety of the underlying disturbances that can cause presbycusis.

About 77 to 84% of cochlear impairments are correctly identified by high SISI scores and 60 to 65% of retrocochlear disorders are correctly revealed by low SISI scores (Buus et al 1982a; Turner et al 1984). Only ~ 5 to 10% of the ears in either group had SISI scores in the "questionable" range (Buus et al 1982a).

The **high-level SISI** attempts to improve the sensitivity of the test by administering it at high intensity levels, typically at 75 to 90 dB HL (Thompson 1963; Harbert, Young, & Weiss 1969; Sanders et al 1974; Cooper & Owen 1976). When administered at high intensity levels, high SISI scores are expected in normal ears and those with cochlear disorders, and low scores are expected with retrocochlear pathology. In actuality, the high-level SISI correctly identifies an average of ~ 90% of cochlear disorders but only 69% of retrocochlear pathologies across studies (Turner et al 1984). This is not much better than what we just saw for the standard (20 dB SL) version of the test.

■ Bekesy Audiometry

Recall from Chapter 5 that Bekesy (1947) audiometry allows the patient to track his own threshold by pressing and releasing a button. The button controls a motor, which in turn controls the attenuator, so that the level increases and decreases at a given rate (usually 2.5 dB/s). The patient is told to hold the button down when he can hear the tone and to release it when he cannot hear the tone. The patient does not press the button whenever the tone is too soft to hear. In this case the motor causes the intensity to rise, so that the tone will eventually become audible. Upon hearing the tone, the patient presses (and holds down) the response button. This causes the motor to reverse so that the intensity decreases. The tone then becomes inaudible and the patient releases the button, which in turn causes the intensity to rise, and so on. This course of events will cause the level of the tone to rise and fall around the patient's threshold. At the same time, the motor also controls a pen that tracks the level of the tone on paper, resulting in a zigzag pattern around the patient's threshold, as shown in **Fig. 5.7** of Chapter 5. The width of the zigzags is often called the excursion width, and the patient's threshold is the midpoint of these excursions.

Conventional Bekesy Audiometry

Bekesy audiograms are obtained either one frequency at a time or while the test frequency slowly changes from low to high. During **sweep-frequency Bekesy audiometry** the patient tracks his threshold while the frequency of the test tone increases smoothly from 100 to 10,000 Hz at a rate of one octave/second. During **fixed-frequency Bekesy audiometry**, the patient tracks his threshold at one frequency for a given period of time, such as 3 minutes. Each Bekesy audiogram is tracked twice, once using a continuous tone and once using a tone that pulses on and off 2.5 times a second, and the results are interpreted by comparing the **continuous** and **pulsed** (or **interrupted**) **tracings**.

Jerger (1960a, 1962) classified Bekesy audiograms into four basic types, although modifications of the original classification system have been described (Owens 1964b; Johnson & House 1964; Hopkinson 1966; Hughes, Winegar, & Crabtree 1967; Ehrlich 1971). The Bekesy types will be described principally in terms of the sweep frequency patterns, examples of which are shown in **Fig. 10.9**. In the **type I** Bekesy audiogram the pulsed and continuous tone tracings are interwoven, following the pattern of the patient's audiogram. This type is associated with those who have normal hearing or conductive hearing losses.

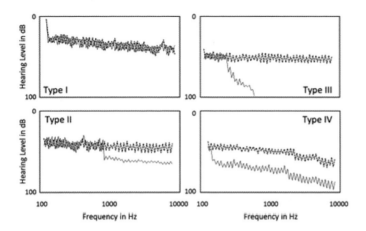

Fig. 10.9 Examples of the classical Bekesy audiogram types. The pulsed tracings are shown as dotted lines and the continuous tracings are shown as solid lines.

Type II is associated with cochlear impairments. Here the pulsed and continuous tracings are interwoven for frequencies up to roughly 1000 Hz. Two things happened at higher frequencies. First, the continuous tracing falls below the pulsed tracing by an amount that is usually less than 20 dB, and then runs parallel to it. In addition, the excursions of the continuous tracing narrow considerably, becoming only ~ 3 to 5 dB wide.

The shifting of the continuous tracing in Bekesy audiograms is generally interpreted as revealing the effects of tone decay (e.g., Harbert & Young 1964; Owens 1965; Parker & Decker 1971; Silman et al 1981). The narrowed excursion widths in the type II Bekesy audiogram reflect how intensity perception is affected by cochlear impairments, but the mechanism is controversial (e.g., Bekesy 1947; Denes & Naunton 1950; Hirsh et al 1954; Owens 1965). It is probably related to the intensity DL around threshold, but it is not a test of loudness recruitment per se.

In the distinctive **type III** pattern, the continuous tracing diverts very quickly from the pulsed tracing, often shifting to the limits of the audiometer. Type III is associated with retrocochlear pathologies.

In **type IV** the continuous tracing quickly falls more than 20 dB below the pulsed audiogram, and then runs parallel to it. Type IV Bekesy audiograms may occur in patients with cochlear or retrocochlear disorders, but they are often taken to suggest the possibility of the latter (e.g., Turner et al 1984).

A fifth Bekesy pattern, called **type V**, was described by Jerger and Herer (1961). It is distinctive because the pulsed tracing falls below the continuous one. The type V Bekesy audiogram is associated with functional (or nonorganic) hearing loss and is described in greater detail in Chapter 14.

Forward-Backward Bekesy Audiometry

Rose (1962) reported that the difference between the continuous and pulsed tracings on sweep-frequency audiograms can be larger when the frequency sweep goes from high to low (backward) compared with the normal direction from low to high (forward). This difference is called the **forward-backward discrepancy**. Large forward-backward discrepancies are associated with retrocochlear pathologies (Kärjä & Palva 1969; Palva, Kärjä, & Palva 1970; Jerger, Jerger, & Mauldin 1972; Jerger & Jerger 1974a; Rose, Kurdziel, Olsen, & Noffsinger 1975).

Fig. 10.10 illustrates how the forward-backward discrepancy using an approach like the one described by Jerger et al (1972) can identify a retrocochlear disorder that would have been missed with standard Bekesy audiometry. There are three Bekesy tracings in each frame, one pulsed and two continuous. The pulsed tracing goes in the forward direction (increasing in frequency from 200 to 8000 Hz). One of the continuous tracings goes in the forward direction (from 200 to 8000 Hz). However, the other continuous tracing goes in the backward direction (decreasing in frequency from 8000 to 200 Hz). All three tracings are superimposed for the patient's normal right ear (upper panel). However, there is a forward-backward discrepancy for her left ear, which has an acoustic neuroma (lower panel). Notice that the backward continuous tracing falls far below the pulsed tracing even though there is much less separation between the tracings for the pulsed tone and the forward continuous sweep (which would have been type II).

Bekesy Comfortable Loudness Testing

Bekesy Comfortable Loudness (BCL) testing is similar to conventional sweep-frequency audiometry except the patient is instructed to press and release the response button to keep the tone "at a comfortable loudness level, neither too loud nor too soft" (Jerger & Jerger 1974a, p. 352). Jerger and Jerger identify three BCL configurations considered to be negative because they were associated with normal hearing and with conductive and cochlear impairments. The pulsed and continuous tracings were interwoven in type N1. The continuous trac-

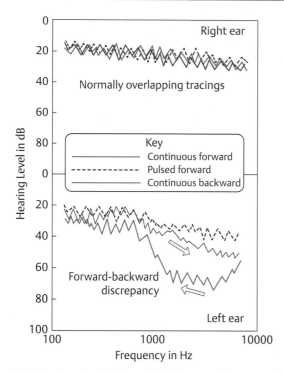

Fig. 10.10 Forward-backward Bekesy audiograms in a patient with an acoustic tumor in the left ear. The upper frame shows normal overlapping of the three tracings in the unaffected right ear. The lower frame shows a forward-backward discrepancy in the pathological left ear.

■ Brief-Tone Audiometry

Brief-tone audiometry involves measuring the thresholds of tones having very short durations. It is the clinical application of **temporal summation (integration)**, which occurs when sounds are shorter than about one third of a second. Recall from Chapter 3 that three normal-hearing people need a 10 dB level change to compensate for a 10-times change in duration; however, a smaller level change is needed for patients with cochlear impairments to offset a 10-times change in duration (Sanders & Honig 1967; Wright 1968, 1978; Hattler & Northern 1970; Barry & Larson 1974; Pedersen 1976; Olsen, Rose, & Noffsinger 1974; Chung & Smith 1980). In other words, the intensity-duration relationship (the temporal integration function) is typically shallower than normal when there is a cochlear impairment. This can be seen by comparing frames a and b in **Fig. 10.11**.

Brief-tone audiometry usually involves Bekesy audiometry, which is why it is discussed at this point. However, other approaches have also been used. The basic testing method is quite simple. Bekesy audiograms are obtained using pulsing tones with various durations, and the resulting thresholds are assessed to determine how much of a threshold change is needed to offset a duration difference. The clinician might test enough durations to plot a diagram such as those in the figure, or test at just two represen-

ing tracked above the pulsed in type N2 and below it in type N3. There were also three positive BCL patterns that were associated with retrocochlear disorders: The continuous tracings fell very far below the pulsed tracings at high frequencies in the type P1 pattern and at low and/or middle frequencies in type P2. The P3 pattern involved a forward-backward discrepancy for the BCL tracings. Nineteen percent of the retrocochlear cases and 8% of the other ears did not fit into the six categories.

Sensitivity and Specificity of Bekesy Audiometry

On average across studies, the correct identification rates for cochlear and retrocochlear disorders, respectively, are ~ 93% and 49% for conventional Bekesy audiometry, 95% and 71% for forward-backward Bekesy, and 92% and 85% for Bekesy Comfortable Loudness (Turner et al 1984).

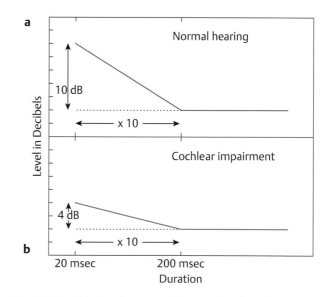

Fig. 10.11 Idealized temporal integration functions showing the trade-off between intensity and duration needed to reach threshold for a tone when there is **(a)** normal hearing and **(b)** cochlear impairment.

tative durations. Wright (1978) suggested that comparing the thresholds for tones having 20 and 500 ms durations is an efficient clinical approach.

Normal and cochlear-impaired ears are typically distinguished with brief-tone audiometry, but the principal clinical question deals with distinguishing between cochlear and retrocochlear disorders. Early findings were optimistic (Sanders, Josey, & Kemker 1971), but subsequent work found too much overlap between the results for cochlear and retrocochlear disorders for brief-tone audiometry to be a viable diagnostic test in this regard (Pedersen 1976; Stephens 1976; Olsen et al 1974; Olsen 1987).

■ Loudness Discomfort and Tolerance Tests

It has been known for a very long time that many patients with recruiting hearing losses complain that high-level sounds are uncomfortably loud. In the past, this relationship was sometimes assessed with a tuning fork test. After establishing the presence of a hearing loss, the clinician would strike the tuning fork very hard (so that it produced a high-intensity sound) and immediately place it near the impaired ear. If the patient perceived the sound to be extremely (uncomfortably) loud in spite of his hearing loss, then the test was considered to reflect "nerve deafness."

The contemporary approach is to determine the patient's **loudness discomfort level (LDL)** or **uncomfortable loudness level (UCL),** which may be used to infer the presence of loudness recruitment, although more important applications of the LDL are in the areas of amplification and the evaluation and management of patients with hyperacusis (Chapter 15). Here, the audiologist obtains the patient's LDL and compares it to normative values. Typically, LDLs occur at ~ 100 dB SPL in normal-hearing individuals, (Hood & Poole 1966; Hood 1969; Morgan, Wilson, & Dirks 1974), although mean LDLs of 102 to 104 dB HL (or ~ 111–115 dB SPL) were found by Sherlock and Formby (2005). Loudness recruitment would be considered present if LDL is found at these normal levels, in which case the result would be interpreted as consistent with a cochlear impairment. Obtaining the LDL at higher levels would be considered to indicate no recruitment, which would be expected if the sensorineural loss is of retrocochlear origin. Another version of the test is to obtain the most comfortable listening level (MCL) as well as the LDL.

In spite of tradition, the LDL has several serious limitations when it is applied as a test of recruitment. First, large LDL differences have been reported between people, so that the normal range of LDLs is very wide (Sherlock & Formby 2005). Second, the LDL reflects the patient's tolerance level rather than abnormally rapid loudness growth. Third, its use in this way rests on the faulty assumption that the LDL is not related to the amount of hearing loss. In fact, however, LDLs get higher as the amount of sensorineural hearing loss increases above ~ 50 dB HL (Kamm, Dirks, & Mickey 1978).

Loudness Scaling

While uncomfortable loudness measurements are ubiquitous, there is no universal method for their measurement (Punch, Joseph, & Rakerd 2004). Clinical loudness measurements can also be accomplished using *direct scaling* methods such as magnitude estimation and magnitude production, as well as by cross-modality matching (e.g., Geller & Margolis 1984; Knight & Margolis 1984; Hellman & Meiselman 1988, 1990). However, *category rating* methods are more commonly used in contemporary audiological practice. In category rating, the patient listens to sounds presented at different levels one at a time, and rates the loudness of each of them based on a list that provides a choice of descriptive categories from very soft to very loud (e.g., Allen, Hall, & Jeng 1990; Hawkins, Walden, Montgomery, & Prosek 1987; Cox 1995; Cox, Alexander, Taylor, & Gray 1997). For example, the **Contour Test** (Cox 1995; Cox et al 1997) uses pulsed warble tone stimuli in response to which the patient gives numerical loudness ratings based on a seven-point scale, as follows: (1) *very soft*, (2) *soft*, (3) *comfortable but slightly soft*, (4) *comfortable*, (5) *comfortable but slightly loud*, (6) *loud but OK*, and (7) *uncomfortably loud*. Sherlock and Formby (2005) found no significant differences between directly measured LDLs and "uncomfortably loud" levels obtained with the Contour Test.

Loudness category rating methods have been adapted for use with children by having them choose ratings from a card showing various descriptive line drawings corresponding to the loudness categories (e.g., Kawell, Kopun, & Stelmachowicz 1988; Skinner 1988).

■ Assessment of Cochlear Dead Regions

Recall from Chapter 6 that **dead regions** are locations along the cochlear spiral without functioning inner hair cells (IHCs) and/or auditory neurons. We would expect there to be no response to a test tone that activates such a dead region. Yet it is still possible for the patient to detect it due to **off-frequency listen-**

ing, which means that part of the vibration pattern caused by the test tone is picked up by functioning IHCs at nearby locations along the basilar membrane (e.g., Moore 2004). For example, a patient with a dead zone at the 2000 Hz place might still respond to a 2000 Hz test tone if part of its excitation pattern activates healthy IHCs at the 1800 Hz location (**Fig. 10.12**). We often need to know about dead regions because they have implications for pitch, loudness and speech perception, hearing aids and other instruments, and patient counseling (McDermott, Lech, Kornblum, & Irvine 1998; Baer, Moore, & Kluk 2002; Moore 2004; Huss & Moore 2005; Kluk & Moore 2006).

Dead regions are suspected when patients have sensorineural hearing losses with steeply sloping audiograms and/or frequencies with thresholds of 70 dB HL or more; however, it is important to remember that the audiogram itself is not a reliable indicator of whether or not dead regions are actually present (e.g., Vinay & Moore 2007). Hence, special techniques may be used to identify dead regions when they are suspected. One approach is to obtain **psychoacoustic tuning curves (PTCs)** for the suspect frequencies (e.g., Summers et al 2003; Kluk & Moore 2005; Sek, Alcántara, Moore, Kluk, & Wicher 2005). Recall from Chapter 3 that the peak of a PTC normally occurs at the frequency of the signal tone. When there is a cochlear dead region, the PTC peak is found to be shifted to the edge of the dead region. However, PTCs involve several technical considerations (e.g., Kluk & Moore 2004, 2005) that make them somewhat cumbersome for regular clinical use.

Another (and clinically more feasible) test for identifying cochlear dead regions is the **TEN Test** (Moore, Huss, Vickers, Glasberg, & Alcántara 2000; Moore, Glasberg, & Stone 2004), so named because it uses **threshold-equalizing noise (TEN)**. Threshold-equalizing noise is a masking noise designed to produce the same masked thresholds at all frequencies (i.e., an 80 dB TEN level should produce an 80 dB masked threshold at every frequency tested). The test originally used sound pressure levels (**TEN-SPL**; Moore et al 2000), but it now uses hearing level (HL) measurements in 2 dB steps at audiometric frequencies between 500 and 4000 Hz (**TEN-HL**; Moore et al 2004).

Testing involves obtaining unmasked thresholds for the test tones followed by masked thresholds using the TEN. If the test tone is *not* in a dead region, then the masked threshold will be about equal to the TEN level, or *less than* 10 dB above it. If the test tone *is* in a dead region, then the masked threshold will be *at least* 10 dB higher than the TEN level. For example, suppose a patient's unmasked threshold is 70 dB HL at 2000 Hz, and the TEN is presented at 80 dB HL (to produce a threshold shift). The masked threshold would be *less than 90 dB HL* if there is *no* dead region (because the 2000 Hz tone is detected at the 2000 Hz place; see **Fig. 10.12a**). However, the masked threshold would be *90 dB HL or higher* if there *is* a dead region (because the 2000 Hz tone is actually detected at the 1800 Hz place, where the vibration amplitude is weaker (see **Fig. 10.12b**).

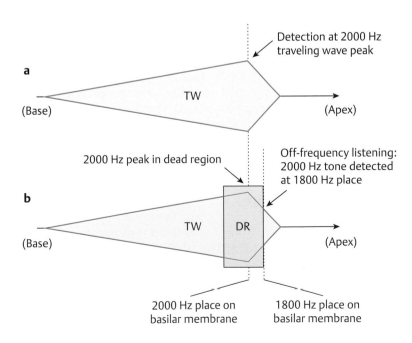

Fig. 10.12 **(a)** A test tone is typically detected at the location of the traveling wave (TW) peak. **(b)** If the traveling wave peaks in a dead region (DR), then the test tone might still be detected by off-frequency listening at a nearby location that has functional inner hair cells.

■ (Central) Auditory Processing Evaluation

Recall from Chapter 6 that (central) auditory processing disorders [(C)APDs] involve a wide variety of sound perception difficulties other than those due to hearing losses per se that result from sensorineural and/or conductive (peripheral) disorders. Many (C)APD tests have been associated with organic lesions or diseases affecting identifiable regions of the brain, and these associations will be mentioned for the tests described below. However, the preponderance of auditory processing disorders are not associated with clearly identifiable organic causes. Thus, (C)APD evaluations frequently focus on identifying and describing the existence and nature of the patient's auditory perceptual problems and how they present challenges for the patient, and leading to interventions that will improve her situation.

The (central) auditory processing evaluation itself involves assessing perceptual functions using a battery composed of behavioral and physiological measures (e.g., Jerger & Musiek 2000; ASHA 2005; Musiek & Chermak 2006; AAA 2010). However, specific test choices are typically left to the clinician, and notable differences do exist among the various specific batteries that have been proposed, at least in terms of the basic groups of tests that are always included (see, e.g., Jerger & Musiek 2000; Medwetsky 2002; ASHA 2005; Bellis 2006; Keith 2009a,b; AAA 2010; Musiek, Chermak, Weihing, Zappulla, & Nagle 2011; Martin, Billiet, & Bellis 2013; Katz n.d.).

Complicating matters is the fact that (C)APDs have behavioral manifestations in common with many other problems, and often coexist with them as comorbid conditions, especially in children. These include speech-language and learning disorders, autistic spectrum disorders, attention deficit hyperactivity disorder, and auditory neuropathy spectrum disorder, as well as problems with memory, attention, and other aspects of cognitive function.

In addition, considerable controversy exists about whether *modality specificity* is necessary for a valid diagnosis of (C)APD to be made, that is, whether the patient's problems must be particular to the auditory realm rather than being manifested in other modalities as well (e.g., Cacace & McFarland 2005a,b, 2008, 2013; Katz & Tillery 2005; Musiek, Bellis, & Chermak 2005; Rosen 2005). There appears to be general agreement that functioning in other modalities should at least be considered in some way. However, the recommendations for how to do this include such widely disparate approaches as considering cognitive and attention issues when auditory test results disagree, assessments by a multidisciplinary team, and the use of specially designed tests that compare performance on analogous auditory and nonauditory (e.g., visual) tasks (e.g., AAA 2010; Bellis & Ross 2011; Bellis, Billiet, & Ross 2011; Cacace & McFarland 2013; Weihing, Bellis, Chermak, & Musiek 2013). All things considered, *absolute* modality specificity does not appear to be a viable requirement, so (C)APD is an appropriate diagnosis when the patient's difficulties are *primarily* auditory in nature (e.g., ASHA 2005).

The major categories of these behavioral tests are enumerated in **Table 10.2**, along with examples of the kinds of tasks involved. Notice that both speech and non-speech materials are used. Many of the specific tests are discussed below or elsewhere in this chap-

Table 10.2 Categories of behavioral auditory perceptual tests and examples of the tasks involved in each category (ASHA 2005; AAA 2010)

Test category	Examples of tasks
Auditory discrimination	• Difference limens for frequency, level, temporal characteristics • Psychoacoustic tuning curves • Phoneme discrimination
Binaural interactions	• Masking level differences • Lateralization and/or localization • Tracking of fused images
Dichotic speech	• Dichotic digit, word, CV, and/or sentence tests
Monaural low-redundancy speech recognition	• Recognition of monaurally presented speech degraded by low- or high-pass filtering; noise, babble, or competing speech; time alterations like speeding, etc.
Temporal processing	• Frequency and/or duration sequences and/or patterns; gap detection • Temporal resolution, integration • Fusion discrimination • Temporal masking

ter, and the physiological assessment techniques are addressed in Chapters 7 and 11. Before proceeding, however, it is important to point out that patients being seen for auditory processing assessments also require complete audiological evaluations, and it is assumed that this has been done.

Non-Speech Tests

Although many commonly used central auditory processing tests involve the use of speech materials, tests using tonal or noise signals are also used. These kinds of signals are used when they are the most appropriate stimuli for testing the perceptual skills of interest. In addition, they have the advantage of minimizing (or at least reducing) the complicating effects of linguistic factors when trying to focus on auditory processing skills. Three examples of non-speech measures of auditory processing are included here, including tests of temporal gap detection, pitch pattern sequences, and masking level differences.

Recall from Chapter 3 that the **gap detection threshold** is simply the briefest silent gap that can be heard between two signals, and is a measure of auditory *temporal resolution*. Several clinical tests of gap detection have been introduced. In the **Random Gap Detection Test** (**RGDT**; Keith 2000), the listener is presented with a series of noise bursts (or tone bursts) containing various gap durations, and must indicate whether the gap was heard in each case. In contrast, the **Adaptive Test of Temporal Resolution** (**ATTR**; Lister, Roberts, Shackelford, & Roberts 2006) presents the listener with a choice of two noise bursts, and he must indicate which of them contains the gap. The test is adaptive because the duration of the silent gap is increased and decreased until the gap detection threshold has been found. The **Gaps-in-Noise (GIN) test** (Musiek et al 2005) uses a different strategy. Here, the patient listens to a series of white noise signals, each lasting a total of 6 seconds. Each noise signal is interrupted by one, two, or three silent gaps, and each gap might last from as little as 2 ms to as long as 20 ms. The patient's task is to push a response button whenever she detects a gap. Musiek et al (2005) showed that patients with confirmed disorders of the central auditory nervous system have significantly longer gap detection thresholds on the GIN test compared with normal individuals.

In the **Pitch Pattern Sequence Test** (Pinheiro 1977; Pinheiro & Musiek 1985), the patient is presented with "high" (1430 Hz) and "low" (880 Hz) brief tones at a readily audible level in groups of three. After hearing each sequence, the patient indicates the *temporal order* of the tones (e.g., *high-low-low*, *high-low-high*, etc.) verbally or manually, and/

or by humming the tonal sequence. It appears that patients with auditory cortex lesions on either side perform poorly for all response modes, while those with inter-hemispheric lesions perform relatively better with the humming response. Musiek, Baran, and Pinheiro (1990) also described a test that uses sequences of longer (500 ms) and shorter (250 ms) tone bursts instead of different pitches (e.g., *long-long-short, short-long-short*). They found that the duration patterns test is also sensitive to cerebral disorders, and that some patients with these disorders do poorly for duration patterns even if they have normal performance on the pitch patterns test.

Binaural **masking level differences (MLDs)** are useful clinically because they depend on the successful processing of binaural signals at the brainstem level to achieve binaural release from masking. Recall from Chapter 3 that the MLD is obtained by comparing two measurements. One of them is the noise level needed to mask a signal when both the signal and the noise are in-phase at both ears: S_oN_o. The other value is the noise level needed to mask the signal when just the signal is out-of-phase at the two ears, but the noise is in-phase: $S_\pi N_o$ (or vice versa, S_oN_π). The MLD is equal to either $S_\pi N_o$ minus S_oN_o, or S_oN_π minus S_oN_o. Clinical MLDs are usually done with a 500 Hz tone and/or with spondee words, and have been studied extensively (e.g., Noffsinger, Olsen, Carhart, Hart, & Sahgal 1972; Olsen & Noffsinger 1976; Olsen, Noffsinger, & Carhart 1976; Lynn, Gilroy, Taylor, & Leiser 1981; Hendler, Squires, & Emmerich 1990). Masking level differences have been found to be abnormally small or absent when there is multiple sclerosis or other disorders involving the brainstem, but tend to be unaffected by cortical lesions. However, one must be mindful that impaired MLDs are also caused by peripheral hearing losses. In fact, one must always consider the impact of a patient's hearing loss when interpreting central auditory tests because most of them are compromised by peripheral impairments to a greater or lesser extent.

Speech Tests

Monaural central auditory tests involve materials that are presented to just one ear. They are known as **distorted, degraded**, or **low-redundancy speech tests** because the speech materials are degraded in some way to reduce the amount of information that can be derived from the signal (Bocca 1958; Calearo & Lazzaroni 1957; Jerger 1960b; Bocca & Calearo 1963). The speech materials are usually distorted by low-pass filtering, accelerating the speech rate (time compression), rapid interruptions, or presenting the speech against a background of noise. An example of this approach is shown in the left panel of **Fig. 10.13**, which illustrates the **low-pass filtered speech test**. Here, a filter is used to remove the higher frequencies, so the patient must rely on only the lower frequencies (such as those below 750 Hz) to repeat the test words or sentences.

These types of tests are often considered to assess *auditory closure* because to correctly identify the test words the listener must use top-down (central) processes to *fill in* the information that is missing in the stimulus due to filtering, noise, or forms of degradation. In terms of the classical conceptualization by Bocca and Calearo (1963), successful speech recognition takes advantage of both the "intrinsic redundancy" that is built into the central auditory pathways and the "extrinsic redundancy" that is provided by the multiplicity of cues in the speech signal. Intrinsic redundancy is impaired by a central auditory lesion, and extrinsic redundancy is reduced by distorting the speech signal. Even though intrinsic redundancy is impaired in a patient who has a central lesion, he can often perform well with *un*distorted speech materials by relying on extrinsic redundancy. The normal person can perform comparably well on distorted speech tests by relying on intrinsic redundancy. In contrast, patients with auditory processing deficits affecting these skills perform poorly when the extrinsic redundancy is reduced by degrading the speech. When these processes are impaired by frank lesions of the brain, abnormally poor results in a given ear are typically associated with pathologies of the auditory cortex on the *opposite side* of the brain, but can also be associated with brainstem disorders.

In **dichotic tests** different speech signals are simultaneously presented to both ears, and the patient must repeat either one or both of them. The tasks are often described as *free recall* when the patient is asked to repeat what was heard in both ears

in any order, *directed recall* when she must repeat both of them in a designated order (right ear first or left ear first), and *binaural separation* when she is to repeat what was heard in one ear while ignoring the speech presented to other ear.

The most common dichotic techniques include the Dichotic Digits test (Kimura 1961; Musiek 1983), Dichotic Consonant-Vowel (CV) Syllables test (Berlin, Lowe-Bell, Jannetta, & Kline 1972; Speaks, Gray, & Miller 1975; Berlin et al 1975), Willeford's Competing Sentences Test (Ivey 1969), and the Staggered Spondaic Word Test (Katz 1962, 1968). Separate scores are obtained for each ear, and the principal clinical finding is that performance is lower in the ear opposite to a cortical lesion. This is consistent with the opposite ear effect already mentioned for the low-redundancy monaural tests. However, when dealing with frank brain lesions, one must be careful about inferring the location of the disorder because dichotic test scores are also affected by brainstem disorders and by deep lesions of the higher pathways and the corpus callosum.

The test items on the **Dichotic Digits Test** are the numbers from "one" to "ten" (except "seven," which has two syllables). As represented in the left panel of **Fig. 10.14**, each presentation includes one digit that goes to the right ear and a different digit that simultaneously goes to the left ear. The patient must repeat both digits, and receives a separate percent correct score for each ear. A similar approach is involved in the **Dichotic CV Test**, except that competing stimuli are CV monosyllables (usually /pa, ta, ka, ba, da, ga/), as shown in the right panel of **Fig. 10.14**. The **Competing Sentences Test** simultaneously presents different sentences to each ear, as illustrated in **Fig. 10.15**. Separate scores are obtained for each, but two different scoring methods have been used. In one method, the patient is asked to repeat only the sentence presented to the right (or left) ear, while ignoring the

a   Low-pass filtered speech test   **b**   Binaural Fusion Test   **c**   Rapidly alternating speech test

Fig. 10.13   Illustrations of the **(a)** low-pass filtered speech test, **(b)** Binaural Fusion Test, and **(c)** rapidly alternating speech test.

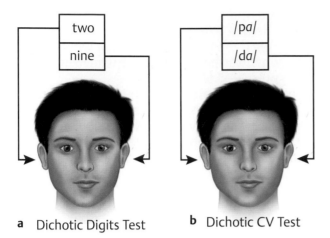

a Dichotic Digits Test   b Dichotic CV Test

Fig. 10.14 Illustrations of **(a)** the Dichotic Digits Test and **(b)** the Dichotic CV Test. In these tests, the patient is asked to repeat both stimuli.

Competing Sentences Test

Fig. 10.15 Illustration of the Competing Sentences Test. In this test, the patient may be asked to repeat both sentences, or to repeat one sentence while ignoring the other one.

sentence in the opposite ear. This is done twice, once for each ear. The alternate method involves having the patient repeat both of the sentences, which are scored separately for each ear.

The **Staggered Spondaic Word (SSW) Test** uses dichotically presented spondee words. However, the two words do not overlap completely in time. Instead, one of the spondees begins earlier than the other one so that (1) the second syllable of the spondee in one ear overlaps with the first syllable of the spondee in the other ear, but (2) the first syllable of one word and the second syllable of the other word are not overlapping. The right and left ears get an equal number of leading and trailing words. This paradigm sounds confusing but it is really quite simple, as shown in **Fig. 10.16**. In effect, only the overlapping syllables ("light" and "lunch" in the figure) are in dichotic competition, whereas the other two ("day" and "time") are noncompeting syllables. Even though we are addressing the SSW simply as a dichotic test in this introductory discussion, a complete interpretation actually considers several test findings, relationships, and nuances that appear to improve its ability to identify the location of a central disorder (see Katz & Ivey 1994).

The **Synthetic Sentence Identification (SSI) Test** (Speaks & Jerger 1965; Jerger, Speaks, & Trammell 1968) involves identifying meaningless but syntactically correct sentences in the presence of a competing message (Chapter 8). The test is referred to as the SSI with an **ipsilateral competing message (SSI-ICM)** when the test sentences and competition (a continuous story) are in the same ear, and as the SSI with a **contralateral competing message (SSI-CCM)**

when the message and competition are in opposite ears. These conditions are illustrated in **Fig. 10.17**. The relative level between the SSI sentences and the competing message is called the **message-to-competition ratio (MCR)**, which is analogous to signal-to-noise ratio. The SSI-ICM and SSI-CCM are done at various MCRs to obtain a performance-intensity function for the SSI (PI-SSI) for both conditions in each ear. The PI-SSI functions are compared with each other and also with the patient's PL-PB

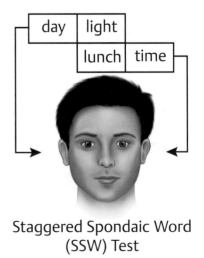

Staggered Spondaic Word
(SSW) Test

Fig. 10.16 Illustration of Staggered Spondaic Word (SSW) Test. Notice how two of the syllables overlap in time ("light" and "lunch"), whereas the other two syllables do not overlap in time ("day" and "time").

Fig. 10.17 Illustration of **(a)** Synthetic Sentence Identification Test with an ipsilateral competing message (SSI-ICM) and **(b)** a contralateral competing message (SSI-CCM). Notice that the SSI-ICM is a monotic test, whereas the SSI-CCM involves a dichotic paradigm.

functions[3] (J. Jerger & S. Jerger 1974a,b, 1975b; Jerger & Hayes 1977; S. Jerger & J. Jerger 1975, 1981). Brainstem disorders are associated with poorer SSI results when the competition is ipsilateral rather than when it is contralateral (SSI-ICM is worse than SSI-CCM). In contrast, temporal lobe lesions are associated with poorer performance when the competing message is in the contralateral ear than when it is in the same ear (SSI-CCM is worse than SSI-ICM). As expected, the abnormally poor results are usually found in the ear on the opposite side of the cortical disorder.

Binaural integration or **resynthesis tests** involve presenting part of the speech signal to one ear and part of it to the other ear. Neither ear gets enough of the signal to allow adequate speech reception. As a result, the signals being presented to the two ears must be "put together," "integrated," or "resynthesized" by the central auditory nervous system. Several types of tests have been used. In the **Binaural Fusion Test** (Matzker 1959; Ivey 1969), filtering is used to produce a low-frequency band (e.g., 500 to 700 Hz) and a high-frequency band (e.g., 1900 to 2100 Hz) for each test word. The low-frequency band of a word goes to one ear and the high-fre-

quency band of the same word simultaneously goes to the other ear, as represented in the middle panel of **Fig. 10.13**. The presentation of a low-pass filtered word to one ear and an unfiltered but very faint version of the same word to the other ear has also been used (e.g., Jerger 1960b). Poor performance on the binaural fusion tests is generally associated with abnormalities affecting the brainstem.

In the **Rapidly Alternating Speech Perception Test** (Bocca & Calearo 1963; Lynn & Gilroy 1977) sentences are switched back and forth between the two ears at a quick rate, e.g., every 300 milliseconds, as illustrated in the right panel of **Fig. 10.13**. At any given moment there is speech in one ear and silence in the other ear, but the whole message is present binaurally. The **Speech With Alternating Masking Index** (**SWAMI**; Jerger 1964) was a variation of this test in which a masking noise (instead of silence) is directed into the ear not receiving the speech at any given time. Difficulty on the rapidly alternating speech test is usually associated with brainstem abnormalities and also with diffuse cortical problems.

When people with normal auditory processing capabilities listen to speech in the presence of noise or competition, they find it easier if the speech and noise are coming from different locations in space compared with when both come from the same location. The **Listening In Spatialized Noise (LISN) Test** (Cameron, Dillon, & Newall 2006a; Cameron & Dillon

---

[3] Review the section on PL-PB functions in Chapter 8 if these terms and concepts are not clear.

2007) assesses the patient's ability to take advantage of spatial separation by comparing speech reception for two loudspeaker arrangements in space, which are *simulated* using binaural signals presented through earphones. In one simulated condition, a speech stimulus comes from a loudspeaker in front of the patient and competing speech comes from the *same* speaker (i.e., both signal and noise from 0° azimuth). In the other simulated condition, the speech comes from a speaker in front of the patient and competing speech comes from two *different* speakers located to his right and left (i.e., signal from 0° azimuth and competition from ± 90° azimuth).

In the *continuous discourse* version of the test (**LISN-CD**; Cameron et al 2006a), the level of a story is kept constant while the level of the competing speech is raised and lowered to find the competition level at which the story is rated "just understandable" by the patient. This is done for both conditions of the test, and the *difference* between them reveals how well the patient is able to take advantage of spatial separation of speech and competition.[4] The LISN-CD can be used with patients who are at least 7 years old (Cameron, Dillon, & Newall 2006b), and performance on the test is impaired in patients with (C)APD (Cameron, Dillon, & Newall 2005, 2006c).

The *sentence* version of the test (**LISN-S**; Cameron & Dillon 2007) uses sentence stimuli that must be repeated by the patient as the level of the competing speech is raised and lowered to find the MCR needed for 50% sentence reception performance (i.e., an SRT). As in the prior version, this is done for (a) both signal and competition at 0° azimuth, and (b) signal at 0° azimuth with competition from ± 90° azimuth; and the *difference* between them shows the advantage provided by spatial separation. The LISN-S may be used with children as young as 6 years of age.

■ Study Questions

1. Define tone decay (or adaptation) and describe the clinical implication of abnormal tone decay.
2. Describe how threshold tone decay testing is performed.
3. Define loudness recruitment.
4. Describe the alternate binaural loudness balance test (ABLB).

5. What are the clinical implications of complete (or hyper-) recruitment versus no recruitment (or decruitment) in a patient who has a sensorineural hearing loss?
6. Describe the short increment sensitivity index (SISI).
7. Describe how Bekesy audiometry is performed.
8. What are cochlear dead regions?
9. What is the masking level difference (MLD) and how is it used as a central auditory test?
10. What are dichotic listening tests and how are they used in central auditory assessment?

References

Allen JB, Hall JL, Jeng PS. Loudness growth in ½-octave bands (LGOB)—a procedure for the assessment of loudness. J Acoust Soc Am 1990;88(2):745–753

American Academy of Audiology (AAA). 2010. Clinical Practice Guidelines: Diagnosis, Treatment and Management of Children and Adults with Central Auditory Processing Disorder. Available at: http://www.audiology.org/resources/documentlibrary/documents/capd%20guidelines%208-2010.pdf

American Speech-Language-Hearing Association (ASHA). 2005. (Central) Auditory Processing Disorders. Rockville Pike, MD: ASHA

Antonelli AR, Bellotto R, Grandori F. Audiologic diagnosis of central versus eighth nerve and cochlear auditory impairment. Audiology 1987;26(4):209–226

Baer T, Moore BCJ, Kluk K. Effects of low pass filtering on the intelligibility of speech in noise for people with and without dead regions at high frequencies. J Acoust Soc Am 2002;112(3 Pt 1):1133–1144

Barry SJ, Larson VD. Brief-tone audiometry with normal and deaf school-age children. J Speech Hear Disord 1974;39:457–464

Bekesy G. A new audiometer. Arch Otolaryngol 1947;35: 411–422

Bellis TJ. 2006. Audiologic behavioral assessment of APD. In: Parthasarathy TK, ed. An Introduction to Auditory Processing Disorders in Children. Mahwah, NJ: Erlbaum; 63–80

Bellis, TJ, Ross J. Performance of normal adults and children on central auditory diagnostic tests and their corresponding visual analogs. J Am Acad Audiol 2011; 22:491–500

Bellis TJ, Billiet C, Ross J. The utility of visual analogs of central auditory tests in the differential diagnosis of (central) auditory processing disorder and attention deficit hyperactivity disorder. J Am Acad Audiol 2011; 22:501–514

Benitez J, Lopez-Rios G, Novon V. Bilateral acoustic tumor: a human temporal bone study. Arch Otolaryngol 1967;86:51–57

Berlin CI, Cullen JK, Hughes LF, Berlin JL, Lowe-Bell SS, Thompson CL. 1975. Dichotic processing of speech: acoustic and phonetic variables. In: Sullivan MD, ed.

---

[4] These measures are actually done for two talker conditions, one with the signal and competition spoken by the same person, and another condition in which the signal and competition are spoken by different people.

Central Auditory Processing Disorders. Omaha, NE: University of Nebraska; 36–46

Berlin CI, Lowe-Bell SS, Jannetta PJ, Kline DG. Central auditory deficits after temporal lobectomy. Arch Otolaryngol 1972;96(1):4–10

Bocca E. Clinical aspects of cortical deafness. Laryngoscope 1958;68(3):301–309

Bocca E, Calearo C. 1963. Central hearing processes. In: Jerger J, ed. Modern Developments in Audiology. New York, NY: Academic Press; 337–370

Buus S, Florentine M, Redden RB. The SISI test: a review. Part I. Audiology 1982a;21(4):273–293

Buus S, Florentine M, Redden RB. The SISI test: a review. Part II. Audiology 1982b;21(5):365–385

Colace AT, McFarland DJ. The importance of modality specificity in diagnosing central auditory processing disorder. Am J Audiol 2005a;14(2):112–123

Cacace AT, McFarland DJ. Response to Katz and Tillery (2005), Musiek, Bellis, and Chermak (2005), and Rosen (2005). Am J Audiol 2005b;14:143–150

Cacace AT, McFarland DJ, eds. 2008. Current Controversies in Central Auditory Processing Disorder. San Diego, CA: Plural

Cacace AT, McFarland DJ. Factors influencing tests of auditory processing: a perspective on current issues and relevant concerns. J Am Acad Audiol 2013;24(7):572–589

Calearo C, Lazzaroni A. Speech intelligibility in relation to the speed of the message. Laryngoscope 1957;67(5):410–419

Cameron S, Dillon H. Development of the Listening in Spatialized Noise—Sentences test (LISN-S). Ear Hear 2007;28(2):196–211

Cameron S, Dillon H, Newall P. Three case studies of children with suspected auditory processing disorder. Aust N Z J Audiol 2005;27:97–112

Cameron S, Dillon H, Newall P. Development and evaluation of the Listening in Spatialized Noise test. Ear Hear 2006a;27(1):30–42

Cameron S, Dillon H, Newall P. The Listening in Spatialized Noise test: normative data for children. Int J Audiol 2006b;45(2):99–108

Cameron S, Dillon H, Newall P. The Listening in Spatialized Noise test: an auditory processing disorder study. J Am Acad Audiol 2006c;17(5):306–320

Carhart R. Clinical determination of abnormal auditory adaptation. AMA Arch Otolaryngol 1957;65(1):32–39

Carver WF. The reliability and precision of a modification of the ABLB test. Ann Otol Rhinol Laryngol 1970;79(2):398–411

Chung DY, Smith F. Quiet and masked brief-tone audiometry in subjects with normal hearing and with noise-induced hearing loss. Scand Audiol 1980;9(1):43–47

Coles RRA, Priede VM. Factors influencing the choice of fixed-level ear in the ABLB test. Audiology 1976;15(6):465–479

Cooper JC Jr, Owen JH. In defense of SISIs. The short increment sensitivity index. Arch Otolaryngol 1976;102(7):396–399

Cox RM. Using loudness data for hearing aid selection: the IHAFF approach. Hear J 1995;47:39–42

Cox RM, Alexander GC, Taylor IM, Gray GA. The contour test of loudness perception. Ear Hear 1997;18(5):388–400

Cueva RA. Auditory brainstem response versus magnetic resonance imaging for the evaluation of asymmetric sensorineural hearing loss. Laryngoscope 2004;114(10):1686–1692

Dallos PJ, Tillman TW. The effects of parameter variations in Bekesy audiometry in a patient with acoustic neuroma. J Speech Hear Res 1966;9:557–572

Davis H, Goodman AC. Subtractive hearing loss, loudness recruitment and decruitment. Ann Otol Rhinol Laryngol 1966;75(1):87–94

Dawes PJD, Jeannon J-P. Audit of regional screening guidelines for vestibular schwannoma. J Laryngol Otol 1998;112(9):860–864

Denes P, Naunton RF. The clinical detection of auditory recruitment. J Laryngol Otol 1950;64(7):375–398

Dix MR, Hallpike CS. The otoneurological diagnosis of tumours of the VIII nerve. Proc R Soc Med 1958;51(11):889–896

Dix MR, Hallpike CS, Hood JD. Observations upon the loudness recruitment phenomenon, with special reference to the differential diagnosis of disorders of the internal ear and eighth nerve. Proc R Soc Med 1948;41(8):516–526

Ehrlich CH. Analysis of selected fixed frequency Bekesy tracings. Arch Otolaryngol 1971;93(1):12–24

Flottorp G. Pathological fatigue in part of the hearing nerve only. Acta Otolaryngol Suppl 1964;188(Suppl):188, 298

Fowler EP. A method for the early detection of otosclerosis: a study of sounds well above threshold. Arch Otolaryngol 1936;24:731–741

Fritze W. A computer-controlled binaural balance test. Acta Otolaryngol 1978;86(1-2):89–92

Gelfand SA. The tracking ABLB in clinical recruitment testing. J Aud Res 1976;16:34–41

Gelfand SA. 2010. Hearing: An Introduction to Psychological and Physical Acoustics, 5th ed. Colchester, Essex, UK: Informa Healthcare

Geller D, Margolis RH. Magnitude estimation of loudness. I: Application to hearing aid selection. J Speech Hear Res 1984;27(1):20–27

Gimsing S. Vestibular schwannoma: when to look for it? J Laryngol Otol 2010;124(3):258–264

Gjaevenes K, Söhoel T. The tone decay test. Acta Otolaryngol 1969;68(1):33–42

Green DS. The modified tone decay test (MTDT) as a screening procedure for eighth nerve lesions. J Speech Hear Disord 1963;28:31–36

Hallpike CS. Clinical otoneurology and its contributions to theory and practice. Proc R Soc Med 1965;58:185–196

Hallpike CS, Hood JD. Some recent work on auditory adaptation and its relationship to the loudness recruitment phenomenon. J Acoust Soc Am 1951;23:270–274

Hallpike CS, Hood JD. Observations upon the neurological mechanism of the loudness recruitment phenomenon. Acta Otolaryngol 1959;50:472–486

Harbert F, Young IM. Threshold auditory adaptation measured by tone decay test and Bekesy audiometry. Ann Otol Rhinol Laryngol 1964;73:48–60

Harbert F, Young IM, Weiss BG. Clinical application of intensity difference limen. Acta Otolaryngol 1969; 67(4):435–443

Harford ER. 1967. Clinical application and significance of the SISI test. In: Graham AB, ed. Sensorineural Hearing Processes and Disorders. Boston, MA: Little, Brown; 223–233

Hattler K, Northern JL. Clinical application of temporal summation. J Aud Res 1970;10:72–78

Hawkins DB, Walden BE, Montgomery A, Prosek RA. Description and validation of an LDL procedure designed to select SSPL90. Ear Hear 1987;8(3):162–169

Hellman RP, Meiselman CH. Prediction of individual loudness exponents from cross-modality matching. J Speech Hear Res 1988;31(4):605–615

Hellman RP, Meiselman CH. Loudness relations for individuals and groups in normal and impaired hearing. J Acoust Soc Am 1990;88(6):2596–2606

Hendler T, Squires NK, Emmerich DS. Psychophysical measures of central auditory dysfunction in multiple sclerosis: neurophysiological and neuroanatomical correlates. Ear Hear 1990;11(6):403–416

Hirsh IJ, Palva T, Goodman A. Difference limen and recruitment. AMA Arch Otolaryngol 1954;60(5):525–540

Hood JD. Auditory fatigue and adaptation in the differential diagnosis of end-organ disease. Ann Otol Rhinol Laryngol 1955;64(2):507–518

Hood JD. Basic audiological requirements in neuro-otology. J Laryngol Otol 1969;83(7):695–711

Hood JD. Loudness balance procedures for the measurement of recruitment. Audiology 1977;16(3): 215–228

Hood JD, Poole JP. Tolerable limit of loudness: its clinical and physiological significance. J Acoust Soc Am 1966;40(1):47–53

Hopkinson NT. Modifications of the four types of Bekesy audiograms. J Speech Hear Disord 1966;31:79–82

Hughes RL, Winegar WJ, Crabtree JA. Békésy audiometry. Type 2 versus type 4 patterns. Arch Otolaryngol 1967;86(4):424–430

Hunter LL, Ries DT, Schlauch RS, Levine SC, Ward WD. Safety and clinical performance of acoustic reflex tests. Ear Hear 1999;20(6):506–514

Huss M, Moore BCJ. Dead regions and pitch perception. J Acoust Soc Am 2005;117(6):3841–3852

Ivey RG. 1969. Tests of CNS auditory function. Unpublished thesis, Colorado State University, Fort Collins

Jerger JF. A difference limen recruitment test and its diagnostic significance. Laryngoscope 1952;62(12): 1316–1332

Jerger JF. DI difference test: improved method for clinical measurement of recruitment. AMA Arch Otolaryngol 1953;57(5):490–500

Jerger J. Bekesy audiometry in the analysis of auditory disorders. J Speech Hear Res 1960a;3:275–287

Jerger JF. Observations on auditory behavior in lesions of the central auditory pathways. AMA Arch Otolaryngol 1960b;71:797–806

Jerger J. Recruitment and allied phenomena in differential diagnosis. J Aud Res 1961;2:145–151

Jerger J. Hearing tests in otologic diagnosis. ASHA 1962; 4:139–145

Jerger J. 1964. Auditory tests for disorders of the central auditory mechanisms. In: Fields WS, Alford BR, eds. Neurological Aspects of Auditory and Vestibular Disorders. Springfield, IL: CC Thomas; 77–93

Jerger JF, Harford ER. Alternate and simultaneous binaural balancing of pure tones. J Speech Hear Res 1960;3: 15–30

Jerger J, Hayes D. Diagnostic speech audiometry. Arch Otolaryngol 1977;103(4):216–222

Jerger J, Herer G. Unexpected dividend in Bekesy audiometry. J Speech Hear Disord 1961;26:390–391

Jerger J, Jerger S. Critical off-time in VIII nerve disorders. J Speech Hear Res 1966;9:573–583

Jerger J, Jerger S. Diagnostic value of Bekesy comfortable loudness tracings. Arch Otolaryngol 1974a;99(5): 351–360

Jerger J, Jerger S. Auditory findings in brain stem disorders. Arch Otolaryngol 1974b;99(5):342–350

Jerger J, Jerger S. A simplified tone decay test. Arch Otolaryngol 1975a;101(7):403–407

Jerger J, Jerger S. Clinical value of central auditory tests. Scand Audiol 1975b;4:147–163

Jerger JF, Jerger S, Mauldin L. The forward-backward discrepancy in Bekesy audiometry. Arch Otolaryngol 1972;96(5):400–406

Jerger J, Musiek F. Report of the consensus conference on the diagnosis of auditory processing disorders in school-aged children. J Am Acad Audiol 2000;11(9):467–474

Jerger J, Shedd JL, Harford E. On the detection of extremely small changes in sound intensity. AMA Arch Otolaryngol 1959;69(2):200–211

Jerger J, Speaks C, Trammell JL. A new approach to speech audiometry. J Speech Hear Disord 1968;33(4): 318–328

Jerger S, Jerger J. Extra- and intra-axial brain stem auditory disorders. Audiology 1975;14(2):93–117

Jerger S, Jerger J. 1981. Auditory Disorders. Boston, MA: Little, Brown

Johnson EW. Confirmed retrocochlear lesions. Auditory test results in 163 patients. Arch Otolaryngol 1966;84(3):247–254

Johnson EW. Auditory test results in 500 cases of acoustic neuroma. Arch Otolaryngol 1977;103(3):152–158

Johnson EW, House WF. Auditory findings in 53 cases of acoustic neuromas. Arch Otolaryngol 1964;80: 667–677

Josey AF. Audiologic manifestations of tumors of the VIIIth nerve. Ear Hear 1987;8(4, Suppl):19S–21S

Kamm C, Dirks DD, Mickey MR. Effect of sensorineural hearing loss on loudness discomfort level and most comfortable loudness judgments. J Speech Hear Res 1978;21(4):668–681

Kärjä J, Palva A. Reverse frequency-sweep Békésy audiometry. Acta Otolaryngol Suppl 1969;263(Suppl):225–228

Katz J. N.d. Buffalo Battery [for auditory processing disorders]. Vancouver, WA: Precision Acoustics. Available at http://www.precisionacoustics.org

Katz J. The use of staggered spondaic words for assessing the integrity of the central auditory nervous system. J Aud Res 1962;2:327–337

Katz J. The SSW test: an interim report. J Speech Hear Disord 1968;33(2):132–146

Katz J, Ivey RG. 1994. Spondaic procedures in central testing. In: Katz J, ed. Handbook of Clinical Audiology, 4th ed. Baltimore, MD: Williams & Wilkins; 239–268

Katz J, Tillery KL. Can central auditory processing tests resist supramodal influences? Am J Audiol 2005;14(2):124–127, discussion 143–150

Kawell ME, Kopun JG, Stelmachowicz PG. Loudness discomfort levels in children. Ear Hear 1988;9(3):133–136

Keith R. 2000. Random Gap Detection Test. St. Louis, MO: Auditec

Keith RW. 2009a. SCAN-3A: Tests for Auditory Processing Disorders in Adolescents and Adults. San Antonio, TX: Pearson

Keith RW. 2009b. SCAN-3C: Tests for Auditory Processing Disorders for Children. San Antonio, TX: Pearson

Kimura D. Some effects of temporal-lobe damage on auditory perception. Can J Psychol 1961;15:156–165

Kluk K, Moore BCJ. Factors affecting psychophysical tuning curves for normally hearing subjects. Hear Res 2004;194(1–2):118–134

Kluk K, Moore BCJ. Factors affecting psychophysical tuning curves for hearing-impaired subjects with high-frequency dead regions. Hear Res 2005;200(1-2):115–131

Kluk K, Moore BCJ. Dead regions in the cochlea and enhancement of frequency discrimination: effects of audiogram slope, unilateral versus bilateral loss, and hearing-aid use. Hear Res 2006;222(1–2):1–15

Knight KK, Margolis RH. Magnitude estimation of loudness. II: Loudness perception in presbycusic listeners. J Speech Hear Res 1984;27(1):28–32

Lamoré JJ, Rodenburg M. Significance of the SISI test and its relation to recruitment. Audiology 1980;19(1):75–85

Lister JJ, Roberts RA, Shackelford J, Rogers CL. An adaptive clinical test of temporal resolution. Am J Audiol 2006;15(2):133–140

Lüscher E. The difference limen of intensity variations of pure tones and its diagnostic significance. J Laryngol Otol 1951;65(7):486–510, passim

Lüscher E, Zwislocki J. A simple method for indirect monaural determination of the recruitment phenomenon (difference limen in intensity in different types of deafness). Acta Otolaryngol 1949;78:156–168

Lynn GE, Gilroy J. 1977. Evaluation of central auditory dysfunction in patients with neurological disorders. In:

Keith RW, ed. Central Auditory Dysfunction. New York, NY: Grune & Stratton; 177–221

Lynn GE, Gilroy J, Taylor PC, Leiser RP. Binaural masking-level differences in neurological disorders. Arch Otolaryngol 1981;107:357–362

Mangham CA. Hearing threshold differences between ears and risk of acoustic tumer. Otolaryngol Head Neck Surg 1991;105:814–817

Margolis RH, Saly GL. Asymmetric hearing loss: definition, validation, and prevalence. Otol Neurotol 2008;29(4):422–431

Marks LE. 1974. Sensory Processes. New York, NY: Academic Press

Martin MJ, Billiet CR, Bellis TJ. 2013. Audiological assessment of (C)APD. In: Geffner D, Ross-Swain D, eds. Auditory Processing Disorders: Assessment, Management, and Treatment, 2nd ed. San Diego, CA: Plural; 117–140

Martin FN, Champlin CA, Chambers JA. Seventh survey of audiometric practices in the United States. J Am Acad Audiol 1998;9(2):95–104

Martin FN, Woodrick Armstrong T, Champlin CA. A survey of audiological practices in the United States. Am J Audiol 1994;3:20–26

Matthies C, Samii M. Management of 1000 vestibular schwannomas (acoustic neuromas): clinical presentation. Neurosurgery 1997;40(1):1–9, discussion 9–10

Matzker J. Two new methods for the assessment of central auditory functions in cases of brain disease. Ann Otol Rhinol Laryngol 1959;68:1185–1197

McDermott HJ, Lech M, Kornblum MS, Irvine DRF. Loudness perception and frequency discrimination in subjects with steeply sloping hearing loss: possible correlates of neural plasticity. J Acoust Soc Am 1998;104(4):2314–2325

Medwetsky L. 2002. Central auditory processing testing: a battery approach. In: Katz J, ed. Handbook of Clinical Audiology, 5th ed. Philadelphia, PA: Lippincott Williams & Wilkins

Miskolczy-Fodor F. Automatically recorded loudness balance testing: a new method. Arch Otolaryngol 1964;79:355–365

Moore BCJ. Dead regions in the cochlea: conceptual foundations, diagnosis, and clinical applications. Ear Hear 2004;25(2):98–116

Moore BCJ, Glasberg BR, Stone MA. New version of the TEN test with calibrations in dB HL. Ear Hear 2004;25(5):478–487

Moore BCJ, Huss M, Vickers DA, Glasberg BR, Alcántara JI. A test for the diagnosis of dead regions in the cochlea. Br J Audiol 2000;34(4):205–224

Morales-Garcia C, Hood JD. Tone decay test in neuro-otological diagnosis. Arch Otolaryngol 1972;96(3):231–247

Morgan DW, Wilson RH, Dirks DD. Loudness discomfort level under earphone and in the free field: the effect of calibration. J Acoust Soc Am 1974;56:577–581

Musiek FE. Assessment of central auditory dysfunction: the dichotic digit test revisited. Ear Hear 1983;4(2):79–83

Musiek FE, Baran JA, Pinheiro ML. Duration pattern recognition in normal subjects and patients with cerebral and cochlear lesions. Audiology 1990;29(6):304–313

Musiek FE, Bellis TJ, Chermak GD. Nonmodularity of the central auditory nervous system: implications for (central) auditory processing disorder. Am J Audiol 2005;14(2):128–138, discussion 143–150

Musiek FE, Chermak GD, eds. 2006. Handbook of (Central) Auditory Processing Disorder. Volume I: Auditory Neuroscience and Diagnosis. San Diego, CA: Plural

Musiek FE, Chermak GD, Weihing J, Zappulla M, Nagle S. Diagnostic accuracy of established central auditory processing test batteries in patients with documented brain lesions. J Am Acad Audiol 2011;22(6):342–358

Musiek FE, Shinn JB, Jirsa R, Bamiou D-E, Baran JA, Zaida E. GIN (Gaps-In-Noise) test performance in subjects with confirmed central auditory nervous system involvement. Ear Hear 2005;26(6):608–618

Noffsinger D, Olsen WO, Carhart R, Hart CW, Sahgal V. Auditory and vestibular aberrations in multiple sclerosis. Acta Otolaryngol Suppl 1972;303(Suppl):1–63

Nouraei SA, Huys QJ, Chatrath P, Powles J, Harcourt JP. Screening patients with sensorineural hearing loss for vestibular schwannoma using a Bayesian classifier. Clin Otolaryngol 2007;32(4):248–254

Obholzer RJ, Rea PA, Harcourt JP. Magnetic resonance imaging screening for vestibular schwannoma: analysis of published protocols. J Laryngol Otol 2004;118(5):329–332

Olsen WO. Brief tone audiometry: a review. Ear Hear 1987;8(4, Suppl):13S–18S

Olsen WO, Kurdziel SA. 1976. Extent and rate of tone decay for cochlear and for VIIIth nerve lesion patients. Paper presented at Convention of American Speech and Hearing Association, Houston

Olsen WO, Noffsinger D. Comparison of one new and three old tests of auditory adaptation. Arch Otolaryngol 1974;99(2):94–99

Olsen WO, Noffsinger D. Masking level differences for cochlear and brain stem lesions. Ann Otol Rhinol Laryngol 1976;85(6 PT. 1):820–825

Olsen WO, Noffsinger D, Carhart R. Masking level differences encountered in clinical populations. Audiology 1976;15(4):287–301

Olsen WO, Rose DE, Noffsinger D. Brief-tone audiometry with normal, cochlear, and eighth nerve tumor patients. Arch Otolaryngol 1974;99(3):185–189

Owens E. Tone decay in VIIIth nerve and cochlear lesions. J Speech Hear Disord 1964a;29:14–22

Owens E. Bekesy tracings and site of lesion. J Speech Hear Disord 1964b;29:456–468

Owens E. Bekesy tracings, tone decay, and loudness recruitment. J Speech Hear Disord 1965;30:50–57

Palva T, Kärjä J, Palva A. Forward vs reversed Bekesy tracings. Arch Otolaryngol 1970;91(5):449–452

Parker W, Decker RL. Detection of abnormal auditory threshold adaptation (ATA). Arch Otolaryngol 1971;94(1):1–7

Pedersen CB. Brief-tone audiometry. Scand Audiol 1976;5:27–33

Perez de Moura L. Inner ear pathology in acoustic neurinomas. J Speech Hear Disord 1967;32:29–35

Pestalozza G, Cioce C. Measuring auditory adaptation: the value of different clinical tests. Laryngoscope 1962;72:240–261

Pinheiro ML. Auditory pattern reversal in auditory perception in patients with left and right hemisphere lesions. Ohio J Speech Hear 1977;12:9–20

Pinheiro ML, Musiek FE. 1985. Sequencing and temporal ordering in the auditory system. In Pinheiro ML, Musiek FE, eds. Assessment of Central Auditory Dysfunction. Baltimore, MD: Williams & Wilkins; 219–238

Priede VM, Coles RRA. Interpretation of loudness recruitment tests—some new concepts and criteria. J Laryngol Otol 1974;88(7):641–662

Punch J, Joseph A, Rakerd B. Most comfortable and uncomfortable loudness levels: six decades of research. Am J Audiol 2004;13(2):144–157

Reger S. Loudness level contours and intensity discrimination of ears with raised auditory threshold. J Acoust Soc Am 1935;7:73 (abstract)

Robinette MS, Bauch CD, Olsen WO, Cevette MJ. Auditory brainstem response and magnetic resonance imaging for acoustic neuromas: costs by prevalence. Arch Otolaryngol Head Neck Surg 2000;126(8):963–966

Rose DE. Some effects and case histories of reversed frequency sweep in Bekesy audiometry. J Aud Res 1962;2:267–278

Rose DE, Kurdziel S, Olsen WO, Noffsinger D. Bekesy test results in patients with eighth-nerve lesions. Forward reverse- and fixed-frequency tracings. Arch Otolaryngol 1975;101(6):373–375

Rosen S. "A riddle wrapped in a mystery inside an enigma": defining central auditory processing disorder. Am J Audiol 2005;14(2):139–142, discussion 143–150

Rosenberg PE. 1958. Rapid clinical measurement of tone decay. Paper presented at Convention of American Speech and Hearing Association, New York

Rosenberg PE. 1969. Tone Decay. Maico Audiological Library Series, VII, report 6.

Ruckenstein MJ, Cueva RA, Morrison DH, Press G. A prospective study of ABR and MRI in the screening for vestibular schwannomas. Am J Otol 1996;17(2):317–320

Saliba I, Martineau G, Chagnon M. Asymmetric hearing loss: rule 3,000 for screening vestibular schwannoma. Otol Neurotol 2009;30(4):515–521

Sanders JW, Honig EA. Brief tone audiometry. Results in normal and impaired ears. Arch Otolaryngol 1967;85(6):640–647

Sanders JW, Josey AF, Glasscock ME III. Audiologic evaluation in cochlear and eighth nerve disorders. Arch Otolaryngol 1974;100(4):283–289

Sanders JW, Josey AF, Kemker FJ. Brief-tone audiometry in patients with 8th nerve tumor. J Speech Hear Res 1971;14(1):172–178

Schlauch RS, Levine S, Li Y, Haines S. Evaluating hearing threshold differences between ears as a screen for acoustic neuroma. J Speech Hear Res 1995;38(5):1168–1175

Sek A, Alcántara J, Moore BCJ, Kluk K, Wicher A. Development of a fast method for determining psychophysical tuning curves. Int J Audiol 2005;44(7):408–420

Sheppard IJ, Milford CAM, Anslow P. MRI in the detection of acoustic neuromas—a suggested protocol for screening. Clin Otolaryngol Allied Sci 1996;21(4):301–304

Sherlock LP, Formby C. Estimates of loudness, loudness discomfort, and the auditory dynamic range: normative estimates, comparison of procedures, and test-retest reliability. J Am Acad Audiol 2005;16(2):85–100

Silman S, Gelfand SA, Lutolf J, Chun TH. A response to Wiley and Lilly. J Speech Hear Disord 1981;46(2):217

Silman S, Silverman CA. 1991. Auditory Diagnosis: Principles and Applications. San Diego, CA: Academic Press

Skinner M. 1988. Hearing Aid Evaluation. Englewood-Cliffs, NJ: Prentice Hall

Sorensen H. A threshold tone decay test. Acta Otolaryngol 1960;158(Suppl):356–360

Sorensen H. Clinical applications of continuous threshold recording. Acta Otolaryngol 1962;54:403–422

Speaks C, Gray T, Miller J. Central auditory deficits and temporal-lobe lesions. J Speech Hear Disord 1975;40(2):192–205

Speaks C, Jerger J. Method for measurement of speech identification. J Speech Hear Res 1965;8:185–194

Stephens SDG. 1976. Auditory temporal summation in patients with central nervous system lesions. In: Stephens SDG, ed. Disorders of Auditory Function, Vol. II. London, UK: Academic Press; 231–243

Summers V, Molis MR, Müsch H, Walden BE, Surr RK, Cord MT. Identifying dead regions in the cochlea: psychophysical tuning curves and tone detection in threshold-equalizing noise. Ear Hear 2003;24(2):133–142

Sung RJ, Sung GS. Study of the classical and modified alternate binaural loudness balance tests in normal and pathological ears. J Am Audiol Soc 1976;2(2):49–53

Sung SS, Goetzinger CP, Knox AW. The sensitivity and reliability of three tone-decay tests. J Aud Res 1969;9:167–177

Suzuki M, Hashimoto S, Kano S, Okitsu T. Prevalence of acoustic neuroma associated with each configuration of pure tone audiogram in patients with asymmetric sensorineural hearing loss. Ann Otol Rhinol Laryngol 2010;119(9):615–618

Thompson G. A modified SISI technique for selected cases with suspected acoustic neurinoma. J Speech Hear Disord 1963;28:299–302

Tillman TW. Audiologic diagnosis of acoustic tumors. Arch Otolaryngol 1966;83(6):574–581

Tillman TW. Special hearing tests in otoneurologic diagnosis. Arch Otolaryngol 1969;89(1):25–30

Turner RG, Shepard NT, Frazer GJ. Clinical performance of audiological and related diagnostic tests. Ear Hear 1984;5(4):187–194

Vinay, Moore BC. Prevalence of dead regions in subjects with sensorineural hearing loss. Ear Hear 2007;28(2):231–241

Weihing J, Bellis TJ, Chermak GD, Musiek FE. 2013. Current issues in the diagnosis and treatment of CAPD in children. In: Geffner D, Ross-Swain D, eds. Auditory Processing Disorders: Assessment, Management, and Treatment, 2nd ed. San Diego, CA: Plural; 3–32

Welling DB, Glasscock ME III, Woods CI, Jackson CG. Acoustic neuroma: a cost-effective approach. Otolaryngol Head Neck Surg 1990;103(3):364–370

Wiley TL, Lilly DJ. Temporal characteristics of auditory adaptation: a case report. J Speech Hear Disord 1980;45(2):209–215

Wright HN. Clinical measurement of temporal auditory summation. J Speech Hear Res 1968;11(1):109–127

Wright HN. 1978. Brief tone audiometry. In: Katz J, ed. Handbook of Clinical Audiology. Baltimore, MD: Williams & Wilkins; 218–232

Yantis PA. Clinical applications of the temporary threshold shift. Arch Otolaryngol 1959;70:779–787

Zapala DA, Criter RE, Bogle JM, Lundy LB, Cevette MJ, Bauch CD. Pure-tone hearing asymmetry: a logistic approach modeling age, sex, and noise exposure history. J Am Acad Audiol 2012;23(7):553–570

11 Physiological Methods in Audiology

An important aspect of audiology deals with the use of physiological tests in addition to the use of behavioral measurements. Physiological measurements provide powerful diagnostic tools that supplement the information obtained from the patient interview and behavioral tests, and make it possible to test patients who are too young or otherwise incapable of responding behaviorally. This chapter introduces the student to three types of physiological assessment approaches that are used in audiology: auditory evoked potentials, otoacoustic emissions, and vestibular assessment. Acoustic immittance methods are discussed in considerable detail in Chapter 7. Physiological techniques that are no longer used (such as psychogalvanic, respiration, and cardiac responses) are not covered; but the inquisitive reader may find discussions of these methods in Bradford (1975). In addition, the student should be aware that audiologists perform physiological monitoring during surgical procedures (ASHA 1992, 2004), and they may also use nonauditory physiological measurements such as facial nerve testing and the use of somatosensory evoked potentials. While intraoperative monitoring will not covered at this introductory level, several lucid discussions of the topic are readily available (Dennis 1988; Beck 1993; Jacobson 1999; Møller 2000; Hall 2007; Martin & Shi 2007, 2009).

■ Auditory Evoked Potentials

The activity of the nervous system produces electrical signals that can be picked up by electrodes placed on the head, and can then be displayed on the screen of a recording device and/or plotted on paper. A change in the activity of the nervous system occurs when it reacts to a stimulus (such as a sound). This change in neural activity also produces a change in the electrical signals picked up by the electrodes. As a result, the nervous system's reaction to a stimulus can be seen as a change in the electrical signals that are displayed on the recording device. These electrical responses of the nervous system that are elicited by a stimulus are called **evoked potentials**. When the stimulus is sound, they are called **auditory evoked potentials (AEPs)**. These auditory evoked potentials can be used to test the integrity of the auditory system and to make inferences about hearing. One of the great advantages of AEPs is that they are usually noninvasive, almost always being measured from outside the body with electrodes on the surface of the skin. The block diagram in **Fig. 11.1** illustrates a typical arrangement involved in recording AEPs from a patient. An example of an instrument used for evoked potentials testing is illustrated in **Fig. 11.2**.

The nature and use of auditory evoked potentials have been described in considerable detail (e.g., Moore 1983; Jacobson 1985; Glattke 1993; Chiappa 1997; Burkhard & Don 2007; Burkhard, Don, & Eggermont 2007; Hall 2007; Abbas & Brown 2009; Burkhard & McNerney 2009; Don & Kwong 2009; Cacace & McFarland 2009; Cone-Wesson & Dimitrinjevic 2009; Kraus 2011; Kraus & Hornickel 2013). **Fig. 11.3** shows the three major AEPs in the form of a single composite picture. The time scale in the figure is labeled **latency**, which is simply the amount of time that has elapsed (or the delay) since the stimulus was presented. Each of the AEPs shown is made up of a characteristic grouping of peaks and troughs that occur within a certain range of latencies, and are for this reason identified as the short, middle, and long latency responses. Notice that a logarithmic time scale is used in this figure so that all three ranges of latencies can be shown. Each of these time frames is called a **time window** or **epoch**, and the ability to observe a given evoked potential is optimized by using the time window best suited for that response.

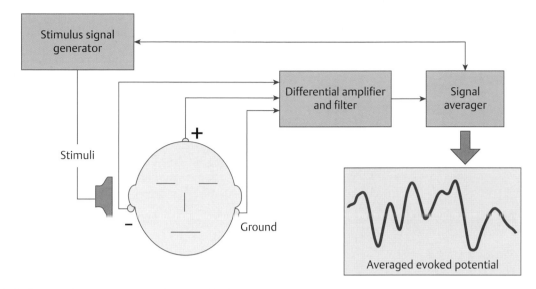

Fig. 11.1 Block diagram for measuring auditory evoked potentials, using the auditory brainstem response as an example.

Fig. 11.2 Example of a clinical instrument used for auditory brainstem responses and other evoked potentials tests. (Courtesy of Grason-Stadler Inc.)

We will first briefly review some aspects of electrocochleography, and then concentrate on the auditory brainstem response (ABR), which is by far the most widely used of the various auditory evoked potentials. We will then go over some aspects of the later evoked potentials.

The electrodes are usually located at some distance from the structures that produce the signals. In addition, the electrodes will pick up all electrical signals that reach them, regardless of why they are there or where they are from. This means that the recording device receives all kinds of signals from the nervous system, muscles, and other physiological sources, as well as signals from electrical sources in the environment. All of these other signals are **noise**. As a result, we need to extract tiny evoked potential responses from an extraordinarily noisy background; for example, the auditory brainstem response is *less than* 1 microvolt (mV) but the noise is often around 10 mV. This goal is accomplished with filtering, differential amplification, and averaging.

Filtering can be used to remove some low-frequency noises such as direct current (DC) signals from electronic equipment, 60 Hz hum from alternating current (AC) power sources, and background electroencephalographic (EEG) activity. **Differential amplification** is used to boost the level of the evoked potential response while at the same time removing noise. It involves using the signals picked up by two separate electrodes at different locations, such as the earlobe of the stimulated (ipsilateral) ear and the vertex of the skull. The differential amplifier then cancels ("rejects") noises that are similar ("in common") at the two electrodes. This process is called **common mode rejection** and is widely used in physiological measurements. A ground or common electrode is also necessary, and is usually located on the mastoid of the opposite ear or at midline on the lower forehead.

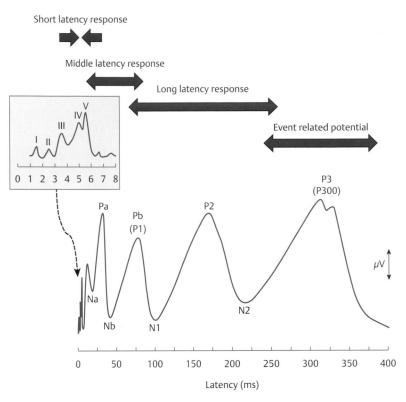

Fig. 11.3 An idealized composite representation of the major auditory evoked potentials. The insert provides an expanded view of the short latency response because it occurs within a time period that is too small to be seen clearly in the main picture.

Recall that the responses we are looking for are tiny signals embedded in all kinds of noise. A great deal of noise still remains after filtering and differential amplification. **Averaging** is a technique that allows the responses (evoked potentials) to be extracted from the noise, and is a central principle of many physiological methods. Averaging relies on a few fundamental notions. The first principle is that the evoked potential responses are *time-locked* to (or *synchronized* with) the stimulus. This means that the response will consistently appear in a certain way at the same latency, or point in time after the stimulus. On the other hand, noise is *random*. Suppose a certain evoked potential is positive in direction 3 ms after a click is presented to the ear, and is negative at a latency of 4 ms. In other words, the electrical response due to that click will be positive when measured 3 ms later and negative when measured 4 ms later. Now, suppose we present 1000 clicks, and measure the electrical signals picked up by the electrodes for a period lasting 10 ms following each one. A computer could be used to keep a "tally" of the electrical signals at 1 ms intervals after each click. More specifically, the computer will algebraically add the voltages in 1-ms intervals for all 1000 clicks. Thus, there would be an algebraic sum at latencies of l ms, 2 ms, 3 ms, 4 ms, etc. Even though any one of the responses might be very small, it will almost

always be positive at a latency of 3 ms and negative at a latency of 4 ms. When these values are added algebraically (averaged) over a large number of trials (samples), a relatively large *positive value will build up at 3 ms* and a relatively large *negative value will build up at 4 ms*, as illustrated in **Fig. 11.4**. On the other hand, the electrical signals due to noise are random. Random events are as likely to be positive as negative, so that they will "average out" ("add up to zero" algebraically) over the long run, which is what happens when we add up a large number of samples. As a result of these principles, the averaging process causes the real response to build up because it is consistent over time, and causes the noise to "cancel out" (actually add up to zero) because it is random over time.

Electrocochleography

Electrocochleography (ECochG) is the measurement of electrical potentials that are derived from the cochlear hair cells and the auditory nerve (ASHA 1987; Ruth, Lambert, & Ferraro 1988; Ferraro 2000; Hall 2007; Schoonhoven 2007; Abbas & Brown 2009). The basic methodology of ECochG involves presenting clicks to the ear and monitoring the resulting electrical responses within a time frame of ~ 5 ms after each

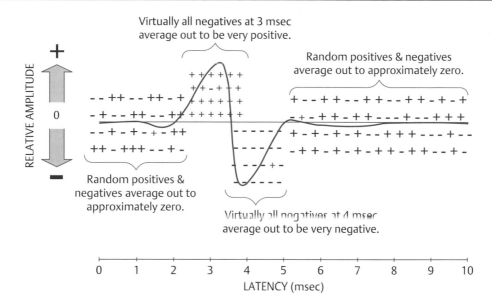

Virtually all negatives at 3 msec
average out to be very positive.

Random positives & negatives
average out to approximately zero.

Random positives &
negatives average out to
approximately zero.

Virtually all negatives at 4 msec
average out to be very negative.

RELATIVE AMPLITUDE

LATENCY (msec)

Fig. 11.4   Illustration of the averaging concept (see text).

click. Averaging the responses to a large number of stimuli results in a waveform like the one illustrated in **Fig. 11.5**, which will be described momentarily.

Electrocochleography typically uses click stimuli, although tone bursts are also used for various applications. The reason for using transient stimuli like clicks is that many neurons must be made to fire, or discharge, at essentially the same time (synchronously) to elicit a measurable action potential. This goal is accomplished by using stimuli that have abrupt onsets, very short durations, and broad spectra, such as clicks. These characteristics enable clicks to almost simultaneously activate a large number of hair cells along the basal part of the cochlea, where the speed of the traveling wave is very fast. This, in turn, causes essentially simultaneous firing of the auditory nerve fibers associated with these basal turn hair cells.

Electrode location is a very important factor in ECochG because the magnitude and quality of the measured response deteriorates significantly with distance from the cochlea and auditory nerve. The highest-quality clinical responses are obtained with an electrode on the cochlear promontory. This method is called the transtympanic approach because it involves using a needle electrode that must penetrate the tympanic membrane to get to the promontory, requiring medical participation. The **transtympanic approach** is thus an invasive procedure, which is its principal limitation. Less pristine but perfectly usable ECochG results are obtained with the alternative, *noninvasive* **extratympanic approach**. It uses various kinds of electrodes that are placed as close as possible to the tympanic membrane in the ear canal

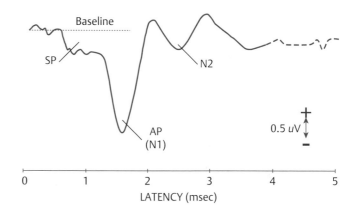

Fig. 11.5   An idealized electrocochleogram. Negative voltage values are plotted downward. Abbreviations: SP, summating potential; AP (N1), auditory nerve action potential; N2, second peak of auditory nerve action potential.

or on the eardrum itself. The extratympanic method avoids the limitations and potential complications of piercing the eardrum, and is the most common ECochG approach used in the United States.

The **electrocochleogram** (also abbreviated **ECochG**) is shown in **Fig. 11.5**. It includes two major components, the **summating potential (SP)** derived from the cochlear hair cells, and the compound **action potential (AP)** of the auditory nerve. It is also possible to show a third component, the **cochlear microphonic**, which is an alternating current (AC) electrical response from the hair cells, although this is not always done clinically. The summating potential is a shift of the electrical baseline (a direct current, or DC, shift) that occurs when the hair cells are activated. This is followed by activation of auditory neurons, which produces the action potential. Notice in **Fig. 11.5** that the ongoing activity before the ECochG response is used as a *baseline*. The figure follows the convention of recording negative peaks downward, although some clinicians show negative values upward. The summating potential is usually seen as a displacement from the baseline just prior to the action potential, or as a hump on its leading edge, as shown in the figure. The AP is seen as a negative peak at a latency of roughly 1.5 ms after the click. It can include up to three peaks (**N1**, **N2**, and **N3**), but the term *AP* usually refers to just the first peak (N1) for clinical purposes.

The ECochG response increases in amplitude (gets larger) and decreases in latency (occurs sooner) as the level of the stimulus is raised. In spite of this relationship, ECochG has not been found to be a reliable physiological method for estimating hearing thresholds, especially with extratympanic electrodes. On the other hand, ECochG has been shown to have at least three valuable clinical applications: (1) Electrocochleography is often used to help identify the first peak of the auditory brainstem response, which will be described in the next section. (2) It also can be used to monitor the status of the inner ear and auditory nerve during surgical procedures that place these structures at risk, such as acoustic tumor removal and endolymphatic sac surgery. (3) Electrocochleography is very useful in the diagnosis of Meniere's disease (e.g., Ferraro & Krishnan 1997; Sass 1998; Ferraro & Tibbils 1999; Chung, Cho, Choi, & Hong 2004). In particular, an abnormally large **SP/AP amplitude ratio** (which is simply the SP amplitude relative to the AP amplitude) is a good indicator of Meniere's disease, in contrast to cases of hair cell loss (which have low SP/AP ratios). The SP/AP ratio has roughly 60 to 70% sensitivity for the identification of Meniere's disease, and ~ 95% specificity (e.g., Sass 1998; Chung et al 2004). A potentially more sensitive measurement for detecting endolymphatic hydrops is the **SP/AP area ratio**, which compares the areas of the SP and the AP instead of their amplitudes (Devaiah, Dawson, Ferraro, & Ator 2003). The area of the SP is basically its amplitude (vertical size) times its duration (horizontal size), and the area of the AP is also its amplitude times its duration.

Auditory Brainstem Response

The group of waves identified as the *short latency response* in **Fig. 11.3** was originally described in detail by Jewett, Romano, and Williston (1970), as well as by Sohmer and Feinmesser (1967). They include up to seven peaks that normally occur within ~ 8 ms following the onset of a click stimulus. It is tempting to attribute these peaks to successive neural sites along the auditory pathway. However, while it does appear that the first two peaks are produced by the auditory nerve, the subsequent peaks actually have *multiple generators*, meaning that they are due to the combined electrical activity of several nuclei in the auditory brainstem (Møller & Jannetta 1985; Scherg & von Cramon 1985; Moore 1987; Rudell 1987; Hall 2007; Møller 2007). These short-latency evoked potentials are generally known as the **auditory brainstem response (ABR)** or the **brainstem auditory evoked response (BAER)**, and are sometimes referred to as the **brainstem evoked response (BSER)** or the **brainstem auditory evoked potential (BAEP)**.

Test Signals

The auditory brainstem response is most commonly obtained using click stimuli for the same reason described above for electrocochleography. As a result, the ABR depends to a considerable extent on the status of the basal turn of the cochlea and principally involves the high frequencies. While their abruptness and broad spectra make clicks optimal stimuli for eliciting synchronous neural firings, these features also cause the ABR to be lacking in the ability to test on a frequency-by-frequency basis. The ability to distinguish among frequencies is often called **frequency specificity**, and this lack of frequency specificity in click-evoked ABR testing must always be kept in mind. Frequency specificity is usually achieved in ABR testing by using **tone bursts** instead of clicks, either alone or in combination with masking techniques.[1] A tone burst is basically a very brief tone that rapidly rises to 100% of its intended amplitude in a few periods of the fundamental fre-

---

[1] Various masking techniques have also been used. For example, one method masks the high frequencies so the response is more likely to come from lower frequencies (e.g., Kileny 1981). The notched-noise method masks all frequencies except a certain narrow range where there is a "hole" or "notch" in the noise; thus, the response is from the frequency range where the masking noise is missing (e.g., Stapells et al 1990; Stapells & Kurtzberg 1991). The derived band method involves combining ABRs obtained from various combinations of noises and signals; and the responses are, in effect, subtracted from one another to derive a frequency-specific response (e.g., Parker & Thornton 1978; Don et al 1979).

quency and then rapidly dies out after a few periods. For example, each tone burst might rise in amplitude for two periods, have one period at 100% amplitude, and then fall to zero in two periods (Fedtke & Richter 2007; ISO 389-6 2007). Tone burst ABRs are used when estimating a patient's hearing thresholds at different frequencies, and are thus often used in the audiological assessment of babies and others who are difficult to test using behavioral methods (see Chapter 12).

The very brief signals used with the ABR, ECochG, and otoacoustic emissions (discussed later) may be calibrated in physical or behavioral terms. *Physical* calibration values describe the level of the click or tone burst in terms of the SPL of a steady pure tone that has the same amplitude. The value is given in decibels of **peak-to-peak** (or just **peak**) **equivalent sound pressure level (peSPL)**. The basic method involves a few steps: First, the click or tone burst from the earphone is displayed on an oscilloscope, and its peak-to-peak amplitude is noted on the oscilloscope screen. The next step is to replace the click (tone burst) with a steady pure tone, and we adjust the level of the tone until its amplitude on the oscilloscope screen is the same as what was found for the click (tone burst). We then read the tone's SPL on the sound level meter. The level of the tone that has the same amplitude on the screen as the peak amplitude of the click (tone burst) becomes the peSPL of the click (tone burst). For example, 40 dB peSPL means the peak level of the click or tone burst has the same amplitude (on the oscilloscope screen) as that produced by a 40 dB SPL pure tone.

An international standard (ISO 389-6 2007) contains reference values that have been developed for clicks (Richter & Fedtke 2005) and tone bursts (Fedtke & Richter 2007) that are analogous to ones described for audiometers in Chapter 4. The reference value for a click and each tone burst is expressed as its **peak-to-peak reference equivalent threshold sound pressure level (peRETSPL)** for use with earphones, and its **peak-to-peak reference equivalent threshold vibratory force level (peRETVFL)** for use with bone-conduction vibrators. Examples of peRETSPLs for clicks and several commonly used tone bursts are illustrated in **Table 11.1**.

Another physical approach involves measuring the click's **peak sound pressure level (peakSPL)**. This is done by directing the click from the earphone through the appropriate calibration coupler into a precision sound level meter that is capable of measuring the *true peak* level of a transient signal. However, sound level meters of this type are not available in most clinical settings.

Table 11.1 Examples of peak-to-peak reference equivalent threshold sound pressure levels (peRETSPLs) for clicks and tone bursts[a]

Signal	peRETSPL in dB (re: 20 µPa)	
	Telephonics TDH-39 supra-aural earphone	Etymotic research ER-3A insert receiver
Clicks	31.0	35.5
250 Hz tone bursts	32.0	28.0
500 Hz tone bursts	23.0	23.5
1000 Hz tone bursts	18.5	21.5
2000 Hz tone bursts	25.0	28.5
4000 Hz tone bursts	27.5	32.5

[a]Based on ISO 389-6 (2007), Richter & Fedtke (2005), and Fedtke & Richter (2007) for 1-second trains of clicks and tone bursts repeating at a rate of 20 Hz. Correction values are required for faster and slower repetition rates.

It is also common to find the stimulus levels expressed in *behavioral* terms. A widely used approach expresses click intensity in decibels of **normal Hearing Level (nHL)**, which is based on a local norm corresponding to 0 dB HL for each click and tone burst. The procedure involves obtaining behavioral thresholds for each signal for a group of young, normal-hearing individuals. Each person is tested to find the lowest hearing level dial level on the ABR instrument where the clicks or tone bursts are just audible. This dial setting constitutes that person's threshold for that click or tone burst, and the average for the group becomes 0 dB nHL.

Another behavior approach is done on an individual-patient basis by determining the patient's own behavioral threshold for clicks, and then expressing the click intensity in **sensation level (dB SL)**. However, this approach is limited because it is difficult, at best, to assess hearing without knowing the physical level of the stimulus. Moreover, ABR testing is often done on patients who cannot be tested behaviorally, in which case the sensation level of the stimulus cannot be determined.

The ABR Waveform

An idealized ABR waveform is shown in **Fig. 11.6**. This figure shows positive peaks that are recorded in the upward direction and numbered from I to VII,

Fig. 11.6 An idealized auditory brainstem response (ABR). Arrows indicate the wave I, II, and III absolute latencies and amplitudes, and the interwave latencies between waves I and V, I and III, and III and V.

which is the most common convention in the United States. However, other recording conventions also exist. As already mentioned, waves I and II are generated by the auditory nerve and correspond to the N1 (AP) and N2 peaks of the electrocochleogram. Even though these first two peaks were plotted downward in the ECochG, they are now flipped upward so they appear in the same direction as the rest of the ABR peaks. This inversion of waves I and II occurs during the process of differential amplification, and is very convenient because it causes all of the ABR peaks to be plotted in the same direction. Before proceeding, notice that only one curve is shown. In actual practice, two sets of tracings would be done because evoked potentials must be *replicated* to confirm that the results obtained are real.

Clinical ABR measurements are concerned with the first five peaks (I to V), and concentrate on peaks I, III, and V. The ABR waveform is usually described and interpreted in terms of the latencies and amplitudes of these peaks, as well as by its **morphology**, or the overall configuration and appearance of the waveform. A given wave's **absolute latency** is simply the time delay from 0 ms (when the click is presented) until its peak occurs.

Electrocochleography is sometimes used to locate wave I when it is not identifiable on the ABR. The time interval between two peaks is called an **interwave latency** or **relative latency**. Interwave latencies are usually measured between waves I and V, I and III, and III and V. These latency measurements are illustrated in the figure by the horizontal arrows.

The vertical arrows show how to measure the **amplitudes** for waves I, II, and V. Wave V is the most prominent and robust of these peaks, and is so closely associated with wave IV that one must speak of a **IV/V complex**. There is, however, considerable variability in the morphology of normal ABR waveforms, particularly with respect to the configuration of the IV/V complex.

The ABR waveforms shown in the two previous figures were all obtained with clicks presented at fairly high intensity levels. They would have looked different if the clicks had been presented at progressively lower intensities, and would eventually disappear when the clicks went below threshold. In other words, the characteristics of the ABR depend on the level of the stimulus.

Fig. 11.7 shows a series of ABR results obtained from a normal individual with clicks presented at 80, 60, 40, and 20 dB nHL. Notice that the characteristics of the ABR waveform change considerably as the intensity of the clicks is decreased. Another series of ABR waveforms is shown across the upper part of **Fig. 11.8**, where intensity increases from left to right along the x-axis. *As the stimulus intensity gets lower, the peak latencies become longer and their amplitudes become smaller.* The latency shift is seen most vividly by the rightward shift of wave V as the intensity drops progressively from 80 dB nHL down to 20 dB nHL in **Fig. 11.7**. Also, the earlier peaks become less distinctive and eventually disappear with progressively lower stimulus levels. Even though wave V becomes progressively smaller and later with decreasing intensity, it is generally still discernible at

Fig. 11.7 A series of click-evoked auditory brainstem responses from a normal adult obtained at various stimulus levels. Wave V indicated on each tracing. (From Arnold [2000], with permission.)

levels as low as the behavioral threshold for the click, which is typically down to 0 dB SL or 0 dB nHL, or roughly 35 dB peakSPL, for a normal person. The ABR is finally undetectable at levels below the behavioral threshold. **Fig. 11.8** also shows a graph that plots the manner in which wave V latency changes as a function of stimulus (click) level. Such a graph is called a latency-intensity function, and it reveals the manner in which the wave V latency changes as a function of stimulus (click) level. Such a graph is called a latency-intensity function, and it reveals the manner latency decreases as stimulus intensity increases.

Clinical Use of the Auditory Brainstem Response

The ABR is a very valuable clinical tool for several reasons. (1) Auditory brainstem responses are measurable in everyone who is normal, including newborns. (2) The ABR is not affected by the patient's state of arousal, or by the use of sedation or anesthesia. As a result, ABR testing can be done with or without the cooperation of the patient, and even when the patient is unconscious or under general anesthesia. The ability to perform the ABR on a patient under sedation makes it possible to assess young and/or difficult-to-test children who could not otherwise be evaluated. It should be stressed, of course, that sedation is a medical responsibility. In addition, the ABR is also used in intraoperative monitoring during surgical procedures that jeopardize the eighth nerve, such as acoustic tumor removal. (3) The ABR can be used to assess hearing because it is affected by hearing loss. (4) Different abnormalities affect the ABR in different ways, so that it can be used for differential diagnosis.

Just because the ABR is ubiquitous does not mean that its characteristics are the same for everyone. On the contrary, maturation, gender, and aging need to be considered when developing norms and interpreting the results.

The ABR is present but not adult-like in newborns, and its character changes with the infant's maturation (Hecox & Galambos 1974; Fria 1980; Chiappa 1997; Hurley, Hurley, & Berlin 2005; Hall 2007; Sininger 2007). For example, waves I, III, and V are observable in newborns, but the absolute latencies of waves III and V are prolonged relative to adult values, as are the interwave latencies. As the infant matures, the other peaks emerge, the latencies of the waves shorten, and their amplitudes change, eventually achieving adult characteristics by roughly 18 months of age.

Among adults, the ABR is affected by gender and aging (Stockard, Stockard, Westmoreland, & Corfits 1979; Jerger & Hall 1980; Jerger & Johnson 1988).

Fig. 11.8 A latency intensity function corresponding to the series of click-evoked ABRs shown in **Fig. 11.7**. The waveforms are superimposed on the graph to highlight the manner in which waveform morphology, latency, and intensity change with the level of the stimulus. (Adapted from Arnold SA [2007]. The auditory brain stem response. In: Roeser RJ, Valente M, Hosford-Dunn H, eds. *Audiology Diagnosis*, 2nd ed. New York, NY: Thieme; 426–442.)

Compared with males, females tend to have shorter absolute latencies and larger amplitudes for waves III, IV, and V, as well as shorter interwave latencies. Also, it appears that the degree of cochlear impairment has a greater effect on wave V latencies for men than for women (Jerger & Johnson 1988). The effect of aging is not as clear-cut, but its absolute latencies appear to become slightly longer with advancing age.

The earlier discussion about how the ABR is affected by stimulus intensity also reveals the procedure for estimating a patient's thresholds with the ABR. The basic procedure is to obtain a series of ABRs at progressively lower intensities until the level is reached where a replicable response is no longer discernible. This usually involves finding the lowest level where wave V can be identified. Normal hearing is implied when a response can be identified at stimulus levels as low as ~ 0 dB nHL. The word *implied* is used because physiological measures are not direct hearing tests in the sense that they do not reveal whether the patient is able to respond to sounds behaviorally. Rather, they are tests of the integrity of the structures and processes involved in hearing, and in the case of the ABR, these responses are coming from just the lower portions of the auditory pathways. In spite of these caveats, it is clear that ABR thresholds provide valuable information about the hearing of patients who cannot respond behaviorally, such as infants and the difficult-to-test. In fact, the ABR is widely used for infant screening purposes as well as for the diagnostic assessment of this population (Chapters 12 and 13). *Click* ABR thresholds are related to *high*-frequency behavioral thresholds. However, the *tone burst* ABR is used to estimate patients' hearing sensitivity because it provides *frequency-specific* thresholds. Tone burst ABR thresholds are typically within ~ 10 to 15 dB of behavioral thresholds at various audiometric frequencies, and correction factors are often applied to the ABR thresholds to achieve better estimates (Stapells, Gravel, & Martin 1995; Stapells 2000; Gorga et al 2006; Rance, Tomlin, & Rickards 2006; Sininger, Abdala, & Cone-Wesson 1997; Vander Werff, Prieve, & Georgantas 2009).

An individual patient's latency-intensity functions are compared with normative values to make inferences about the nature and degree of her hearing loss. Several examples are shown in **Fig. 11.9**. The normal range of wave V latencies is shown by a pair of curved lines in each panel. Each facility should develop a set of normal ranges that applies to its own equipment and procedures. The leftmost symbol of each individual latency-intensity function is obtained from the lowest click level that produces a replicable ABR, and therefore also represents the threshold for clicks. These points occur at 5 dB nHL for the normal case and 45 dB nHL for conductive loss in the upper panel of the figure, and at 30, 35, and 45 dB nHL for the examples of cochlear impairments in the lower panel.

The typical **wave V latency-intensity functions** associated with normal hearing, conductive losses, and sensorineural losses of cochlear origin are quite different. As we would expect, the *normal* latency-intensity function falls within the normal limit lines (*orange circles* in **Fig. 11.9a**). *Conductive losses* reduce the amount of signal intensity reaching the cochlea. For this reason, they tend to have latency-intensity functions that are essentially displaced horizontally to the right (higher click levels) by roughly the amount of the conductive loss (*green circles* in **Fig. 11.9a**). On the other hand, *cochlear impairments* typically have wave V latencies that are elevated at and slightly above threshold, and then converge to the normal latency range as the click intensity is raised (circles in **Fig. 11.9b**). However, whether this pattern occurs depends on the configuration of the hearing loss because the ABR relies heavily on the basal (high-frequency) portion of the cochlea

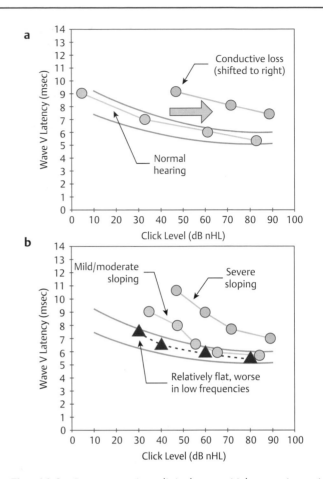

Fig. 11.9 Representative clinical wave V latency-intensity functions. The paired curved lines in each panel are normal confidence limits. **(a)** Results for a normal ear and a case of conductive loss. Notice the conductive function is shifted to the right, represented by the arrow. **(b)** Functions for cochlear sensorineural loss generally converge toward the normal latency range as click intensity is raised, but this is affected by the shape and degree of loss.

(Yamada, Kodera, & Yagi 1979). Notice in **Fig. 11.9b** that the wave V latency-intensity function is abnormal when the sensorineural hearing loss involves the high frequencies (circles), but can actually be within the normal range in cases of low frequency and relatively mild flat sensorineural loss, where the high frequencies are preserved (triangles).

The different latency-intensity functions associated with conductive and cochlear impairments allow the ABR to help us discriminate between these two kinds of hearing losses. However, conductive losses may have to exceed 35 dB to be reliably distinguished from sensorineural impairments with the ABR (van der Drift, Brocaar, & van Zanten 1988a,b).

Another way to use the ABR to identify the type of loss is to compare the results obtained when the clicks are presented by air-conduction versus bone-conduction. When bone-conduction ABRs are done, one must be mindful that (1) the highest usable click levels for bone-conduction ABR testing are limited to ~ 50 dB nHL, (2) bone-conduction wave V latencies are roughly 0.5 ms longer than they are by air-conduction, and (3) appropriate masking of the contralateral ear should be employed (Mauldin & Jerger 1979; Weber 1983; Schwartz, Larson, & De Chicchis 1985; Gorga & Thornton 1989).

Because the ABR reflects the activity of the auditory nerve and brainstem pathways, it is not surprising that it can be used to identify *retrocochlear pathologies* like acoustic tumors. The identification of retrocochlear disorders from the ABR has an overall sensitivity of ~ 95% (Turner, Shepard, & Frazer 1984). The identification of retrocochlear disorders from the ABR involves interpreting peak measurements and waveform morphology. The following ABR findings are associated with retrocochlear abnormalities, several of which may be found in **Fig. 11.10**:

- *Prolonged latency* for wave V.
- *Prolonged interwave latency* for I to V (as well as for I to III and/or III to V).
- *Interaural latency differences*. Significant differences between the patient's two ears are considered for both the wave V latency and the interwave latencies.
- *Absence of the later waves.*
- *Absence of an ABR* even though hearing is normal or only mildly impaired.
- An ABR waveform that is *not replicable.*
- Abnormally low V:I amplitude ratio. The V:I amplitude ratio is simply the amplitude of wave V over the amplitude of wave I, and is expected to be ≥ 1.0 because wave V is normally larger. One becomes suspicious of a retrocochlear disorder when the V:I ratio is less than 1.0, but this criterion is not as sensitive as the latency measurements.
- Significant shifting of wave V latency when the clicks are presented at a faster rate, although the usefulness of this criterion is controversial.

An absent or grossly abnormal ABR with normal outer hair cell functioning demonstrated by otoacoustic emissions and/or cochlear microphonics (discussed elsewhere in this chapter) is also associated with *auditory neuropathy spectrum disorder* (e.g., Starr, Picton, Sininger, Hood, & Berlin 1996; Hood 2007; see Chapter 6).

Although standard ABR testing has excellent sensitivity for acoustic tumors overall, it has been disappointing when trying to identify small tumors (those ≤ 1 cm in size; e.g., Chandrasekhar, Brackmann, & Devgan 1995; Schmidt, Sataloff, Newman, Spiegel,

& Myers 2001). However, an approach called the stacked **auditory brainstem response (stacked ABR)** has been quite successful at identifying these small tumors even when they are missed by the standard ABR (e.g., Don, Masuda, Nelson, & Brackmann 1997; Don & Kwong 2002; Don, Kwong, Tanaka, Brackmann, & Nelson 2005). For example, Don et al (2005) found that the stacked ABR had 95% sensitivity for a group of 54 patients with acoustic tumors that were missed by the standard ABR or were ≤ 1 cm in size, as well as 88% specificity for 78 tumor-free control subjects with normal hearing. The stacked ABR method uses the derived-band approach described earlier to obtain several ABRs derived from different frequency locations along the cochlea. These derived ABR waveforms are then shifted so that they are aligned at the wave V peak, and summed to arrive at the stacked ABR. The wave V amplitude of this stacked response is then measured and can then be compared with normative values.

Later Auditory Evoked Potentials

The ABR is by far the class of auditory evoked potentials that is most widely used by audiologists, sometimes to the exclusion of all others. Yet other kinds of AEPs are not only available but also provide information not obtainable with the ABR. **Fig. 11.3** identifies these as the **middle latency response (MLR)** and the **long latency response (LLR)** (McPherson & Ballachanda 2000; Hall 2007; Pratt 2007; Martin, Tremblay, & Stapells 2007; Cacace & McFarland 2009). The major advantage of these responses is that they can provide frequency-specific information about hearing sensitivity. Their major disadvantage is that they are significantly affected by the state of the patient and are altered or obliterated by drugs (including sedatives and anesthetics), which curtails their usefulness with young children and other difficult-to-test patients.

The middle latency response is a series of negative (N) and positive (P) waves occurring at latencies between 15 and 50 ms, identified as **Na, Pa, Nb**, and **Pb (Fig. 11.3)**. It appears to reflect neural activity originating from several cortical and subcortical locations involving the midbrain, reticular formation, and the thalamocortical pathways. The principal clinical contribution of the MLR is that it can be elicited by relatively low-frequency tone bursts, such as 500 or 1000 Hz, which would not be successful stimuli with the ABR. As a result, the MLR can be used successfully to assess low-frequency hearing sensitivity. It is also useful in the diagnosis of central auditory nervous system abnormalities.

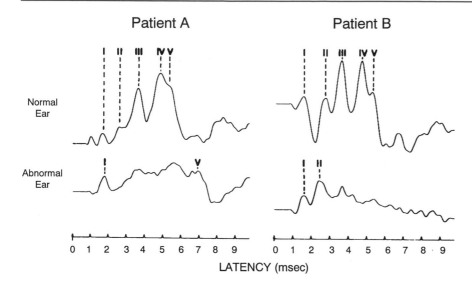

Patient A   Patient B

Normal
Ear

Abnormal
Ear

LATENCY (msec)

Fig. 11.10 Two examples of abnormal ABR results in cases of retrocochlear pathology. (Adapted from ASHA [1987], with permission of American Speech-Language-Hearing Association.)

The long latency responses occur at latencies beyond ~ 75 ms and have also been known as the **cortical evoked potentials**. The major LLR components are shown in **Fig. 11.3** as waves **N1**, **P2**, and **N2**. (Wave **P1** is generally considered to be the latest peak of the middle response, Pb.) It appears that the P2 and N2 components of the LLR are largely derived from activity from the auditory cortex, and that contributions are also made by the limbic system. Even though it is possible to obtain frequency-specific evoked response thresholds with the LLR, its susceptibility to the state of arousal and drugs means that its use is largely limited to awake and cooperative patients.

Event-Related Potentials

Other kinds of late responses also occur that involve discriminations and various levels of processing for all kinds of signals from tones to speech (Hall 2007; Starr & Golob 2007). For example, **P3** (or **P300**) is a large positive wave that occurs at a latency of ~ 300 ms when the patient attends to and elicits a cognitive response to an atypical stimulus (e.g., Sutton, Braren, Zubin, & John 1965; Burkhard, et al 2007; Hall 2007). Testing for the P3 wave involves an **odd-ball procedure** that uses two different signals, one that occurs frequently (the "frequent" signal) and another that occurs infrequently (the "rare" signal). The rare signal is also called an "odd-ball" because it differs from the frequent signal in some way, such as frequency. Different sets of evoked potentials are then obtained. "Frequent" test conditions have signals that are all the same. "Rare" test conditions include a relatively small percentage of odd-ball sig-

nals distributed randomly among the frequent signals. If the patient *ignores* the test stimuli, then the result will be a routine LLR regardless of whether the odd-ball was present or absent **(Fig. 11.11a,b)**. The situation is different if the patient *pays attention to the signals, listening particularly for the odd-balls*. Here the AEP is unchanged for the frequent-only signals **(Fig. 11.11c)**; however, a clear P3 wave appears for the rarely included signals **(Fig. 11.11d)**. In contrast, **mismatch negativity (MMN)** is a physiological measure of discrimination that occurs even *without attending* to the stimulus (Näätänen & Kraus 1995), and is affected by a variety of central disorders as well as the aging process (Näätänen, Kujala, Escera,

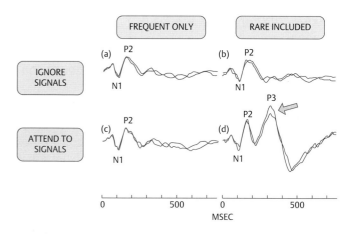

Fig. 11.11 A P3 wave (*arrow*) is obtained when odd-ball signals are present and attended to by the patient. (Modified from "Electrophysiological evaluation of higher level auditory processing" by Squires and Hecox [1983], with permission.)

et al 2012). It appears as a negative deflection that occurs at latencies between roughly 150 and 275 ms when the patient detects a signal that is different from those that came before it.

As one might expect, these and other event-related potentials are produced by neural activity extending well beyond just the auditory cortex, and provide us with physiological windows into the patient's ability to deal with almost every level of processing, from detecting and discriminating signals to processing them linguistically and cognitively.

Auditory Steady-State Response (ASSR)

The **auditory steady-state response (ASSR)** is an AEP that is elicited by a tone that fluctuates (modulates) periodically over time. An example of **amplitude modulation (AM)** is shown in **Fig. 11.12a**. It represents a 1000 Hz tone that fluctuates in level at a rate of 80 times per second. In this case, 1000 Hz is the *carrier frequency* and 80 Hz is the *modulation rate* or *frequency*. (The fluctuations in the figure have a *modulation depth* of 100% because the amplitude drops to 0 during the troughs.) If the tone fluctuates 40 times per second, then the modulation rate would be 40 Hz. Other kinds of modulation are also possible, such as **frequency modulation (FM)**, where the frequency of the carrier tone fluctuates over time, or a combination of both AM and FM. However, we will limit our discussion to AM tones for clarity.

The spectra of four representative AM tones (500, 1000, 2000, and 4000 Hz) are illustrated on the same set of axes in **Fig. 11.12b**. Notice that the spectrum of each AM tone contains just the carrier frequency and a couple of relatively weaker components at nearby frequencies just above and below it.[2] As a result, an AM tone is a stimulus that is fairly specific in frequency. This means that the ASSR can give information about hearing in a narrow range around each test frequency, and thus provide us with approximations of a patient's thresholds at a variety of audiometric frequencies, such as 500 Hz, 1000 Hz, 2000 Hz, and 4000 Hz .

When presented with an AM (or other type of modulated) tone (**Fig. 11.12**), the auditory nervous

Fig. 11.12 Idealized drawings of the **(a)** waveform of an AM tone with a 1000 Hz carrier frequency and an 80 Hz modulation rate; **(b)** spectra of 500 Hz, 1000 Hz, 2000 Hz, and 4000 Hz AM tones with an 80 Hz modulation rate (logarithmic scale); **(c)** envelope of an amplitude modulation tone (stimulus); **(d)** ASSR (response) waveform in which the EEG activity is synchronized to the modulation rate of the stimulus, with a slight delay (*arrows*). (Graphic **(d)** adapted from Grason-Stadler, Inc. [2001] with permission.)

system responds in a way that is synchronized (phase-locked) with the temporal pattern of the modulating pattern (**Fig. 11.12d**), although with a slight delay as shown by the arrows in the figure. In other words, the EEG activity in response to the AM tone will be seen at the modulation frequency. This is the ASSR. For example, the ASSR would be seen at 80 Hz when the modulation rate is 80 Hz, and at 40 Hz when the modulation rate is 40 Hz. The ASSR reflects activity from both the brainstem and the auditory cortices, with the response being dominated by the brainstem at higher modulation rates and the cortex at lower modulation rates (Herdman et al 2002). Thus, we are not surprised that the ASSR is differently affected by state of arousal at low versus high modulation rates: Specifically, sleep and anesthesia affect the ASSR at *lower* modulation rates like 40 Hz, similar to the longer-latency potentials (Jerger, Chmiel, Frost, & Coker 1986; Picton, John, Purcell, & Plourde 2003); but state of arousal does not substantially affect the ASSR at *higher* modulation rates like 80 Hz, similar to the ABR (Cohen, Rickards, & Clark 1991; Levi, Folsom, & Dobie 1993; Aoyagi et al 1993).

---

[2] Specifically, it contains energy at the carrier frequency and smaller amounts of energy at frequencies equal to the carrier plus and minus the modulation frequency. So, a 1000 Hz tone being modulated at 80 Hz has energy at 1000 Hz and smaller amounts at 920 Hz and 1080 Hz, and a 1000 Hz tone being modulated at 40 Hz has energy at 1000 Hz and smaller amounts at 960 and 1040 Hz. Similarly, a 500 Hz tone being modulated at 40 Hz has energy at 500 Hz, and weaker amounts at 460 and 540 Hz.

Although approaches differ (e.g., Rance, Rickards, Cohen, De Vidi, & Clark 1995; Dimitrijevic, John, Van Roon, et al 2002), ASSR measurement fundamentally involves presenting modulated tones to a patient while monitoring his EEG activity. An ASSR is considered present if the amplitude and/or phase (delay) of the response is reliably related to the modulated tone, which is determined based on a statistical analysis. This sounds complicated, but the decision is actually automated, being reached according to objective criteria programmed into the measurement instrumentation.

The ASSR has several assets as a clinical tool in audiology. The ASSR is present from infancy through adulthood (e.g., Lins et al 1996; Cone-Wesson, Parker, Swiderski, & Rickards 2002; Rance et al 2006), which combined with its resistance to sleep and anesthesia makes it a valuable tool for pediatric evaluation (Chapter 12). The ASSR probably has potential in neonatal screening (Chapter 13) as well. However, responses are small in newborns and thresholds decrease with age during the first 12 months (Savio, Cárdenas, Pérez Abalo, González, & Valdés 2001; John, Brown, Muir, & Picton 2004; Rance & Tomlin 2006). Thus, more information is needed before deciding about its applicability in neonatal screening.

We have already seen that the ASSR provides for frequency-specific testing. Average ASSR thresholds are within about ≤ 15 dB of behavioral thresholds in normal-hearing listeners, which is also true among those with hearing loss (e.g., Lins et al 1996; Herdman & Stapells 2001, 2003; Dimitrijevic et al 2002; Picton, Dimitrijevic, Perez-Abalo, & Van Roon 2005; Vander Werff & Brown 2005). However, ASSR thresholds are somewhat higher among infants (e.g., Lins et al 1996), as illustrated in **Table 11.2**. Thresholds obtained by ASSR are comparable to those obtained by ABR (e.g., Cone-Wesson, Dowell, Tomlin, Rance, & Ming 2002; Rance et al 2006; Cone-Wesson & Dimitrinjevic 2009). Moreover, ASSR testing appears to be feasible at higher levels than are possible with the ABR, which makes it possible to test patients with much more severe hearing losses; but there have been some concerns about distortions and artifacts at these high levels (Gorga et al 2004).

Topographical Brain Mapping

It is possible to record a particular potential, such as the P3 wave or a component of the MLR, simultaneously from many different locations on the head. As one would expect, the amplitude of these responses will vary according to where they are picked up, being largest where the underlying neural activity is greatest and smallest at locations that are inactive. A

Table 11.2 Means (standard deviations) for the difference between ASSR and behavioral thresholds (dB) in normal-hearing adults and for ASSR thresholds (dB HL) in well (presumably normal-hearing) babies[a]

Carrier frequency (Hz)	Adults: ASSR-behavioral differences (dB)	Well babies: ASSR thresholds (dB HL)
500	14 (11)	33 (103)
1000	12 (11)	22 (10)
2000	11 (8)	19 (8)
4000	13 (11)	19 (10)

[a]Based on Lins et al (1996).

computer program can then be used to "fill in" the amplitudes that should occur between these sampled locations. The result can be drawn as contour lines or differently shaded areas depicting equally active locations on the scalp, just as geographical maps use contours to show equal land elevations. Other programs show equally active locations with different colors. We see the same kinds of pictures on television weather reports every day, representing regions of equal temperature or rainfall. Just as red means hot weather and other colors mean progressively lower temperatures, red areas on a topographical brain map are "hot" from the standpoint of neurologic brain activity and other colors represent progressively less active locations. Clinically, a patient's topographical brain map may be compared with normal patterns for such purposes as evaluating the physiological aspects of processing disorders and determining disordered anatomical sites.

■ Otoacoustic Emissions

One of the most fascinating characteristics of the cochlea is that it can produce sounds as well as receive them. These sounds that are elicited by the ear are called **otoacoustic emissions (OAEs)**, and can be measured with a sensitive microphone in the ear canal. Kemp (1978, 1979) demonstrated that OAEs are produced in response to signals presented to the ear, as well as spontaneously without any stimulation. The concept is best understood by imagining a simple experiment in which an OAE is produced as a result of presenting a click to the ear. We will need a probe assembly similar to the kind used for acoustic immittance testing (Chapter 7). For convenience, we will call this assembly the "probe tip." It contains a tiny loudspeaker ("receiver" or "earphone") to present the click stimulus, and a sensitive microphone to record the sounds in the ear canal, including the OAE. The method involves measuring the sounds in the ear canal for a period of ~ 20 ms, beginning with the presentation of a click.

First, let us see what happens when the click is directed into an *inanimate cavity*. To do this, the probe tip is inserted into a Zwislocki coupler, which is a metal cavity that mimics the acoustics of the ear. The result is a damped oscillation lasting several milliseconds, as shown in the top frame of **Fig. 11.13**. This damped oscillation is the acoustic waveform of the click itself. In contrast, presenting a click into a real ear results in the waveform shown in the middle frame of the figure. The most obvious aspects of this waveform are the same large, damped oscillations due to the click seen in the inert cavity. However, notice that this waveform, measured in a real ear canal, also contains a second group of tiny oscillations that begin several milliseconds later. These oscillations constitute the OAE or **cochlear echo**

(Kemp echo) produced in the cochlea, transmitted back into the ear canal, and picked up by the probe tip microphone. The lower panel of the figure shows the OAE after it has been amplified, with the earlier click waveform removed. This kind of OAE is called a transient-evoked otoacoustic emission because it occurs in response to a click (transient) stimulus, and will be covered in greater detail below.

Otoacoustic emissions are generally interpreted as being the result of microscopic biomechanical activity (motility) associated with healthy outer hair cells. This activity produces a signal within the cochlea that is transmitted "backward" through the middle ear and into the ear canal, where it can be picked up by a microphone. The cochlear events that produce OAEs are said to be "preneural" because they occur before the signal is transmitted to the auditory nerve, and are related to the physiological processes underlying the sensitivity and the "fine tuning" of the normal cochlea (e.g., Kiang, Liberman, Sewell, & Guinan 1986; Probst, Lonsbury-Martin, & Martin 1991; Norton 1992; Robinette & Glattke 2007a,b; Gelfand 2010). Our interest in OAEs is practical as well as theoretical because they are also useful clinical tools. Otoacoustic emissions are valuable clinically because

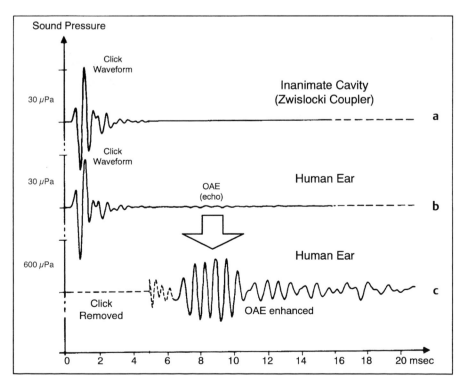

Fig. 11.13 **(a)** Waveform of a click in an inanimate cavity (Zwislocki coupler). **(b)** Click waveform and resulting otoacoustic emission (OAE) or cochlear echo in a human ear canal. **(c)** Same as middle panel, but with click waveform removed and the otoacoustic emission enhanced. (Adapted from Johnsen and Elberling [1982], with permission of *Scandinavian Audiology*.)

they are (1) sensitive to the presence of hearing loss, (2) sensitive to problems affecting the integrity of the cochlea, particularly the outer hair cells, and (3) preneural in nature, which makes them different from measurements that involve neural activity—for example, the auditory brainstem response. In addition, OAEs are very practical because they are quick and easy to obtain without any invasive procedures. Otoacoustic emissions are the subject of extensive, ongoing research, and their clinical attributes and applications are provided in several contemporary reviews (e.g., Glattke & Robinette 2007; Robinette & Glattke 2007a,b; Prieve & Fitzgerald 2009; Dhar & Hall 2011).

As anticipated from the example just described, the equipment needed to measure OAEs includes a probe tip assembly that contains a microphone to measure sounds in the ear canal, as well as receivers to present various kinds of stimuli. The faint sounds picked up by the measurement microphone are amplified and filtered to minimize noises, and are then analyzed in one of several ways depending on what kind of OAE is being examined. The microphone is involved in all OAE measurements, regardless of whether the emissions are evoked by some kind of stimulus or occur spontaneously in the absence of stimulation. The receivers present the stimuli used to elicit the various kinds of evoked OAEs. The characteristics of OAE equipment are given in an International Electrotechnical Commission standard (IEC 60645-6-2009), and examples of clinical OAE instruments are shown in **Fig. 11.14**. Block diagrams describing the instrumentation involved in measuring various kinds of OAEs appear later in this chapter.

Spontaneous Otoacoustic Emissions

Spontaneous otoacoustic emissions (SOAEs) are narrow-band sounds emitted from the ear in the absence of stimulation. They are identified by examining the spectrum of the sound monitored by a probe microphone in the ear canal. The spectrum is the result of a spectral analysis performed by the OAE analysis system, as illustrated in the upper part of **Fig. 11.15**. The lower part of the figure shows an example of the averaged spectrum from an ear with SOAEs at 1140, 1680, and 2255 Hz. The SOAEs are seen as narrow peaks extending above the background noise in the spectrum. They usually occur at one or several frequencies between 1000 and 3000 Hz, and occasionally as low as ~ 500 Hz. As indicated in the figure, SOAEs are very faint, typically ranging in size from roughly −10 to +20 dB SPL. For this reason, several spectra are averaged so that we are able to see the SOAEs above the background noise. This

Fig. 11.14 Example of **(a)** desktop and **(b)** hand-held otoacoustic emissions instruments (Courtesy of Otodynamics Audiology Systems.)

spectral averaging procedure is based on the same principles that were explained for auditory evoked potentials, except that averaging is done as a function of frequency instead of over time.

It was originally thought that SOAEs would be a useful clinical tool because they are relatively simple to measure, tend to occur at the same frequencies over time for a given ear, do not appear to be age related, and may be present at frequencies where thresholds are in the normal range *but* are absent in frequency regions where the hearing loss exceeds 20 to 30 dB HL. However, the clinical usefulness of SOAEs is actually rather limited because of two different kinds of drawbacks. One set of restrictions

Spontaneous otoacoustic emissions

Fig. 11.15 Instrumentation block diagram and an example of spontaneous otoacoustic emissions (SOAEs). These are seen as narrow peaks in the spectrum monitored in the ear canal. This idealized example shows SOAEs at 1140, 1680, and 2255 Hz.

involves the relatively low prevalence of SOAEs. Specifically, SOAEs occur in only about half of the normal-hearing population and are also less likely to occur in males than in females. The other clinical weaknesses of SOAEs pertain to the ears where they are found. These limitations are that (1) just a few (or only one) SOAEs are found in an ear; (2) they occur at different frequencies in different ears; (3) SOAEs are found in a relatively restricted range of frequencies; and (4) their amplitudes can vary over time.

Although it is inviting to wonder whether SOAEs are the cause of tinnitus (or are at least a physiological manifestation of it), this is unlikely in most cases for several reasons. For example, tinnitus is more likely to be associated with hearing loss and/or disordered ears, whereas SOAEs are associated with normality. In fact, most people who have SOAEs are not aware of them. Thus, we are not surprised that although an association with SOAEs has been reported in up to perhaps 12% of tinnitus patients (Norton, Schmidt, & Stover 1990; Penner 1990), the common finding is that tinnitus and SOAEs are generally unrelated (e.g., Penner & Burns 1987; Probst, Lonsburry-Martin, Martin, & Coats 1987; Bonfils 1989; Penner 1990).

Evoked Otoacoustic Emissions

Evoked otoacoustic emissions are sounds emitted from the ear as a result of stimulation. There are basically three different kinds of evoked otoacoustic emissions. **Stimulus-frequency otoacoustic emissions (SFOAEs)** are elicited by presenting a sweep-frequency tone to the ear. This class of OAEs may provide useful information, but complications in terms of technology and interpretation have prevented it from being a viable clinical tool at this point in time. We shall therefore concentrate on the two other types of evoked OAEs, which have considerable clinical utility and promise. These include transient evoked otoacoustic emissions and distortion product otoacoustic emissions.

Transient-Evoked Otoacoustic Emissions

Transient-evoked otoacoustic emissions (TEOAEs) are produced in response to very brief stimuli, such as clicks. The TEOAE is also known as the **click-evoked otoacoustic emission**, **Kemp echo**, or **cochlear echo**. (Although not discussed here, more frequency-specific stimuli such as tone bursts can also be used.) Recall from the example used to introduce the concept of otoacoustic emissions earlier in this section that the TEOAE is seen as a waveform that is picked up in the ear canal several milliseconds after a click has been presented. The upper part of **Fig. 11.16** shows a block diagram of the equipment used to elicit and measure TEOAEs. The probe tip includes a loudspeaker to present the clicks and a microphone to monitor the sounds in the ear canal. The signals picked up by the microphone then go through an amplifier and filter to a signal analysis system. Because the OAEs have very small amplitudes that must be distinguished from background noise, a large number of clicks are presented in succession, and the sounds in the ear canal are monitored for a period of time (e.g., 20 ms) after each click. These responses are then averaged using the same basic approach described for auditory evoked potentials earlier in this chapter.

Clinical TEOAEs are usually elicited using clicks presented at ~ 82 to 83 dB peSPL. An example of a normal TEOAE waveform is shown in the lower portion of **Fig. 11.16**. The large frame shows the waveform of the TEOAE response. The time scale shows the latency of the response from when the click was presented. The first several milliseconds of the response appear flat so as to remove the waveform of the click stimulus, which is shown in a separate box (above left). Notice that two separate waveforms (A and B) were obtained and superimposed to establish

Transient-evoked otoacoustic emissions

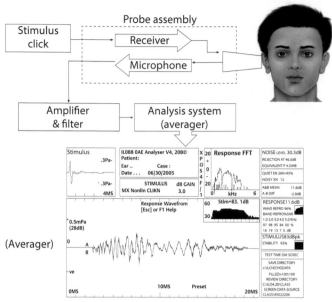

Fig. 11.16 Instrumentation block diagram and an example of transient evoked otoacoustic emissions (TEOAEs; see text). (From Glattke TJ, Robinette MS [2007]. Transient evoked optoacoustic emissions in populations with normal hearing sensitivity. In: Robinette MS, Glattke TJ, eds. *Otoacoustic Emissions: Clinical Applications*, 3rd ed. New York, NY: Thieme; 87–105, with permission.)

the reliability of the results. The TEOAE waveform has latencies between ~ 5 and 20 ms. A given latency on this waveform reflects the "round trip" time it takes for the click to reach a particular location along the cochlear duct and for the returning TEOAE (cochlear echo) to be picked up by the probe microphone in the ear canal. This travel time is shortest for locations near the base of the cochlea and increases toward the apex. Hence, it appears that (1) the earlier parts of the TEOAE waveform (i.e., those at shorter latencies) are from locations toward the base of the cochlea, where higher frequencies are represented; and (2) the parts of the waveform at successively longer latencies are from locations successively closer to the apex, where lower frequencies are represented. The spectrum of this TEOAE is shown in the box above and to the right of the waveform. Normal TEOAEs are generally obtained at frequencies from ~ 400 to 500 Hz up to ~ 4500 Hz in adults and ~ 5000 to 6000 Hz in babies and young children. The decision about whether a TEOAE is present often depends on a visual assessment of the response along with certain objective criteria, such as the reproducibility of the waveform (in percent) and the signal-to-noise ratio (in decibels) of the response compared with the noise floor.

It is possible to point out several generalities about TEOAEs that have considerable clinical relevance. Transient-evoked OAEs can be obtained in almost all normal-hearing individuals, including newborns. In fact, responses are larger in babies than they are in adults. Reduced or obliterated TEOAEs result from the same factors that are known to cause cochlear hearing losses, such as ototoxic agents, hypoxia, and noise exposure. Similarly, TEOAEs are absent in patients with cochlear sensorineural losses greater than ~ 30 to 50 dB HL, depending on the details of the test parameters. Conductive abnormalities can also interfere with the ability to obtain TEOAEs because they interfere with the ability of the OAE to be transmitted back to the probe microphone. These factors make TEOAEs very useful for detecting the presence of hearing loss, even in newborns. As a result, newborn hearing screening programs have been one of the most rapidly growing applications of TEOAEs, as discussed in Chapter 13. Because otoacoustic emissions are preneural events, it is not surprising that TEOAEs are usually not a particularly useful test for acoustic tumors per se (Bonfils & Uziel 1988). However, they do contribute to differential diagnosis, improving the ability to distinguish cochlear and neural involvement, when used with tests that involve neural transmission, such as acoustic reflexes and the ABR (e.g., Robinette, Bauch, Olsen, Hamer, & Beatty 1992; Starr et al 1996; Robinette & Glattke 2007a,b; Lonsbury-Martin, Martin, & Telischi 1999).

Distortion Product Otoacoustic Emissions

Distortion product otoacoustic emissions (DPOAEs) are elicited by simultaneously presenting to the ear two stimulus tones with different frequencies, as shown in the block diagram at the top of **Fig. 11.17**. The lower stimulus tone is called f_1 and the higher tone is called f_2. As a result of its normal nonlinear response to the two stimulus tones, the cochlea will generate another tone "of its own" at a different frequency, called a **distortion product**. The distortion product is then transmitted back to the ear canal as an otoacoustic emission. (This is why it is called a distortion product otoacoustic emission.) The probe microphone thus picks up three tones: the two original stimulus tones (often called primaries) plus the DPOAE that was produced in the cochlea. The OAE instrument then performs a spectral analysis similar to that described earlier for SOAEs, the result of which is exemplified in the lower part of **Fig. 11.17**. Here we see the two original tones (f_1 and f_2) along with the much fainter DPOAE. The DPOAE is typically ~ 60 dB weaker than the primary tones. The frequency at which the DPOAE will be found is

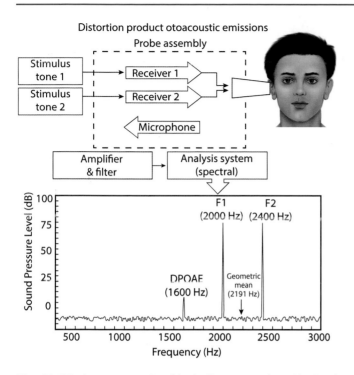

Distortion product otoacoustic emissions

Fig. 11.17 Instrumentation block diagram and an idealized example of a distortion product otoacoustic emission (DPOAE) at 1600 Hz in response to stimulus tones of 2000 and 2400 Hz (see text).

equal to twice the frequency of the lower stimulus tone minus the frequency of the higher one, or **$2f_1 - f_2$**. The two stimulus tones shown in the figure are 2000 and 2400 Hz; thus the DPOAE occurs at 1600 Hz. The arithmetic is as follows:

$$2f1 - f2 = (2 \times 2000) - 2400$$

$$= 4000 - 2400$$

$$= 1600 \text{ Hz}$$

As with other OAEs, DPOAEs are affected by various stimulus parameters. It appears that the strongest DPOAEs are obtained when f_1 and f_2 are between 1000 and 4000 Hz, and when the ratio of their frequencies (f_2/f_1) is ~ 1.2. In our example, this ratio is exactly 1.2 because 2400/2000 = 1.2. Even though the DPOAE occurs at a frequency of $2f_1 - f_2$, the location in the cochlea and thus the frequency actually being tested is in the vicinity of the primary tones, and is usually taken to be the *geometric mean* of f_1 and f_2. The geometric mean is found by multiplying the two stimulus frequencies and then finding the square root of their product, or $\sqrt{(f_1 \times f_2)}$. In our example, this

frequency is $\sqrt{(2000 \times 2400)} = \sqrt{4,800,000} = 2190.9$ Hz, and is shown in the figure by the arrow at 2191 Hz.

The DPOAE is also affected by the levels of the two primary tones (L_1 and L_2), and are often presented so that L_1 is 10 higher than L_2, such as $L_1 = 65$ dB and $L_2 = 55$ dB. However, it is sometimes desirable for the two primary tones to be equal when using overall higher levels of stimulation (e.g., 75 dB SPL), and for L_1 to be ~ 10 dB higher than L_2 when testing at somewhat lower levels (e.g., L_1 at 60 dB SPL and L_2 at 50 dB SPL).

In addition to stimulus parameters like the ones just mentioned, the ability to measure OAE also can be affected by negative middle ear pressure (see Keefe 2007; Sun & Shaver 2009 for reviews). For example, OAEs can be affected by negative middle ear pressure. Sun and Shaver (2009) have shown that this problem may be corrected when testing DPOAEs by adjusting the pressure in the outer ear to counterbalance the negative middle ear pressure. This is analogous to what is done when measuring peak-compensated static acoustic immittance (see Chapter 7).

Distortion product OAEs are found in essentially all normal ears and are typically absent when there is a sensorineural loss of ~ 50 to 60 dB HL. The size of the DPOAE increases with the level of the primaries. In addition, DPOAEs can be obtained as a function of frequency.

Two kinds of DPOAE measures based on these properties are the **DPOAE input/output function** and the DP-gram. The DPOAE input/output function is obtained by measuring DPOAE amplitude as a function of stimulus level at a particular frequency (given as either F2 or the geometric mean of F1 and F2). **The DP-gram** (sometimes called the DP audiogram or DPOAE audiogram) is obtained by presenting the stimulus tones at fixed levels (e.g., L1 at 65 SPL and L2 at 55 dB SPL) across a range of frequencies (expressed as either F2 or the geometric mean of F1 and F2). In other words, it shows DPOAE amplitude as a function of frequency.

Fig. 11.18 shows an example of a DPOAE input/output function at an F2 frequency of 1000 Hz obtained from an individual with normal hearing. Abnormal results would be displaced rightward on the graph (shown by arrow labeled "hearing loss" in the figure), indicating that stronger sound pressure levels are needed to obtain the DPOAEs.

The filled circles connected by zigzag lines in **Fig. 11.19** show an example of a normal DP-gram, and it is from the same person whose normal I/O function is in the previous figure. Here, the filled circles show the DPOAE amplitudes at various F2 frequencies between 1000 Hz and 6000 Hz when the stimulus levels were kept fixed at L1 = 65 dB SPL and L2 = 55 dB SPL. The graph is divided into white, pink-

Fig. 11.18   Example of normal results on the distortion product otoacoustic emission (DPOAE) input/output function. It depicts DPOAE amplitude as a function of stimulus level for an F2 frequency of 1000 Hz. The arrow shows that results from ears with hearing loss would be displaced rightward (represented by the arrow). (Adapted from Lonsbury-Martin BL, Martin GK. 2007. Distortion-product otoacoustic emissions in populations with normal hearing sensitivity. In Robinette MS, Glattke TJ, eds. *Otoacoustic Emissions: Clinical Applications*, 3rd ed. New York, NY: Thieme; 107–130. Used with permission.)

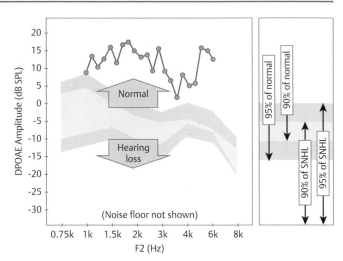

Fig. 11.19   The left panel shows an example of normal results on the DP-gram (Lonsbury-Martin & Martin 2007). Distortion product otoacoustic emission (DPOAE) amplitudes are shown as a function of F2 frequencies between 1000 and 6000 Hz when the stimulus levels were kept fixed at 65 dB SPL for F1 and 55 dB SPL for F2. (Lonsbury-Martin & Martin 2007). It also shows normative information that might be used to distinguish normal and hearing loss ears based on DPOAE amplitudes (Gorga et al 2007). The upper white region of the graph is associated with DPOAEs from ears with normal hearing and the lower white region is associated with ears having sensorineural hearing loss (SNLH). The shaded areas represent ranges where DPOAEs overlap for normal and hearing-impaired ears. Specifically, 90% of normal ears have DPOAE amplitudes extending down to the bottom of the green-shaded area, and 95% of them have DPOAEs extending down to the bottom of the lower pink-shaded area. Similarly, 90% of ears with SNHL have DPOAEs extending up to the top of the green-shaded area, and 95% have DPOAEs up to the top of the upper pink-shaded area. These distributions are illustrated schematically by the arrows in the right-hand frame. (Adapted from Lonsbury-Martin BL, Martin GK. 2007. Distortion-product otoacoustic emissions in populations with normal hearing sensitivity (pp. 107–130); and Gorga MP, Neely ST, Johnson TA, Dierking DM, Garner CA. 2007. Distortion-product otoacoustic emissions in relation to hearing loss. In: Robinette MS, Glattke TJ, eds. *Otoacoustic Emissions: Clinical Applications*, 3rd ed. New York, NY: Thieme; 197–225. Used with permission.)

shaded, and green-shaded areas that were developed by Gorga and colleagues (2007) to help distinguish between normal ears and those with sensorineural hearing loss. Notice that the normal DP-gram example is in the upper white area of the graph, which is associated with normal ears. In contrast, ears with sensorineural hearing loss have lower DPOAE amplitudes and would be found in the lower white region of the graph. These "normal" (upper) and "hearing loss" (lower) regions are separated by the shaded areas, where there are various amounts of overlapping between the DPOAE amplitudes of normal and hearing-impaired ears. (Interested students should see the right pane of **Fig. 11.19** and its legend for how the different areas on the graph are related to the distributions of DPOAE amplitudes from ears with normal hearing versus hearing loss.) Even though both normal and impaired ears have DP-grams in the shaded areas, there is a better chance that DP-grams falling into the upper pink one are from ears with normal hearing, whereas there is a better chance

that those falling into the lower pink-shaded area are from ears with hearing impairment. On the other hand, there is too much overlap in the green-shaded region to distinguish between those with normal hearing and hearing loss.

Before leaving our discussion of otoacoustic emissions, it is worth pointing out even at this introductory level that evoked OAEs are normally suppressed by the presentation of a noise to either one or both ears, reflecting the **medial olivocochlear bundle reflex** (e.g., Collet et al 1990; Berlin, Hood, Hurley,

Wen, & Kemp 1995; Hood, Berlin, Hurley, Cecola, & Bell 1996; De Ceulaer, Yperman, & Daemers, et al 2001; Killan & Kapadia 2006; Wagner, Heppelmann, Müller, Janssen, & Zenner 2007).

■ Vestibular and Balance Assessment

Audiologists are interested in the vestibular (balance) system because of its close association with the auditory system. The inner ear houses the sensory receptor organs for both hearing (the cochlea) and balance (the semicircular canals, utricle, and saccule). In addition, the auditory and vestibular systems both use the eighth nerve to send their signals to the central nervous system. It is therefore not surprising that at least some auditory problems are often accompanied by dizziness.

Vestibular disorders are associated with a kind of dizziness called **vertigo**, which is a sensation of rotation. The patient with vertigo feels as though he is spinning or that the environment is spinning around him. Vertigo is accompanied by a kind of eye movement called **nystagmus**, in which the eyes move to one side and then bounce back to the center very rapidly. Nystagmus reflects what is going on in the vestibular system and is easily measured. Thus, vestibular evaluation to a large extent involves measuring and interpreting the nystagmus. **Electronystagmography (ENG)** measures nystagmus and other eye movements with electrodes placed around the eyes. **Videonystagmography (VNG)** measures nystagmus and other eye movements using goggles fitted with infrared-equipped video cameras.

Even though VNG is the newer technology, it is easy to imagine how tiny video cameras in goggles can be used to register eye movements. On the other hand, it is necessary to explain how eye movements are recorded by the electrodes used in ENG. Actually, the electrodes monitor an electrical signal from the eyes and how it changes when the eyes move. Specifically, the electrodes pick up the **corneoretinal potential**, which is an electrical difference between the front and back of the eye. The front of the eye (cornea) has a positive electrical charge and the back of the eye (retina) has a negative charge. The orientation of the positive and negative "ends" changes according to which way the eyes are facing. Looking rightward makes the electrical signal positive toward the right and negative toward the left, and vice versa for looking leftward. Looking upward makes the signal positive above the eyes and negative below, and vice versa for looking downward. The resulting electrical signals are picked up by electrodes near the eyes and transmitted to the ENG recorder, as illustrated in **Fig. 11.20**. *Horizontal* eye movements are measured by a pair of electrodes placed to the right of the right eye and to the left of the left eye. These electrodes are connected to one channel of an ENG recorder, which draws the right–left position of the eyes on a moving strip of graph paper or on a computer screen. The recorder pen moves *upward* when the eyes move to the *right* and *downward* when the eyes move to the *left* (frames a and b). *Vertical* eye movements are picked up by a second pair of electrodes above and below one of the eyes, which lead to a second channel of the recorder. Here, *upward* eye movement is drawn *upward* on the recorder and *downward* eye motion is drawn *downward* (frames c and d).

Recall that nystagmus involves a pattern of eye movement that first goes in one direction and then

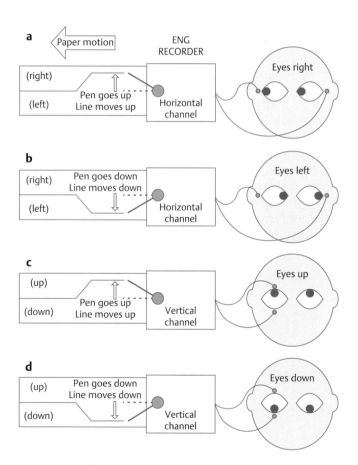

Fig. 11.20 Electronystagmography (ENG) involves monitoring horizontal eye movements with the right and left electrodes, and vertical eye movements with the electrodes above and below one eye. On the horizontal channel, the recorder pen moves **(a)** up when the eyes move rightward and **(b)** down when the eyes move leftward. On the vertical channel, the recorder pen moves **(c)** up when the eyes move upward, and **(d)** down when the eyes move downward.

rapidly bounces back in the opposite direction. Thus, we say that nystagmus occurs in **beats**. The relatively slower motion is called the **slow component** or **slow phase** and is due to the activity of the *vestibular system*. The very rapid movement back to the center is called the **fast component** or **fast phase** and is due to activity arising from within the *central nervous system*. The more traditional term is *phase*, but *component* is preferred when describing nystagmus because *phase* has a different meaning with rotational tests of vestibular function (ANSI S3.45 2009). Each complete set of eye movements to the side and back is a beat, and nystagmus is generally composed of a succession of beats one after the other. The *direction* of nystagmus is the direction of the *fast* component. Its magnitude or strength is determined from the *slow* component and is expressed in degrees of eye rotation per second. **Fig. 11.21** shows examples of right-beating and left-beating nystagmus.

The vestibular evaluation is clearly beyond the scope of a basic text, but it is worthwhile for even a beginning student to have a rudimentary idea of what the most commonly used tests are and what the various outcomes imply. Many informative sources are available for students interested in more detailed coverage of this topic (e.g., Coats 1975, 1986; Barber & Stockwell 1980; Stockwell 1983; Yellin 2000; Gans & Roberts 2005; Shepard & Telian 1996; Desmond 2004; Shepard 2007, 2009; Zapala 2007; ANSI S3.45 2009; Barin 2009).

The outcomes of vestibular tests are often interpreted as normal or abnormal. Abnormal results may be further delineated as (1) peripheral; (2) central; or (3) "nonlocalizing," which indicates that the abnormal result can be associated with either peripheral or central disorders.

The first procedure during an ENG/VNG evaluation is to calibrate the recorder to the patient's eye movements. The recorder paper is a strip of graph paper with 1 mm square boxes. The paper comes out of the recorder at 10 mm/s, so that time is easily read horizontally. However, we want each millimeter vertically to represent 1° of eye rotation. This is easier than it sounds. The patient is asked to look back and forth between two points that are 10° to the right and left of center (a total of 20° of eye rotation). At the same time, the tester adjusts a control on the equipment so that the recording moves up or down a total of 20 mm every time the eyes cover the 20° arc. The calibration procedure is also a clinical test. Normal people can do the task quite accurately. However, patients with pathologies of the cerebellum often overshoot the mark when trying to look back and forth between the two target points. Such a finding is called **calibration overshoot** or **ocular dysmetria**.

Gaze testing involves having the patient stare at a fixed point, and should not result in nystagmus. If it does, the result is called **gaze nystagmus**, which is associated with central involvement.

Two more tasks involve following a visual target, and both of them are tests of central dysfunctions. One of these is a **smooth pursuit test,** in which the patient's eyes must follow a smoothly moving target, such as a pendulum. The motion of the target is sinusoidal, so that the normal eye motion should cause a smooth sine wave to be drawn on the ENG/VNG recording. The abnormal response, in which the sine wave pattern is distorted and irregular, is called sinusoidal break-up or cog-wheeling.

The other procedure that involves following a visual target is called the **optokinetic nystagmus test**. The basic test involves having the patient follow a series of vertical bands moving from left to right, and then from right to left. The test mimics what happens when a passenger watches the rapid progression of telephone poles while looking out the window of a speeding train. This causes nystagmus in which the slow component goes in the same direction as the moving bands. The normal result is for the nystagmus induced by the rightward-moving bands to be a mirror image of the nystagmus induced by the leftward-moving bands. The result is considered abnormal when the nystagmus is grossly asymmetric for the two different directions.

Nystagmus induced by being in a given position is called **positional nystagmus**. One test for this determines whether nystagmus is present on the ENG/VNG record while the patient is kept in each of several positions. The most typical positions tested are lying down supine, on the right and left sides, and supine with the head hanging off the end of

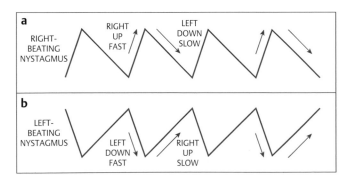

Fig. 11.21 Horizontal nystagmus is **(a)** right-beating when the fast component is drawn upward and **(b)** left-beating when the fast component is drawn downward. If these were vertical channel recordings, then **(a)** would be up-beating and **(b)** would be down-beating nystagmus.

the table, and sitting erect. **Spontaneous nystagmus** is said to occur if nystagmus is present when the patient is in a "neutral" position, that is, sitting erect (Coats 1975), or if the nystagmus has the same characteristics in several different positions (Barber & Stockwell 1980). Both positional and spontaneous nystagmus are abnormal, but are most conservatively interpreted as nonlocalizing.

Many patients complain of vertigo associated with such quick movements as bending over, called paroxysmal vertigo. The clinical test for **paroxysmal vertigo** involves performing the **Dix-Hallpike maneuver**, which is basically as follows: The patient begins by sitting erect. Under the control of the clinician, she is then rapidly moved down to a supine position with her head hanging off the end of the table and turned to one side or the other. One determines whether this manipulation results in nystagmus with particular characteristics. The maneuver may be repeated one or more times depending on whether the patient experiences vertigo and if there is nystagmus with a particular set of characteristics. The interpretation depends on the resulting constellation of findings.

The **bithermal** (two-temperature) **caloric test** is used to stimulate the right and left semicircular canals separately, so that their responses can be compared. The patient lies supine with her head elevated 30°, which causes the horizontal semicircular canals to be in a vertical position. Then each ear canal is separately stimulated with cool water and then with warm water. Irrigating[3] with *warm* water heats the endolymph in that ear, causing it to flow upward and thus deflect the cupula. The result should be nystagmus that beats in the direction of the stimulated ear. Irrigating the ear with *cool* water will cool the endolymph, causing it to flow downward and thus deflect the cupula in the other direction, causing nystagmus that beats away from the stimulated ear.

The strength of the nystagmus caused by stimulating the right ear (right cool and right warm) is compared with the nystagmus due to stimulating the left ear (left cool and left warm). A difference of more than 20 to 25% between the ears is called a **unilateral weakness** or **reduced vestibular response**, implying a peripheral disorder on the side with the smaller response. The strength of the bithermal caloric test is that we can recombine the nystagmus results into those that "beat toward the right ear" (right warm and left cool) and those that "beat toward the left ear" (left warm and right cool). We can thus distinguish between results due to a unilateral weakness and those due to a greater propensity for the eyes to beat in one direction relative to the other, called a **directional preponderance**.

A test for **fixation suppression** is performed during at least one of the caloric tests. Here, we ask the patient to open her eyes and look at (fixate upon) a specified point. This is done while she is experiencing nystagmus due to the caloric stimulus. The normal response to visual fixation is a large reduction in the strength of the nystagmus. If the nystagmus does not get much weaker during fixation, the result is called **failure of fixation suppression**, which suggests central pathology.

Other balance system tests may also be done, such as sinusoidal harmonic acceleration testing, posturography, and vestibular evoked myogenic potentials. **Sinusoidal harmonic acceleration** (or **rotating chair**) testing involves a variety of nystagmus measurements on a patient who is rotated from side to side in a computer-controlled chair. **Computerized dynamic posturography** involves assessing the patient's ability to maintain balance while standing. This is done by placing the patient on a platform in a booth and measuring her responses while the platform is still or moves (which manipulates proprioceptive cues) and/or the surrounding booth stays still or moves (which manipulates visual cues).

As its name implies, the **vestibular evoked myogenic potential (VEMP)** is an evoked potential coming from a muscle in response to vestibular stimulation. To elicit the VEMP, we use high-level sounds (e.g., clicks) to activate the saccule. This is possible because the saccule is located in close proximity to the oval window within the vestibule. The saccule's response leads to reflexive contractions of the sternocleidomastoid muscle; and we pick up the resulting electrical activity with electrodes, one of which is placed on the side of the neck over the muscle. As with the evoked potentials discussed earlier in the chapter, these electrodes lead to an averaging computer, resulting in a response waveform called the VEMP.

■ Study Questions

1. What are auditory evoked potentials?
2. Describe the electrocochleogram (ECochG).
3. What is the auditory brainstem response (ABR)?
4. How is the ABR used to assess hearing sensitivity?
5. How is the ABR used to identify retrocochlear disorders?

---

[3] Directing the water into the ear canal constitutes an "open loop" system. "Closed loop" systems direct the heated or cooled water into a plastic balloon located in the ear canal. Other systems use air instead of water.

6. Describe the auditory steady-state response (ASSR).
7. What are otoacoustic emissions?
8. What are the clinical implications of normal versus abnormal transient-evoked or distortion product otoacoustic emissions?
9. Define vertigo and nystagmus, and explain how they are related.
10. Describe how electronystagmography or videonystagmography is used to measure the integrity of the vestibular system.

References

Abbas PJ, Brown CJ. 2009. Electrocochleography. In: Katz J, Burkard RF, Medwetsky L, eds. Handbook of Clinical Audiology, 6th ed. Philadelphia, PA: Lippincott Williams & Wilkins; 265–292

American National Standards Institute (ANSI). 2009. American National Standard Procedures for Testing Basic Vestibular Function. ANSI S3.45-2009. New York, NY: ANSI

American Speech-Language-Hearing Association (ASHA). 1987. The Short Latency Auditory Evoked Potentials. Rockville Pike, MD: ASHA

American Speech-Language-Hearing Association (ASHA). Neurophysiologic intraoperative monitoring. ASHA 1992;34(Suppl 7):34–36

American Speech-Language-Hearing Association (ASHA). 2004. Scope of Practice in Audiology. Rockville Pike, MD: ASHA

Aoyagi M, Kiren T, Kim Y, Suzuki Y, Fuse T, Koike Y. Optimal modulation frequency for amplitude-modulation following response in young children during sleep. Hear Res 1993;65(1-2):253–261

Arnold SA. 2000. The auditory brain stem response. In: Roeser RJ, Valente M, Hosford-Dunn H, eds. Audiology Diagnosis. New York, NY: Thieme; 451–470

Barber HO, Stockwell CW. 1980. Manual of Electronystagmography, 2nd ed. St. Louis, MO: Mosby

Barin K. 2009. Clinical neurophysiology of the vestibular system. In: Katz J, Burkard RF, Medwetsky L. eds. Handbook of Clinical Audiology, 6th ed. Philadelphia, PA: Lippincott Williams & Wilkins; 431–466

Beck DL, ed. Audiology: beyond the sound booth. Sem Hear 193;14:1–214

Berlin CI, Hood LJ, Hurley AE, Wen H, Kemp DT. Binaural noise suppresses linear click-evoked otoacoustic emissions more than ipsilateral or contralateral noise. Hear Res 1995;87(1-2):96–103

Bonfils P. Spontaneous otoacoustic emissions: clinical interest. Laryngoscope 1989;99(7 Pt 1):752–756

Bonfils P, Uziel A. Evoked otoacoustic emissions in patients with acoustic neuromas. Am J Otol 1988;9(5):412–417

Bradford LJ. 1975. Physiological Measures of the Audio-Vestibular System. New York, NY: Academic Press

Burkhard R. McNerney. 2009. Introduction to auditory evoked potentials. In: Katz J, Burkard RF, Medwetsky L, eds. Handbook of Clinical Audiology, 6th ed. Philadelphia, PA: Lippincott Williams & Wilkins; 222–264

Burkhard RF, Don M. 2007. The auditory brainstem response. In: Burkhard RF, Don M, Eggermont JJ, eds. Auditory Evoked Potentials: Basic Principles and Clinical Applications. Philadelphia, PA: Lippincott Williams & Wilkins; 229–253

Burkhard RF, Don M, Eggermont JJ, eds. 2007. Auditory Evoked Potentials: Basic Principles and Clinical Applications. Philadelphia, PA: Lippincott Williams & Wilkins

Cacace AT, McFarland DJ. 2009. Middle latency auditory evoked potentials: update. In Katz J, Burkard RF, Medwetsky L, eds. Handbook of Clinical Audiology, 6th ed. Philadelphia, PA: Lippincott Williams & Wilkins; 373–394

Chandrasekhar SS, Brackmann DE, Devgan KK. Utility of auditory brainstem response audiometry in diagnosis of acoustic neuromas. Am J Otol 1995;16(1):63–67

Chiappa KH, ed. 1997. Evoked Potentials in Clinical Medicine, 3rd ed. New York, NY: Lippincott-Raven

Chung WH, Cho DY, Choi JY, Hong SH. Clinical usefulness of extratympanic electrocochleography in the diagnosis of Ménière's disease. Otol Neurotol 2004;25(2):144–149

Coats AC. 1975. Electronystagmography. In: Bradford IJ, ed. Physiological Measures of the Audio-Vestibular System. New York, NY: Academic Press; 37–85

Coats AC. ENG examination technique. Ear Hear 1986;7(3):143–150

Cohen LT, Rickards FW, Clark GM. A comparison of steady-state evoked potentials to modulated tones in awake and sleeping humans. J Acoust Soc Am 1991;90(5):2467–2479

Collet L, Kemp DT, Veuillet E, Duclaux R, Moulin A, Morgon A. Effect of contralateral auditory stimuli on active cochlear micro-mechanical properties in human subjects. Hear Res 1990;43(2-3):251–261

Cone-Wesson B, Dimitrinjevic A. 2009. The auditory steady-state response. In: Katz J, Burkard RF, Medwetsky L, eds. Handbook of Clinical Audiology, 6th ed. Philadelphia, PA: Lippincott Williams & Wilkins; 322–350

Cone-Wesson B, Dowell RC, Tomlin D, Rance G, Ming WJ. The auditory steady-state response: comparisons with the auditory brainstem response. J Am Acad Audiol 2002;13(4):173–187, quiz 225–226

Cone-Wesson B, Parker J, Swiderski N, Rickards F. The auditory steady-state response: full-term and premature neonates. J Am Acad Audiol 2002;13(5):260–269

De Ceulaer G, Yperman M, Daemers K, et al. Contralateral suppression of transient evoked otoacoustic emissions: normative data for a clinical test set-up. Otol Neurotol 2001;22(3):350–355

Dennis JM, ed. Intraoperative monitoring with evoked potentials. Sem Hear 1988;9:1–164

Desmond AL. 2004. Vestibular Function: Evaluation & Treatment. New York, NY: Thieme

Devaiah AK, Dawson KL, Ferraro JA, Ator GA. Utility of area curve ratio electrocochleography in early Meniere disease. Arch Otolaryngol Head Neck Surg 2003;129(5):547–551

Dhar S, Hall JW. 2011. Otoacoustic Emissions: Principles, Procedures, and Protocols. San Diego, CA: Plural

Dimitrijevic A, John MS, Van Roon P, et al. Estimating the audiogram using multiple auditory steady-state responses. J Am Acad Audiol 2002;13(4):205–224

Don M, Eggermont JJ, Brackmann DE. Reconstruction of the audiogram using brain stem responses and high-pass noise masking. Ann Otol Rhinol Laryngol Suppl 1979;57(3 Pt 2, Suppl 57)1–20

Don M, Kwong B. 2009. Auditory brainstem response: differential diagnosis. In: Katz J, Burkard RF, Medwetsky L, eds. Handbook of Clinical Audiology, 6th ed. Philadelphia, PA: Lippincott Williams & Wilkins; 265–292

Don M, Kwong B, Tanaka C, Brackmann D, Nelson R. The stacked ABR: a sensitive and specific screening tool for detecting small acoustic tumors. Audiol Neurootol 2005;10(5):274–290

Don M, Masuda A, Nelson RA, Brackmann DE. Successful detection of small acoustic tumors using the stacked derived-band ABR amplitude. Am J Otol 1997;18:608–621

Fedtke T, Richter U. Reference zero for the calibration of air-conduction audiometric equipment using "tone bursts" as test signals. Int J Audiol 2007;46(1):1–10

Ferraro JA. 2000. Electrocochleography. In: Roeser RJ, Valente M, Hosford-Dunn H, eds. Audiology Diagnosis. New York, NY: Thieme; 425–450

Ferraro JA, Krishnan G. Cochlear potentials in clinical audiology. Audiol Neurootol 1997;2(5):241–256

Ferraro JA, Tibbils RP. SP/AP area ratio in the diagnosis of Ménière's disease. Am J Audiol 1999;8(1):21–28

Fria TJ. The auditory brainstem response: background and clinical applications. Monogr Contemp Audiol 1980;2:1–44

Gans RE, Roberts RA. Understanding vestibular-evoked myogenic potentials (VEMPs). Audiol Today 2005;17(1):23–25

Gelfand SA. 2010. Hearing: An Introduction to Psychological and Physiological Acoustics, 5th ed. Colcheter, Essex, UK: Informa Healthcare

Glattke TJ. 1993. Short-Latency Auditory Evoked Potentials. Austin, TX: Pro-Ed

Glattke TJ, Robinette MS. 2007. Transient evoked otoacoustic emissions in populations with normal hearing sensitivity. In: Robinette MS, Glattke TJ, eds. Otoacoustic Emissions: Clinical Applications, 3rd ed. New York, NY: Thieme; 87–105

Gorga MP, Johnson TA, Kaminski JR, Beauchaine KL, Garner CA, Neely ST. Using a combination of click- and tone burst-evoked auditory brain stem response measurements to estimate pure-tone thresholds. Ear Hear 2006;27(1):60–74

Gorga MP, Neely ST, Hoover BM, Dierking DM, Beauchaine KL, Manning C. Determining the upper limits of stimulation for auditory steady-state response measurements. Ear Hear 2004;25(3):302–307

Gorga MP, Neely ST, Johnson TA, Dierking DM, Garner CA. 2007. Distortion-product otoacoustic emissions in relation to hearing loss. In: Robinette MS, Glattke TJ, eds. Otoacoustic Emissions: Clinical Applications, 3rd ed. New York, NY: Thieme; 197–225

Gorga MP, Thornton AR. The choice of stimuli for ABR measurements. Ear Hear 1989;10(4):217–230

Grason-Stadler, Inc. (GSI). 2001. Auditory Steady-State Response: A New Tool for Frequency-Specific Hearing Assessment in Infants and Children. Madison, WI: Viasys NeuroCare/GSI

Hall JW. 2007. New Handbook for Auditory Evoked Responses. Boston, MA: Allyn & Bacon

Hecox K, Galambos R. Brain stem auditory evoked responses in human infants and adults. Arch Otolaryngol 1974;99(1):30–33

Herdman AT, Lins O, Van Roon P, Stapells DR, Scherg M, Picton TW. Intracerebral sources of human auditory steady-state responses. Brain Topogr 2002;15(2):69–86

Herdman AT, Stapells DR. Thresholds determined using the monotic and dichotic multiple auditory steady-state response technique in normal-hearing subjects. Scand Audiol 2001;30(1):41–49

Herdman AT, Stapells DR. Auditory steady-state response thresholds of adults with sensorineural hearing impairments. Int J Audiol 2003;42(5):237–248

Hood LJ. 2007. Auditory neuropathy and dys-synchrony. In: Burkhard RF, Don M, Eggermont JJ, eds. Auditory Evoked Potentials: Basic Principles and Clinical Applications. Philadelphia, PA: Lippincott Williams & Wilkins; 275–290

Hood LJ, Berlin CI, Hurley A, Cecola RP, Bell B. Contralateral suppression of transient-evoked otoacoustic emissions in humans: intensity effects. Hear Res 1996;101(1-2):113–118

Hurley RM, Hurley A, Berlin CI. Development of low-frequency tone burst versus the click auditory brainstem response. J Am Acad Audiol 2005;16(2):114–121, Quiz 122

International Electrotechnical Commission (IEC). 2009. Electroacoustics—Audiometric Equipment—Part 6: Instruments for the Measurement of Otoacoustic Emissions. Standard IEC 60645-6-2009. Geneva: IEC

International Organization for Standardization (ISO). 2007. Acoustics—Reference Zero for Calibration of Audiometric Equipment—Part 6: Reference Threshold of Hearing for Test Signals of Short Duration. ISO 389-6. Geneva: ISO

Jacobson GP. 1999. Otoacoustic emissions in clinical practice. In: Musiek FE, Rintelmann WF, eds. Contemporary Perspectives in Hearing Assessment. Needham Heights, MA: Allyn & Bacon; 273–303

Jacobson JT. 1985. The Auditory Brainstem Response. San Diego, CA: College-Hill

Jerger J, Chmiel R, Frost JD Jr, Coker N. Effect of sleep on the auditory steady state evoked potential. Ear Hear 1986;7(4):240–245

Jerger J, Hall J. Effects of age and sex on auditory brainstem response. Arch Otolaryngol 1980;106(7):387–391

Jerger J, Johnson K. Interactions of age, gender, and sensorineural hearing loss on ABR latency. Ear Hear 1988;9(4):168–176

Jewett DL, Romano MN, Williston JS. Human auditory evoked potentials: possible brain stem components detected on the scalp. Science 1970;167(3924): 1517–1518

John MS, Brown DK, Muir PJ, Picton TW. Recording auditory steady-state responses in young infants. Ear Hear 2004;25(6):539–553

Johnsen NJ, Elberling C. Evoked acoustic emissions from the human ear. I. Equipment and response parameters. Scand Audiol 1982;11(1):3–12

Keefe DH. 2007. Influence of middle-ear function and pathology on otoacoustic emissions. In: Robinette MS, Glattke TJ, eds. Otoacoustic Emissions: Clinical Applications, 3rd ed. New York, NY: Thieme; 163–196

Kemp DT. Stimulated acoustic emissions from within the human auditory system. J Acoust Soc Am 1978; 64(5):1386–1391

Kemp DT. Evidence of mechanical nonlinearity and frequency selective wave amplification in the cochlea. Arch Otorhinolaryngol 1979;224(1-2):37–45

Kiang NYS, Liberman MC, Sewell WF, Guinan JJ. Single unit clues to cochlear mechanisms. Hear Res 1986;22: 171–182

Kileny P. The frequency specificity of tone-pip evoked auditory brain stem responses. Ear Hear 1981;2(6): 270–275

Killan EC, Kapadia S. Simultaneous suppression of tone burst–evoked otoacoustic emissions—effect of level and presentation paradigm. Hear Res 2006;212(1-2): 65–73

Kraus N. Listening in on the listening brain. Phys Today 2011;64(6):40–45

Kraus N, Hornickel J. 2013. cABR: A biological probe of auditory processing. In: Geffner D, Ross-Swain D, eds. Auditory Processing Disorders, 2nd ed. San Diego, CA: Plural

Levi EC, Folsom RC, Dobie RA. Amplitude-modulation following response (AMFR): effects of modulation rate, carrier frequency, age, and state. Hear Res 1993;68(1):42–52

Lins OG, Picton TW, Boucher BL, et al. Frequency-specific audiometry using steady-state responses. Ear Hear 1996;17(2):81–96

Lonsbury-Martin BL, Martin GK. 2007. Distortion-product otoacoustic emissions in populations with normal hearing sensitivity. In: Robinette MS, Glattke TJ, eds. Otoacoustic Emissions: Clinical Applications, 3rd ed. New York, NY: Thieme; 107–130

Lonsbury-Martin BL, Martin GK, Telischi FF. 1999. Otoacoustic emissions in clinical practice. In: Musiek FE, Rintelmann WF, eds. Contemporary Perspectives in Hearing Assessment. Needham Heights, MA: Allyn & Bacon; 167–196

Lonsbury-Martin BL, Whitehead ML, Martin GK. Clinical applications of otoacoustic emissions. J Speech Hear Res 1991;34(5):964–981

Martin BA, Tremblay KL, Stapells DR. 2007. Principles and applications of cortical auditory evoked potentials. In: Burkhard RF, Don M, Eggermont JJ, eds. Auditory Evoked Potentials: Basic Principles and Clinical Applications. Philadelphia, PA: Lippincott Williams & Wilkins; 482–507

Martin M, Shi BY. 2007. Intraoperative monitoring. In: Burkhard RF, Don, M, Eggermont JJ, eds. Auditory Evoked Potentials: Basic Principles and Clinical Applications. Philadelphia, PA: Lippincott Williams & Wilkins; 355–384

Martin M, Shi BY. 2009. Intraoperative neurophysiology: monitoring auditory evoked potentials. In: Katz J, Medwetsky L, Burkhard RF, Hood H, eds. Handbook of Clinical Audiology, 6th ed. Philadelphia, PA: Lippincott Williams & Wilkins; 351–372

Mauldin L, Jerger J. Auditory brain stem evoked responses to bone-conducted signals. Arch Otolaryngol 1979; 105(11):656–661

McPherson DL, Ballachanda B. 2000. Middle and long latency auditory evoked potentials. In: Roeser RJ, Valente M, Hosford-Dunn H, eds. Audiology Diagnosis. New York, NY: Thieme; 471–502

Møller AR. 2000. Intraoperative neurophysiological monitoring. In: Roeser RJ, Valente M, Hosford-Dunn H, eds. Audiology Diagnosis. New York, NY: Thieme; 545–570

Møller AR. 2007. Neural generators for auditory brainstem evoked potentials. In: Burkhard RF, Don M, Eggermont JJ, eds. Auditory Evoked Potentials: Basic Principles and Clinical Applications. Philadelphia, PA: Lippincott Williams & Wilkins; 336–354

Møller AR, Janetta PJ. 1985. Neural generators of the auditory brainstem response. In: Jacobson JT, ed. The Auditory Brainstem Response. San Diego, CA: College Hill; 13–31

Moore EJ. 1983. Bases of Auditory Brain-Stem Evoked Responses. New York, NY: Grune & Stratton

Moore JK. The human auditory brain stem as a generator of auditory evoked potentials. Hear Res 1987;29(1): 33–43

Näätänen R, Kraus N, Eds. Special issue: Mismatch negativity as an index of central auditory function. Ear Hear 1995;16:1–146

Näätänen R, Kujala T, Escera C, et al. The mismatch negativity (MMN)—a unique window to disturbed central auditory processing in ageing and different clinical conditions. Clin Neurophysiol 2012;123(3):424–458

Norton SJ. Cochlear function and otoacoustic emissions. Semin Hear 1992;13:1–14

Norton SJ, Schmidt AR, Stover LJ. Tinnitus and otoacoustic emissions: is there a link? Ear Hear 1990;11(2): 159–166

Parker DJ, Thornton ARD. Derived cochlear nerve and brainstem evoked responses of the human auditory system. The effect of masking in the derived band. Scand Audiol 1978;7(2):73–80

Penner MJ. An estimate of the prevalence of tinnitus caused by spontaneous otoacoustic emissions. Arch Otolaryngol Head Neck Surg 1990;116(4):418–423

Penner MJ, Burns EM. The dissociation of SOAEs and tinnitus. J Speech Hear Res 1987;30(3):396–403

Picton TW, Dimitrijevic A, Perez-Abalo MC, Van Roon P. Estimating audiometric thresholds using auditory steady-state responses. J Am Acad Audiol 2005;16(3): 140–156

Picton TW, John MS, Purcell DW, Plourde G. Human auditory steady-state responses: the effects of recording technique and state of arousal. Anesth Analg 2003; 97(5):1396–1402

Pratt H. 2007. Middle-latency responses. In: Burkhard RF, Don M, Eggermont JJ, eds. Auditory Evoked Potentials: Basic Principles and Clinical Applications. Philadelphia, PA: Lippincott Williams & Wilkins; 463–481

Prieve B, Fitzgerald T. 2009. Otoacoustic emissions. In: Katz J, Medwetsky L, Burkhard RF, Hood H, eds. Handbook of Clinical Audiology, 6th ed. Philadelphia, PA: Lippincott Williams & Wilkins; 497–528

Probst R, Lonsbury-Martin BL, Martin GK. A review of otoacoustic emissions. J Acoust Soc Am 1991;89(5): 2027–2067

Probst R, Lonsbury-Martin BL, Martin GK, Coats AC. Otoacoustic emissions in ears with hearing loss. Am J Otolaryngol 1987;8(2):73–81

Rance G, Rickards FW, Cohen LT, De Vidi S, Clark GM. The automated prediction of hearing thresholds in sleeping subjects using auditory steady-state evoked potentials. Ear Hear 1995;16(5):499–507

Rance G, Tomlin D. Maturation of auditory steady-state responses in normal babies. Ear Hear 2006;27(1): 20–29

Rance G, Tomlin D, Rickards FW. Comparison of auditory steady-state responses and tone-burst auditory brainstem responses in normal babies. Ear Hear 2006;27(6):751–762

Richter U, Fedtke T. Reference zero for the calibration of audiometric equipment using 'clicks' as test signals. Int J Audiol 2005;44(8):478–487

Robinette MS, Bauch CD, Olsen WO, Hamer SG, Beatty CW. Use of TEOAE, ABR and acoustic reflex measures to assess auditory function in patients with acoustic neuroma. Am J Audiol 1992;1:66–72

Robinette MS, Glattke TJ, eds. 2007a. Otoacoustic Emissions: Clinical Applications, 3rd ed. New York, NY: Thieme

Robinette MS, Glattke TJ. 2007b. Otoacoustic emissions. In: Roeser RJ, Valente M, Hosford-Dunn H, eds. Audiology Diagnosis, 2nd ed. New York, NY: Thieme; 478–496

Rudell AP. A fiber tract model of auditory brainstem responses. EEG Clin Neurophysiol 1987;62:53–62

Ruth RA, Lambert PR, Ferraro JA. Electrocochleography: methods and clinical applications. Am J Otol 1988; 9(Suppl):1–11

Sass K. Sensitivity and specificity of transtympanic electrocochleography in Meniere's disease. Acta Otolaryngol 1998;118(2):150–156

Savio G, Cárdenas J, Pérez Abalo M, González A, Valdés J. The low and high frequency auditory steady state responses mature at different rates. Audiol Neurootol 2001;6(5):279–287

Scherg M, von Cramon D. A new interpretation of the generators of BAEP waves I-V: results of a spatio-temporal dipole model. Electroencephalogr Clin Neurophysiol 1985;62(4):290–299

Schmidt RJ, Sataloff RT, Newman J, Spiegel JR, Myers DL. The sensitivity of auditory brainstem response testing for the diagnosis of acoustic neuromas. Arch Otolaryngol Head Neck Surg 2001;127(1):19–22

Schoonhoven R. 2007. Responses from the cochlea. In: Burkhard RF, Don M, Eggermont JJ, eds. Auditory Evoked Potentials: Basic Principles and Clinical Applications. Philadelphia, PA: Lippincott Williams & Wilkins; 180–198

Schwartz DM, Larson VD, De Chicchis AR. Spectral characteristics of air and bone conduction transducers used to record the auditory brain stem response. Ear Hear 1985;6(5):274–277

Shepard NT. Dizziness and balance disorders: the role of history and laboratory studies in diagnosis and management. ASHA Leader 2007;12(7):6-7,16–17

Shepard NT. 2009. Evaluation of the patient with dizziness and balance disorder. In: Katz J, Burkard RF, Medwetsky L, eds. Handbook of Clinical Audiology, 6th ed. Philadelphia, PA: Lippincott Williams & Wilkins; 467–496

Shepard NT, Telian SA. 1996. Practical Management of the Balance Disorder Patient. San Diego, CA: Singular

Sininger YS. 2007. The use of auditory brainstem response in screening for hearing loss and audiometric threshold prediction. In: Burkhard RF, Don M, Eggermont JJ, eds. Auditory Evoked Potentials: Basic Principles and Clinical Applications. Philadelphia, PA: Lippincott Williams & Wilkins; 254–274

Sininger YS, Abdala C, Cone-Wesson B. Auditory threshold sensitivity of the human neonate as measured by the auditory brainstem response. Hear Res 1997;104(1-2): 27–38

Sohmer H, Feinmesser M. Cochlear action potentials recorded from the external ear in man. Ann Otol Rhinol Laryngol 1967;76(2):427–435

Squires KC, Hecox KE. Electrophysiological evaluation of higher level auditory processing. Semin Hear 1983; 4:415–433

Stapells DR. Threshold estimation of the tone-evoked auditory brainstem response: a literature meta-analysis. J Speech Lang Pathol Audiol 2000;24:74–83

Stapells DR, Gravel JS, Martin BA. Thresholds for auditory brain stem responses to tones in notched noise from infants and young children with normal hearing or sensorineural hearing loss. Ear Hear 1995;16(4): 361–371

Stapells DR, Kurtzberg D. Evoked potential assessment of auditory system integrity in infants. Clin Perinatol 1991;18(3):497–518

Stapells DR, Picton TW, Durieux-Smith A, Edwards CG, Moran LM. Thresholds for short-latency auditory-evoked potentials to tones in notched noise in normal-hearing and hearing-impaired subjects. Audiology 1990;29(5):262–274

Starr A, Golob EJ. 2007. Cognitive factors modulating auditory cortical potentials. In: Burkhard RF, Don M, Eggermont JJ, eds. Auditory Evoked Potentials: Basic Principles and Clinical Applications. Philadelphia, PA: Lippincott Williams & Wilkins; 508–524

Starr A, Picton TW, Sininger Y, Hood LJ, Berlin CI. Auditory neuropathy. Brain 1996;119(Pt 3):741–753

Stockard JE, Stockard JJ, Westmoreland BF, Corfits JL. Brainstem auditory-evoked responses. Normal variation as a function of stimulus and subject characteristics. Arch Neurol 1979;36(13):823–831

Stockwell CW. 1983. ENG Workbook. Austin, TX: Pro-Ed

Sun X-M, Shaver MD. Effects of negative middle ear pressure on distortion product otoacoustic emissions and application of a compensation procedure in humans. Ear Hear 2009;30(2):191–202

Sutton S, Braren M, Zubin J, John ER. Evoked-potential correlates of stimulus uncertainty. Science 1965;150(3700):1187–1188

Turner RG, Shepard NT, Frazer GJ. Clinical performance of audiological and related diagnostic tests. Ear Hear 1984;5(4):187–194

van der Drift JF, Brocaar MP, van Zanten GA. Brainstem response audiometry. I. Its use in distinguishing between conductive and cochlear hearing loss. Audiology 1988a;27(5):260–270

van der Drift JF, Brocaar MP, van Zanten GA. Brainstem response audiometry. II. Classification of hearing loss by discriminant analysis. Audiology 1988b;27(5):271–278

Vander Werff KR, Brown CJ. Effect of audiometric configuration on threshold and suprathreshold auditory steady-state responses. Ear Hear 2005;26(3):310–326

Vander Werff KR, Prieve BA, Georgantas LM. Infant air and bone conduction tone burst auditory brain stem responses for classification of hearing loss and the relationship to behavioral thresholds. Ear Hear 2009;30(3):350–368

Wagner W, Heppelmann G, Müller J, Janssen T, Zenner H-P. Olivocochlear reflex effect on human distortion product otoacoustic emissions is largest at frequencies with distinct fine structure dips. Hear Res 2007;223(1-2):83–92

Weber BA. Pitfalls in auditory brain stem response audiometry. Ear Hear 1983;4(4):179–184

Yamada O, Kodera K, Yagi T. Cochlear processes affecting wave V latency of the auditory evoked brain stem response. A study of patients with sensory hearing loss. Scand Audiol 1979;8(2):67–70

Yellin MW. 2000. Assessment of vestibular function. In: Roeser RJ, Valente M, Hosford-Dunn H, eds. Audiology Diagnosis. New York, NY: Thieme; 571–592

Zapala D. The VEMP: ready for the clinic. Hear J 2007;60(3):10–18

12 Assessment of Infants and Children

This chapter is concerned with the audiological evaluation of children. Here, we are concerned with audiological procedures that have been modified or specially developed for use with infants and children at various levels of development, and with the clinical considerations that pertain to this population. The student should notice more than a few similarities between what is discussed here and what is covered in the context of audiological screening for children in Chapter 13. This is not surprising because screening tests are usually simplified and/or abbreviated clinical procedures. In fact, some procedures used for screening purposes are equally useful clinically. For example, the acoustic immittance methods used to screen for the presence of middle ear fluid are also used as part of the clinical immittance assessment and are often used to monitor a patient's middle ear status over time. However, the greater depth and scope involved in clinical assessment and the knowledge and expertise demanded of those who accomplish it should be readily apparent as well. For example, the auditory brainstem response is used on a "pass/fail" basis for screening purposes, but its clinical use involves extensive and sophisticated testing procedures. Similarly, the screening use of the hearing loss risk factors enumerated in Chapter 13 is to indicate the need for a referral, but they are also used clinically as part of the case history that contributes to the diagnostic assessment of the child.

By convention, children are considered *infants* from birth to 3 years old. The first 28 days of life are generally referred to as the *neonatal* period. They are *preschoolers* from ages 3 to 5, and *school-age* from then through high school. We will use these terms loosely because phrases like *2-week-old infant* and *14-month-old child* are self-explanatory. However, we must be aware of certain *kinds* of ages that have specific meanings and that are pertinent when dealing with children. For example, we are all aware that **chronological age** means age since birth, and that **mental age** expresses an individual's cognitive abil-

ity (usually as measured on an intelligence test) in terms of the age when an average normal person achieves the same level of performance. **Gestational age** is the time period between conception and birth, and is conventionally measured from the time of the last menstruation until the time when the baby is born. **Conceptional age** is the child's age measured from the date of conception; in other words, it includes the gestational age plus the time since the baby was born. Consider two babies born on the same day, one following a full-term pregnancy, and the other who was born one month early. Even though their chronological ages will be the same on the day when they eat their first birthday cakes, they will be 1 month apart in conceptional age (21 and 20 months). This difference brings us to the notion of **developmental age**, which is the individual's age in terms of his level of maturation; for example, if a 12-month-old (chronologically) functions in a manner that is typical of the average normal 8-month-old, then his developmental age would be 8 months. For audiological purposes, it is often helpful to consider an infant's **prematurity-adjusted** or **corrected age**, which is determined by subtracting the number of weeks of prematurity from his chronological age (e.g., Moore, Wilson, & Thompson 1977; Moore, Thompson, & Folsom 1992; ASHA 2004).

The initial aspects of the audiological evaluation of a child involve obtaining a case history, carrying out a physical inspection of the ears and related structures, and taking the time to observe and informally interact with the child to develop a clinical impression of her developmental level and communicative abilities. The physical inspection of the ears and related structures is necessary to identify anomalies that affect audiological procedures, suggest the possibility of hearing-related abnormalities, and/or indicate the need for medical referral. The child's case history is generally obtained from the parents or other caregivers, and should address the child's medical history, her physical and neuromotor development, and her communicative behavior and development. As pointed out in Chapter 6, the specific material to be covered in the case history should come from a knowledge and understanding of auditory and related disorders (Chapter 6) and risk indicators (JCIH 2007; see Chapter 13, **Table 13.2**), and a firm background in child development in general and in speech-language in particular (e.g., Linder 1990; Nelson 1993). In addition to providing diagnostic insight, the history is used in combination with an informal observation of and interaction with the child to help determine what kinds of audiological testing methods might be most appropriate to use with her.

■ Behavioral Assessment

It is so obvious that nobody expects an infant to raise her hand every time she hears a tone, that it seems ridiculous to say so. Yet what makes such a state-

ment preposterous or humorous is a common albeit general understanding that there is a developmental sequence for *what* sounds babies will respond to and *how* they will go about responding. The details of this developmental sequence form the foundation for the audiological evaluation of infants and young children.

Table 12.1 is an **Auditory Behavior Index** (Northern & Downs 1991) that summarizes many of the responses to sound expected from infants during the first 2+ years of life, along with the levels of various kinds of sounds expected to elicit these responses. Before proceeding to the details, it is a good idea to peruse this chart for several important general principles. First, notice that the earliest responses are gross, reflexive behaviors and that they become finer and more specific with the infant's development. The behavioral assessment of hearing depends on knowing which responses to look for at which age range in the child's development. In addition, the audiologist must also be alert for responses that are characteristic of children who are appreciably younger

Table 12.1   Responses to sounds from developmentally normal infants at various ages, and typical stimulus levels expected to elicit these responses in behavioral observation audiometry[a]

Age range	Types of behavioral responses	Warble Tones (dB HL)	Speech[b] (dB HL)	Noisemakers (dB SPL, approximate)
0 to 6 weeks	Eye blink Eye widening Startle Arousal/stirring from sleep	78	40–60	50–70
6 weeks to 4 months	Eye blink Eye widening Eye shift Quieting Rudimentary head turn starts by 4 months	70	47	50–60
4 to 7 months	Head turn laterally toward sound Listening attitude	51	21	40–50
7 to 9 months	Directly localizes to side Indirectly localizes below ear level	45	15	30–40
9 to 13 months	Directly localizes to side and below ear level Indirectly localizes above ear level	38	8	25–35
13 to 16 months	Directly localizes to side/below/above ear level	32	5	25–30
16 to 21 months	Directly localizes to side/below/above ear level	25	5	25
21 to 24 months	Directly localizes to side/below/above ear level	26	3	25

[a]Adapted from Northern JL, Downs MP. 1991. Hearing in Children, 4th edition. Baltimore, MD: Williams and Wilkins, with permission.
[b]A startle response to speech is typically expected at 65 dB HL for all of the age groups shown.

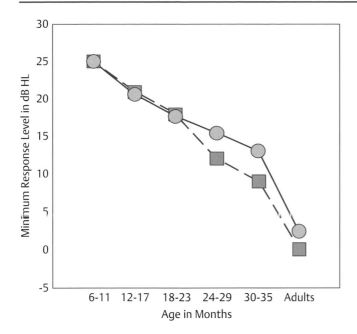

Fig. 12.1 The improvement of infants' minimum response levels with maturation from 6 to 35 months of age using visual reinforcement audiometry and adult thresholds for comparison. (Based on data by Matkin [1977].)

than the one being tested, indicating the possibility of developmental intellectual disorders or other developmental issue and the need for an appropriate referral. An example of such a developmentally delayed response would be an 18-month-old who can localize sounds to one side or the other, but not above or below eye level.

Second, comparing the stimulus intensities needed for a normal infant to respond to warble tones versus speech or noisemakers reveals that infants are not equally responsive to all kinds of sounds. Third, looking down any of the three representative stimulus columns shows that normal infants elicit developmentally appropriate responses to sounds at progressively lower intensity levels with increasing age. This does *not* mean that the normal infant's hearing sensitivity improves with age. Rather, it highlights the fact that we are often looking at the infant's responsiveness to the *presence* of a sound, which must be distinguished from the *threshold* of hearing for that sound. Similarly, the lowest levels at which infants respond also tend to improve with increasing age, as shown in **Fig. 12.1**. In recognition of these points, the lowest level at which an infant produces a behavioral response at a given time is often called the **minimum response level (MRL)** rather than the threshold (Matkin 1977).

Behavioral Observation

Behavioral observation (or **behavior observation audiometry, BOA**) involves watching the baby's responses to relatively sudden and intense stimulus sounds presented in the sound field, such as a speech signal (e.g., "bah-bah-bah"), warble tones, narrow band noises, and various hand-held noise-makers. *Behavioral observation* is preferred over the older term *behavior observation audiometry*, because it helps provide insight about the development of global auditory skills but does not actually involve hearing assessment (AAA 2012).

Remember that sound field testing means that we do not know whether a response resulted from hearing in both ears or just one of them. The stimulus levels expected to elicit responses from normal infants at various ages are shown in **Table 12.1**. Because wide-band stimuli are being used, any information we might get about hearing in different frequency regions is limited at best. In addition, we must keep in mind that many of the toys used as noisemakers for behavioral observation are unstandardized sound sources, the characteristics of which are unknown to us unless we actually measure their spectra (which is done with embarrassing rarity). This is not a minor point because, for example, an apparently "high-frequency" toy may have a very complex spectrum including considerable energy at much lower frequencies than we might think.

Behavioral observation should involve two examiners, typically one with the infant and the other in the control room with the audiometer, who observes the patient through the control room window. It is preferable for both examiners to be audiologists, but one audiologist and a knowledgeable and experienced assistant is a commonly used alternative. The infant should be placed on an examining table so that his whole body is clearly seen by both examiners. Depending on the infant's age and state, it may be necessary for him to be held by a parent or an assistant, but it is essential for the person holding the child to not respond during testing.

During the first 4 months of life the infant's response may include any of several reflexes and a change in its state, either alone or in combination. **Startle reflexes** are often seen as a body shudder and/or considerable gross movements of the arms, legs, and/or the body. The startle response is often called the **Moro reflex** when the body is thrown into a hugging or embracing posture. Eye-related reflexes are often seen as well, and include eye blinks and opening or widening of the eyes. The reflexive contraction of the muscles around the eyes, producing a blink, is known as the **auropalpebral reflex (APR)**. The startle and APR reflexes habituate rather quickly with repeated presentations of the stimulus sounds. **Habituation** means that the child stops responding after several stimulus presentations. The most typical changes in state that we watch for are arousal from sleep or stirring in response to the stimulus sound. Later during this period (between roughly 6 weeks and 4 months), we can observe quieting in response to the stimulus, eye shifts toward the sound source (the **cochleo-oculogyric** or **auro-oculogyric reflex**), and some rudimentary head turning toward the sound source.

Although behavioral assessments provide insights about the infant's auditory behavior and help us corroborate parent or caregiver reports, it is well established that they are simply too variable to provide reliable estimates of hearing sensitivity during the birth to 4 month period (Thompson & Weber 1974; Widen 1993; Hicks, Tharpe, & Ashmead 2000; ASHA 2004). Several sources of variability and subjectivity in behavioral observation have been outlined by Widen (1993). First, examiner judgments are subject to bias because the response itself can be elusive in the sense that it varies depending on such factors as the infant's state and age, and with the nature of the stimulus. For example, decisions about the infant's responses are biased by whether the examiner knows when the stimulus was presented (Ling, Ling, & Doehring 1970; Gans & Flexer 1982). Second, it is the infant's responsiveness to the presence of sound rather than his threshold that is being measured, and this responsiveness differs for different kinds of sounds. Third, the intensity levels at which responses occur and the nature of those responses vary with the age of the infant. The fourth issue is that habituation leads to variability in the responses obtained from the same child. The fifth source of variability is that normal infants respond over such a wide range of levels that the examiner can be hard-pressed to tell when a given child's responses are within or beyond the normal range.

Visual Reinforcement Audiometry

During the 4- to 7-month age period, the infant becomes more interested in softer sounds, an active listening attitude becomes apparent, and her neuro-motor control matures to the extent that she begins to develop a localization response that involves turning her head toward the sound source. As shown in **Table 12.1**, these responses begin as horizontal localizations at ear level, and then mature to include localizations below (at ~ 9 to 13 months) and finally above ear level around 13 to 16 months. Testing approaches that make use of these localization responses are sometimes referred to as "localization audiometry."

When the infant reaches about 5 to 6 months of age, the localization responses are robust enough for us to move from behavioral observation, which involves the observation of *unconditioned* behaviors, to the use of *conditioned* responses.

Hearing measurement using a conditioned localization response and a visual reinforcer is generally known as **visual reinforcement audiometry (VRA)** (Lidén & Kankkunen 1969). The basic approach was described by Suzuki and Obiga (1961), who called it the **conditioned orientation reflex (COR)**. In their method, the child is placed in the test room with loudspeakers off to each side, as shown schematically in **Fig. 12.2**. Presenting a sound from one of the loudspeakers elicits an orientation or localization response from the child, which involves turning toward the stimulus speaker. This response is followed by the illumination of a visually appealing object that is associated with that loudspeaker, which serves as a reward or **reinforcer**. An example is shown in **Fig. 12.3**, where the visual reinforcer is mounted on top of each speaker. This process constitutes **conditioning** because the visual reinforcer increases the chances that the child will continue responding to subsequent stimulus presentations.

Various visual reinforcement audiometry approaches and testing protocols are available (e.g., AAA 2012; Day, Green, Munro, et al 2008; Haug, Baccaro, & Guilford 1967; Lidén & Kankkunen 1969;

Fig. 12.2 Typical testing arrangement for visual reinforcement audiometry, with the child sitting on its parent's lap at a table. The reinforcer devices in this diagram are on top of the two corner loudspeakers. Some methods, like COR, use loudspeakers and reinforcers on one side, but many (though not all) contemporary VRA approaches place the loudspeaker and reinforcer(s) on just one side, which is represented by the brightly-filled star (representing that it is being illuminated).

Moore, Thompson, & Thompson 1975; Matkin 1977; Diefendorf & Gravel 1996; Gravel & Hood 1999; Gravel & Wallace 2000; Widen, Folsom, Cone-Wesson, et al 2000; Widen, Johnson, White, et al 2005), of which the one developed by Moore et al (1975) is one of the most extensively documented and studied. The major characteristics of this VRA method are as follows:

1. A single loudspeaker and associated visual reinforcer(s) on one side are used; although it should be known that speakers and reinforcers on both sides are often used as well. The loudspeakers and reinforcers are often placed at 45° angles, as shown in **Fig. 12.2**, but 90° angles have been recommended so that the child's head turn will be clearly observable (AAA 2012).

2. The reinforcement device usually is a toy that is illuminated *and* moves in place. Typical examples of these animated reinforcers include mechanical stuffed animals or a clown that plays the drums or cymbals (silently) when activated. The same switch activates the mechanical toy and the light. (Keep in mind that some children are frightened by clowns, so it is wise to ask the parents about this issue before using them as reinforcers.) The toy is mounted inside a dark Plexiglas box so that it is not visible until it is lit up for reinforcement purposes. A selection of several different animated toy reinforcers may be used instead of just one (e.g., Merer & Gravel 1997; Gravel & Wallace 2000; Widen et al 2005).

3. To be acceptable, the infant's response must be a clear head turn toward the loudspeaker/reinforcer.

4. Responses are judged by two examiners.

5. There are clearly defined criteria for when the patient is considered to be conditioned (e.g., three correct responses in a row) and habituated (e.g., four nonresponses out of five consecutive trials).

Depending on the infant's age, neuromotor status, and state, she is seated on a chair (or on a parent's lap), held, or placed on an examining table. The examiner with the infant usually manipulates quiet toys or pictures on a table in front of the child, which are used as midline distractors (AAA 2012) to keep her passively attendant and facing forward. The person holding the child should not respond during testing, and parents in particular must be instructed not to participate in the testing process.

Thresholds may be obtained using modifications of conventional threshold search approaches, or with

Fig. 12.3 An example of a typical illuminated visual reinforcer used in VRA.

sophisticated programmed approaches (e.g., Bernstein & Gravel 1990). Unlike the usual "up 5 dB/down 10 dB" threshold method used in routine pure tone audiometry, visual reinforcement audiometry often involves an "up 10 dB/down 10 dB" or an "up 10 dB/down 20 dB" approach, or more sophisticated computer-assisted techniques (e.g., Gravel 1989; Eilers, Miskiel, Ozdamar, Urbano, & Widen 1991; Eilers, Widen, Urbano, Hudson, & Gonzales 1991; Gravel & Hood 1999; Tharpe & Ashmead 1993). On the basis of findings obtained using computer simulations, for example, Tharpe and Ashmead (1993) suggested that an efficient threshold testing strategy for visual reinforcement audiometry involves the following characteristics: (1) beginning the test without conditioning (i.e., training) trials in which the test tone and reinforcer are paired, (2) an initial test level of 30 dB HL (which is raised in 20 dB steps if there is no response at 30 dB HL), and (3) the use of an "up 10 dB/ down 20 dB" technique.

The characteristics of effective reinforcers were investigated by Moore et al (1977). They found that the highest rate of responses among 12- to 18-month-old infants occurs when using complex visual reinforcers such as toys that were lit up and moved in place. Progressively lower response rates are obtained with a simple visual reinforcer such as a flashing light; social reinforcers such as verbal praise, a pat on the shoulder, and/or smiling; and without any reinforcement at all. Video clips from movies or television shows that are appealing to young children provide another useful class of visual reinforcers (Schmida, Peterson, & Tharpe 2003; Lowery, von Hapsburg, Plyler, & Johnstone 2009; Karzon & Banerjee 2010).

Visual reinforcement audiometry can be effective with full-term infants who are at least 5 to 6 months old (Moore et al 1977) and is typically recommended up to roughly 24 months of age (ASHA 2004; AAA 2012). Babies who were born prematurely can be expected to respond effectively to VRA at a corrected age of 8 months (Moore et al 1992). Recall that the corrected age is the child's chronological age minus the estimated number of weeks of prematurity. One- and 2-year-olds tend to be conditioned for visual reinforcement audiometry quickly and easily, and are similar in terms of the rate of conditioning (how quickly they learn to perform the task) and the consistency of their responses (Primus & Thompson 1985). Unfortunately, however, infants do not continue responding to the stimulus forever. Instead, their responses habituate, or die out, as the stimulus trials are repeated over the course of the testing session. Habituation occurs more quickly for 2-year-olds than for 1-year-olds (Primus & Thompson 1985; Thompson, Thompson, & McCall 1992).

Habituation is a major consideration with young children because the amount of information we can get about the child's hearing depends on how many times he will respond. The number of responses obtained before habituation occurs can be increased by using different reinforcers instead of using just one (e.g., Primus & Thompson 1985; Thompson et al 1992). Giving the child a 10-minute break after habituation has occurred and then beginning a second test session significantly increases the total number of responses obtained from 1-year-olds, but not from 2-year-olds (Thompson et al 1992). Culpepper and Thompson (1994) showed the number of responses from 2-year-olds before habituation increased as the duration of the reinforcer was reduced from 4 seconds to a half-second.

Tangible and Visual Reinforcement Operant Conditioning Audiometry

Tangible reinforcement operant conditioning audiometry (TROCA) (Lloyd, Spradlin, & Reid 1968) is a highly structured testing approach originally described for use with **difficult-to-test** patients, such

as those with developmental disabilities. *Difficult-to-test* is a general term used to mean those who cannot be readily assessed with conventional behavioral tests, so that special methods are needed. Patients may be difficult to test due to physical, developmental, perceptual, cognitive, emotional, or other problems, or to any combination of these factors. Approaches like TROCA, which were developed for the difficult to test, are also effective with normal young children. Upon hearing a tone (or other test signal), the child is required to push a response button or to make another simple but specific motor response within his range of neuromotor capabilities. Correct responses are reinforced by the delivery of a tangible reward, which might be cereal, candy, tokens, or other small trinkets. False-positive responses are discouraged because they are followed by time-out periods. The entire procedure is accomplished with instrumentation programmed to present the stimuli, monitor the responses, and deliver the reinforcers according to a predefined operant conditioning schedule.

In **visual reinforcement operant conditioning audiometry (VROCA)** (Wilson & Thompson 1984; Thompson, Thompson, & Vethivelu 1989) the child is required to press a response button (which is a large, bright box) instead of turning toward the loudspeaker, after which a visual reinforcer is presented. The visual reinforcer itself is the same kind used in visual reinforcement audiometry. When VROCA is employed with sound field testing, the loudspeaker is kept in front of the child so he is not distracted from the response box, as opposed to being placed off to one side as is done for a head turning response.

Conditioned Play Audiometry

Conditioned play audiometry, or play audiometry, involves training the child to listen for stimuli and then make a specific motor response within the framework of a game, usually in combination with social reinforcement such as smiles, praise, etc. For example, the child might be trained to place a peg into a pegboard after each test sound. Other commonly used games include stacking blocks or cups, placing small items into a container (or taking them out), or just about any other simple activity that can be repeated over and over again. Play audiometry is often appropriate for children between about 2 and 5 years of age (Northern & Downs 1991; AAA 2012). However, one should keep in mind that this is a wide age range as far as child development is concerned; and it is not surprising to find that the successful use of conditioned play audiometry improves with age, especially beyond the second year (e.g., Nielsen & Olsen 1997). Hence, we should not expect that all youngsters will be ready to be conditioned for play audiometry at age 2 (Thompson et al 1989).

If at all possible, the mother or father should not be in the room during play audiometry. Parents in the control room are also undesirable, especially if the child can see them through the observation window. A parent who simply must be in the room should be seated quietly out of the child's direct line of sight, and instructed not to interact with the child or participate in the testing process in any way.

Play audiometry employs two clinicians who communicate by intercom and visually through the window between the control and test rooms. One of them operates the audiometer and the other stays with the child. The child is generally seated at a small table, which is the play surface, either next to or opposite one of the examiners. A collection of games should be kept on hand so that when the child gets bored with one activity you can quickly and smoothly replace it with another. Keep the backup games out of sight so they do not distract the child from the task at hand. If accepted by the child, earphone testing may be attempted at the start, or at least as soon as possible. Some children accept earphones immediately. In other cases, getting the child to accept earphones is a challenge in which the audiologist's personal "way with kids" comes to the fore. A knowledge of the most current children's cartoon series and action toy fads is a valuable asset in this context. Earphone acceptance is sometimes facilitated if the clinician first puts on her own headset (which houses the intercom and permits her to monitor the test signals). A reasonable amount of good-natured firmness and confident tenacity often works, but keep in mind that "winning" means getting the child to cooperate sufficiently that valid and reliable audiological information can be obtained, which will not happen if he is crying hysterically. If earphones are simply out of the question, then in the most matter-of-fact manner try the bone-conduction vibrator or insert earphones. If all reasonable attempts fail, simply place the headset on the table where the child can see it, and start the test in sound field.

The goal is to condition the child to perform a specific, observable action every time he hears a tone, and then to manipulate the level of the tone to find the child's threshold. The basic game used in conditioned play audiometry involves having the child hold a peg up to his ear while listening for a tone, and then placing it into a hole in the pegboard when a tone is heard (or adding it to a pile, etc.). *Tell and demonstrate* what to do. Then tell the child it is now his turn. It is often necessary to take the child's hand and *lead him through* the task physically at first while verbalizing what he is doing. Then let him try. *Praise* the child for doing the task correctly. Reinstruct the child if necessary (this usually involves reminding him to wait for the tone before responding), but keep the emphasis on reinforcing the desired behavior.

Once the child has learned the task, we need to obtain thresholds efficiently before habituation occurs. Northern and Downs (1991) recommend starting in the 40 dB HL to 50 dB HL range and descending in 10 or 15 dB steps, and then using ascending presentations to find the threshold, with two responses as the criterion; or one may use the threshold search methods described earlier in the section on visual reinforcement audiometry. Habituation will most likely limit the number of thresholds that can be obtained in any one session, which means we must begin testing at the frequencies that will provide the most information about the child's audiogram as quickly as possible. For this reason it is usually desirable to obtain thresholds at 500 and 2000 Hz for both ears first. The other frequencies can then be filled in as long as the child remains "on task." Northern and Downs recommended that these frequencies generally be added in the following order: 1000 Hz, 250 Hz, and 4000 Hz.

■ Physiological Measures

Physiological methods are playing an increasing role in the audiological evaluation of infants and young children. These allow us to assess neonates and younger infants in ways that cannot be done by behavioral observation audiometry because they (1) do not require the child's cooperation, (2) allow us to test each ear individually, and (3) directly assess the physiological integrity of at least the lower portions of the auditory system. On the other hand, we must keep in mind that physiological measurements give us a limited perspective of the infant's world of sound because they do not involve a behavioral response. As previously indicated, physiological tests are often useful even with children who can be tested with behavioral methods, because they provide us with valuable cross-checks on the behavioral results (Jerger & Hayes 1976; ASHA 2004; JCIH 2007; AAA 2012) and also provide additional differential diagnostic information.

The physiological tests regularly used in pediatric audiology include the auditory brainstem response (ABR), auditory steady-state response (ASSR), otoacoustic emissions (OAEs), and acoustic immittance tests. The later evoked potentials (see Chapter 11) are not routinely used with infants and younger children because they are affected by sleep and sedation. This is a significant factor because it is often necessary for young children and difficult-to-test patients to be asleep or sedated for results to be obtained. (This involves the participation of a physician because sedation and other forms of anesthesia are medical activities.) However, the later evoked responses cannot be totally discarded for use with young children. For example, Shimizu (1992) pointed out that it is possible to obtain cortical evoked potentials from young children during certain sleep stages, and that this can provide important information, particularly in children with absent ABRs. Other physiological approaches have also been used in the past. Examples include the monitoring of respiratory and/or cardiac responses to sound (Bradford 1975; Eisenberg 1975) and the psychogalvanic skin response (PGSR) (Ventry 1975). These methods were more cumbersome and less practical than modern approaches, in addition to which the PGSR was unnecessarily traumatic for the child.

Auditory Evoked Potentials

Although there are maturational effects that must be considered, the **auditory brainstem response (ABR)** and the **auditory steady-state response (ASSR)** are particularly well suited for use in pediatric audiology (Jacobson 1985; Dimitrijevic, John, Van Roon, et al 2002; Stapells 2002; Hall 2006; ASHA 2004; Rance, Tomlin, & Rickards 2006; Picton 2007; Sininger 2007; JCIH 2007; AAA 2012; see Chapter 11). Very young as well as seriously disabled children can be tested by ABR and ASSR because they do not involve a behavioral response and they are reasonably unaffected by sleep and sedation. Both techniques provide separate results for each ear. *Frequency-specific* results are needed to estimate the audiogram, and are provided by the ABR using tone burst stimuli or with the ASSR. Diagnostic information about the child's neurological integrity at the brainstem level is provided by the ABR when click stimuli are used. Moreover, ABR and ASSR testing with bone-conduction stimuli in addition to air-conduction signals allows us to assess the type of hearing loss.

Otoacoustic Emissions

Distortion product (DPOAE) and transient-evoked (TEOAE) otoacoustic emissions, described in Chapter 11, have considerable value in pediatric audiological assessment (e.g., ASHA 2004; JCIH 2007; AAA 2012). In contrast to the ABR, acoustic reflexes, and other tests that rely on both sensory and neural activity, otoacoustic emissions are "preneural," relying only on the integrity of the cochlea before the auditory nervous system gets involved in the processing of a signal; hence, they can be measured even when there are neurological deficits that affect other measures. Otoacoustic emissions do not require a behavioral response, are reliably obtained in normal infants and young children, are very sensitive to hearing loss, are obtained separately for each ear, and can provide information at different frequencies.

Acoustic Immittance

Tympanometry and acoustic reflex tests are a central part of the evaluation of infants and young children. The use of acoustic immittance tests with infants and children is covered in Chapter 7. Acoustic immittance measurements allow us to monitor middle ear conditions over time, and also can provide us with information about the status of the middle ear when reliable masked thresholds cannot be obtained, as is often the case with very young children. Acoustic reflex measurements provide information about the integrity of several aspects of the peripheral ears and lower parts of the auditory pathway, and also help us distinguish between the presence and absence of significant amounts of hearing loss.

◼ Speech Audiometry

Threshold for Speech

Speech signals are used in the behavioral assessment of infants and children from birth onward. The initial use of speech may be to elicit a startle response from a neonate; months later, speech signals may be used to elicit localizing behavior.

Olsen and Matkin (1991) have suggested some guidelines for determining the threshold for speech depending on the child's overall level of functioning, which is effectively her developmental age. As with other aspects of assessment in pediatric audiology, there is no clear line of demarcation between the times when one type of method or the other should be used, which is implied by Olsen and Matkin's subtle use of overlapping age ranges. They recommended that a **speech detection threshold (SDT)** using a repetitive speech utterance be obtained from children who are functioning below the 3-year-old level. The speech detection threshold is obtained using the same kinds of techniques described earlier in this chapter. Unconditioned responses are used for those functioning at the lowest developmental levels, whereas conditioned responses can be obtained from children who can be tested by VRA, play audiometry, TROCA, or VROCA.

A modified speech recognition (reception) threshold (SRT) can be obtained from many children from ~ 30 months to roughly 6 years old. This can be accomplished by, for example, presenting a group of easily recognizable objects or pictures that depict words selected to be within the child's receptive vocabulary (e.g., a toy airplane, baseball, cowboy, toothbrush, etc.) and having her identify them as they are named by the examiner. It is also possible to have a child respond by pointing with an eye gaze in the direction of a selected picture (Byers & Bristow 1990). This kind of technique can be used for testing either speech thresholds or word recognition performance, and is useful with some children regardless of age (and adults, for that matter) who have cerebral palsy or other disorders that prevent them from pointing manually. Older children within this range are often able to give a verbal response to selected spondee words.

A conventional SRT can often be obtained from children who function in the 5- to 10-year-old range, although a children's spondee list is recommended for them. A list of spondee words considered to be within the receptive vocabularies of most children (ASHA 1988) is included in Appendix B. A conventional SRT based on standard spondee word lists is expected from children functioning at the level of 10 years and above.

Testing the speech recognition threshold by bone-conduction and comparing it to the air-conduction SRT can provide insights about the type of hearing loss, which can be quite valuable if reliable tonal results have yet to be obtained (Olsen & Matkin 1991; Northern & Downs 1991). However, calibration values for speech presented via the bone-conduction vibrator must be determined empirically before this procedure is used.

Speech Recognition

In general, speech recognition tests (Chapter 8) are used to reveal the accuracy of the patient's auditory reception and processing of speech material, usually in terms of a percent correct score for monosyllabic words. This can be problematic when testing children because their speech recognition scores are affected by their level of language development as well as by their auditory capabilities. As a result, normal children's speech recognition scores on many tests increase as they get older, eventually becoming comparable to adult scores at roughly 10 to 12 years of age, when they are familiar with most if not all of the test words. The situation is exacerbated in patients who have speech-language disorders, or other problems that impair either the level of linguistic functioning or the ability to respond during the test. In addition, we must remember that speech-language disorders are common among children with significant amounts of hearing impairment. Consequently, we should try to use speech recognition tests that include words within the child's receptive vocabulary and employ responses that she is capable of

making, at least to the extent that this is possible. Moreover, in light of the fact that practical tests often cannot realize these lofty goals, we must consider the individual child's receptive vocabulary and response limitations when interpreting and reporting speech recognition test results.

Open-Set Tests

Several open-set tests are available for children who are not ready for adult speech recognition measures. Recall from Chapter 8 that the open-set format is essentially the same as a fill-in test. The speech recognition ability of children who are ~ 6 to 9 years old can often be tested with the **Phonetically-Balanced Kindergarten** or **PBK-50 lists** (Haskins 1949). The PBK-50 test is made up of 50-word lists based on a kindergarten-level vocabulary, and the word recognition score is simply the percent of the words that were repeated correctly. The four PBK-50 lists are included in Appendix K. Although PBK-50 lists 1, 3, and 4 are usually considered to be equivalent, list 2 is rarely used clinically because Haskins found it to be easier than the other three. Meyer and Pisoni (1999) demonstrated that compared with the words in the other three "equivalent" lists, the words in the easier list 2 have a higher frequency of occurrence and are less likely to be confused with other words.

Boothroyd's **isophonemic word lists** (Boothroyd 1968, 1970, 1984; Boothroyd & Nittrouer 1988) can also be used with children in this age range. The isophonemic word test was discussed in Chapter 8, and may also be found in Appendix H. Each isophonemic word test list includes 10 consonant-vowel-consonant (CVC) words that are scored on a phoneme-by-phoneme basis. In other words, scores on the isophonemic word test are based on 30 phonemes.

The **Lexical Neighborhood Test (LNT)** and the **Multisyllabic Lexical Neighborhood Test (MLNT)** were developed to facilitate the assessment of children with profound hearing losses with cochlear implants (Kirk, Pisoni & Osberger 1995; Kirk 1999; Kirk, Eisenberg, Martinez, & Hay-McCutcheon 1999). Because many of these children have limited vocabularies, the words on these tests were chosen from those known to be familiar to 3- to 5-year-olds based on Logan's (1992) analysis of the Child Language Data Exchange System (CHILDS) database (MacWhinney & Snow 1985). The LNT includes 25 lexically hard monosyllabic words and 25 lexically easy monosyllabic words. (Recall that words with a high frequency of occurrence and few similar-sounding alternatives are lexically easy, whereas low-frequency words with many alternatives are lexically hard.) Instead of using monosyllabic words, the MLNT involves presenting 24 two- and three-syllable words. As with the LNT, half of the words on the MLNT are lexically hard and half are lexically easy. The two LNT and MLNT lists are shown in Appendices I and J.

Closed-Set Tests

Several closed-set or multiple-choice format monosyllabic word recognition tests are available for children who are at least about 3 years of age. The most widely used tests of this type are the **Word Intelligibility by Picture Identification (WIPI) Test** (Ross & Lerman 1970, 1971), the **Northwestern University Children's Perception of Speech (NU-CHIPS) Test** (Kalikow, Stevens, & Elliott 1977; Elliott & Katz 1980), and the **Pediatric Speech Intelligibility (PSI) Test** (Jerger, Lewis, Hawkins, & Jerger 1980; Jerger, Jerger, & Lewis 1981; Jerger & Jerger 1984), although others are also available. In the WIPI test, the child points to a picture that corresponds to the stimulus word from a choice of six color pictures. Each set of six pictures is arranged on the same page of a test book. An administration of the WIPI includes 25 items, and there are four test lists. **Fig. 12.4** shows an example of a response plate from the WIPI test, and the test words are listed in Appendix L.

The NU-CHIPS test is made up of 50 words that are within the receptive vocabularies of inner-city 3-year-olds, which are listed in Appendix M, including four recorded randomizations of these words. The child is presented with a page showing four picture choices for each test word, as in **Fig. 12.5**, and responds by pointing to the picture that corresponds to the test word.

The material in the PSI test was derived from the vocabularies and sentence structures used by normal 3- to 6-year-old children. The test words are 20 monosyllabic nouns. The child responds by pointing at the picture corresponding to the test word or sentence. Two sentence formats may be used on the PSI test, depending on the child's language level, which are referred to as Format I (e.g., "Show me a bear combing his hair") and Format II (e.g., "A bear is combing his hair").

Other speech recognition tests have also been developed for use with children. For example, the **Auditory Perception of Alphabet Letters (APAL) Test** can be used for younger children who are familiar with the alphabet even if their vocabularies are inadequate for word recognition testing (Ross & Randolf 1988). Robbins and Kirk (1996) described a technique for assessing speech recognition in preschoolers with limited vocabularies by having them follow verbal directions to assemble the familiar Mr. Potato Head toy.

Sentence Tests

A number of speech recognition tests for children employ a sentence format. Weber and Redell (1976) devised a modification of the WIPI test in which the test items are presented in a sentence format. Another children's sentence test was developed by Bench, Kowal, and Bamford (1979) and is called the **BKB Sentences Test**. One version of the BKB test is composed of 16 sentences that are presented to older children in an open-set format, and the test is graded on the basis of how many key words are

Fig. 12.4 An example of a WIPI test response plate. (From Ross and Lerman [1971], with permission.)

Fig. 12.5 An example of a NU-CHIPS test response plate. (From Elliott and Katz [1980], with permission.)

repeated correctly. The other version is intended for use with younger children and involves a picture pointing response. The **Hearing in Noise Test for Children (HINT-C)** (Nilsson, Soli, & Gelnett 1996) is a pediatric version of the Hearing in Noise Test (HINT) (described in Chapter 8) and is used to measure the SRT for sentences.

An interesting approach to sentence-based speech recognition assessment in children is provided by the **Pediatric AzBio Sentence Lists** (Spahr, Dorman, Litvak, et al 2014). The Pediatric AzBio has 16 test lists with equivalent difficulty, and is similar in overall format to the adult AzBio test (Spahr, Dorman, Litvak, et al 2012) described in Chapter 8. As in the adult version, each Pediatric AzBio list contains 20 sentences varying in length from 3 to 12 words, and the test score is simply the percentage of the correctly repeated words based on the total number of words in the whole list. However, unlike the adult test, the sentences in the pediatric version were taken from utterances produced by 5 to 12 year olds (with slight grammatical corrections) that were recorded by one adult female talker.[1] Moreover, Spahr and colleagues found that normal-hearing kindergarteners and the first graders were able to accurately repeat the sentences in the test. As a result, the Pediatric AzBio appears to be well-suited for evaluating speech recognition skills in a sentence context for children as young as about 5 years of age.

Special Tests and Techniques

Other speech recognition testing approaches for children are also available that are different from those already described. Several tests involve the **change/ no change** or **go/no go task**, in which the child is trained to respond to a *change* in the stimulus. The **Visual Reinforcement Infant Speech Discrimination (VRISD) Test** uses *visual reinforcement audiometry* with the change/no change task to test an infant's ability to discriminate between pairs of syllables (Eilers, Wilson, & Moore 1977). Instead of being conditioned to respond to the presence of a stimulus sound, the infant is trained to respond when a train of syllables that are all the same (e.g., /va va va ... va/) *changes* to another, contrasting syllable (e.g., (/sa sa ... /). A modification of the VRISD method, using real words instead of syllables and pointing instead of head turning, has been used to test speech discrimination in 4-year-olds (Menary, Trehub, & McNutt 1982). The **Speech Feature Test (SFT)**

uses *conditioned play audiometry* with the change/ no change task to test discrimination between pairs of syllables, and can be employed successfully with many 3- and 4-year-olds, as well as some 2-year-olds (Dawson, Nott, Clark, & Cowan 1998).

Recall from Chapter 8 that the **Speech Pattern Contrast (SPAC) Test** provides information about the patient's ability to correctly perceive the acoustic information needed to make phonologically relevant distinctions (Boothroyd 1984, 1988). Similar information is often needed for young children who do not have the vocabulary or reading ability required for the SPAC test, and may be obtained with the **Three-Interval Forced-Choice Test of Speech Pattern Contrast Perception (THRIFT)** (Boothroyd, Springer, Smith, & Schulman 1988). On the THRIFT the child must simply identify the location of the "**odd-ball**" in a sequence like "pea–*bee*–pea" or "*sue*–zoo–zoo." The odd-ball is distinguished from the other two stimuli based on the same kinds of contrasts used in the SPAC test. The THRIFT can be used with prelingually deaf children because it does not require the child to have any pre-existing phonological knowledge, vocabulary, or reading skills, but the motivational demands of the test limit its use to children who are at least 7 years old (Boothroyd 1991). The imitative version of the SPAC test (**IMSPAC**) makes it possible to test children too young for the THRIFT (perhaps as young as 2 to 3 years of age) because the response mode involves imitating the stimuli, although performance does improve with increasing age (Boothroyd 1991; Boothroyd, Hanin, Yeung, & Eran 1996). A video game variation of the speech contrast test (**VIDSPAC**) appears to be useful with children as young as 3 years of age (Boothroyd 1991; Boothroyd, Hanin, Yeung, & Chen 1992). On this test an animated character says a stimulus sound and then hides. The following scene shows two hiding places. Two sounds are produced in sequence; one of them matches the sound produced by the animated character and the other is a contrasting sound. One of these sounds is represented as coming from a hideout on the left side of the computer screen and the other coming from a hideout on the right. The child then points to where the character is hiding. A tangible reinforcer is provided after a certain number of correct responses.

The **Ling Five and Six Sounds Tests** (Ling 1976, 1989; Ling & Ling 1978) employ an informal approach to obtain information about the child's ability to make use of spectral cues in speech reception. Although these tests are typically administered by live voice, a recorded version of the Six Sounds Test has been developed by Scollie, Glista, Tenhaaf, and colleagues (2012). In the **Five Sounds Test**, the child is asked to detect the five sounds, /a, u, i, s, ʃ/,

---

[1] Recordings by additional talkers are planned (Spahr et al, 2014).

that are presented separately by the examiner. Hearing the vowels implies that the child has usable residual hearing up to roughly 1000 Hz and that she can also hear the suprasegmental features of speech. If /ʃ/ is also audible, it is inferred that the child's usable residual hearing extends up to ~ 2000 Hz and at least several vowel discriminations are possible. The ability to hear /s/ implies usable residual hearing as high as ~ 4000 Hz. The **Six Sounds Test** adds the /m/ sound and is used to assess residual hearing for the lower frequencies.

Other types of tests are also needed under certain circumstances. Consider, for example, the case of a child with a severe to profound hearing loss whose conventional speech recognition score is very low or even zero, or "chance" on a closed-set test. Chance performance means that the score could have occurred from random guessing. For example, guessing would yield the "right" answer one fifth of the time on a closed-set test with five alternatives per item, so that chance performance in this case would be 20%. In these cases, useful information might be obtained by determining how well the child is able to recognize words containing more than one syllable, which is done with tests such as the **Multisyllabic Lexical Neighborhood Test (MLNT)** (Kirk, Pisoni, & Osberger 1995; Kirk 1999; Kirk et al 1999), described earlier in the chapter.

When dealing with very limited speech recognition ability, it often becomes important to know whether the child can at least recognize differences in the temporal or rhythmic patterns of speech. This type of information is provided by the **Monosyllable-Trochee-Spondee (MTS) test**, which was originally described as the **Children's Auditory Test (CT)** (Erber & Alencewicz 1976), which is frequently used along with, or as part of, speech perception batteries for those with profound hearing impairments. The MTS test involves three categories of words that are distinguishable on the basis of the number of syllables and the stress pattern: (1) **monosyllables** (e.g., "bed"); (2) **spondees**, which have two syllables with equal emphasis on both of them (e.g., "baseball"); and (3) **trochees**, which have two syllables with unequal emphasis on the first syllable (e.g., "button"). In this test, a test word is presented to the patient, who responds by making a selection from a choice of alternative words.

The stimuli and responses can be tallied on a matrix like the one in **Fig. 12.6**. Examining the relationships between the stimulus words and responses reveals whether the patient can correctly identify words with different levels of difficulty, and also whether she is able to take advantage of temporal and/or stress patterns in speech. Let us consider several kinds of responses on the MTS test. We might

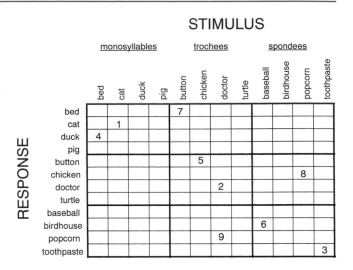

Fig. 12.6 The MTS test allows us to analyze confusions among monosyllabic, trochaic, and spondaic words. Responses 1, 2, and 3 are correct word identifications; 4, 5, and 6 indicate incorrect word recognition but correct identification of the temporal patterns (i.e., monosyllable for monosyllable, trochee for trochee, spondee for spondee); 7, 8, and 9 are examples of word recognition errors that also involve temporal pattern errors: In 7, two syllables are identified as only one; in 8, equally stressed syllables are identified as unequal; and in 9, unequally stressed syllables are identified as having similar stress. (Adapted from Erber and Alencewicz [1976], with permission of American Speech Language-Hearing Association.)

find that a patient who cannot identify monosyllables (the conventional speech recognition stimuli) may still be able to correctly identify less difficult material such as two-syllable words. Errors like pointing to "popcorn" in response to "baseball" (both spondees) suggest that the patient correctly identified the stress pattern even though the word itself was not heard correctly. On the other hand, pointing to "duck" (a monosyllable) or "birdhouse" (a spondee) in response to "turtle" (a trochee) shows that the patient also has difficulty identifying temporal or stress patterns. The fundamental approach of the MTS test has been modified and expanded in various ways, such as increasing the number of words tested in each category (Geers & Moog 1992) and the addition of three-syllable words (Erber 1982).

Similar information may be obtained with the **Early Speech-Perception (ESP) Test** (Geers & Moog 1989; Moog & Geers 1990), which employs pointing responses to pictures and toys with children as young as 3 years of age. The **Auditory Numbers Test (ANT)** is a simplified approach designed to obtain information about the ability to use spectral versus temporal patterns of speech in young children whose vocabularies are too limited for the MTS test; it can be used with 3-year-olds who can count from 1 to 5 (Erber 1980). Here the examiner says a number and the child points to the corresponding one of five cards that illustrates the number in the form of numerals and pictures of groups of ants. Analyzing the nature of errors provides insight about whether the child can make use of spectral cues and temporal patterns.

Tests such as the **Sound Effects Recognition Test (SERT)** (Finitzo-Hieber, Matkin, Cherow-Skalka, & Rice 1975; Finitzo-Hieber, Matkin, Cherow-Skalka, & Gerling 1977) can often be used with children who cannot respond adequately to verbal stimuli. On the SERT, the child listens to a familiar environmental sound and then points to the corresponding picture from a choice of four alternatives. Some examples of the test stimuli used include a dog barking, splashing water, a father's voice, and a doorbell. This kind of information reveals how well a child can make use of spectral and temporal information to identify complex stimuli.

The tests outlined in this section are by no means the only ones available to assess the speech reception abilities of children; neither do they represent the only approaches that can be used. They do, however, reveal the diversity of approaches available to us as we try to construct a picture of the child's auditory ability.

Because of the differences among the test instruments, the meaning of a given speech recognition score is unclear unless the clinician also specifies which test instrument was used and the conditions of testing. These differences are quite substantial even for "conventional" tests such as the PBK-50, WIPI, and NU-CHIPS. This notion is illustrated in **Fig. 12.7**, which shows the average speech recognition scores of normal children who took these three tests under the same conditions. It is clear that the three tests yield three different speech recognition scores. In addition, closed-set tests like the WIPI and NU-CHIPS result in considerably higher scores than the PBK-50, which is an open-set test. Also notice that the 10-year-olds have higher scores than the 5-year-olds, which highlights the importance of considering the effects of language development when interpreting children's speech recognition scores. Differences among the test instruments are complicated when the clinician must modify the "standard" procedures to test a particular child.

■ Testing Approaches at Various Ages

In this section we will review the kinds of testing procedures that are typically appropriate at different stages of the child's development. Several sets

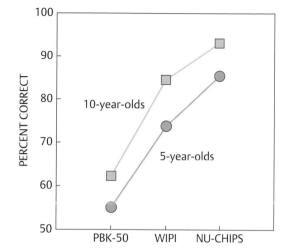

Fig. 12.7 Different speech recognition tests result in different speech recognition scores. The graph compares the mean speech recognition scores obtained by normal 5- and 10-year-old children on three different tests (PBK-50, WIPI, and NU-CHIPS) presented at 12 dB sensation level. (Based on data reported by Elliott and Katz [1980].)

of pediatric assessment guidelines are available, such as the ones by the American Speech-Language-Hearing Association (ASHA 2004) and the American Academy of Audiology (AAA 2012). The ASHA (2004) guidelines are presented in terms of three age ranges from birth to 60 months, but other age breakdowns are also available. For example, the Joint Committee on Infant Hearing (JCIH 2007) outlines evaluation procedures appropriate for the birth to 6 months and 6 to 36 months age ranges. The AAA (2012) guidelines provide pediatric assessment protocols that are arranged according to techniques, and are summarized with their appropriate age ranges in **Table 12.2**. Although the first three age ranges described in this section (birth to 4 months, 5 to 24 months, and 25 to 60 months) are presented according to the ASHA (2004) guidelines, referring to **Table 12.2** will reveal that they essentially comport with the AAA (2012) guidelines as well.

From the earliest stages, the assessment approach includes a case history, consideration of risk indicators (see Chapter 13), otoscopy, and measurement techniques intended to provide frequency-specific information for each age group (ASHA 2004; AAA 2012). In addition to speech threshold and recognition testing, ASHA (2004) recommends assessing the child's development of speech perception skills with an eye toward management, focusing on such levels of function as detection, discrimination, and comprehension. Moreover, functional auditory assessments and developmental screening are included,

Table 12.2 Recommended age ranges for the use of pediatric assessment methods based on American Academy of Audiology guidelines (AAA 2012)

Assessment method	Approximate age range	Comments
Behavioral observation	0–6 months	Also for others who cannot be tested behaviorally. To assess "global auditory skill development" (AAA 2012, p. 9)
Visual reinforcement audiometry	5–24 months	
Conditioned play audiometry	2–5 years	
Speech audiometry	≥6 months	
Immittance (tympanometry; acoustic reflex thresholds)	All ages	678 or 1000 Hz probe < 6 months 226 Hz probe ≥ 6 months
Otoacoustic emissions	All ages	
Auditory brainstem response; auditory steady-state response	Newborns/infants	Also others if behavioral results are untestable/incomplete/unreliable

not only as supplements to the diagnostic process, but also because they provide valuable information for intervention and referral. Examples of developmental screening and functional auditory assessment instruments appropriate for various age ranges are listed in **Table 12.3**. Additional instruments are discussed in Chapter 16.

Before proceeding, it is wise to mention that a central principle in pediatric audiology is that no single test should be used to define a child's auditory status (e.g., Jerger & Hayes 1976; Gravel, Kurtzberg, Stapells, Vaughan, & Wallace 1989; Stach, Wolf, & Bland 1993; Hall 2006; AAA 2012). Instead, we often employ the judicious use of both behavioral and physiological testing methods to complement and supplement one another. The use of one type of measure to corroborate the results of another is often called the **cross-check principle** (Jerger & Hayes 1976).

Birth to 4 Months

The assessment of infants' hearing during the first 4 months of life (adjusted for prematurity) is principally based on physiological tests, focusing on the auditory brainstem response (ABR) and the auditory steady-state response (ASSR). Behavioral assessment is not used for the purpose of estimating hearing sensitivity with infants in the birth to 4 months age range; but rather to assess the qualitative aspects of the infant's auditory behavior, and to corroborate what has been reported by the parents or caregiver.

Table 12.3 Examples of developmental screening and functional auditory assessment instruments (based on ASHA 2004)

Developmental screening
Birth to 24 months
Early Language Milestone Scale (EML Scale-2; Coplan & Gleason 1993)
25 to 60 months
Meadow-Kendal Socio-Emotional Assessment Inventories for Deaf and Hearing Impaired Students (Meadow-Orlans 1983)[a]

Functional auditory assessment
5 to 24 months
Early Listening Function (ELF; Anderson 2002)
Functional Auditory Performance Indicators (FAPI; Stredler-Brown & Johnson 2003)
Infant-Toddler Meaningful Auditory Integration Scale (IT-MAIS; Zimmerman-Phillips, Robbins, & Osberger 2000)[b]
Early Listening Function (ELF; Anderson 2002)
25 to 60 months
Screening Instrument for Targeting Educational Risk in Preschool Children (Preschool SIFTER; Anderson & Matkin 1993)[c]
Meaningful Auditory Integration Scale (MAIS; Robbins, Renshaw, & Berry 1991)[b]

[a] For ages ≥ 36 months.
[b] For those with severe to profound hearing loss.
[c] For those with minimal and mild hearing losses.

To obtain frequency-specific information about the infant's audiometric configuration separately for each ear, air-conduction testing using insert receivers (whenever possible) is done by tone burst ABR and/ or ASSR at frequencies of at least 500 and 2000 Hz. Bone-conduction testing is also done if the air-conduction thresholds are elevated (worse than normal). Comparing the physiological thresholds for air-conduction and bone-conduction permits us to determine whether there is an air-bone-gap, and hence identify the type of hearing loss. Auditory brainstem response testing with clicks is used to assess auditory nerve integrity. In fact, the JCIH (2007) position statement specifies that click-evoked ABRs must be done whenever an infant has no response with tone burst ABR testing.

During the neonatal period, acoustic immittance and otoacoustic emissions are used to augment and corroborate the ABR/ASSR findings. Recall from Chapter 7 that low-frequency probe tones are problematic during the neonatal period; hence, immittance assessment during this period should be done with higher probe tone frequencies (i.e., 660/678 Hz or 1000 Hz). Otoacoustic emissions provide complementary information because they reflect preneural cochlear integrity.

Five to 24 Months

The audiological evaluation approach changes from physiological testing to a behavioral focus when the child is approximately 5 or 6 months old. At this stage, the infant's neuromotor development has matured to the extent that visual reinforcement audiometry is feasible. Hence, audiological evaluations for infants in the 5 to 24 months corrected age range concentrate on behavioral methods combined with acoustic immittance tests. According to the ASHA (2004) guidelines, ABR and OAE testing are now reserved for cases in which the behavioral results are questionable or inadequate, or when there are reasons to question the integrity of the lower auditory pathways. However, the JCIH (2007) recommends including OAEs in the regular audiological evaluation of 6- to 36-month-olds.

The behavioral testing battery recommended by ASHA (2004) involves visual reinforcement audiometry to find minimum response levels in the 500 to 4000 Hz range and for speech signals. It is desirable to obtain results for each ear using insert receivers, if possible, although sound field testing may be necessary. An attempt should be made to obtain bone-conduction thresholds if the air-conduction thresholds are elevated, but the limitations of unmasked bone-conduction thresholds should be kept in mind. An

estimate of speech recognition ability should be made as early as possible, albeit informally, within the constraints imposed by the infant's language abilities.

Acoustic immittance testing is now done using a low-frequency (i.e., 226 Hz) probe tone for tympanometry and acoustic reflex testing. The ASHA protocol recommends ipsilateral acoustic reflex thresholds at 500, 1000, and 2000 Hz, with contralateral reflex testing added "if there is a question of neural pathology" (ASHA 2004, p. 11). The AAA protocol also includes ipsilateral reflexes and points out that adding the "contralateral reflex is useful for assessment of auditory pathway integrity" (AAA 2012, p. 24). The author prefers both ipsilateral and contralateral reflex testing whenever possible because their combined use provides useful diagnostic information (see Chapter 7).

Twenty-Five to 60 Months

The audiological evaluation of children in the 25 to 60 months age range is principally composed of behavioral methods combined with acoustic immittance tests. The indications and testing protocols for physiological measures are the same as they were for 5- to 24-month-olds. The type of behavioral testing used during this period depends on the developmental and other individual characteristics of the child, and may involve VRA, TROCA, VROCA, conditioned play audiometry, and even conventional testing methods. Thus, the audiologist must take the time to interact with the child, not only to establish a sense of rapport but also to estimate the child's developmental level and ability to perform the tasks involved with each of the behavioral approaches being considered.

The findings of Thompson, Thompson, and Vethivelu, (1989) are very instructive in this context. They compared the performance of 2-year-olds using visual reinforcement audiometry, VROCA, and play audiometry. All of the children could be conditioned to respond for VRA, compared with 83% for VROCA and only 68% for play audiometry. However, among the 2-year-olds who could be conditioned, the average number of responses given before habituation was highest (28.3) for play audiometry and smallest (11.4) for VRA, with VROCA occupying the position between them.

Regardless of the methodology used, or whether the testing can be completed within a single session or must be spread over several visits, the goal is to obtain an audiological picture of the child that is as complete as possible. As before, we hope to obtain air-conduction thresholds for each ear between at least 500 and 4000 Hz, bone-conduction thresholds where the air-conduction thresholds are elevated, and acoustic immittance measurements.

Speech audiometry for children in this age range should include a measure of the threshold for speech, usually with a closed-set approach such as pointing to the named picture or object, or by repeating the words. Whenever possible, speech recognition scores should be obtained using an age-appropriate standardized test, such as the WIPI (Ross & Lerman 1971), NU-CHIPS (Elliott & Katz 1980), and the PSI (Jerger & Jerger 1984). If standardized tests are not appropriate for a child, then her speech recognition ability should be assessed informally. However, the results of informal testing should be expressed in the form of a descriptive statement about the child's speech recognition performance instead of using a percentage score.

Six Years and Beyond

Children become candidates for more standard audiometric testing procedures (Chapter 5) somewhere in the vicinity of 5 or 6 years old. However, just because a child can perform the task does not mean she will be a self-motivated responder. If anything, this is a period when the audiologist must provide the child with encouragement, direction, and praise to keep the child "on task." Open-set speech recognition testing using a vocabulary within the child's range, such as the PBK-50 (Haskins 1949), can also be used around this time. Otherwise, normal children are responding in an almost adult-like manner by roughly 10 to 12 years old, and standard speech recognition tests (Chapter 8) can be used provided the material is within the child's receptive vocabulary.

■ Study Questions

1. Define behavior observation audiometry.
2. Describe some commonly encountered reflexive responses to sound during the first months of life.
3. Define and describe visual reinforcement audiometry.
4. Define and describe conditioned play audiometry.
5. Describe the preferred approach for the audiological assessment of infants during the first several months of life.
6. Describe the preferred approach for the audiological assessment of infants between approximately 5 and 24 months of age.
7. Describe the preferred approach for the audiological assessment of infants between approximately 2 and 5 years of age.
8. How does the approach for measuring speech thresholds change as young children develop?
9. Describe the considerations involved in assessing speech recognition in young children.
10. Describe two speech recognition tests commonly used with young children.

References

American Academy of Audiology (AAA). 2012. Audiologic Guidelines for the Assessment of Hearing in Infants and Young Children. Available at: http://www.audiology.org/resources/documentlibrary/Pages/Pediatric-Diagnostics.aspx

American Speech-Language-Hearing Association (ASHA). Guidelines for determining threshold level for speech. ASHA 1988;30(3):85–89

American Speech-Language-Hearing Association (ASHA). 2004. Guidelines for the Audiologic Assessment of Children from Birth to 5 Years of Age. Rockville Pike, MD: ASHA

Anderson KL. 2002. Early Listening Function: Discovery Tool for Parents and Caregivers of Infants and Toddlers (available from: www.phonak.com).

Anderson KL, Matkin N. 1993. Screening Instrument for Targeting Educational Risk in Preschool Children, Age 3–Kindergarten (Preschool SIFTER). Tampa, FL: Educational Audiology Association

Bench J, Kowal A, Bamford J. The BKB (Bamford-Kowal-Bench) sentence lists for partially-hearing children. Br J Audiol 1979;13(3):108–112

Bernstein RS, Gravel JS. A method for determining hearing sensitivity in infants: the interweaving staircase procedure (ISP). J Am Acad Audiol 1990;1(3):138–145

Boothroyd A. Developments in speech audiometry. Sound 1968;2:3–10

Boothroyd A. Developmental factors in speech recognition. Int Audiol 1970;9:30–38

Boothroyd A. Auditory perception of speech contrasts by subjects with sensorineural hearing loss. J Speech Hear Res 1984;27(1):134–144

Boothroyd A. Perception of speech pattern contrasts from auditory presentation of voice fundamental frequency. Ear Hear 1988;9(6):313–321

Boothroyd A. 1991. Speech perception measures and their role in the evaluation of hearing aid performance in a pediatric population. In: Feigin J, Stelmachowicz P, eds. Pediatric Amplification. Omaha, NE: Boys Town National Research Hospital; 78–91

Boothroyd A, Hanin L, Yeung E, Chen Q. 1992. Video-game for speech perception testing and training of young hearing-impaired children. Proceedings of the Johns Hopkins National Search for Computing Applications to Assist Persons with Disabilities, Laurel, MD; 25–28

Boothroyd A, Hanin L, Yeung E, Eran O. 1996. Speech perception and production in hearing-impaired children. In: Bess FH, Gravel JS, Tharpe AM, eds. Amplification for Children with Auditory Deficits. Nashville, TN: Billy Wilkerson Center Press; 55–74

Boothroyd A, Nittrouer S. Mathematical treatment of context effects in phoneme and word recognition. J Acoust Soc Am 1988;84(1):101–114

Boothroyd A, Springer N, Smith L, Schulman J. Amplitude compression and profound hearing loss. J Speech Hear Res 1988;31(3):362–376

Bradford LJ. 1975. Respiration audiometry. In: Bradford LJ, ed. Physiological Measures of the Audio-Vestibular System. New York, NY: Academic Press; 249–317

Byers VW, Bristow DC. Audiological evaluation of nonspeaking, physically challenged populations. Ear Hear 1990;11(5):382–386

Coplan J, Gleason JR. Test-retest and inter-observer reliability of the Early Language Milestone Scale, Second Ed. J Ped Health Care 1993;7:212–219

Culpepper B, Thompson G. Effects of reinforcer duration on the response behavior of preterm 2-year-olds in visual reinforcement audiometry. Ear Hear 1994;15(2): 161–167

Dawson PW, Nott PE, Clark GM, Cowan RSC. A modification of play audiometry to assess speech discrimination ability in severe–profoundly deaf 2- to 4-year-old children. Ear Hear 1998;19(5):371–384

Day J, Green R, Munro K, et al. 2008. Visual reinforcement audiometry testing of infants: A recommended test protocol, Version 2.0. Newborn Health Screening Program, National Health Service (England). Available online at http://hearing.screening.nhs.uk/audiologyprotocols

Diefendorf AO, Gravel JS. 1996. Behavioral observation and visual reinforcement audiometry. In: Gerber S, ed. Handbook of Pediatric Audiology. Washington, DC: Gallaudet University Press; 55–83

Dimitrijevic A, John MS, Van Roon P, et al. Estimating the audiogram using multiple auditory steady-state responses. J Am Acad Audiol 2002;13(4):205–224

Eilers RE, Miskiel E, Ozdamar O, Urbano R, Widen JE. Optimization of automated hearing test algorithms: simulations using an infant response model. Ear Hear 1991;12(3):191–198

Eilers RE, Widen JE, Urbano R, Hudson T, Gonzales L. Optimization of automated hearing test algorithms: a comparison of data from simulations and young children. Ear Hear 1991;12(3):199–204

Eilers RE, Wilson WR, Moore JM. Developmental changes in speech discrimination in infants. J Speech Hear Res 1977;20(4):766–780

Eisenberg RB. 1975. Cardiotachometry. In: Bradford LJ, ed. Physiological Measures of the Audio-Vestibular System. New York, NY: Academic Press; 319–347

Elliott L, Katz D. 1980. Northwestern University Children's Perception Speech (NU-CHIPS). St. Louis, MO: Auditec

Erber NP. Use of the auditory numbers test to evaluate speech perception abilities of hearing-impaired children. J Speech Hear Disord 1980;45(4):527–532

Erber NP. 1982. Auditory Training. Washington, DC: AG Bell Association for the Deaf

Erber NP, Alencewicz CM. Audiologic evaluation of deaf children. J Speech Hear Disord 1976;41(2):256–267

Finitzo-Hieber T, Matkin ND, Cherow-Skalka E, Gerling IJ. 1977. Sound Effects Recognition Test. St. Louis, MO: Auditec

Finitzo-Hieber T, Matkin ND, Cherow-Skalka E, Rice C. 1975. A preliminary investigation of a sound effects recognition test. Paper presented at American Speech and Hearing Association Convention, Washington, DC

Gans DP, Flexer C. Observer bias in the hearing testing of profoundly involved multiply handicapped children. Ear Hear 1982;3(6):309–313

Geers AE, Moog JS. 1989. Evaluating speech perception skills: tools for measuring benefits of cochlear implants, tactile aids and hearing aids. In: Owens E, Kessler D, eds. Cochlear Implants in Children. Boston, MA: College-Hill

Geers AE, Moog JS. Speech perception and production skills of students with impaired hearing from oral and total communication education settings. J Speech Hear Res 1992;35(6):1384–1393

Gravel JS. Behavioral assessment of auditory function. Semin Hear 1989;10:216–228

Gravel JS, Hood LJ. 1999. Pediatric audiologic assessment. In: Musiek FE, Rintelmann WF, eds. Contemporary Perspectives in Hearing Assessment. Needham Heights, MA: Allyn & Bacon; 305–326

Gravel JS, Kurtzberg D, Stapells D, Vaughan H, Wallace IF. Case studies. Semin Hear 1989;10:272–286

Gravel JS, Wallace IF. Effects of otitis media with effusion on hearing in the first 3 years of life. J Speech Lang Hear Res 2000;43(3):631–644

Hall JW. 2006. New Handbook for Auditory Evoked Responses. Boston, MA: Allyn & Bacon

Haskins HA. 1949. A phonetically balanced test of speech discrimination for children. Master's thesis, Northwestern University, Evanston, IL

Haug O, Baccaro P, Guilford FR. A pure-tone audiogram on the infant. The PIWI technique. Arch Otolaryngol 1967;86(4):435–440

Hicks CB, Tharpe AM, Ashmead DH. Behavioral auditory assessment of young infants: methodological limitations or natural lack of auditory responsiveness? Am J Audiol 2000;9(2):124–130

Jacobson JT, ed. 1985. The Auditory Brainstem Response. San Diego, CA: College-Hill

Jerger JF, Hayes D. The cross-check principle in pediatric audiometry. Arch Otolaryngol 1976;102(10): 614–620

Jerger S, Jerger J. 1984. Pediatric Speech Intelligibility Test—PSI. St. Louis, MO: Auditec

Jerger S, Jerger J, Lewis S. Pediatric speech intelligibility test. II. Effect of receptive language age and chronological age. Int J Pediatr Otorhinolaryngol 1981;3(2): 101–118

Jerger S, Lewis S, Hawkins J, Jerger J. Pediatric speech intelligibility test. I. Generation of test materials. Int J Pediatr Otorhinolaryngol 1980;2(3):217–230

Joint Committee on Infant Hearing (JCIH), American Academy of Pediatrics. Year 2007 position statement: Principles and guidelines for early hearing detection and intervention programs. Pediatrics 2007;120(4): 898–921

Kalikow DN, Stevens KN, Elliott LL. Development of a test of speech intelligibility in noise using sentence materials with controlled word predictability. J Acoust Soc Am 1977;61(5):1337–1351

Karzon RK, Banerjee P. Animated toys versus video reinforcement in 16–24-month-old children in a clinical setting. Am J Audiol 2010;19(2):91–99

Kirk KI. Assessing speech perception in listeners with cochlear implants: the development of the Lexical Neighborhood Test. Colta Rev 1999;100:63–85

Kirk KI, Eisenberg LS, Martinez AS, Hay-McCutcheon M. Lexical Neighborhood Test: test-retest reliability and interlist equivalency. J Am Acad Audiol 1999; 10:113–123

Kirk KI, Pisoni DB, Osberger MJ. Lexical effects on spoken word recognition by pediatric cochlear implant users. Ear Hear 1995;16(5):470–481

Lidén G, Kankkunen A. Visual reinforcement audiometry. Arch Otolaryngol 1969;89(6):865–872

Linder TW. 1990. Transdisciplinary Play-Based Assessment: A Functional Approach to Working with Young Children. Baltimore, MD: Brooks

Ling D. 1976. Speech for the Deaf Child. Washington, DC: AG Bell Association for the Deaf

Ling D. 1989. Foundations of Spoken Language for Hearing-Impaired Children. Washington, DC: AG Bell Association for the Deaf

Ling D, Ling AH. 1978. Aural Habilitation. Washington, DC: AG Bell Association for the Deaf

Ling D, Ling AH, Doehring DG. Stimulus, response, and observer variables in the auditory screening of newborn infants. J Speech Hear Res 1970;13(1):9–18

Lloyd LL, Spradlin JE, Reid MJ. An operant audiometric procedure for difficult-to-test patients. J Speech Hear Disord 1968;33(3):236–245

Logan, JS. 1992. A Computational Analysis of Young Children's Lexicons (Speech Research Laboratory Technical report No. 8). Bloomington, IN: Indiana University. Available as http://www.iu.edu/~srlweb/pr/Technical_Report_8_A_Computational_Analysis_of_Young_Childrens_Lexicons.pdf

Lowery KJ, von Hapsburg D, Plyler EL, Johnstone P. A comparison of video versus conventional visual reinforcement in 7- to 16-month-old infants. J Speech Lang Hear Res 2009;52(3):723–731

MacWhinney B, Snow C. The child language data exchange system. J Child Lang 1985;12(2):271–295

Matkin N. 1977. Assessment of hearing sensitivity during the preschool years. In: Bess F, ed. Childhood Deafness. New York, NY: Grune & Stratton; 127–134

Meadow-Orlans KP. 1983. Meadow-Kendal Social-Emotional Assessment Inventories for Deaf and Hearing Impaired Students. Washington, DC: Gallaudet University

Menary S, Trehub SE, McNutt J. Speech discrimination in preschool children: a comparison of two tasks. J Speech Hear Res 1982;25(2):202–207

Merer DM, Gravel JS. Screening infants and young children for hearing loss: examination of the CAST procedure. J Am Acad Audiol 1997;8(4):233–242

Meyer TA, Pisoni DB. Some computational analyses of the PBK test: effects of frequency and lexical density on spoken word recognition. Ear Hear 1999;20(4): 363–371

Moog JS, Geers AE. 1990. Early Speech Perception Test. St. Louis, MO: Central Institute for the Deaf Publications

Moore JM, Thompson G, Folsom RC. Auditory responsiveness of premature infants utilizing visual reinforcement audiometry (VRA). Ear Hear 1992;13(3):187–194

Moore JM, Thompson G, Thompson M. Auditory localization of infants as a function of reinforcement conditions. J Speech Hear Disord 1975;40(1):29–34

Moore JM, Wilson WR, Thompson G. Visual reinforcement of head-turn responses in infants under 12 months of age. J Speech Hear Disord 1977;42(3):328–334

Nelson NW. 1993. Childhood Language Disorders in Context: Infancy through Adolescence. New York, NY: Merrill

Nielsen SE, Olsen SØ. Validation of play-conditioned audiometry in a clinical setting. Scand Audiol 1997; 26(3):187–191

Nilsson MJ, Soli SD, Gelnett D. 1996. Development of the Hearing in Noise Test for Children. Los Angeles, CA: House Ear Institute

Northern JL, Downs MP. 1991. Hearing in Children, 4th ed. Baltimore, MD: Williams & Wilkins

Olsen WO, Matkin ND. 1991. Speech audiometry. In: Rintelmann WF, ed. Hearing Assessment, 2nd ed. Austin, TX: Pro-Ed; 39–140

Picton TW. 2007. Audiometry using auditory steady-state responses. In: Burkhard RF, Don, M, Eggermont JJ, eds. Auditory Evoked Potentials: Basic Principles and Clinical Applications. Philadelphia, PA: Lippincott Williams & Wilkins; 441–462

Primus MA, Thompson G. Response strength of young children in operant audiometry. J Speech Hear Res 1985;28(4):539–547

Rance G, Tomlin D, Rickards FW. Comparison of auditory steady-state responses and tone-burst auditory brainstem responses in normal babies. Ear Hear 2006; 27(6):751–762

Robbins AM, Kirk KI. Speech perception assessment performance in pediatric cochlear implant users. Semin Hear 1996;17:353–369

Robbins AM, Renshaw JJ, Berry SW. Evaluating meaningful auditory integration in profoundly hearing-impaired children. Am J Otol 1991;12(Suppl):144–150

Ross M, Lerman J. A picture identification test for hearing-impaired children. J Speech Hear Res 1970;13(1): 44–53

Ross M, Lerman J. 1971. Word Intelligibility by Picture Identification (WIPI). St. Louis, MO: Auditec

Ross M, Randolf K. 1988. Auditory Perception of Alphabet Letters Test (APAL). St. Louis, MO: Auditec

Schmida MJ, Peterson HJ, Tharpe AM. Visual reinforcement audiometry using digital video disc and conventional reinforcers. Am J Audiol 2003;12(1):35–40

Scollie S, Glista D, Tenhaaf J, et al. Stimuli and normative data for detection of Ling-6 sounds in hearing level. Am J Audiol 2012;21(2):232–241

Shimizu H. Childhood hearing impairment: issues and thoughts on diagnostic approaches. AAS Bull 1992; 17:15–37

Sininger YS. 2007. The use of auditory brainstem response in screening for hearing loss and audiometric threshold prediction. In: Burkhard RF, Don, M, Eggermont JJ, eds. Auditory Evoked Potentials: Basic Principles and Clinical Applications. Philadelphia, PA: Lippincott Williams & Wilkins; 254–274

Spahr AJ, Dorman MF, Litvak LM, et al. Development and validation of the AzBio sentence lists. Ear Hear 2012;33(1):112–117

Spahr AJ, Dorman MF, Litvak LM, et al. Development and validation of the pediatric AzBio sentence lists. Ear Hear 2014;35(4):418–422

Stach BA, Wolf SJ, Bland L. Otoacoustic emissions as a cross-check in pediatric hearing assessment: case report. J Am Acad Audiol 1993;4(6):392–398

Stapells DR. The tone-evoked ABR: why it's the measure of choice for young infants. Hear J 2002;55(11):14–18

Stredler-Brown A, Johnson DC. 2003. Functional auditory performance indicators: an integrated approach to auditory development (available from www.cde.state.co.us/cdesped/SpecificDisability-Hearing.htm)

Suzuki T, Obiga Y. Conditioned orientation audiometry. Arch Otolaryngol 1961;74:192–198

Tharpe AM, Ashmead DH. Computer simulation technique for assessing pediatric auditory test protocols. J Am Acad Audiol 1993;4(2):80–90

Thompson G, Thompson M, McCall A. Strategies for increasing response behavior of 1- and 2-year-old children during visual reinforcement audiometry (VRA). Ear Hear 1992;13(4):236–240

Thompson G, Weber BA. Responses of infants and young children to behavior observation audiometry (BOA). J Speech Hear Disord 1974;39(2):140–147

Thompson M, Thompson G, Vethivelu S. A comparison of audiometric test methods for 2-year-old children. J Speech Hear Disord 1989;54(2):174–179

Ventry IM. 1975. Conditioned galvanic skin response audiometry. In: Bradford LJ, ed. Physiological Measures of the Audio-Vestibular System. New York, NY: Academic Press; 215–247

Weber S, Redell RC. A sentence test for measuring speech discrimination in children. Audiol Hear Educ 1976;2:25–30

Widen JE. Adding objectivity to infant behavioral audiometry. Ear Hear 1993;14(1):49–57

Widen JE, Folsom RC, Cone-Wesson B, et al. Identification of neonatal hearing impairment: hearing status at 8 to 12 months corrected age using a visual reinforcement audiometry protocol. Ear Hear 2000;21(5):471–487

Widen JE, Johnson JL, White KR, et al. A multisite study to examine the efficacy of the otoacoustic emission/automated auditory brainstem response newborn hearing screening protocol: results of visual reinforcement audiometry. Am J Audiol 2005;14(2):S200–S216

Wilson WR, Thompson G. 1984. Behavioral audiometry. In: Jerger J, ed. Pediatric Audiology. San Diego, CA: College-Hill; 1–44

Zimmerman-Phillips S, Robbins AM, Osberger MJ. Assessing cochlear implant benefit in very young children. Ann Otol Rhinol Laryngol Suppl 2000;185(Suppl 185): 42–43

13 Audiological Screening

■ Screening Principles

Screening programs are used to identify those individuals who have a particular disorder or group of disorders. Screening is warranted when a disorder has appreciable adverse effects on those who have it, and if it can be treated once it has been identified. In addition, the problem should be reasonably widespread in its occurrence, and there must be a test for it that is quick, reliable, and acceptable to those who receive it. These criteria are undeniably met by hearing impairments, disorders, and disabilities, which may be defined as follows (ASHA 1997).[1] A **disorder** is an anatomical *abnormality* (e.g., an ear deformity) or a *pathology* (e.g., a middle ear infection). An **impairment** means that physiological and/or psychological *functioning* is lost or abnormal (e.g., a hearing loss). A **disability** occurs when a person's *ability to perform* is adversely affected (e.g., when a hearing loss impedes academic performance or social interactions). These areas are addressed by **audiological screening** programs (AAA 1997a,b; ASHA 1997; NIH 1993; Mauk & Behrens 1993; JCIH 2007). (The term **identification audiometry** is sometimes used to refer to screening for hearing impairment, and is often encountered in the older literature.)

Hearing screening programs must be supervised by a qualified audiologist, but it is generally agreed that cost-effective mass screening programs entail testing procedures that do not require an audiologist's expertise (NIH 1993; AAA 1997a,b; ASHA 1997; JCIH 2007). Thus, the goal is for the day-to-day screening activities to be performed by support personnel hired for this purpose, or by non-audiologist professionals who are in the right place at the right time to perform the tests.

Although we will not directly address financial factors in detail here, one must also be aware that the costs of personnel, instrumentation, space, etc., cannot be overlooked, and often play a central role in real-world decisions about screening programs. For these reasons, the clinician may be asked to provide such information as the cost of a screening program on a per-child basis. An example of a typical formula that might be used for this purpose (Copper, Gates, Owen, & Dickson 1975) is

$$\text{Cost per child} = \frac{S}{R} + \frac{C + (M\,L)}{(N\,L)}$$

Here, S is the hourly salary of the screening personnel, R is the rate of screening (children tested per hour), C is the cost of the equipment, M is the annual equipment maintenance cost, N is the number of children screened in a year, and L is the expected lifetime (in years) of the equipment.

The fundamental goal of a screening test is to identify the individuals in a population who have a specified disorder or group of disorders. People who actually have the targeted disorder are said to be "abnormal" and those who really do not have that disorder are "normal." It is important to remember that normality or abnormality here pertains only to the particular disorder(s) being screened. In a perfect screening test every abnormal person would fail and every normal case would pass. In spite of our best intentions, no screening test (or any test, for that matter) can separate all normal and abnormal individuals with complete accuracy. For this reason we must consider the screening process in terms of the percentages of correct and incorrect results. Complicating matters is the issue of what constitutes the "**gold standard**" used to determine the patient's "real status." This is often established by another test, which itself may not be perfect.

To understand the principles involved in assessing a screening test, let us make up a population to be

---

[1] For consistency, these terms as defined in the ASHA (1997) screening guidelines will be employed throughout this chapter.

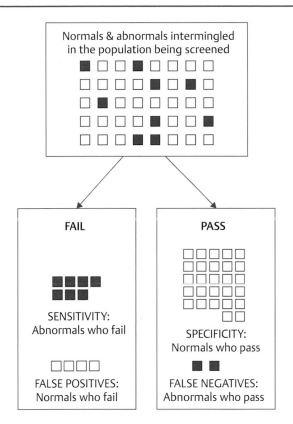

Fig. 13.1 The upper box represents a hypothetical population being screened for some disorder, and the two lower boxes represent those who pass and fail the screening test. Open squares represent people who are actually normal; filled squares are those who really have the disorder (see text).

screened for a particular disorder. It is represented by the upper box of **Fig. 13.1**, and includes 9 individuals who really have the disorder (filled squares) and who are intermingled with 31 people who are actually normal (open squares). This disorder has a **prevalence** of 22.5% because it occurs in 9 out of 40 people (9/40 = 0.225).

A person who *passes* a screening test is considered to be free of the problem, whereas one who *fails* is thought to have the problem. For example, a hearing screening test might involve listening for a tone. People who *can hear* the tone will *pass* the screening test, but those who *cannot hear* the tone will *fail*. Hence, on a perfect screening test, everyone who is really normal would pass and everyone who is really abnormal would fail. The results of our hypothetical screening test are represented by the two lower boxes in the figure, labeled "pass" and "fail." Notice that the screening test outcome is not perfect: 27 of the 31 normal people passed the screening, but 4 of them failed; and 7 of the 9 abnormal individuals failed, but 2 of them passed. Hence, even though screening tests seem to have two results (pass and fail), there are

really four possible outcomes from the standpoint of whether the pass and fail results are right or wrong.

The four possible outcomes of a screening test are often shown in the form of a matrix such as the one shown in **Fig. 13.2**. The two correct outcomes are called sensitivity and specificity. **Sensitivity** is the proportion of *abnormal* people who *fail* the screening test, and is also known as the **hit rate**. It is obtained by dividing the number of abnormals who fail by the total number of abnormals. The sensitivity of our hypothetical screening test is 7/9 = 0.78, or 78%. **Fig. 13.3** shows the sensitivity and other values obtained in our hypothetical example. **Specificity** is the proportion of *normal* individuals who *pass* the screening test. It is calculated by dividing the number of normals who pass by the total number of normal cases, which is 27/31 = 0.87, or 87%, in our example.

The two incorrect screening outcomes are false negatives and false positives. A **false-negative** result, or a **miss**, occurs when an *abnormal* person *passes* the screening test. In contrast, a **false-positive** result occurs when a *normal* person *fails*. Passing the screening test is a "negative" result because it implies the person does *not* have the problem, and failing the screening test is a "positive" result because it suggests the person *does* have the problem. The false-negative rate is the proportion of abnormal cases who pass the test, that is, the number of misses divided by the total number of abnormals. For our hypothetical data the false-negative rate is 2/9 = 0.22, or 22%. The false-positive rate is the proportion of normals who fail the screening test. It is obtained by dividing the number of false positives by the total number of normals, which is 4/31 = 0.13, or 13%.

In summary, sensitivity (or the hit rate) tells us how well the screening test correctly identifies peo-

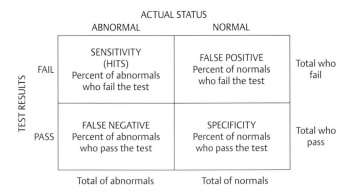

Fig. 13.2 The outcomes of screening tests are shown as a matrix that plots the test results (passes or failures) against the true condition of the patient (normal or abnormal).

Fig. 13.3   **(a)** Number of patients in each category from the screening test example in **Fig. 13.1**. **(b)** Sensitivity, specificity, false-positive, and false-negative rates for this example.

ple who have the problem, and specificity shows how well the test correctly identifies those who are normal. The false-negative (miss) and false-positive rates are the errors associated with sensitivity and specificity, respectively. The goal is to have a screening test with both good sensitivity and good specificity. Even a very sensitive screening test would be useless if it is also failed by too many people who are normal, and a test with great specificity would be useless if it is also passed by too many people who are abnormal.

■ Prevalence of Hearing Impairment

Newborns The need for hearing screening in infants and children becomes clear when we consider the high prevalence of hearing loss, the impact of hearing impairment, and the importance of early intervention. Prevalence estimates for infant hearing loss from the 1990s ranged from about 1 to 6 per 1000 births depending on the degree of loss and whether one or two ears were involved, rising to ~ 2 to 4% among at-risk babies like those in the neonatal intensive care unit (NICU; e.g., Mauk & Behrens 1993; Stein 1999). More recent findings place the prevalence of infants in the United States with diagnosed hearing loss among those who were screened during 2011 at 1.5 per 1000 (CDC 2013).

Children and adolescents Estimates of the prevalence of hearing loss among children, adoles-

cents, and young adults have varied widely between roughly 3 and 33%, depending on how "hearing loss" is defined and a host of differences in methodology, sampling, and how confounding influences were addressed (e.g., Sarff 1981; Axelsson, Aniansson, & Costa 1987; Lundeen 1991; Montgomery & Fujikawa 1992; Bess, Dodd-Murphy, & Parker 1998; Niskar et al 1998; Augustsson & Engstrand 2006; Rabinowitz, Slade, Galusha, Dixon-Ernst, & Cullen 2006; Henderson, Testa, & Hartnick 2011; Schlauch & Carney 2011, 2012; Schlauch 2013).

An analysis of the 1988–1994 National Health and Nutrition Examination Survey (NHANES)[2] by Niskar et al (1998) and a large-sample study by Bess et al (1998) suggested that the overall prevalence among American school children is ~ 11 to 15%. Niskar et al (1998) categorized losses as slight, mild/moderate, and severe/profound based on a low-frequency average (500, 1000, 2000 Hz) and a high-frequency average (3000, 4000, 6000 Hz). Bess et al (1998) distinguished between *minimal sensorineural hearing losses* and other types and degrees of hearing loss (**Table 13.1**). Niskar et al (1998) found that *slight losses* (16–25 dB HL) are more prevalent than greater degrees of hearing loss (**Fig. 13.4**); and Bess et al (1998) found a prevalence of 5.4% for various types of

[2] The NHANESs are available on line from the Centers for Disease Control and Prevention at http://www.cdc.gov/nchs/nhanes.htm.

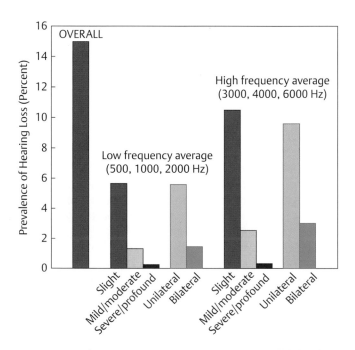

Fig. 13.4   Prevalence of average hearing losses of ³16 dB HL for low frequencies (500, 1000, and 2000 Hz) and high frequencies (3000, 4000, and 6000 Hz) among 6166 children between 6 and 19 years old. (Based on Niskar et al [1998]).

Table 13.1 Characteristics of minimal and other hearing loss categories used in **Fig. 13.5**[a]

Minimal sensorineural hearing loss (SNHL) categories[b]

Bilateral minimal SNHL	• 500–2000 Hz pure tone-average (PTA) 20–40 dB HL in both ears
Unilateral minimal SNHL	• 500–2000 Hz PTA ≥ 20–40 dB HL in poorer ear • 500–2000 Hz PTA ≤ 15 dB HL in better ear
High-frequency SNHL	• ≥ 2 thresholds ≥ 25 dB HL among 3000, 4000, 6000, and 8000 Hz • One or both ears

Other hearing loss categories[c]

Conductive hearing loss	• Average air conduction thresholds ≥ 25 Hz • Average air-bone-gap ≥ 10 dB HL • Type B tympanogram • One or both ears
Other hearing loss	• Hearing losses not falling into the other groups (e.g., greater than minimal sensorineural losses, mixed losses)

[a]As defined by Bess, Dodd-Murphy, and Parker (1998).
[b]Normal hearing defined as average thresholds ≤ 15 dB HL in both ears and no more than one threshold > 25 dB HL in either ear.
[c]Combined in **Fig. 13.5**.

minimal sensorineural hearing loss and 5.9% for other categories of hearing loss **(Fig. 13.5)**. In addition, both studies also found high-frequency hearing losses among school-age children, although there were different prevalence rates at 3% by Bess et al (1998) and 12.7% by Niskar et al (1998).[3]

A comparison of the 1988–1994 and 2005–2006 NHANES results by Shargorodsky, Curhan, Curhan, & Eavey (2010) revealed that the prevalence of hearing loss among American 12- to 19-year-olds between these two time periods rose from 14.9 to 19.5% for losses that were > 16 dB HL (slight or worse) and from 3.5 to 5.3% for losses ≥ 25 dB HL (mild or worse). Of particular importance is that the increase was more common and statistically significant for the *high* frequencies (12.8 to 16.4%), but less common and not significant for the *low* frequencies (6.1 to 9.0%). Since noise exposure is associated with high-frequency hearing loss (see Chapter 17), one compelling implication of this increase is that the impact of excessive noise exposure is growing among adolescents.

It is no surprise that the findings just described precipitated a considerable amount of media attention.[4] However, subsequent analyses of the same survey data indicated that the prevalence of high-frequency hearing loss among American adolescents

Fig. 13.5 Prevalence of hearing losses among 1218 children in the third, sixth, and ninth grades according to the categories defined in **Table 13.1**. (Based on Bess, Dodd-Murphy, & Parker [1998].)

[3] Let's use this difference as an opportunity to illustrate why it is important to pay attention to how terms are defined and how subjects are placed into groups. The Niskar et al (1998) prevalence figures for high-frequency losses are close to those for older children and teenagers by Axelsson, Aniansson, & Costa (1987) and by Montgomery and Fujikawa (1992). However, those studies found prevalence rates of ~ 6% for 7-year-olds and second graders, whereas Niskar et al found similar percentages for 6- to 11-year-olds (12.2%) and 12- to 19-year-olds (13%). The Niskar et al 6–11-year-old age range included 7-year-olds (who had a lower prevalence in the earlier studies) and 10-year-olds (who had a high prevalence rate). Also, Bess et al (1998) commented that their prevalence rates were similar to or higher than the ones by Axelsson et al and by Montgomery and Fujikawa when they recalculated their data using the definitions of high-frequency loss from those studies. Thus, some of the discrepancies may be related to differences in how high-frequency hearing loss was defined and possibly to how the children were grouped by age. See Schlauch and Carney (2011, 2012) for additional information about confounding influences in hearing surveys and how they affect hearing loss prevalence rates.

[4] For example, a *Washington Post* headline read, "Study shows sharp increase in hearing loss among U.S. teens, especially boys" (available at http://www.washingtonpost.com/wp-dyn/content/article/2010/08/17/AR2010081705861.html). The headline points out that the analysis by Shargorodsky et al (2010) revealed a larger increase in high-frequency loss for boys. Ironically, even though the analysis by Henderson et al (2011) showed no prevalence increase overall, it did reveal a prevalence increase for girls.

actually did not increase between the 1988–1994 and 2005–2006 surveys (Henderson et al 2011; Schlauch & Carney 2012). The analysis by Schlauch and Carney (2012; see also Schlauch 2013) is of particular interest because it excluded cases with any evidence of outer or middle ear disorders, and accounted for other confounds such as hearing losses involving both the low and high frequencies as opposed to just the highs. The resulting analysis revealed that the prevalence of high-frequency losses for teenagers in the 2005–2006 survey was only 7.4 to 7.9% (depending on whether 8000 Hz was included in the average), which is, of course, much more optimistic than the 12.8 to 16.4% rates calculated in the other studies (Niskar et al 1998; Shargorodsky et al 2010). In a similar vein, the prevalence of high-frequency hearing loss did not increase for 18-year-old Swedish males tested during 1969–1977 compared with those tested in 1998 (Augustsson & Engstrand 2006), or for American 17- to 25-year-olds tested between 1985 and 2004 (Rabinowitz et al 2006). This does not mean that the prevalence of high-frequency hearing loss will remain steady into the future, particularly in light of what appear to be increasing opportunities for environmental, recreational, and workplace noise exposure (see Chapter 17). On the contrary, hearing loss prevalence throughout childhood and adolescence certainly bears monitoring over time.

Adults The prevalence of hearing impairments among adults increases with age from roughly 5% among young adults to over 40% among the elderly. **Fig. 13.6** illustrates this trend in terms of both self-

identified hearing difficulty (Pleis, Lucas, & Ward 2009), as well as better-ear thresholds exceeding 25 dB HL for the frequencies between 500 and 4000 Hz (Mitchell, Gopinath, Wang, et al 2011).

It is heartening to note, however, that comparing the NHANES results obtained over the years shows that the hearing status of American adults appears to be better now than it was in the past. In particular, the overall prevalence of hearing loss (≥ 25 dB HL) among 25- to 69-year-old adults without diabetes fell from 27.9% during 1971–1973 to 19.1% during 1999–2004 (Cheng et al 2009); and adults' median thresholds were better in 1999–2004 than they were in 1959–1962 (Hoffman, Dobie, Ko, Themann, & Murphy 2010).

■ Audiological Screening in Infants and Children

Prevalence rates like those just described make it clear that we need a strategy to identify hearing-impaired infants as early as possible and to continue screening efforts in children through the school years.

The adverse impact of hearing impairment on speech and language, literacy and academic performance, and psychosocial factors is substantial and well established (see, e.g., AAA 1997a,b; ASHA 1997; JCIH 2007; Tye-Murray 2009). Even children with minimal sensorineural hearing loss and unilateral hearing loss experience educational and psychosocial difficulties (e.g., Bess et al 1998). The key to mitigating these effects lies in early identification leading to early intervention. Particularly impressive is the finding of significantly better language skills among hearing-impaired children who were identified by the time they were 6 months old compared with those who were identified later than this (Yoshinaga-Itano, Sedey, Coulter, & Mehl 1998).

■ Newborn Hearing Screening

Early hearing detection and intervention (EHDI) refers to the systematic identification of babies with hearing loss and the provision to them of comprehensive habilitative approaches as early as possible. It has been endorsed by major professional organizations, state and federal legislation, and international groups, and is the subject of extensive clinical and research efforts.[5] **Universal newborn hearing screening (UNHS)** by 1 month of age, diagnosis by 3 months, and commencement of an intervention program by 6 months (the "1-3-6 rule") is viewed as the goal throughout the United States (e.g., White, Vohr, Meyer, et al 2005; JCIH 2007). In fact, 98.4% of babies

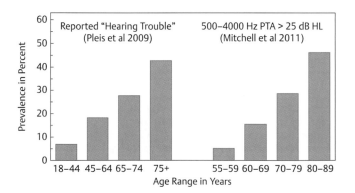

Fig. 13.6 Estimated prevalence of hearing impairments through the adult years based on those reporting "hearing trouble" in the U.S. National Health Interview Survey (left panel; Pleis et al 2009), and those in the Australian Blue Mountains Hearing Study with pure tone averages for 500, 1000, 2000, and 4000 Hz greater than 25 dB HL in the better ear (right panel; Mitchell et al [2011]).

born in the United States[6] were screened for hearing loss in 2011, with 94.9% being screened by 1 month of age (CDC 2013).

A variety of approaches and techniques for identifying hearing loss in infants have been used over the years. In the broadest terms, these include (a) public awareness campaigns, (b) high-risk registers, and (c) screening programs employing behavioral and/or physiological tests, often combined with the use of risk indicators.

Public Awareness Campaigns

The public awareness approach uses such methods as mass media campaigns, brochures, and checklists to educate the public about the danger signs of hearing loss in children. The idea is to make parents and other caregivers aware of the problem and able to identify it so they can refer the child for diagnosis and treatment. Although public awareness campaigns are a valuable adjunct to hearing loss identification in general, they are not effective by themselves because there is great uncertainty about who actually receives and responds to these efforts, and concerns that many primary care health providers might tend to discount parental suspicions (Elssmann, Matkin, & Sabo 1987; Mauk, White, Mortensen, & Behrens 1991).

High-Risk Registers

Another approach that has been used in the early identification of hearing-impaired babies involves determining whether the child meets any of several criteria associated with hearing loss. Infants identified by this **high-risk register** are then referred for evaluation and their cases are followed over time. **Table 13.2** summarizes a contemporary list of **risk indicators** (JCIH 2007), although they are actually part of a comprehensive early identification program as opposed to being a stand-alone high-risk register. Hearing loss identification programs based on high-

Table 13.2 Risk indicators for congenital, progressive, and delayed-onset hearing loss based on the JCIH (2007) position statement

Familial history of permanent hearing loss in childhood (delayed-onset risk)

Prenatal infections, especially
- Cytomegalovirus (delayed-onset risk)
- Herpes
- Rubella
- Toxoplasmosis
- Herpes
- Syphilis

Craniofacial anomalies (e.g., anomalies of pinna, external auditory meatus, temporal bone, ear pits and/or tags)

Syndromes involving congenital hearing loss, delayed-onset or progressive hearing loss (delayed-onset risk) *Examples:* Alport syndrome, Jervell syndrome, Lange-Nielsen syndrome, neurofibromatosis, osteopetrosis, Pendred syndrome, Usher syndrome, Waardenburg syndrome

Physical characteristics associated with syndromes involving sensorineural (e.g., white forelock) or permanent conductive hearing loss

Neonatal intensive care exceeding 5 days

Neonatal intensive care of any duration involving
- Extracorporeal membrane oxygenation (delayed-onset risk)
- Assisted ventilation
- Hyperbilirubinemia with exchange transfusion
- Ototoxic drugs (e.g., gentimycin, tobramycin, loop diuretics)

Neurodegenerative disorders (delayed-onset risk) *Examples:* Charcot-Marie-Tooth syndrome, Friedreich ataxia, Hunter syndrome

Postnatal infections associated with sensorineural hearing loss (delayed-onset risk)
- Bacterial meningitis
- Viral meningitis (especially herpes, varicella)

Chemotherapy (delayed-onset risk)

Head trauma, especially fracture of temporal bone/skull base (delayed-onset risk)

Caregiver concerns (delayed-onset risk) about
- Hearing
- Speech
- Language
- Developmental delay

---

[5] The interested student will find up-to-date information, reference material, internet links, etc., pertaining to all aspects of newborn screening and related matters at web sites like the ones maintained by the Centers for Disease Control and Prevention (www.cdc.gov/nceh/programs/CDDH/ehdi.htm), American Speech-Language-Hearing Association (www.asha.org), American Academy of Audiology (www.audiolog.org), Joint Committee on Infant Hearing (www.jcih.org), and the National Center for Hearing Assessment and Management (www.infanthearing.org).

[6] Excluding infant deaths and cases in which the parents refused to allow the screening.

risk registers are relatively inexpensive to administer, but they were found to be subject to significant problems (e.g., Pappas 1983; Elssmann, Matkin, & Sabo 1987; Mauk et al 1991; NIH 1993): There were difficulties involved in gathering the needed information. For example, the information used to decide whether a baby should be placed on the high-risk register was usually based on birth certificate information or maternal questionnaires. Moreover, it has been shown that high-risk registers miss about half of all hearing-impaired newborns, and many children have been lost to follow-up.

Screening Approaches

Behavioral Screening

Behavioral methods (e.g., Wedenberg 1956; Downs & Sterritt 1967) were used for infant hearing screening in the past. Recall from Chapter 12 that behavioral observation (or "behavior observation audiometry") involves presenting a stimulus to the child and watching for changes in behavior appropriate for her stage of development. With newborns, this involves determining whether rather intense stimuli (typically 60 dB SPL or more) evoke responses such as a startle reflex, an auropalpebral reflex, or arousal from sleep. Automated approaches were also used to identify behavioral responses to high-level stimuli, such as the *Crib-O-Gram* (Simmons & Russ 1974), which employed a crib fitted with motion detectors that monitored the infant's movements, and the *Neonatal Auditory Response Cradle* (Bennett 1975; Shepard 1983), which monitored respiratory changes as well as body movements.

Behavioral observation approaches are no longer used in neonatal screening because of several serious limitations (e.g., Northern & Gerkin 1989; Durieux-Smith & Jacobson 1985; Durieux-Smith, Picton, Edwards, Goodman, & MacMurray 1985; Shimizu et al 1990; Mauk & Behrens 1993). They involve subjective judgments that are highly susceptible to bias; there are considerable reliability problems as well as many false-positive and false-negative results; and the use of high-level stimuli presented from a loudspeaker, so that mild and moderate losses cannot be identified, and it is impossible to tell whether a response was due to hearing the sound in one or both ears. However, *conditioned* behavioral methods can be used with older infants and toddlers, as described below.

Physiological Screening

Physiological measures have become the standard means of testing in neonatal hearing screening programs. The principal techniques are the auditory brainstem response (ABR), the auditory steady-state responses (ASSR) and otoacoustic emissions (OAE) (e.g., NIH 1993; ASHA 1997; JCIH 2007; Gravel, White, Johnson, et al 2005; Johnson, White, Widen, et al 2005a,b; White et al 2005; Widen, Johnson, White, et al 2005); and auditory steady-state responses (ASSR) are also being used as an infant screening method (e.g., Savio, Perez-Abalo, Gaya, Hernandez, & Mijares 2006). In addition to good sensitivity and objectivity, the physiological methods can be used when the infant is sleeping, and permit us to screen each ear separately. These methods require more costly instrumentation than behavioral approaches, tend to be limited in their ability to detect low-frequency hearing losses, and reflect the integrity of the peripheral and lower auditory system rather than the notion of "hearing" that is inferred from a behavioral response.

The auditory brainstem response is well established as a neonatal hearing screening test and has impressive rates of sensitivity, specificity, and reliability (e.g., Mauk & Behrens 1993; Finitzo, Albright, & O'Neil 1998; Vohr, Carty, Moore, & Letourneau 1998; Norton, Gorga, Widen, et al 2000; Hall 2007; Sininger 2007). Successful screening outcomes have been found for both **transient-evoked otoacoustic emissions** (**TEOAEs**; e.g., Bonfils, Uziel, & Pujol 1988; Uziel & Piron 1991; Maxon, White, Behrens, & Vohr 1995; Prieve 1997; Thompson 1997; Finitzo et al 1998; Vohr et al 1998; Gravel, Berg, Bradley, et al 2000; Dalzell, Orlando, MacDonald, et al 2000; Norton et al 2000; Prieve, Dalzell, Berg, et al 2000; Prieve & Stevens 2000; Spivak, Dalzell, Berg, et al 2000) and **distortion product otoacoustic emissions** (**DPOAEs**; e.g., Bonfils, Avan, Francois, Trotoux, & Narcy 1992; Lafreniere, Smurzynski, Jung, Leonard, & Kim 1993; Brown, Sheppard, & Russell 1994; Bergman et al 1995; Norton et al 2000). The EOAE shares excellent sensitivity with the ABR for detecting hearing loss in infants, although its specificity may not be quite as high as that obtained with the auditory brainstem response. Moreover, the ABR can be used to screen for auditory neuropathy spectrum disorder, whereas the preneural nature of OAEs makes them inappropriate for this purpose (e.g., JCIH 2007). The use of OAEs as a screening tool has also been reported in preschoolers (Sideris & Glattke 2006; Eiserman et al 2007), school-age children (Nozza, Sabo, & Mandel 1997), and adults (Engdahl, Woxen, Arnesen, & Mair 1996; Scudder, Culbertson, Waldron, & Stewart 2003; Seixas et al 2005).

Universal newborn hearing screening becomes simpler, quicker, and more cost-efficient when *automated* auditory brainstem response (A-ABR) or otoacoustic emissions screening devices are used in place of clinical instrumentation. These instruments employ statistical criteria to determine if an acceptable response is present, leading to a "pass" versus "refer" recommendation instead of an ABR or OAE record that must be professionally interpreted. As a result, the routine aspects of carrying out the screening program do not require highly trained professionals to perform the tests. Thus, it is not surprising that automated ABR and/or OAE devices are widely used in neonatal screening programs (e.g., Jacobson, Jacobson, & Spahr 1990; Herrmann, Thornton, & Joseph 1995; Prieve 1997; Thompson 1997; Mason & Herrmann 1998; Mason, Davis, Wood, & Farnsworth 1998; Gravel et al 2005; Johnson et al 2005a,b; White et al 2005; Widen et al 2005; Uus & Bamford 2006; Lévêque, Schmidt, Leroux, et al 2007; Lin, Shu, Lee, Lin, & Lin 2007).

Numerous proposed guidelines and position statements have been published over the years in an evolutionary attempt to arrive at the optimal strategy for identifying hearing-impaired infants. Let us briefly outline some of the approaches to the issue, being mindful that (1) we are dealing with an evolutionary process in the development of strategies for the early identification of hearing impairment, and (2) no single protocol can be expected to be the best one for every screening program and setting. These caveats are not limited to hearing screening in babies; they also apply to screening approaches used for children and adults, discussed later in this chapter.

NIH Consensus Statement (1993)

A consensus statement on the early identification of hearing impairment prepared by a National Institutes of Health multidisciplinary panel (NIH 1993) calls for the universal screening for hearing impairment of all neonates regardless of whether they are at high risk or low risk for hearing impairment. This screening should occur within 3 months of birth, and preferably before the infant has been discharged from the hospital because accessibility is greatest while babies are in the newborn nursery. Recognizing that many hearing losses develop or worsen after the neonatal period, the NIH panel also recommended that surveillance for hearing impairment continue through early childhood. They also pointed out that another opportunity for universal screening presents itself when children enter school.

The newborn screening approach suggested by the NIH panel is a two-tier protocol involving TEOAE screening for all babies followed by ABR screening for those who fail the TEOAE screen. The TEOAE screening is done first because it is very sensitive to hearing loss, is fast, and does not require the use of electrodes. Neonates who pass the OAE screen are

considered normal. Those who fail the OAE screening proceed to the next step (ABR screening) to minimize over-referrals (i.e., false-positive results). Babies who fail the ABR screen are referred for diagnostic evaluations. Those who pass the ABR screen are discharged, but they should be rescreened in 3 to 6 months. Although the NIH panel estimated that the two-tier TEOAE/ABR protocol is more cost-effective, it encouraged institutions that have been successfully using the ABR alone for universal newborn screening to continuing doing so.

An important multi-state study involving seven hospitals with high quality neonatal screening programs concentrated on babies who *failed* the *OAE* but were *passed* by the *two-tier screening protocol* because they were *missed* by the *A-ABR* (Gravel et al 2005; Johnson et al 2005a,b; White et al 2005; Widen et al 2005). These babies were then seen for diagnostic evaluations when they were 8 to 12 months old. Of the 973 babies who met various selection requirements and returned for diagnosis, a PHL was found in 30 ears of 21 infants. In other words, 21 infants with PHLs failed the OAE but were passed (missed) by the two-tier screening protocol. Considering these cases along with 158 infants with PHL who failed the two-tier screen, the investigators estimated that ~ 23% of the babies with PHL were missed by the A-ABR.[7] Before reacting to the 23% miss rate, we must be aware that (a) the A-ABR used a 35 dB nHL stimulus, and (b) most (71.4%) of the missed PHL cases had mild hearing losses (pure tone averages less than 40 dB HL). In contrast, most of the babies with PHL who were identified by the two-tier protocol (i.e., failed the A-ABR) had losses in the moderate-to-profound range. Certainly, fewer ears with mild hearing losses would be missed if the A-ABR used a lower screening level, such as 25 dB nHL. This is not to diminish the considerable implications of mild hearing losses. On the contrary, it highlights the need for screening programs to specify what degrees of hearing loss are being targeted for identification, and then to use techniques (e.g., screening levels) that address them. It also reveals the importance of continued surveillance of children's hearing beyond the newborn period. Interested students should see the informa-

---

[7] Of 86,634 infants screened, 158 with PHL failed the two-tier protocol, for a prevalence per 1000 of 1.82. Adding the 21 with PHL who passed the A-ABR gives 179 cases with PHL, for a prevalence of 2.6, and the 0.24 increase means that 12% of those with PHL are missed by the A-ABR. The investigators adjusted this value to 0.55 because the 0.24 rise in prevalence was based on 44% of those who failed the OAE and passed the A-ABR (0.24/0.44 = 0.55). Thus, the estimated prevalence of PHL was 1.82 + 0.55 = 2.37, of which 0.55 is 23%.

tive and insightful discussions of these and other considerations by Gravel et al (2005) and Johnson et al (2005a).

An important suggestion made by the NIH panel is that primary caregivers and health care providers need to be educated about hearing loss and its identification in young children. These educational efforts should highlight (1) neonatal risk factors, (2) acquired hearing impairment risk factors, (3) the early behavioral signs of hearing loss, and (4) the fact that crude "measures" of hearing ability (e.g., hand clapping) do not work and are misleading.

ASHA (1997) Infant Screening Guidelines

The American Speech-Language-Hearing Association (ASHA 1997) infant screening guidelines cite the JCIH goal of hearing impairment detection by 3 months old and intervention under way by 6 months of age. The ASHA guidelines call for newborns and younger infants up to 6 months of age to be screened for hearing impairment using ABR *and/or* otoacoustic emissions testing. The OAE test may use either transient-evoked or distortion product otoacoustic emissions. Passing the ABR test requires a response at 35 dB nHL in both ears; and passing the OAE test requires an acceptable TEOAE or DPOAE in both ears. In addition to these screening tests, the ASHA guidelines also call for surveillance based on the kinds of indicators listed in **Table 13.2**, which continue to be considered as the child gets older.

JCIH (2007) Infant Screening Guidelines

The Joint Committee on Infant Hearing (JCIH) has provided position statements on hearing loss identification in infants since 1982, and has revised them to reflect accumulating knowledge and scientific advances over the years. The current position statement (JCIH 2007) calls for (a) physiological hearing screening of all infants before they are 1 month old, (b) confirmation of the hearing loss before 3 months of age, and (c) commencement of an interdisciplinary intervention program before the infant is 6 months old. Moreover, the scope of disorders targeted for identification been expanded to include neural hearing loss (i.e., auditory neuropathy spectrum disorder) in addition to sensorineural (cochlear) and permanent conductive hearing losses.

In general, the JCIH protocol calls for physiological screening (and rescreening for those who fail the initial screen) before discharge from the hospital, and comprehensive diagnostic evaluations for infants

who fail the screening protocol. However, different screening protocols are recommended for infants in well-baby nurseries and those in the NICU.

Neonates in the *well-baby nursery* may be screened using A-ABR or OAEs, and those who fail an initial screen must be prescreened before discharge with the same technology that was used initially. (Babies discharged before screening or born outside of the hospital should have an outpatient screening by 1 month of age.) Regardless of whether the initial screening is failed in one or both ears, rescreenings should always be done for both ears. Two-tier screening is permitted as long as those who fail an initial OAE screen are rescreened by A/ABR; in which case passing the A/ABR rescreen constitutes a "pass." On the other hand, those who fail an initial A/ABR screen should not be rescreened by OAE, because passing the OAE rescreen would not change the fact that the baby has been identified as being at risk for auditory neuropathy spectrum disorder. Infants failing the rescreening are referred for comprehensive audiological evaluations.

Because babies in the *NICU* are considered to be at risk for auditory neuropathy spectrum disorder, they should be screened with ABR techniques. In addition, NICU babies who fail the initial screen should be rescreened by an audiologist, and have a comprehensive audiological evaluation if they fail the rescreen.[8] The Guidelines Development Conference (GDC 2008) has endorsed ABR screenings for NICU babies, and added that infants in the well-baby nursery should also be screened by ABR whenever the family history includes "childhood hearing loss or sensory motor neuropathy" (GDC 2008, p. 7).

Risk indicators are used to help identify children with delayed-onset or progressive hearing losses, as well as those with mild losses, who are likely to have passed the newborn screening protocol. **Table 13.2** summarizes the hearing loss risk indicators recommended by the JCIH (2007). Notice that it includes items targeting *progressive* and *delayed-onset* hearing losses as well as congenital losses. Many of the indicators are observable during or soon after birth (e.g., structural anomalies) or become apparent during the postnatal hospital stay, such as those related to care in the NICU. Some rely to a greater or lesser extent upon historical information (e.g., family history of hearing loss and, to some extent, infections

---

[8] Outpatient rescreenings to avoid over-referrals for diagnostic evaluations may be done for infants in the well-baby nursery as long as the rescreening occurs before 1 month of age; but not for NICU babies.

during pregnancy). Others may not become apparent for quite some time, perhaps years later (e.g., head trauma, meningitis). Children with risk indicators should have at least one audiological evaluation by the time they are 30 months old, and more frequent evaluations are recommended for those with indicators for delayed-onset hearing loss.

In addition, the JCIH (2007) recommends *ongoing surveillance for all children in the child's medical home* (typically the pediatrician or family practitioner) according to the pediatric periodicity schedule (AAP 2000) during regularly scheduled well-care visits; as well as the administration of a validated screening tool at 9, 18, and 24 or 30 months (AAP 2006), or sooner if there are caretaker concerns or suspicions based on the physician's observations. The American Academy of Pediatrics calls for neonatal screening and hearing screenings in the pediatric office at certain ages up to 10 years old (AAP 2008; Harlor & Bower 2009). During these visits, attention is given to the risk indicators in **Table 13.2**, developmental milestones, and other factors such as persistent middle ear fluid.

Screening Babies Beyond 6 Months of Age (ASHA 1997)

There are many reasons to screen babies after the sixth month. Regardless of our goals and efforts to effect universal screening within the newborn period, there will always be at least some infants who have not been screened by the time they reach 6 months old. Other babies will require rescreening based on risk indicators (often at regular intervals), suspicions that develop over time, and various screening mandates that might apply. In fact, phrases like "as needed, requested, or mandated" appear as screening indicators throughout the guidelines.

The ASHA (1997) screening guidelines recommend that *pure tone screening* should be done at 1000, 2000, and *4000 Hz* using *conditioned response methods* for children in the age range from 7 months to 2 years. The test tones should be presented at a screening level of *30 dB HL* using *visual reinforcement audiometry (VRA)* or at *20 dB HL* using *conditioned play audiometry* (**Table 13.3**). These methods require the screening to be done by audiologists rather than by support personnel. The inability to hear any tone in either ear constitutes a failure, leading to rescreening or an audiological evaluation. Sound field testing may be an acceptable modification for children who refuse earphones, keeping in mind that we do not know which ear(s) are responsible for a response to a sound field stimulus. However, unconditioned methods like behavioral observation are not considered acceptable. Of course, there will be children in this age range who cannot be reliably tested with conditioned audiometric techniques, in which case ABR and OAE should be used.

■ Screening in Preschool and School-Age Children

Hearing screening through the childhood years is important because many hearing losses cannot be identified during the newborn screening processes. These are not just cases of false negative newborn screening outcomes. Many hearing losses become apparent during childhood because they are of delayed onset or progressive in nature, or are caused by such things as illness, physical trauma, noise exposure, or ototoxicity (ASHA 1997; Bamford, Fortnum, Bristow, et al 2005; JCIH 2007; Harlor & Bower 2009; AAA 2011; see also **Table 13.2**). Several examples of the recommended timing of routine hearing screenings are shown in **Table 13.4**. Two of them are from the comprehensive school hearing screening guidelines we will discuss in some detail below (ASHA 1997; AAA 2011), and the third one is recommended by the

Table 13.3 Summary of the ASHA (1997) hearing impairment screening protocols for infants and young children under 3 years of age

Age	Frequencies	Level	Pass criteria
Newborn–6 months			ABR at ≤ 35 dB nHL, or TEOAE or DPOAE in *both* ears
7 months–2 years (VRA[a])	1000 Hz 2000 Hz 4000 Hz	30 dB HL	Respond at *all* frequencies in *both* ears
7 months–2 years (CPA[b])		20 dB HL	

[a]Visual response audiometry.
[b]Conditioned play audiometry.

Table 13.4 Routine childhood hearing screening schedules recommended in three sets of guidelines

ASHA (1997)[a]	AAA (2011)[a,b]	AAP (2008)[c]
Enter school	Preschool	4 years old
Kindergarten	Kindergarten	5 years old
First grade	First grade	6 years old
Second grade		
Third grade	Third grade	8 years old
	Fifth grade	10 years old
Seventh grade	Seventh or ninth grade	
Eleventh grade		

[a]School screenings.
[b]The guideline calls for these times as a *minimum* requirement.
[c]Preventive pediatric health care visits for otherwise healthy children.

American Academy of Pediatrics as part of regular preventive pediatric health care visits for otherwise healthy children (AAP 2008; Harlor & Bower 2009). Notice that the recommended screening schedules are similar up to the first grade or ~ 6 years old, but differ afterward, especially for those during pediatric visits that do not continue after age 10.

Before proceeding, it is wise to point out that there will be many references to **otitis media with effusion (OME)** and **middle ear effusion (MEE)**. We will use these terms interchangeably here to refer to the presence of *fluid* in the middle ear *without* any signs or symptoms an *infection* (e.g., Stool, Berg, Berman, et al 1994; AAA 2011).

ASHA (1997) Screening Guidelines

The screening guidelines recommended by ASHA (1997) call for hearing screenings to be administered when the child enters school; annually in kindergarten (K) through the third grade; and then in grades 7 and 11. The screening protocol involves determining whether the child can hear pure tones of *1000, 2000, and 4000 Hz* presented at a screening level of *20 dB HL.* Each ear is tested separately by air-conduction. To pass the screen, the child must respond to *all* of the tones presented in *both* ears. Missing one or more of the tones in either ear constitutes a failure. Those failing the screening test should be *rescreened* during the same session. Children who fail the rescreening

(or could not be conditioned for the screening test) should be referred for audiological evaluations, to be followed by the appropriate kind of management.

In addition to the regularly scheduled screenings in grades K–3, 7, and 11, additional screenings are recommended when special circumstances or risk factors exist. In particular, hearing screenings should take place are when a child

- initiates special education;
- repeats a grade;
- was absent for the last "regularly scheduled" screening; or
- enters a new school system without evidence of having passed the previous scheduled hearing screening.

The risk factors indicating the need for a hearing screen include

- concern about the child's hearing, speech, language, or learning;
- history of delayed and/or late-onset hearing loss in the family;
- signs of syndrome that includes hearing loss;
- craniofacial and/or ear anomalies;
- persistent or recurrent otitis media with effusion;
- head trauma with unconsciousness;
- exposure to ototoxic drugs; and
- exposure to potentially harmful noise levels.

The ASHA (1997) screening guidelines also include procedures to screen for outer and middle ear disorders in children: The protocol includes (1) a *case history* obtained from the child's parent or guardian; (2) *otoscopic inspection* for obvious structural anomalies and obstructions of the ear canal and tympanic membrane; and (3) low-frequency (220 or 226 Hz) *tympanometry. Pure tone* screening is *not* employed by contemporary protocols for identifying disorders of the outer and middle ear (ASHA 1997; AAA 1997a,b, 2011).

The child should be referred for a medical examination if any of the following conditions are identified for either ear:

- drainage from the ear (otorrhea);
- ear pain (otalgia);
- structural anomalies of the ear that were not previously identified;
- ear canal abnormalities (e.g., impacted cerumen, foreign body, blood or other secretion, atresia, stenosis, otitis externa); or
- eardrum abnormalities or perforations.

A medical referral is also indicated if there is a flat tympanogram when the ear volume exceeds 1.0 cm^3 (suggesting perforation of the tympanic membrane)

Table 13.5 AAA (2011) minimum screening protocol for children 3 years of age and older

Pure tone screening (all children)

Frequencies[a]	Level	Failure criteria
1000 Hz 2000 Hz 4000 Hz	20 dB HL	Does not respond to *all* frequencies in *both* ears[b]

Otoacoustic emissions screening (preschool, kindergarten if pure tone screening is not feasible)

Test	Levels	Failure criteria
DPOAE	L$_1$: 65 dB SPL L$_2$: 55 dB SPL	Does not meet appropriately chosen cutoff criteria
TEOAE	80 dB SPL	

Immittance screening (if failure on pure tone/OAE rescreening)

Test	Failure criteria
Tympanometry	Tympanometric width ≥ 250 daPa *or* Static admittance < 0.2 mmho *or* Tympanometric peak (middle ear) pressure more negative than −200 daPa[c]

[a]High-frequency screening protocol starting in fifth grade if noise-induced hearing loss program.
[b]Up to four tries allowed for each test tone.
[c]Tympanometric peak pressure below −200 daPa should *not* be used as an isolated referral criterion.

unless the excessive volume is explained by the presence of a tympanostomy tube and/or the child has a perforation that is under medical care. The tympanograms are also evaluated in terms of *static acoustic admittance* (Y$_{TM}$ in mmhos) and *tympanometric width* (TW, which is the pressure interval, or how wide the tympanogram is in daPa, when measured halfway down from its peak). The criteria for failure are static acoustic admittance that is too low and/or tympanometric width that is too wide. The specific failure criteria recommended by ASHA (1997) were: (1) static admittance < 0.2 mmho and/or TW > 235 daPa for infants (Roush, Bryant, Mundy, Zeisel, & Roberts 1995), and (2) static admittance < 0.3 mmho and/or TW > 200 daPa for those 1 year old through school age (Nozza, Bluestone, Kardatzke, & Bachman 1992, 1994). Screening failures on this basis should result in referral for a rescreening, and failure of the rescreening should result in a referral for a medical examination.

The ASHA (1997) guidelines also point out that different screening guidelines may sometimes be appropriate depending on the nature of the population being screened. For example, Nozza et al (1992, 1994) found different 5 to 95% normal ranges for the general population of children and those from a subpopulation who were at risk for middle ear effusion. Several examples of these differences are shown in **Table 13.6**. Thus, different pass/fail criteria may be appropriate depending on whether the children being screened are from the general ("unselected") population or from a subgroup known ("selected") to have a higher than average risk for middle ear effusion.

AAA (2011) Screening Guidelines

The most current childhood hearing screening guidelines were introduced by the American Academy of Audiology (AAA) in 2011. They share several features with the ASHA (1997) screening guidelines, but they are by no means identical. The AAA screening guidelines were developed to identify children with permanent sensorineural hearing losses and/or persistent otitis media with effusion during the preschool and school years. An overview of the AAA screening protocol is illustrated as a flowchart in **Fig. 13.7**. We will discuss the details of each component later.

Table 13.6 Ranges (5–95%) for several tympanometric measures from an unselected group of children with normal otoscopy versus a group of at-risk children found to have no middle ear effusion during surgery[a]

	Static admittance (mmhos)	Tympanometric width (daPa)	Tympanometric peak pressure (daPa)
Unselected children/no effusion by otoscopy	0.4 to 1.4	60 to 168	−207 to +15
At-risk children/no effusion at surgery	0.2 to 1.2	84 to 394	−325 to +30

[a]Based on Nozza et al (1992, 1994).

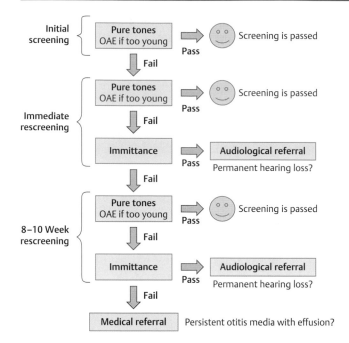

Fig. 13.7 The AAA (2011) screening protocol includes an initial screening, an immediate rescreening, and a second-tier rescreening 8 to 10 weeks later. Notice that the immittance component is a second-level procedure that is administered after failing pure tone rescreenings.

Initial Screening

If the child passes the initial *pure tone* screening (or OAEs), then she has passed the screening test (represented by the "smiley face" in the figure), and we are done. If the child fails the initial screening, then she is given an immediate pure tone rescreening on the same day.

Immediate Rescreening

The same-day rescreening should involve a different tester and audiometer if possible, but should always include reinstructing the child as well as removing and reseating the earphones. The first phase of the immediate rescreening is to repeat the *pure tone* screening (or OAEs). If the child passes it this time, then she has passed the screening test (another "smiley" in the figure), and we are done.

Failing the pure tone rescreening is followed by an immediate *immittance* screening as a secondary procedure. If the child *passes* the immittance screening, then she is referred for an audiological evaluation. Here is why. Failing the pure tones suggests a hearing loss, and passing the immittance test suggests that OME did not cause it. Thus, an audiological evalua-

tion is needed to determine if the child has a sensorineural hearing loss. The child is not called back for a follow-up screening to avoid delaying the diagnosis and management of a sensorineural hearing loss. A child who *fails* the immittance screening is scheduled for a second-tier rescreening in 8 to 10 weeks to identify cases of persistent middle ear effusion.

8–10-Week Rescreening

The follow-up rescreening employs the same testing protocol that was used for the immediate rescreening. The first phase is a *pure tone* screening (or OAEs). *Passing* it this time constitutes passing the screening protocol (yet another "smiley" in the figure) and we are done. The implication here is that whatever caused the original failure has been resolved.[9] *Failing* the *pure tones* again leads to an immittance screening. *Passing* the *immittance* phase suggests that the hearing problem is persistent even though the conductive issue appears to have been resolved, and thus leads to an audiological evaluation to determine if the child has a permanent hearing loss. However, failing the immittance test suggests that the child has persistent conductive condition such as middle ear effusion, and therefore leads to a medical referral.

The AAA (2011) screening protocol calls for all children to be screened beginning at age 3 in *preschool*, in *kindergarten* and in the *first*, *third*, *fifth*, and *seventh* or *ninth grades* (**Table 13.4**). It is important to remember that is the *minimum* recommendation. Based on an analysis of outcomes from several large school districts, the guidelines point out that *adding* a *second-grade* screening to the protocol yields a substantial improvement to its ability to discover new hearing losses. (However, this benefit is not expected if more screenings are added in high school.) In addition, a *high-frequency screening protocol* should be considered starting in the fifth grade to address concerns about noise-induced hearing loss. The main components of the testing protocol are summarized in **Table 13.5**.

Pure Tone Screening

The primary stage of the protocol is a pure tone hearing screening. Children are screened separately by air-conduction using *1000-, 2000-, and 4000-Hz pure tones*

---

[9] The author's bias would be to repeat the immittance even if the 8–10-week pure tone screen is passed. A child returning for this rescreening was already identified as at risk for OME by the original immittance screen, and pure tone screening is not a sensitive measure of OME. Hence, such a child might pass the follow-up pure tone screen and still have persistent OME.

presented at a *fixed* level of *20 dB HL*. To pass the pure tone screening, the child must respond at *all* three frequencies in *both* ears. Missing even one frequency in either ear constitutes a failure. However, *up to four tries* are permitted for each tone since a child may not respond to a particular presentation due to such factors as ambient noise in the screening room, attention, etc.

Otoacoustic Emissions

Behavioral pure tone screening often is not feasible with young children or those functioning below approximately the 3-year developmental level. Consequently, the guidelines allow the pure tone screening to be replaced with *otoacoustic emission* measurements as needed with children in *preschool, kindergarten,* and the *first grade.* Either distortion product or transient-evoked OAEs may be used, with recommended screening levels of ≤ 65 dB SPL for DPOAEs and 80 dB SPL for TEOAEs. When OAEs are employed, it is important to be cognizant of measurement technicalities and ambient noise levels, and to use appropriately chosen pass/fail criteria.

Immittance Screening

As discussed earlier, the AAA protocol includes acoustic immittance measurements as a second-stage screening that is done if the child has failed the pure tone (or OAE) screening. Its purpose is to identify conductive disorders, principally otitis media with effusion. Recall that failing the immittance screening as part of the initial screening triggers a follow-up screening 8 to 10 weeks later to determine whether the problem has been resolved or is persistent. On the other hand, failing the follow-up immittance screening implies that the effusion is persistent, and leads to a medical referral.

The immittance screening involves obtaining tympanograms with a 220 or 226 Hz probe. The principal criteria for failing the immittance screening are (1) tympanometric width that is ≥ 250 daPa, and/or (2) peak-compensated static acoustic admittance that is < 0.2 mmho. Negative tympanometric peak pressure (middle ear pressure) of more than −200 daPa constitutes a third failure criterion; but it should not be used as a basis for a medical referral all by itself.

Tympanometric Peak Pressure and Acoustic Reflexes in Screening for Middle Ear Effusion

The ASHA (1997) screening guidelines do not include the use of tympanometric peak pressure (TPP) because it was judged to have little value

in the identification of middle ear effusion (e.g., Nozza et al 1992; ASHA 1997). The AAA (2011) guidelines do include TPPs lower than −250 daPa with the caveat that this should not be used as a basis for referral all by itself. They omit ipsilateral acoustic reflex testing because it is associated with unacceptably high false-positive rates, that is, over-referrals due to absent reflexes in normal ears (e.g., Lucker 1980; Lous 1983; Roush & Tait 1985; ASHA 1997; AAA 1997a,b, 2011).

In contrast, Silman, Silverman, and Arick (1992) reported 90% sensitivity and 92.5% specificity for a middle ear effusion immittance screening protocol that includes both TPP and the ipsilateral acoustic reflex. Their protocol uses the following referral criteria:

- *Either*
  - TW > 180 daPa and/or Y_{TM} < 0.35 mmho, *plus*
  - Absent 1000 Hz ipsilateral acoustic reflex at 110 dB HL
- *Or*
  - TPP ≤ 100 daPa, *plus*
  - Absent 1000 Hz ipsilateral acoustic reflex at 110 dB HL

It is important to stress that this protocol assumes the use of an immittance device with a circuit that alternates the probe and stimulus tones to minimize artifact responses during ipsilateral acoustic reflex testing, and a pump speed of 50 daPa/s during tympanometry.

At least one reason for the inconsistencies about ipsilateral acoustic reflexes in screening for middle ear effusion appears to have been identified by Sells, Hurley, Morehouse, and Douglas (1997). Using the same subjects, they found a 31% false-positive rate for ipsilateral acoustic reflexes when the immittance device was set to its "screening mode" compared with its "diagnostic mode." The high false-positive rate for ipsilateral reflex screening has to do with how the screening mode differs from the diagnostic mode. In the diagnostic mode (1) the probe and stimulus tones are rapidly alternated so they are less likely to interact and produce artifacts, and (2) the clinician can use small immittance changes to determine whether a reflex has occurred. In the screening mode, however, (1) the probe and stimulus tones can interact and produce artifacts because they are on at the same time, and (2) the criterion for a reflex response is a relatively large preset immittance change. The implication of these findings is that screening protocols might include ipsilateral reflex testing using the appropriate instrumentation and measurement parameters.

Effect of the Gold Standard

Before proceeding with the next topic, it is important to emphasize that the success of a screening protocol for middle ear effusion is affected by the validity of the eventual diagnosis. A conclusive diagnosis of middle ear effusion depends on whether fluid is actually found surgically (by myringotomy)—a true gold standard for effusion (Stool et al 1994). However, real-world screening outcomes are usually judged by whether they are validated by otoscopic examinations—an assumed gold standard. The problem is that middle ear effusion is not reliably diagnosed by regular otoscopy (e.g., Roeser, Soh, Dunckel, & Adams 1978; Stool 1984; Nozza et al 1994; Stool et al 1994), and that otoscopic errors will affect both the apparent sensitivity and false-positive rate of the screening program. Otoscopic errors may be minimized with pneumatic and/or microscopic otoscopy. The Agency for Health Care Policy and Research Clinical Practice Guideline specifies the use of pneumatic otoscopy in the diagnosis of otitis media with effusion in young children (Stool et al 1994), although it too is far from infallible (e.g., Toner & Mains 1990; Kaleida & Stool 1992).

■ Screening for Hearing Disability in Children

A distinction is drawn between hearing disorders and impairments on the one hand and *hearing disability* on the other. As a result, current philosophy also encourages screening for audiologically relevant disabilities, such as problems in speech and language development, academic progress, and behavior and adjustment. The ASHA (1997) audiological screening guidelines recommend disability screening as part of all pediatric well-care visits and audiological evaluations for children up to 5 years of age, as well as for children with hearing impairments and those with risk factors, and when concerns arise. The AAA (1997b) position statement on audiological screening encourages audiologists to refer a child to a speech-language pathologist if delays in speech/language development are suggested by the case history, results from developmental screening instruments, or direct observation.

Disability screening may employ any of a wide variety of age-appropriate measures having published data about their validity, reliability, and pass/fail criteria. Several examples of tests that might be used for this purpose are listed in **Table 13.7**. Obviously, the criteria for what constitutes a "pass" or "refer" decision depends on the specific instrument

used, and the nature of the problem will determine the kind of professional to whom the referral should be made.

■ Follow-up Diagnosis and Intervention

Few things are more disturbing than to find that a hearing-impaired infant or child has been "lost to follow-up." It is universally accepted that infants and children who are identified by a hearing screening program should be referred for diagnostic evaluation and a comprehensive program of early intervention (e.g., NIH 1993; ASHA 1997; JCIH 2007, 2013). The assessment and management program for the hearing-impaired infant or child should be multidisciplinary, and the child's parents or other caregivers should be integrated into the process from the start. The professionals involved in the diagnostic and management team will depend on many individual aspects, but will always include the audiologist and physician, and often the speech-language pathologist, special and/or deaf educators, genetic counselor, and family support counselors. These details of diagnosis and intervention are discussed elsewhere throughout the text.

■ Audiological Screening in Adults

In spite of the high prevalence of hearing impairment among adults, discussed earlier in the chapter, there has long been a lack of ongoing, formal hearing screening programs for adults in the general public, except for occasional community health fairs and similar events. Moreover, the common omission of hearing from routine medical examinations has been a disturbing reality. Happily, attention to hearing screening for adults is increasing, and it appears to be attracting at least some interest among primary care physicians (Bogardus, Yueh, & Shekelle 2003; Yueh, Shapiro, MacLean, & Shekelle 2003).

Hearing Disorders Screening in Adults

The ASHA (1997) guidelines call for screening adults for hearing disorders using case history information and visual inspection, pure tone screening for hearing impairment, and the use of hearing disability measures (typically self-assessment instruments) to screen for hearing disability.

Table 13.7 Examples of instruments that may be used for disability screening for different age groups

Infants and toddlers	
Physician's Developmental Quick Screen for Speech Disorders	Kulig & Bakler (1973)
Fluharty Preschool Speech & Language Screening Test	Fluharty (1974)
Communication Screen	Striffler & Willis (1981)
Early Language Mildstone (ELM) Scale	Coplan (1983)
Preschool children	
Physician's Developmental Quick Screen for Speech Disorders	Kulig & Bakler (1973)
Compton Speech & Language Screening Evaluation	Compton (1978)
Fluharty Preschool Speech & Language Screening Test	Fluharty (1974)
Communication Screen	Striffler & Willis (1981)
Texas Preschool Screening Inventory	Haber & Norris (1983)
Preschool SIFTER	Anderson & Matkin (1996)
School-age children	
Revised Behavior Problem Checklist (RBPC)	Quay (1983)
Screening Instrument for Targeting Educational Risk (SIFTER)	Anderson (1989)
Dartmouth COOP Functional Health Assessment Charts	Nelson, Wasson, Johnson & Hays (1996)
Adults	
Self-Assessment for Communication (SAC)	Schow & Nerbonne (1982)
Hearing Handicap Inventory for the Elderly/Screening Version (HHIE-S)	Ventry & Weinstein (1983)

The case history portion of the ASHA (1997) hearing disorders screening protocol for adults involves asking whether the individual has any of the following problems, and whether he has received medical attention:

- hearing loss
- unilateral hearing loss
- sudden-onset or rapidly progressing hearing loss
- dizziness
- unilateral tinnitus
- recent ear pain or discomfort
- recent ear drainage

In addition to case history information, hearing disorders screening in adults also includes identifying outer ear and ear canal abnormalities, and impacted cerumen, by visual inspection and otoscopy. The screening is passed if no problems are identified by the case history and physical inspection. An immediate medical examination or cerumen management should be recommended if any problems are detected.[10]

Hearing Impairment Screening in Adults

The ASHA (1997) guidelines recommend pure tone screening for hearing impairment and for hearing disability (see below) in adults at least every 10 years up to age 50 and every 3 years thereafter. Pure tone screening for adults is done at *25 dB HL* at *1000, 2000,* and *4000 Hz* separately for *both* ears. The inability to hear any tone in either ear constitutes a failure, and leads to a referral in the form of a brief counseling session about hearing impairment. Other considerations are discussed below in the context of the hearing disability screening.

---

[10] The ASHA (1997) guidelines exclude immittance screening for adults, citing a low incidence of middle ear disorders and a negligible diagnostic yield.

Notice that the adult screening level is 25 dB HL rather than 20 dB HL, as recommended for use with children. Screening for hearing impairments in the adult population is not a straightforward problem and involves controversial practical and theoretical considerations. Much of the difficulty is related to the fact that the prevalence and degree of hearing loss increases with increasing age. The problem might be stated this way: A 20 or 25 dB HL screening criterion is needed to identify hearing losses that adversely affect communication. Yet so many older adults will fail at these levels that the very use of a screening test to identify those who are hearing impaired could become a superfluous exercise. However, just because hearing problems are common among the elderly does not mean they are any less impairing (Gelfand & Silman 1985). Happily, the current ASHA (1997) screening guidelines for adults indicate that a 25 dB screening level is appropriate for adults because hearing losses greater than this level "can affect communication regardless of age."

Hearing Disability Screening in Adults

The ASHA (1997) screening proposal for hearing disability involves the administration of disability measures with known validity, reliability, and pass/fail criteria. These measures are also known as functional assessment and self-assessment scales. The **Self-Assessment for Communication (SAC)** (Schow & Nerbonne 1982) and the **Hearing Handicap Inventory for the Elderly/Screening Version (HHIE-S)** (Ventry & Weinstein 1983) are included in the screening guidelines, and are shown in **Table 13.8** and **Table 13.9**. (See Chapter 16 for other functional assessment scales commonly used with adults.) The scores based on the patient's responses are associated with various degrees of handicap[11] or disability, as illustrated in **Table 13.10**. Higher scores indicate greater degrees of self-assessed disability, and scores outside the normal range (≥ 19 on the SAC or ≥ 10 on the HHIE-S) are considered screening failures. Those who fail the disability screening are counseled so that they understand that their responses fall outside of the norms that are established for the screening scale.

The outcomes of the hearing impairment and the hearing disability screenings are considered together for the purpose of making follow-up recommendations. Audiological evaluations are recommended for those who fail both the impairment and disability

screenings. Discharge may be recommended if the individual fails the impairment screening and passes the disability screening (or vice versa) *and* declines an audiological evaluation.

■ Ambient Noise Levels in the Screening Environment

Recall from Chapter 4 that the lowest stimulus levels that can be used in a hearing test depend on the ambient noise levels in the testing environment. This is so because ambient noise can prevent the test signals from being heard due to **masking** (Chapter 3). Hearing screening tests are usually done in rooms or offices that were not designed for hearing testing. Even though the quietest available room should be used, it is not realistic to expect the sound isolation provided by an audiometric chamber. As a result, ambient noise is always a major consideration in hearing screening programs. Clearly, we cannot legitimately test hearing in a room unless its noise levels are known.

We have seen that the AAA (2011) guidelines involve screening with 1000 to 4000 Hz pure tones presented at 20 Hz, and that the ASHA (1997) guidelines recommend 20, 25, or 30 dB HL depending on the individual's age and the testing method used. The maximum allowable ambient noise octave-band levels appropriate for these screening levels were calculated based on the ANSI (2003) standard, and are shown in section a of **Table 13.11**. Maximum allowable noise levels for the 125, 250, and 500 Hz octave-bands are included because of the upward spread of masking, which effectively means that lower-frequency noises in the room can potentially mask higher-frequency test tones (Chapter 3). Section b of the table shows how these maximum allowable levels are calculated, using a 20 dB HL screening level as an example. Section c of the table gives the maximum allowable room noise as sound pressure levels at 1000, 2000, and 4000 Hz as provided in the AAA (2011) screening guidelines.

The ambient noise issue has several practical considerations that interact with the intended goals of a screening program. Once we decide on the test level that accomplishes the intended goals of our screening program, we must find a room in which the noise levels are low enough to permit testing at that level. What if the quietest available room has noise levels too high to permit screening at the level appropriate for our purposes? Then we must (1) consider changing the screening levels and/or frequencies so that they are testable in that room; and (2) grapple with the question of whether these practical, compromised screening criteria are justifiable within the goals of our screening program.

---

[11] As in the ASHA (1997) guidelines, the term *handicap* is employed here to be consistent with the terminology used in the research references.

Table 13.8   Self-assessment of communication (SAC) (Schow & Nerbonne 1982)[a]

Please respond by circling the appropriate number, ranging from 1 to 5, to the following questions:

(**1**) almost never (or never)

(**2**) occasionally (about ¼ of the time)

(**3**) about half of the time

(**4**) frequently (about ¾ of the time)

(**5**) practically always (or always).

If you have a hearing aid, please fill out the form according to how you communicate when the hearing aid *is not* in use.

Various communication situations

1. Do you experience communication difficulties in situations when speaking with one other person? (For example: at home, at work, in a social situation, with a waitress, a store clerk, a spouse, a boss, etc.)

1 2 3 4 5

2. Do you experience communication difficulties in situations when conversing with a small group of several persons? (For example: with friends or family, coworkers, in meetings or casual conversations, over dinner or while playing cards, etc.)

1 2 3 4 5

3. Do you experience communication difficulties while listening to someone speak to a large group? (For example, at church or in a civic meeting, in a fraternal or women's club, at an educational lecture, etc.)

1 2 3 4 5

4. Do you experience communication difficulties while participating in various types of entertainment? (For example: TV, radio, plays, night clubs, musical entertainment, etc.)

1 2 3 4 5

5. Do you experience communication difficulties when you are in an unfavorable listening environment? (For example: at a noisy party, where there is background music, when riding in an auto or a bus, when someone whispers or talks from across the room, etc.)

1 2 3 4 5

6. Do you experience communication difficulties when using or listening to various communication devices? (For example: telephone, telephone ring, doorbell, public address system, warning signals, alarms, etc.)

1 2 3 4 5

Feelings about communication

7. Do you feel that any difficulty with your hearing limits or hampers your personal or social life?

1 2 3 4 5

8. Does any problem or difficulty with your hearing upset you?

1 2 3 4 5

Other people

9. Do others suggest that you have a hearing problem?

1 2 3 4 5

10. Do others leave you out of conversations or become annoyed because of your hearing?

1 2 3 4 5

Raw score (total of circled numbers): _____ (Normal range: 10–18)

[a]Adapted from Considerations in screening adults/older persons for handicapping hearing impairments. *ASHA* 34, 81–87 (1992), with permission.

Table 13.9 Hearing Handicap Inventory for the Elderly/Screening version (HHIE-S)[a]

Please check "yes," no," or "sometimes" in response to each of the following items. Do not skip a question if you avoid a situation because of a hearing problem. If you use a hearing aid, please answer the way you hear without the aid.

		Yes	Sometimes	No
E1.	Does a hearing problem cause you to feel embarrassed when you meet new people?			
E2.	Does a hearing problem cause you to feel frustrated when talking to members of your family?			
S3.	Do you have difficulty hearing when someone speaks in a whisper?			
E4.	Do you feel handicapped by a hearing problem?			
S5.	Does a hearing problem cause you difficulty when visiting friends, relatives, or neighbors?			
S6.	Does a hearing problem cause you to attend religious services less often than you would like?			
E7.	Does a hearing problem cause you to have arguments with family members?			
S8.	Does a hearing problem cause you difficulty when listening to TV or radio?			
E9.	Do you feel that any difficulty with your hearing limits or hampers your personal or social life?			
S10.	Does a hearing problem cause you difficulty when in a restaurant with relatives or friends?			

S, social-situational; **E**, emotional.
"No" = 0, "sometimes" = 2, "yes" = 4. To score, count the number of "yes" responses and multiply by 4; count the number of "sometimes" responses and multiply by 2; then add the two products:
"*Yes*" responses _____ × 4 = _____ (a)
"*Sometimes*" responses _____ × 2 = _____ (b)
Score equals sum of (a) + (b): _____ (normal range 0–8)

[a]Adapted from Ventry I, Weinstein B. Identification of elderly people with hearing problems. ASHA 1983;25:37–47, with permission.

Table 13.10 Handicap interpretations for raw scores on the SAC and the HHIE-S[a]

	SAC raw score	HHIE-S raw score
Normal/no handicap/no referral	10–18	0–8
Disability screening referral criterion (ASHA, 1997)	≥ 19	≥10
Slight handicap	19–26	
Mild-to-moderate handicap	27–38	10–24
Severe handicap	39–50	26–40

[a]Based on Schow, Smedley, and Longhurst (1990) for SAC, and Lichtenstein, Bess, and Logan (1988) for HHIE-S.

Table 13.11 Examples of maximum permissible ambient noise levels in the testing room for air-conduction screening tests with supra-aural earphones

	Frequency (Hz)					
	125	250	500	1000	2000	4000
a. Maximum allowable octave-band noise levels (OBLs) in dB calculated based on ANSI S3.1 (1999-R2003) for screening at 500–4000 Hz or 1000–4000 Hz						
20 dB HL screening level	69	55	41	46	54	57
25 dB HL screening level	74	60	46	51	59	62
30 dB HL screening level	79	65	51	56	64	67
b. Examples of how the maximum allowable OBLs shown in (a) were calculated (for a 20 dB HL screening level)						
ANSI (2003) value for 0 dB HL	49	35	21	26	34	37
+ 20 dB screening level	20	20	20	20	20	20
= Maximum allowable noise level	69	55	41	46	54	57
c. Maximum allowable sound pressure levels (SPLs) in dB for screening at 1000–4000 Hz based on AAA (2011) screening guidelines						
20 dB HL screening level				50	58	76

■ Study Questions

1. Explain the considerations involved in assessing the effectiveness of a screening test.
2. Describe the implications of minimal and unilateral hearing loss in children.
3. What are the JCIH goals for physiological screening, confirmation of hearing losses, and the commencement of intervention in infants?
4. Describe the techniques used in universal newborn hearing screening programs.
5. What are risk indicators and how are they used in hearing loss identification?
6. How do the JCIH screening guidelines address the issue of identifying children with auditory neuropathy spectrum disorder?
7. Describe the pure tone hearing screening criteria recommended by ASHA for children in preschool through high school.
8. Describe the approach suggested by ASHA and AAA to screen for outer and middle ear disorders in school children.
9. Describe the pure tone hearing screening criteria recommended by ASHA for adults.
10. Describe how self-assessment instruments are used in hearing disability screening.

References

American Academy of Audiology (AAA). Position Statement: Identification of hearing loss and middle-ear dysfunction in children. Audiology Today 1997a;9(3):18–20

American Academy of Audiology (AAA). Position Statement: Identification of hearing loss and middle-ear dysfunction in preschool and school-age children. Audiology Today 1997b;9(3):21–23

American Academy of Audiology (AAA). 2011. Clinical Practice Guidelines: Childhood Hearing Screening. Available at http://www.audiology.org/resources/documentlibrary/Documents/ChildhoodScreeningGuidelines.pdf

American Academy of Pediatrics (AAP). Recommendations for preventive pediatric health care. Pediatrics 2000;105:645–646

American Academy of Pediatrics (AAP). Council on Children with Disabilities; Section on Developmental Behavioral Pediatrics; Bright Futures Steering Committee; Medical Home Initiatives for Children with Special Needs Project Advisory Committee. Identifying infants and young children with developmental disorders in the medical home: an algorithm for developmental surveillance and screening. Pediatrics 2006;118(1):405–420

American Academy of Pediatrics/Bright Futures (AAP). 2008. Recommendations for Preventive Pediatric Health Care. Available at http://brightfutures.aap.org/pdfs/aap%20bright%20futures%20periodicity%20sched%20101107.pdf

American National Standards Institute (ANSI). 2003. Maximum Permissible Ambient Noise Levels for Audiometric Test Rooms. ANSI S3.1-1999 (R2003). New York, NY: ANSI

American Speech-Language-Hearing Association (ASHA). Considerations in screening adults/older persons for handicapping hearing impairments. ASHA 1992;34(8):81–87

American Speech-Language-Hearing Association (ASHA). 1997. Guidelines for Audiologic Screening. Rockville Pike, MD: ASHA

Anderson KL. 1989. Screening Instrument for Targeting Educational Risk (SIFTER). Austin, TX: Pro-Ed

Anderson KL, Matkin ND. 1996. Preschool SIFTER: Screening Instrument for Targeting Educational Risk in Preschool Children (Age 3-Kindergarten). Tampa, FL: Educational Audiology Assn.

Augustsson I, Engstrand I. Hearing ability according to screening at conscription: comparison with earlier reports and with previous screening results for individuals without known ear disease. Int J Pediatr Otorhinolaryngol 2006;70(5):909–913

Axelsson A, Aniansson G, Costa O. Hearing loss in school children: a longitudinal study of sensorineural hearing impairment. Scand Audiol 1987;16(3):137–143

Bamford J, Fortnum H, Bristow K, et al. 2005. Current practice, accuracy, effectiveness and cost-effectiveness of the school entry hearing screen. Health Technology Assessment 11(32);1–168. Executive summary available at: http://www.hta.ac.uk/pdfexecs/summ1132.pdf

Bennett MJ. The auditory response cradle: a device for the objective assessment of auditory state in the neonate. Symp Zool Soc Lond 1975;37:291–305

Bergman BM, Gorga MP, Neely ST, Kaminski JR, Beauchaine KL, Peters J. Preliminary descriptions of transient-evoked and distortion-product otoacoustic emissions from graduates of an intensive care nursery. J Am Acad Audiol 1995;6(2):150–162

Bess FH, Dodd-Murphy J, Parker RA. Children with minimal sensorineural hearing loss: prevalence, educational performance, and functional status. Ear Hear 1998;19(5):339–354

Bogardus ST Jr, Yueh B, Shekelle PG. Screening and management of adult hearing loss in primary care: clinical applications. JAMA 2003;289(15):1986–1990

Bonfils P, Avan P, Francois M, Trotoux J, Narcy P. Distortion-product otoacoustic emissions in neonates: normative data. Acta Otolaryngol 1992;112(5):739–744

Bonfils P, Uziel A, Pujol R. Screening for auditory dysfunction in infants by evoked oto-acoustic emissions. Arch Otolaryngol Head Neck Surg 1988;114(8):887–890

Brown AM, Sheppard SL, Russell PT. Acoustic distortion products (ADP) from the ears of term infants and young adults using low stimulus levels. Br J Audiol 1994;28(4-5):273–280

Centers for Disease Control and Prevention (CDC). 2013. Preliminary Summary of 2011 National CDC EHDI Data. (April 2013). Available at http://www.cdc.gov/ncbddd/hearingloss/2011-data/2011_ehdi_hsfs_summary_a.pdf

Cheng YJ, Gregg EW, Saaddine JB, Imperatore G, Zhang X, Albright AL. Three decade change in the prevalence of hearing impairment and its association with diabetes in the United States. Prev Med 2009;49(5):360–364

Compton A. 1978. Compton Speech and Language Screening Evaluation. San Francisco, CA: Carousel House

Coplan J. 1983. EML Scale: The Early Language Mildstone Scale. Tulsa, OK: Modern Education Corp

Copper JC Jr, Gates GA, Owen JH, Dickson HD. An abbreviated impedance bridge technique for school screening. J Speech Hear Disord 1975;40(2):260–269

Dalzell L, Orlando M, MacDonald M, et al. The New York State universal newborn hearing screening demonstration project: ages of hearing loss identification, hearing aid fitting, and enrollment in early intervention. Ear Hear 2000;21(2):118–130

Downs MP, Sterritt GM. A guide to newborn and infant hearing screening programs. Arch Otolaryngol 1967;85(1):15–22

Durieux-Smith A, Jacobson JT. Comparison of auditory brainstem response and behavioral screening in neonates. J Otolaryngol Suppl 1985;14:47–53

Durieux-Smith A, Picton T, Edwards C, Goodman JT, MacMurray B. The Crib-O-Gram in the NICU: an evaluation based on brain stem electric response audiometry. Ear Hear 1985;6(1):20–24

Eiserman D, Shisler L, Foust T, Buhrmann J, Winston R, White KR. Screening for hearing loss in early childhood programs. Early Child Res Q 2007;22:105–117

Elssmann S, Matkin N, Sabo M. Early identification of congenital hearing loss. Hear J 1987;40:13–17

Engdahl B, Woxen O, Arnesen AR, Mair IWS. Transient evoked otoacoustic emissions as screening for hearing losses at the school for military training. Scand Audiol 1996;25(1):71–78

Finitzo T, Albright K, O'Neal J. The newborn with hearing loss: detection in the nursery. Pediatrics 1998;102(6):1452–1460

Fluharty NB. 1974. Fluharty Preschool Speech and Language Screening Test. Boston, MA: Teaching Resources

Gelfand SA, Silman S. Future perspectives in hearing and aging: clinical and research needs. Semin Hear 1985;6:207–219

Gravel J, Berg A, Bradley M, et al. New York State universal newborn hearing screening demonstration project: effects of screening protocol on inpatient outcome measures. Ear Hear 2000;21(2):131–140

Gravel JS, White KR, Johnson JL, et al. A multisite study to examine the efficacy of the otoacoustic emission/automated auditory brainstem response newborn hearing screening protocol: recommendations for policy, practice, and research. Am J Audiol 2005;14(2):S217–S228

Guidelines Development Conference (GDC). 2008. Guidelines for Identification and Management of Infants and Young Children with Auditory Neuropathy Spectrum Disorder. Como, Italy. Monograph available at http://www.childrenscolorado.org/pdf/ANSD%20Monograph%20Bill%20Daniels%20Center%20for%20Childrens%20Hearing.pdf

Haber JS, Norris ML. The Texas preschool screening inventory: a simple screening device for language and learning disorders. Child Health Care 1983;12:11–18

Hall JW. 2007. New Handbook of Auditory Evoked Responses. Boston, MA: Allyn & Bacon

Harlor ADB Jr, Bower C; Committee on Practice and Ambulatory Medicine; Section on Otolaryngology–Head and Neck Surgery. Hearing assessment in infants and children: recommendations beyond neonatal screening. Pediatrics 2009;124(4):1252–1263

Henderson E, Testa MA, Hartnick C. Prevalence of noise-induced hearing-threshold shifts and hearing loss among US youths. Pediatrics 2011;127(1):e39–e46

Herrmann BS, Thornton AR, Joseph JM. Automated infant hearing screening using the ABR: Development and validation. Am J Audiol 1995;4:6–14

Hoffman HJ, Dobie RA, Ko C-W, Themann CL, Murphy WJ. Americans hear as well or better today compared with 40 years ago: hearing threshold levels in the unscreened adult population of the United States, 1959–1962 and 1999–2004. Ear Hear 2010;31(6):725–734

Jacobson JT, Jacobson CA, Spahr RC. Automated and conventional ABR screening techniques in high-risk infants. J Am Acad Audiol 1990;1(4):187–195

Johnson JL, White KR, Widen JE, et al. A multicenter evaluation of how many infants with permanent hearing loss pass a two-stage otoacoustic emissions/automated auditory brainstem response newborn hearing screening protocol. Pediatrics 2005a;116(3):663–672

Johnson JL, White KR, Widen JE, et al. A multisite study to examine the efficacy of the otoacoustic emission/automated auditory brainstem response newborn hearing screening protocol: introduction and overview of the study. Am J Audiol 2005b;14(2):S178–S185

Joint Committee on Infant Hearing (JCIH). American Academy of Pediatrics, Year 2007 position statement: Principles and guidelines for early hearing detection and intervention programs. Pediatrics 2007;120(4): 898–921

Joint Committee on Infant Hearing (JCIH). American Academy of Pediatrics. Supplement to the JCIH 2007 position statement: principles and guidelines for early intervention after confirmation that a child is deaf or hard of hearing. Pediatrics 2013;131(4):e1324–e1349

Kaleida PH, Stool SE. Assessment of otoscopists' accuracy regarding middle-ear effusion: otoscopic validation. Am J Dis Child 1992;146(4):433–435

Kulig SG, Bakler K. 1973. Physician's Developmental Quick Screen for Speech Disorders. Galveston, TX: University of Texas Medical Branch

Lafreniere D, Smurzynski J, Jung M, Leonard G, Kim DO. Otoacoustic emissions in full-term newborns at risk for hearing loss. Laryngoscope 1993;103(12): 1334–1341

Lévêque M, Schmidt P, Leroux B, et al. Universal newborn hearing screening: a 27-month experience in the French region of Champagne-Ardenne. Acta Paediatr 2007;96(8):1150–1154

Lichtenstein MJ, Bess FH, Logan SA. Diagnostic performance of the Hearing Handicap Inventory for the Elderly (Screening Version) against differing definitions of hearing loss. Ear Hear 1988;9(4):208–211

Lin H-C, Shu M-T, Lee K-S, Lin H-Y, Lin G. Reducing false positives in newborn hearing screening program: how and why. Otol Neurotol 2007;28(6):788–792

Lous J. Three impedance screening programs on a cohort of seven-year-old children: can serial impedance screening reveal chronic middle ear disease? Scand Audiol Suppl 1983;17:60–64

Lucker JR. Application of pass-fail criteria to middle ear screening results. ASHA 1980;22(10):839–840

Lundeen C. Prevalence of hearing impairment among school children. Lang Speech Hear Serv Sch 1991;22:269–271

Mason JA, Herrmann KR. Universal infant hearing screening by automated auditory brainstem response measurement. Pediatrics 1998;101(2):221–228

Mason S, Davis A, Wood S, Farnsworth A. Field sensitivity of targeted neonatal hearing screening using the Nottingham ABR Screener. Ear Hear 1998;19(2):91–102

Mauk GW, Behrens TR. Historical, political and technological context associated with early identification of hearing loss. Semin Hear 1993;14:1–17

Mauk GW, White KR, Mortensen LB, Behrens TR. The effectiveness of screening programs based on high-risk characteristics in early identification of hearing impairment. Ear Hear 1991;12(5):312–319

Maxon AB, White KR, Behrens TR, Vohr BR. Referral rates and cost efficiency in a universal newborn hearing screening program using transient evoked otoacoustic emissions. J Am Acad Audiol 1995;6(4):271–277

Mitchell P, Gopinath B, Wang JJ, et al. Five-year incidence and progression of hearing impairment in an older population. Ear Hear 2011;32(2):251–257

Montgomery J, Fujikawa S. Hearing thresholds of students in the second, eighth, and twelfth grades. Lang Speech Hear Serv Sch 1992;23:61–63

National Institutes of Health (NIH). Early identification of hearing impairment in infants and young children. NIH Consens Statement 1993;11(1):1–24

Nelson EC, Wasson JH, Johnson D, Hays R. 1996. Dartmouth COOP functional health assessment charts: brief measures for clinical practice. In: Spilker B, ed. Quality of Life and Pharmacoeconomics in Clinical Trials, 2nd ed. Philadelphia, PA: Lippincott-Raven; 161–168

Niskar AS, Kieszak SM, Holmes A, Esteban E, Rubin C, Brody DJ. Prevalence of hearing loss among children 6 to 19 years of age: the Third National Health and Nutrition Examination Survey. JAMA 1998;279(14):1071–1075

Northern JL, Gerkin KP. New technology in infant hearing screening. Otolaryngol Clin North Am 1989;22(1): 75–87

Norton SJ, Gorga MP, Widen JE, et al. Identification of neonatal hearing impairment: evaluation of transient evoked otoacoustic emission, distortion product otoacoustic emission, and auditory brain stem response test performance. Ear Hear 2000;21(5):508–528

Nozza RJ, Bluestone CD, Kardatzke D, Bachman R. Towards the validation of aural acoustic immittance measures for diagnosis of middle ear effusion in children. Ear Hear 1992;13(6):442–453

Nozza RJ, Bluestone CD, Kardatzke D, Bachman R. Identification of middle ear effusion by aural acoustic admittance and otoscopy. Ear Hear 1994;15(4):310–323

Nozza RJ, Sabo DL, Mandel EM. A role for otoacoustic emissions in screening for hearing impairment and middle ear disorders in school-age children. Ear Hear 1997;18(3):227–239

Pappas DG. A study of the high-risk registry for sensorineural hearing impairment. Otolaryngol Head Neck Surg 1983;91(1):41–44

Pleis JR, Lucas JW, Ward BW. Summary Health Statistics for U.S. Adults: National Health Interview Survey, 2008, National Center for Health Statistics. Vital Health Stat 10 2009;242:1–157

Prieve BA. Establishing infant hearing programs in hospitals. Am J Audiol 1997;6(Suppl):84–87

Prieve B, Dalzell L, Berg A, et al. The New York State universal newborn hearing screening demonstration project: outpatient outcome measures. Ear Hear 2000; 21(2):104–117

Prieve BA, Stevens F. The New York State universal newborn hearing screening demonstration project: introduction and overview. Ear Hear 2000;21(2):85–91

Quay HC. A dimensional approach to children's behavioral disorder: the revised behavior problem checklist. School Psych Rev 1983;12:244–249

Rabinowitz PM, Slade MD, Galusha D, Dixon-Ernst C, Cullen MR. Trends in the prevalence of hearing loss among young adults entering an industrial workforce 1985 to 2004. Ear Hear 2006;27(4):369–375

Roeser RJ, Soh J, Dunckel DC, Adams RM. 1978. Comparison of tympanometry and otoscopy in establishing pass/fail referral criteria. In: Harford ER, Bess FH, Bluestone CD, Klein JO, eds. Impedance Screening for Middle Ear Disease in Children. New York, NY: Grune & Stratton; 135–144

Roush J, Bryant K, Mundy M, Zeisel S, Roberts J. Developmental changes in static admittance and tympanometric width in infants and toddlers. J Am Acad Audiol 1995;6(4):334–338

Roush J, Tait CA. Pure-tone and acoustic immittance screening of preschool-aged children: an examination of referral criteria. Ear Hear 1985;6(5):245–250

Sarff CS. 1981. An innovative use of free-field amplification in regular classrooms. In: Roeser RJ, Downs MP, eds. Auditory Disorders in School Children. New York, NY: Thieme; 263–272

Savio G, Perez-Abalo MC, Gaya J, Hernandez O, Mijares E. Test accuracy and prognostic validity of multiple auditory steady state responses for targeted hearing screening. Int J Audiol 2006;45(2):109–120

Schlauch RS. Noise-induced hearing loss in teenagers. Acoustics Today 2013;9(4):14–18

Schlauch RS, Carney E. Are false-positive rates leading to an overestimation of noise-induced hearing loss? J Speech Lang Hear Res 2011;54(2):679–692

Schlauch RS, Carney E. The challenge of detecting minimal hearing loss in audiometric surveys. Am J Audiol 2012;21(1):106–119

Schow RL, Nerbonne MA. Communication screening profile: use with elderly clients. Ear Hear 1982;3(3): 135–147

Schow RL, Smedley TC, Longhurst TM. Self-assessment and impairment in adult/elderly hearing screening—recent data and new perspectives. Ear Hear 1990;11(5, Suppl):17S–27S

Scudder SG, Culbertson DS, Waldron CM, Stewart J. Predictive validity and reliability of adult hearing screening techniques. J Am Acad Audiol 2003;14(1):9–19

Seixas NS, Goldman B, Sheppard L, Neitzel R, Norton S, Kujawa SG. Prospective noise induced changes to hearing among construction industry apprentices. Occup Environ Med 2005;62(5):309–317

Sells JP, Hurley RM, Morehouse CR, Douglas JE. Validity of the ipsilateral acoustic reflex as a screening parameter. J Am Acad Audiol 1997;8(2):132–136

Shargorodsky J, Curhan SG, Curhan GC, Eavey R. Change in prevalence of hearing loss in US adolescents. JAMA 2010;304(7):772–778

Shepard NT. Newborn hearing screening using the Linco-Bennett auditory response cradle: a pilot study. Ear Hear 1983;4(1):5–10

Shimizu H, Walters RJ, Proctor LR, Kennedy DW, Allen MC, Markowitz RK. Identification of hearing impairment in the neonatal intensive care unit population: outcome of a five-year project at the Johns Hopkins Hospital. Semin Hear 1990;11:150–160

Sideris I, Glattke TJ. A comparison of two methods of hearing screening in the preschool population. J Commun Disord 2006;39(6):391–401

Silman S, Silverman CA, Arick DS. Acoustic-immittance screening for detection of middle-ear effusion in children. J Am Acad Audiol 1992;3(4):262–268

Simmons FB, Russ FN. Automated newborn hearing screening: the crib-o-gram. Arch Otolaryngol 1974; 100(1):1–7

Sininger YS. 2007. The use of auditory brainstem response in screening for hearing loss and audiometric threshold prediction. In: Burkhard RF, Don, M, Eggermont JJ, eds. Auditory Evoked Potentials: Basic Principles and Clinical Applications. Philadelphia, PA: Lippincott Williams & Wilkins; 254–274

Spivak L, Dalzell L, Berg A, et al. New York State universal newborn hearing screening demonstration project: inpatient outcome measures. Ear Hear 2000;21(2): 92–103

Stein L. 1999. Factors influencing the efficacy of universal newborn hearing screening. Pediatr Clin North Am 46:95–105

Stool SE. Medical relevancy of immittance measurements. Ear Hear 1984;5(5):309–313

Stool SE, Berg AO, Berman S, et al. 1994. Otitis Media with Effusion in Young Children: Clinical Practice Guideline. AHCPR publ. no. 94-0622. Rockville, MD: Agency for Health Care Policy & Research, Public Health Service, US Department of Health & Human Services

Striffler N, Willis S. 1981. Communication Screen. Tucson, AZ: Communication Skills Builders

Thompson V. The Colorado newborn hearing screening project. Am J Audiol 1997;6(Suppl):74–77

Toner JG, Mains B. Pneumatic otoscopy and tympanometry in the detection of middle ear effusion. Clin Otolaryngol Allied Sci 1990;15(2):121–123

Tye-Murray N. 2009. Foundations of Aural Rehabilitation: Children, Adults, and Their Family Members, 3rd ed. Clifton Park, NY: Delmar

Uus K, Bamford J. Effectiveness of population-based newborn hearing screening in England: ages of interventions and profile of cases. Pediatrics 2006; 117(5):e887–e893

Uziel A, Piron JP. Evoked otoacoustic emissions from normal newborns and babies admitted to an intensive care baby unit. Acta Otolaryngol Suppl 1991;482: 85–91, discussion 92–93

Ventry IM, Weinstein BE. Identification of elderly people with hearing problems. ASHA 1983;25(7):37–42

Vohr BR, Carty LM, Moore PE, Letourneau K. The Rhode Island Hearing Assessment Program: experience with statewide hearing screening (1993–1996). J Pediatr 1998;133(3):353–357

Wedenberg E. Auditory tests on newborn infants. Acta Otolaryngol 1956;46(5):446–461

White KR, Vohr BR, Meyer S, et al. A multisite study to examine the efficacy of the otoacoustic emission/automated auditory brainstem response newborn hearing screening protocol: research design and results of the study. Am J Audiol 2005;14(2):S186–S199

Widen JE, Johnson JL, White KR, et al. A multisite study to examine the efficacy of the otoacoustic emission/automated auditory brainstem response newborn hearing screening protocol: results of visual reinforcement audiometry. Am J Audiol 2005;14(2):S200–S216

Yoshinaga-Itano C, Sedey AL, Coulter DK, Mehl AL. Language of early- and later-identified children with hearing loss. Pediatrics 1998;102(5):1161–1171

Yueh B, Shapiro N, MacLean CH, Shekelle PG. Screening and management of adult hearing loss in primary care: scientific review. JAMA 2003;289(15):1976–1985

14 Nonorganic Hearing Loss

Routine audiological tests rely on the patient's behavioral responses to the stimuli presented to her. If she can hear a tone as soft as 0 dB HL, then she will respond to tones down to 0 dB HL, and if the softest tone she can hear is 50 dB HL then she will respond to all tones down to 50 dB HL. Her thresholds represent her actual hearing sensitivity, and any hearing loss revealed by these thresholds will be due to some kind of real, physical disorder or anomaly. Here we may say that the hearing loss is of *organic origin* because it is the result of anatomical and/or physiological abnormalities. In contrast, another patient might not respond as directed. Instead of responding to the softest sound she can hear, she might wait until the sounds are well above her actual threshold before she is willing to volunteer a response. For example, she might hold off on responding until a tone reaches 55 dB HL even though she could really hear it as low as 0 dB HL. In this case, her 55 dB HL threshold gives the false impression that she has a hearing loss even though she is actually normal. This exaggerated loss is not due to an organic cause, and may therefore be called a **nonorganic hearing loss**. Nonorganic hearing losses are also known as **functional** or **exaggerated hearing losses**, or **pseudohypacusis**, and these terms will be used interchangeably here.

A functional loss involves *questionable test results*. In operational terms, a nonorganic hearing loss is identified on the basis of observable discrepancies in the audiological tests and/or between the patient's behavior and the test results, that are not accounted for by an organic disorder (Ventry & Chaiklin 1965). On the other hand, a functional loss is not indicated by test results that are better than expected from the patient's complaints, or when subjective problems cannot be verified by routine audiological tests. In fact, subjective complaints that are not accounted for by the audiogram may suggest the possibility of abnormalities requiring more advanced diagnostic efforts (e.g., Saunders & Haggard 1989; Baran & Musiek 1994).

Not all patients with exaggerated hearing losses actually have normal hearing. In fact, most adults with functional impairments have at least some degree of underlying organic hearing loss (Chaiklin & Ventry 1963; Coles & Priede 1971; Coles & Mason 1984; Gelfand & Silman 1985, 1993; Gelfand 1994). For example, a functional patient whose real threshold is 35 dB HL might not respond until 65 dB HL. In this case, 35 dB of the loss is organic (real) and the remaining 30 dB is nonorganic. Hence, we often distinguish between (1) the overall nonorganic loss, which is represented by the patient's voluntary thresholds, and (2) the **functional component** or **overlay**, which is the *nonorganic part* of the loss. The nonorganic component is simply the difference between the exaggerated thresholds volunteered by the patient and the underlying organic loss.

The literature is unclear about the relative incidences of bilateral and unilateral nonorganic hearing loss, but clinical experience suggests that it is more common bilaterally. For example, among 88 patients whose nonorganic losses were eventually resolved, 72% were bilateral cases and 28% were unilateral (Gelfand & Silman 1993). Some possible reasons to explain why bilateral functional losses might be more common are (1) an underlying organic loss is more likely to be experienced in both ears, (2) it is easier to respond the same way for both ears, and (3) the belief that "real" hearing losses "should be" bilateral. On the other hand, sensing a difference between the ears might influence the patient to exaggerate the impairment in only one ear. A loss might be exaggerated in the poorer ear to maximize the benefits that can be derived from the loss in that ear. Alternatively, the patient might feign a loss in the good (or "better") ear because he (1) believes that hearing losses "should be" bilateral or (2) envisions greater benefits from an impairment in both ears instead of just one.

◼ Nonorganic Hearing Loss in Adults: Motivating Factors

Because functional losses do not have an organic basis they must be due either to **psychogenic** causes or to **malingering** or **feigning**. The psychogenic explanation says the hearing loss is the result of unconscious psychodynamics, and includes such phenomena as hysterical and conversion reaction deafness. It implies the patient actually experiences impaired hearing and he truly believes the hearing loss is real. Malingering means the patient is faking a hearing loss he does not have, or is falsely exaggerating whatever amount of loss he actually does have. Malingering may be motivated by financial or other benefits that the patient associates with a hearing loss. Financial gain is often an issue with injury-related lawsuits, and with veterans' and workers' compensation claims. Here, worse hearing translates into larger legal settlements, pensions, and/or compensation payments. The other real or perceived benefits to be derived from an exaggerated hearing loss may be summarized as the desire for real or perceived special attention, preferential treatment, considerations, and support in a host of social and occupational life situations.

Goldstein (1966) argued that exaggerated hearing losses are due to malingering because they cannot meet the criteria for a psychogenic disorder, which must include alleviation of the nonorganic hearing loss when the underlying psychiatric disorder is resolved. Others argued that we cannot ascribe a patient's functional loss to malingering (unless he admits feigning) because we really do not know why his responses are exaggerated, which may well include a psychogenic cause (Hopkinson 1967, 1973; Chaiklin & Ventry 1963; Ventry 1968). This is one of the reasons for using nonjudgmental, descriptive terms such as *functional hearing loss*. Noble (1978, 1987) has challenged the concept of "functional *hearing loss*" as a clinical entity and the appropriateness of the term itself to describe the exaggeration of thresholds during compensation evaluations. He argued that we are dealing with faking that is related to a process that is legalistic and adversarial rather than clinical, and that is often itself unfair. This point of view makes sense, but it does not explain why patients should have exaggerated losses when monetary issues are not involved.

Reported cases of psychogenic hearing loss are noticeably sparse. For example, Ventry (1968) presented only one case to make his point, and Coles (1982) reported that he *might* have seen three cases, but was not certain. The author came across only one reasonably convincing case of psychogenic hearing loss among all the patients seen in a Veterans Administration audiology program over ~ 15 years. This patient had psychiatric diagnoses that included an infantile personality and conversion reactions. He had various somatic disorders that responded to placebo treatments, among which was a functional hearing loss that he insisted was helped by a hearing aid. The intangible nature of other people's motivations and the desire to be fair-minded makes it hard to conclude with absolute certainty that psychogenic cases of nonorganic hearing loss do not exist. However, it appears that these cases are few and far between.

Even in the absence of a deeply rooted psychogenic cause, it is still reasonable to ask what psychological factors are associated with nonorganic hearing loss. Most of what we know about the personality and other psychosocial characteristics of individuals with nonorganic hearing loss is based on a fairly small number of studies reported during the 1940s through the 1960s. These culminated with the authoritative and well-known study by Trier and Levy (1965), who compared adult male veterans with functional losses and those with organic hearing impairments. The subjects with nonorganic hearing loss had an average intelligence quotient (IQ) of 98.7, which was slightly but significantly lower than the average IQ of 106.8 in the organic group. Compared with those with organic losses, the functional group were found to exhibit more emotional disturbances, nervousness and submissiveness, hypochondria and preoccupation with their hearing problems, tinnitus, tendencies to exploit their physical symptoms, and variability in the manifestation of the effects of their hearing losses. In addition, the individuals in the functional group earned $1300 less per year than their organic loss counterparts, and their mean family incomes were $2000 per year lower. This reflects a major economic difference between the two groups because the median regional family income at that time was about $7000. Trier and Levy hypothesized that the patients with nonorganic hearing loss experienced general feelings of inadequacy, which included the belief that they were incapable wage earners. These beliefs led to exaggeration of their impairments for monetary compensation to help provide for their families, and doing so caused them to suffer a loss of self-esteem.

◼ Nonorganic Hearing Loss in Children

Nonorganic hearing losses in children have been described by many investigators (Dixon & Newby 1959; Barr 1963; Rintelmann & Harford 1963; Ross

1964; Berger 1965; Lumio, Jauhiainen, & Gelhar 1969; McCanna & DeLupa 1981; Veniar & Salston 1983; Aplin & Rowson 1986, 1990; Bowdler & Rogers 1989; Pracy, Walsh, Mepham, & Bowdler 1996). Nonorganic hearing loss tends to occur in children who fail hearing screening tests at school, but it has also been reported following incidents of head trauma (Radkowski, Cleveland, & Friedman 1998) and in some cases of child abuse (Riedner & Efros 1995). Many of these children do not show any evidence of hearing impairment except for the failed screening tests in school and functional losses on subsequent audiological evaluations, and for the most part their nonorganic hearing losses are usually resolved over time. Different samples of children with nonorganic hearing loss have been described as having normal intelligence and academic performance (e.g., Dixon & Newby 1959); normal intelligence but poor educational achievement (e.g., Barr 1963); and widely ranging (and below-average mean) intelligence with a substantial rate of poor academic achievement (e.g., Aplin & Rowson 1990). These observations suggest that children with nonorganic hearing loss can vary widely in terms of their intellectual abilities and academic performance.

Financial rewards are clearly not the motivation for nonorganic hearing loss in children. Instead, children with pseudohypacusis are usually motivated by the secondary gains of having a hearing impairment. For example, a hearing loss can serve as a justification for underachievement at school, and to lighten the academic demands made upon him by teachers and parents, and can also provide a means to obtain needed attention and emotional support at home or school (Lumio et al 1969; Aplin & Rowson 1986). These gains become apparent to the child who has failed a routine hearing screening test. Ross (1965) recommended that actual hearing losses should be identified as soon as possible, preferably during the screening process before referrals are made, to avoid undue attention and concern that could precipitate pseudohypacusis in children who are actually normal. The majority of children with nonorganic hearing loss do not appear to have significant emotional problems, but this certainly does occur. There is also evidence of psychodynamic origins in at least some cases of childhood nonorganic hearing loss (e.g., Hallewell, Goetzinger, Allen, & Proud 1966; Lumio et al 1969; Broad 1980).

Several modified testing methods can help obtain improved thresholds from children with nonorganic losses. Ross (1964) modified an earlier method used by Dixon and Newby (1959) to arrive at the **variable intensity pulse count method**. The child's task is to count the number of tones that are heard. Groups of tones are then presented, composed of various numbers of tones at different levels. Testing begins above the child's admitted threshold. Once she is responding properly, the tone levels are manipulated until finding the lowest level at which the child is able to respond appropriately three times in a row. The success of this procedure depends on presenting it to the child as a test of *counting rather than hearing*. In the **Yes-No Method** (Miller, Fox, & Chan 1968; Frank 1976) the child is told to immediately say "yes" whenever she hears a tone and "no" whenever she does not hear one. The tones are then presented using an ascending technique. Any response associated with the presentation of a tone indicates that the child heard the tone, regardless of whether she says "yes" or a "no." This technique depends on the immaturity of the child's logic, which allows her to say "no" in response to a supposedly inaudible tone without realizing that any response demonstrates that the tone was actually heard. Rintelmann and Harford (1963) reported that children with nonorganic hearing losses could be identified by atypical findings on the SAL test (Chapter 9). Here, the patients' voluntary thresholds presented a picture of sensorineural hearing loss, but their SAL test results were of the type found with normal hearing or conductive hearing losses.

■ Relation to Organic Hearing Thresholds

Patients with nonorganic hearing loss have functional components that are related to the configuration of the underlying, organic thresholds (Coles & Mason 1984; Gelfand & Silman 1985, 1993; Gelfand 1993). This relationship is seen most clearly in patients who actually have precipitously sloping sensorineural losses, as illustrated in **Fig. 14.1**. Notice how the functional components are relatively large for the frequencies up to 2000 Hz, where the organic thresholds are relatively low, and become abruptly smaller beginning at 4000 Hz, where the organic thresholds get abruptly worse. Similarly, functional patients who really have sloping losses tend to have nonorganic components that become progressively smaller as their real thresholds become progressively worse **(Fig. 14.2)**. However, functional components and underlying organic thresholds are not related in patients who actually have normal hearing and mild losses.

Patients with functional loss seem to use an internalized reference level or "anchor" that has a certain loudness level, which we will call the "target." It appears that they will not respond to a test

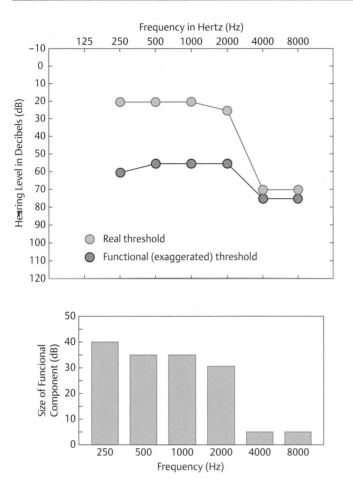

Fig. 14.1 Example of how the configuration of functional components is related to the configuration of the underlying sensorineural hearing loss sloping precipitously at 4000 Hz.

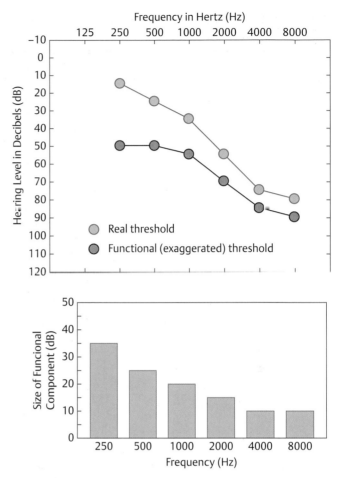

Fig. 14.2 Example of how the configuration of functional components is related to the configuration of the underlying sloping sensorineural hearing loss.

stimulus until its loudness level reaches the target (Gelfand & Silman 1985, 1993; Gelfand 1993). The inverse relationship between the degree of organic loss and the size of the functional component at each frequency appears to be produced by the following mechanism: Because of loudness recruitment, test tones reach the target at lower sensation levels (SLs) for frequencies where the underlying organic thresholds are higher (worse), and at higher SLs where the underlying thresholds are lower (better), within the same ear. This occurs because loudness recruitment is related to the amount of sensorineural loss (Chapter 10). Larger functional components are more common at lower frequencies and smaller ones are more common at higher frequencies because most sensorineural losses tend to worsen with increasing frequency. These relationships cause the exaggerated audiograms of

patients with underlying high-frequency losses to appear relatively flattened (Coles & Mason 1984). Functional components tend not to be systematically related to the underlying organic thresholds in patients who really have normal and mildly impaired hearing because these patients do not experience substantial loudness level differences between test frequencies.

Even though the configurations of functional components are consistently related to the configurations of the underlying losses, patients vary widely in terms of the absolute sizes of their functional components. This variability is probably influenced by differences between patients with respect to (1) the loudness level used as the target, (2) the range between the organic threshold and the highest stimulus level the patient is willing tolerate, and (3) the amount of recruitment.

■ Clinical Signs and Manifestations of Nonorganic Hearing Loss

Presenting and Behavioral Manifestations of Nonorganic Hearing Loss

The first factors that raise the index of suspicion for a possible nonorganic hearing loss involve real-world considerations about who referred the patient and why the evaluation is being done, rather than his clinical behavior or complaints. These include referrals made by attorneys, insurance companies, or compensation boards. Also included are referrals that are in any way related to legal issues, accidents, employment and/or work environment issues, or any form of claim that deals with any kind of pension or compensation.

The characteristics of patients with functional hearing loss are well established in the audiologic literature (Chaiklin & Ventry 1963; Hopkinson 1973; Coles 1982). Many of these patients exaggerate the behaviors and complaints that they associate with people who have real hearing problems. Examples include leaning forward, turning the head to favor the "better side," cupping a hand over one ear to make sounds louder, and obviously gazing at the talker's mouth to demonstrate a reliance on lipreading. Some patients talk loudly in an exaggerated effort to hear their own voices. Many functional patients fail to have the speech and voice aberrations associated with long-standing hearing losses, but the same behavior also occurs in many patients with organic impairments. Functional patients may also constantly ask for repetition and clarification, or even insist on having things written for them. Vague complaints about hearing problems, excessive needs to rely on lipreading, and a lack of knowledge about the use of hearing aids by a patient who "used to own one" also raise the index of suspicion for pseudohypacusis. One might observe the patient conversing effortlessly with others in the waiting room even though his audiometric thresholds would make this impossible. Few adult feigners make this mistake when the clinician is present unless they are caught off guard. However, it is not uncommon for children with nonorganic hearing loss to carry on a conversation in an informal setting but not in a test situation.

Two caveats should be mentioned about the behavioral manifestations of nonorganic hearing loss. First, even though many patients are caricature-like in their portrayal of these behaviors, there are many others whose deportment typifies any patient with a real hearing impairment, or who play the part with practiced subtlety. Subtlety should not be surprising because, after all, patients do talk to other patients and are perfectly capable of reading an audiology textbook. Second, the diagnosis of pseudohypacusis depends on *test results*. Behavioral signs of exaggeration raise the index of suspicion for a nonorganic hearing loss and provide support for any test findings that are obtained, but they do not indicate a functional loss themselves.

Indicators of Nonorganic Hearing Loss in the Routine Evaluation

Several signs of nonorganic hearing loss are obtained during the routine audiological evaluation that is administered to almost every patient. The fact that functional impairments can be revealed by routine testing is important because the clinician does not have to suspect a patient of exaggerating his hearing loss before she is able to test for it. Acoustic reflex tests are covered later along with other physiological measures, even though they are most certainly part of the routine evaluation battery.

Lack of False Alarm Responses

Almost all patients who have normal hearing and organically based hearing losses will occasionally respond even though no tone has been presented. These responses that are made during the silent periods between tone presentations are called **false-positive responses** or **false alarms**. False alarms can be disturbing to the audiologist because they make it more difficult to establish the patient's threshold; however, they do demonstrate that the patient is highly motivated to hear every possible signal, no matter how faint it might be. Patients with functional losses obviously do not share this desire and often fail to elicit any false alarms. For example, Chaiklin and Ventry (1965b) found that false alarms were elicited by 86% of patients with real hearing losses compared with only 22% for those with pseudohypacusis. They recommended that pure tone testing should include 1-minute "silent periods," during which no stimuli are presented, as a check for false alarms. One should consider the possibility of nonorganic hearing loss if the patient does not produce any false alarms, especially during these rather long silent intervals.

Threshold Variability

Pure tone thresholds are usually repeatable within a range of ± 5 dB, and test-retest reliability is certainly expected to be within ± 10 dB. Thresholds that vary by 15 dB or more from test to retest are associated with a nonorganic hearing loss (Chaiklin & Ventry

1965b). On the other hand, good test-retest reliability does not rule out a nonorganic hearing loss because many functional patients are able to produce thresholds that are quite reliable (Berger 1965; Shepherd 1965).

Absence of a Shadow Curve

Recall that cross-hearing means that the test signal is actually heard by the opposite ear instead of by the ear being tested. With this in mind, consider the audiogram in **Fig. 14.3a**, which is from a patient who is unilaterally deaf in the left ear and has normal hearing in the right ear. The unmasked thresholds for the left ear are actually due to cross-hearing in the right ear, and are known as a **shadow curve**.

The hearing levels of the shadow audiogram are in the 50 to 65 dB HL range because they depend on interaural attenuation and the bone-conduction thresholds of the better ear. In this case, the right ear has bone-conduction thresholds of 0 dB HL and interaural attenuation is in the 50 to 65 dB range. Hence, the right cochlea is able to hear the tones presented to the left ear by air-conduction at 50 to 65 dB HL. The shadow curve disappears when the deaf left ear is retested with masking noise in the opposite ear.[1] **Fig. 14.3b** shows the unmasked audiogram of a patient with *nonorganic* unilateral deafness in the

---

[1] If these points are not clear, the student should review the material on crossover, cross-hearing, interaural attenuation, and masking in Chapters 5 and 9.

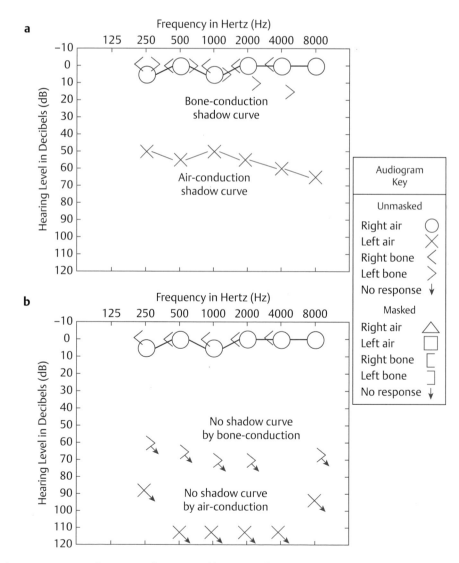

Fig. 14.3 **(a)** Shadow curves occur for air-conduction and bone-conduction in the unmasked audiogram of a patient who is completely deaf in the left ear and normal in the right ear. **(b)** Shadow curves are missing in the unmasked audiogram of a patient who is feigning unilateral deafness in the left ear.

left ear and normal hearing in the right ear. There is *no shadow curve* because the patient refuses to respond to any sound being presented to the left ear, no matter how intense it might be. He is unaware that the normal right ear would have started hearing these tones by the time they reached ~ 50 to 60 dB HL in a genuinely deaf left ear, and it is the absence of the shadow curve that reveals the nonorganic origin of the loss. Similarly, a real unilateral loss has a shadow curve for bone-conduction. However, the "no response" symbols for bone-conduction show that this functional patient would not respond when the bone vibrator was on the left side of his head, in spite of the fact that little interaural attenuation occurs for bone-conduction.

The absence of a shadow curve for air-conduction is a strong indicator of nonorganic hearing loss when there is a unilateral (or asymmetrical) hearing loss so large that it must result in cross-hearing of the signals being presented to the poorer ear. In addition, because there is little interaural attenuation for bone-conduction, the absence of a shadow curve for bone-conduction is a very strong sign of pseudohypacusis. However, we must be mindful of several considerations and caveats in this context: (1) *Unmasked* air- and bone-conduction thresholds from the poorer side are needed to tell whether shadow curves are present or absent. (2) Instead of thinking in terms of specific hearing levels where shadow curves "must be," it is wiser to consider whether the signal being directed to the poorer is likely to reach the bone-conduction threshold of the better ear. (3) Although the prior consideration is similar to the "Do I need to mask?" question, there is one important distinction: The masking decision uses the smallest reasonable amount of interaural attenuation because it is better to mask when it was not necessary rather than to misdiagnose the hearing loss. However, when dealing with a nonorganic hearing loss, we must think in terms of the *largest* amount of interaural attenuation that is reasonably possible because we do not want to classify a loss as exaggerated without good cause. (4) We must be sure that the absence of a bone-conduction shadow curve is not due to problems with the placement of the bone vibrator on the "bad" side.

Atypical Speech Audiometry Responses

Functional patients often give a variety of atypical responses to spondee words during speech recognition threshold (SRT) testing (Chaiklin & Ventry 1965b). They often miss spondee words previously repeated correctly at lower hearing levels. For example, a patient might not repeat "farewell" at 55 dB HL even though she could repeat that word at 45 dB

HL earlier during the same test. They also give many half-word responses to the spondee words (e.g., "cow" for "cowboy," or "well" for "farewell"), and even monosyllabic word responses that are unrelated to the spondee that was presented (e.g., "ball" for "armchair").

Functional patients may also obtain higher than expected speech recognition scores when tested at low sensation levels (SLs) relative to their admitted thresholds (Gold, Lubinsky, & Shahar 1981). This suggests a nonorganic hearing loss because high speech recognition scores are not expected until the presentation level reaches ~ 30 dB SL or even higher (Chapter 8). For example, suppose a patient whose SRT is 50 dB HL is able to score 92% correct for words presented at 60 dB HL, which is only 10 dB SL (re: SRT). Such high scores rarely occur at only 10 dB SL. This implies that 60 dB HL is more than just 10 dB above the SRT, and for this to be true the patient's real SRT must be lower (better) than 50 dB HL.

SRT-PTA Discrepancy

The pure tone average (PTA) of the 500, 1000, and 2000 Hz thresholds and the SRT normally agree within reasonable limits. In contrast to the agreement between the SRT and PTA in patients with real hearing losses, Carhart (1952) observed that the SRT is often better (lower) than the PTA in patients with functional losses. An **SRT-PTA discrepancy** (or **PTA-SRT discrepancy**) of 12 dB or more is considered to indicate a nonorganic hearing loss (Chaiklin & Ventry 1965b). For example, if a patient has a PTA of 47 dB HL and an SRT of 30 dB HL, he would be considered to have a nonorganic hearing loss because his SRT is better than his PTA by ≥ 12 dB. A significant SRT-PTA discrepancy has been shown to be the best audiometric indicator of functional losses (Ventry & Chaiklin 1965).

One must be mindful of the shape of the audiogram when making the SRT-PTA comparison. Suppose a patient has an SRT of 20 dB HL and the pure tone thresholds given in **Table 14.1**. The 2000 Hz threshold is clearly out of line with the thresholds at 500 and 1000 Hz. Hence, the SRT should be compared with the two-frequency PTA of 500 and 1000 Hz, which is (20 + 30)/2 = 25 dB HL. The SRT-PTA discrepancy is only 5 dB, which is perfectly acceptable. In contrast, the three-frequency PTA is (20 + 30 + 65)/3 = 38 dB HL. This results in an 18 dB SRT-PTA discrepancy, giving the false impression of a nonorganic hearing loss. This example shows that the two-frequency PTA should also be considered before labeling a patient as functional. In fact, it is even occasionally appropriate to compare the SRT to the

Table 14.1 Example of possible pure tone thresholds consistent with an SRT of 20 dB HL in an ear with a sloping hearing loss (see text)

Frequency (Hz)	250	500	1000	2000	4000	8000
Threshold (dB HL)	15	20	30	65	70	80

single frequency that has the best tonal threshold, which is usually 500 Hz but can be 250 Hz (Gelfand & Silman 1985, 1993; Silman & Silverman 1991).

The size of the SRT-PTA discrepancy also appears to be affected by how the SRT and pure tone thresholds are tested. Exaggerated losses are more clearly identified (i.e., the discrepancy is bigger) when the SRT is obtained with an ascending testing method compared with a descending method (Conn, Ventry, & Woods 1972; Schlauch, Arnce, Olson, Sanchez, & Doyle 1996). This difference can be seen by comparing the first two bars in **Fig. 14.4**. Schlauch et al (1996) also demonstrated that the SRT-PTA discrepancy can be enhanced considerably by using a descending method for pure tones with an ascending method for the SRT (third bar in **Fig. 14.4**), and they recommended this approach as a screening test for functional loss. The descending pure tone procedure involves (1) presenting the first tone at each frequency at high level (90 dB HL), (2) working downward in 10 dB steps, and (3) then following the standard audiometric method to arrive at a threshold (see Chapter 5).

Audiogram Configuration

The classical literature described nonorganic hearing loss as "saucer-shaped" or "flat," but it has been shown that no particular audiometric configurations are characteristic of functional losses (Chaiklin, Ventry, Barrett, & Skalbeck 1959; Chaiklin & Ventry 1965a). On the other hand, the *functional components* of exaggerated audiograms are related to the configuration of the *underlying, organic thresholds* (Coles & Mason 1984; Gelfand & Silman 1985, 1993; Gelfand 1993). This relationship is seen most clearly in patients who actually have precipitously sloping sensorineural losses, as illustrated in **Fig. 14.1**. Notice how the functional components are relatively large for the frequencies up to 2000 Hz, where the underlying thresholds are relatively good, and become abruptly smaller beginning at 4000 Hz, where the organic thresholds get abruptly worse. Similarly, functional patients who really have sloping losses

tend to have nonorganic components that become progressively smaller as their real thresholds worsen with increasing frequency (**Fig. 14.2**). In general, the functional components are (1) bigger at the lower frequencies where the organic thresholds are better, and (2) smaller at the higher frequencies where the organic thresholds are worse.

As explained earlier, this appears to happen because patients with functional impairments use an internalized reference level or "anchor" that has a certain loudness level; they will not respond to a test tone (or other test stimulus) until its loudness level reaches that of the anchor (Gelfand & Silman 1985, 1993; Gelfand 1993). Within an ear, functional components are smaller at the frequencies where the actual losses are worse and larger at the frequencies where the real thresholds are better because loudness recruitment is related to the degree of hearing loss (Chapter 10). As a result, the majority of functional components tend to be wider at lower frequencies and narrower at higher frequencies simply because high-frequency losses are so common.

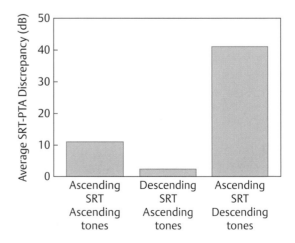

Fig. 14.4 The size of the discrepancy between the speech recognition threshold (SRT) and pure tone average (PTA) depends on whether ascending or descending methods were used to arrive at the SRT and the pure tone thresholds. (Based on data of Schlauch, Arnce, Olson, Sanchez, and Doyle [1996].)

■ Tests for Nonorganic Hearing Loss

Many tests for nonorganic hearing loss have been developed over the years. Most of them identify the presence of an exaggerated hearing loss, but some of these tests can be used to make an estimate of the patient's actual organic hearing levels.

Behavioral Tests

Ascending-Descending Gap Tests

Recall that an unusual amount of threshold variability is often but not always found among functional patients. One way to help identify patients with functional losses is to use techniques that cause their exaggerated thresholds to be even more variable. This can be done by testing the threshold for the same tone separately with an ascending approach and with a descending approach (Harris 1958; Hood, Campbell, & Hutton 1964; Kerr, Gillespie, & Easton 1975). The difference between these two thresholds is usually called the **ascending-descending gap**, and the testing itself can be done by either manual or Bekesy audiometry. When Bekesy audiometry is used, the method is known as **Bekesy Ascending-Descending Gap Evaluation (BADGE)** (Hood et al 1964). The common feature of these methods is that one threshold is obtained by starting at a low hearing level and increasing the intensity, whereas the other threshold is obtained by starting at a high hearing level and decreasing the intensity. As illustrated in **Fig. 14.5**, the ascending-descending gap is narrow for real thresholds and wide for exaggerated hearing losses. Functional patients have wide ascending-descending gaps because it is hard to maintain the same frame of reference for the exaggerated threshold "target" when it is being approached from below as when it is being approached from above.

Bekesy Audiometry

Type V Bekesy pattern In the four conventional Bekesy audiogram patterns, either the continuous and pulsed tone tracings are interleaved, or the continuous tracings are tracked below the pulsed tone tracings (Chapter 10). These configurations occur because (1) continuous tone thresholds may be either the same as or worse than the pulsed tone thresholds, and (2) higher (poorer) thresholds are plotted downward on the audiogram. In contrast, patients with nonorganic hearing loss have the opposite arrangement—*their pulsed tracings are tracked*

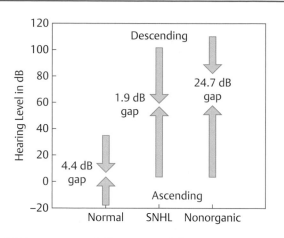

Fig. 14.5 Conceptual illustration of the ascending-descending gaps associated with real thresholds (normal and sensorineural hearing loss) and exaggerated hearing losses. (Values based on data reported by Cherry and Ventry [1976].)

below the continuous tracings, which is known as the **type V Bekesy** pattern (Jerger & Herer 1961). A typical example of a type V Bekesy audiogram is shown in **Fig. 14.6**. Sweep frequency tracings are preferred over the fixed-frequency method when conventional Bekesy audiometry is being used to identify nonorganic hearing loss (Rintelmann & Harford 1967).

Why does the pulsed tracing fall below the continuous one on the type V Bekesy audiogram? It appears that this pattern is due to the effects of loudness memory as the functional patient attempts to keep the continuous and pulsed tones at a targeted loudness above his real thresholds. This notion is based on findings by Rintelmann and Carhart (1964).

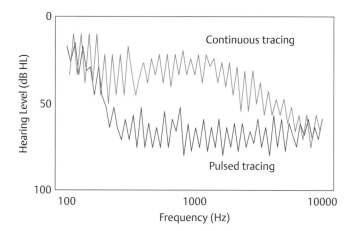

Fig. 14.6 Unlike other Bekesy audiograms, the Type V pattern is distinguished by a pulsed tracing that falls below the continuous tracing.

Their subjects heard a 1000 Hz "target" tone at a certain level immediately before doing a sweep-frequency Bekesy tracing. The task was to keep the sweep-frequency tone at the same loudness as recalled for the target tone. To do this, more intensity was needed when the sweep-frequency tone was pulsed and less intensity was needed when it was continuous. In other words, the pulsed tone needed more intensity than the continuous tone to reach the same recalled loudness. Consequently, the pulsed tracing was tracked below the continuous tracing (recall again that "more intensity" is "lower down" on the audiogram).

Lengthened Off-Time (LOT) test Conventional Bekesy audiometry uses pulsed tones that are *on* and *off* for equal amounts of time (200 ms *on* and 200 ms *off*). The **Lengthened Off-Time (LOT) test** (Hattler 1968, 1970, 1971) is a test for nonorganic hearing loss that uses Bekesy audiometry in which the pulsed tones have an *off-time* that is lengthened from 200 to 800 ms.[2] In addition, the LOT test uses fixed-frequency rather than sweep frequency tracings. Procedurally, the LOT test is just like standard fixed-frequency Bekesy audiometry except that the continuous tracing is compared with a pulsed tracing that is obtained with a tone that pulses at a rate of 200 ms *on* and 800 ms *off*. The LOT test increases the degree to which the pulsed tracing falls below the continuous tracing in functional patients, thereby improving the identification of functional impairments with the type V Bekesy pattern. This can be seen by comparing the conventional pulsed and LOT tracings in **Fig. 14.7**.

DELOT test The **Descending-LOT (DELOT) test** (Chaiklin 1990) combines the LOT with the BADGE. Recall that the BADGE (Hood et al 1964) is an ascending-descending gap test that uses Bekesy audiometry. The DELOT test begins with the same ascending continuous and 200 ms *on*/800 ms *off* pulsed tracings that are used in the LOT test. It then adds a *third* 200 ms *on*/800 ms *off* pulsed tracing that begins 25 dB above the worst (highest) threshold found on the LOT test. This will be a descending tracing because it starts from above the patient's apparent threshold. Functional patients tend to produce DELOT tracings that fall below the LOT tracing on the Bekesy audiogram (i.e., at higher hearing levels). This widens the gap between the continuous and pulsed

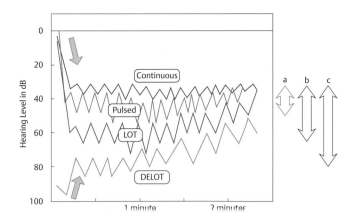

Fig. 14.7 Type V fixed-frequency Bekesy tracings using a standard pulsed tone, lengthened off-time (LOT), and descending lengthened off-time (DELOT). Notice how the separation between the continuous and pulsed tracings for the conventional Bekesy **(a)** gets wider for the LOT **(b)** and even wider for the DELOT **(c)**.

tracings, making the type V pattern even clearer, as can be seen in **Fig. 14.7**. Chaiklin (1990) recommended screening for nonorganic hearing loss with the DELOT at 500 Hz, which is supported by what we know about the configuration of functional components (Coles & Mason 1984; Gelfand & Silman 1985, 1993; Gelfand 1993).

Stenger Test

A tone presented from the right earphone is heard in the right ear, and a tone presented from the left earphone is heard in the left ear. However, a tone presented from both earphones is heard as a single, fused image that seems to be located somewhere in the head. This phenomenon is called **binaural fusion**. The image is heard in the middle of the head if the tone has the same sensation level in both ears. This is a midline lateralization. Small differences in the SLs at the two ears will cause the tone to be perceived toward the side with the higher sensation level, that is, it will be lateralized to the right or to the left. Consider the following example, which is broken down into three parts:

1. A 1000 Hz tone presented *only* to the *right* ear at *10 dB SL* is heard in the *right* ear.
2. A 1000 Hz tone presented *only* to the *left* ear at *20 dB SL* is heard in the *left* ear.
3. If *both* of these tones are presented *simultaneously*, then the listener hears *one tone* in her *left* ear.

---

[2] The ratio of the on-time to the on-time plus off-time is often called the **duty cycle**. In these terms, conventional Bekesy pulsed tones have a duty cycle of 200/(200 + 200) = 200/400 = 0.5, or 50%, and the duty cycle for the LOT Bekesy is 200/(200 + 800) = 200/1000 = 0.2, or 20%.

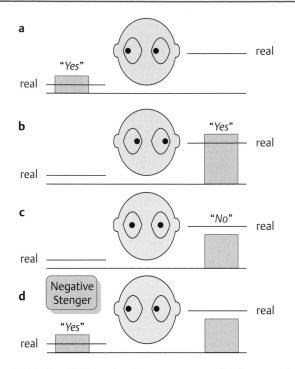

Fig. 14.8 (a–d) Negative Stenger test results for a patient with a real unilateral hearing loss. "Real" represents a true, organically based threshold (see text).

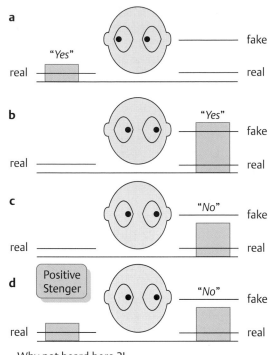

Why not heard here ?!

Fig. 14.9 (a–d) Positive Stenger test results for a patient with a nonorganic unilateral hearing loss. "Real" represents a true, organically based threshold; "fake" indicates the exaggerated voluntary threshold (see text).

The third part of this example illustrates the lateralization of the fused image to the (left) ear where the SL is higher. We could also say that the sound is *audible* in both ears, but that the patient is only *aware* of it in the left ear (where the SL is higher), in which case the situation is called the **Stenger phenomenon (effect)**. More formally, the Stenger effect states that when a sound is presented to both ears, the listener is aware of its presence only in the ear where it has a higher sensation level (or more loosely, where it is "louder").

The **Stenger test** makes use of the Stenger effect in a clinical test for *unilateral* functional hearing loss. It was first described by Stenger in 1900 as a tuning fork procedure and is now performed audiometrically in a variety of ways (Watson & Tolan 1949; Altshuler 1970). The Stenger test can be used to identify a unilateral nonorganic hearing loss, and to also estimate the patient's real thresholds in that ear. It is called the **pure tone Stenger test** when testing is done with pure tones, and the **speech Stenger test** when spondee words are used as the stimuli. There must be a unilateral or asymmetrical hearing loss in which the two ears differ by *at least 30 dB* (preferably ≥ 40 dB) at each frequency where the pure tone Stenger test is performed. The speech

Stenger test requires a similar difference between the two SRTs.

The Stenger can be administered immediately after finding the voluntary thresholds for both ears. As far as the patient is concerned, the Stenger is part of the pure tone threshold test, during which she is to respond whenever a tone is heard. In fact, the patient should not even be aware a special test is being administered. The question is whether she will or will not respond to various tones presented slightly above and/or below the voluntary thresholds of the two ears, either alone or in combination. The easiest way to learn the Stenger test is to work through the procedure itself. We will do this for two patients who have voluntary thresholds of 0 dB HL in the right ear and 50 dB HL in the left ear. The unilateral hearing loss in the left ear will be real in the first example and functional in the second example. Even though the Stenger test has numerous variations, most experts agree that test tones should be presented at 5 to 10 dB HL above and/or below the voluntary thresholds. We will use 10 dB.

Fig. 14.8 illustrates the results of a Stenger test for a patient with a *real* unilateral hearing loss in her left ear. Her thresholds are represented by the reference lines on each side of the head. The patient responds ("yes") when a 10 dB tone is presented to her right ear because it is above her threshold (**Fig. 14.8a**). She also responds ("yes") when a 60 dB HL tone is presented to her left ear because it too is above her threshold (**Fig. 14.8b**). In **Fig. 14.8c** she does not respond ("no") when a 40 dB HL tone is presented to her left ear because it is 10 dB below her threshold (i.e., she does not respond because she really cannot hear it). Two tones are presented simultaneously in panel (d). One of them is 10 dB *above* the better ear's threshold, just like **Fig. 14.8a**, and the other one is 10 dB *below* the poor ear's threshold, just like **Fig. 14.8c**. The patient responds ("yes") because she can hear the tone in her better, right ear. She is not influenced by the below-threshold 40 dB tone in her left ear because she cannot hear it. This is called a *negative Stenger test result* and suggests the threshold in the poorer ear is real.

Now let us see what happens when the same Stenger test is given to a patient who has a *nonorganic* unilateral loss, as illustrated in **Fig. 14.9**. Here, the left ear's 50 dB HL threshold is represented by a line labeled "fake" because it is exaggerated. His real thresholds are 0 dB HL in both ears, and these are represented by the lines labeled "real." The patient responds ("yes") to a 10 dB HL tone in his right ear because it is above his threshold (**Fig. 14.9a**). He also responds ("yes") when a 60 dB HL tone is presented to his left ear because it is loud enough to be higher than his exaggerated threshold (**Fig. 14.9b**). The 40 dB HL tone in **Fig. 14.9c** is well above his real threshold, but he fails to respond ("no") because the tone is lower than his exaggerated threshold (i.e., he denies hearing the tone even though he really can hear it). The stimulus combination in **Fig. 14.9d** is the same as it was in **Fig. 14.8d**: two tones are presented simultaneously; one *is 10 dB above the better ear's threshold,* just like **Fig. 14.9a**, and the other one is *10 dB below the poor ear's threshold,* just like **Fig. 14.9c**. A patient with a real loss would not hear the below-threshold tone in the left ear, and would thus respond to the above-threshold tone in the right ear. However, even though 40 dB HL is 10 dB below the exaggerated threshold, it is also 40 dB *above the real threshold* (0 dB HL). Here comes the Stenger effect: A 1000 Hz tone is in the right ear at 10 dB SL and also in the left ear at 40 dB SL. The fused image of these two tones is heard only in the left ear. Hence, all the patient knows about is the 40 dB HL tone in the left ear, which is lower than his exaggerated loss. He therefore refuses to respond ("no"). This is a *positive Stenger test result*, indicating a functional loss in the poorer ear. Why? Because if the hearing loss in his left ear were real, he still would hear the above-threshold tone in the right ear! The only thing that could prevent him from hearing the 10 dB SL tone in

the right ear would be a tone that is heard at an even higher sensation level in the left ear.

The speech Stenger test is done in the same way as the pure tone Stenger, except spondee words are used instead of pure tones, and the test is done at sensation levels relative to the SRTs of the two ears.

When it is performed as just described, the Stenger test only shows that a unilateral nonorganic hearing loss is present. The Stenger test can also be used to approximate the organic thresholds of the poorer ear. Threshold determination with the Stenger test goes well beyond our current scope, but the basic idea is to vary the level of the tone presented to the "bad" ear until the Stenger test result changes from positive to negative. The **Fusion Inferred Threshold (FIT) Test** (Bergman 1964) is another advanced technique that relies on binaural fusion to estimate organic thresholds in patients with functional hearing loss. Interested students will find a contemporary description of the test procedure and several interesting case studies in Pope (1998).

Delayed Auditory Feedback Tests

DAF speech test People expect to hear what they are saying simultaneously as they are talking. If a person speaks into a microphone and hears himself through earphones, then it is possible to insert a time delay between when he says something and when he hears it. This phenomenon is called **delayed auditory feedback (DAF)** or **delayed side tone for speech**, and it causes disruptions of the talker's speech production in terms of such characteristics as rate, fluency, intensity, and vocal quality. It is a simple matter to apply DAF for speech as a test for nonorganic hearing loss (Tiffany & Hanley 1952; Hanley & Tiffany 1954): The patient is asked to read a passage. His speech is picked up by a microphone, subjected to a time delay of ~ 180 ms, and then directed to his earphones. Pseudohypacusis is indicated if the patient's speech production can be disrupted by DAF at hearing levels below the patient's SRT.

Delayed feedback audiometry A more effective application of DAF for the assessment of functional loss is **delayed feedback audiometry (DFA)** (Ruhm & Cooper 1964; Cooper, Stokinger, & Billings 1976), which might also be called the **tonal DAF tapping test**. The patient is asked to tap out a simple rhythmic pattern on a key or button. The tapping pattern is "4 taps-pause-2 taps," and is repeated over and over again:

◆◆◆◆ ◆◆, ◆◆◆◆ ◆◆, ◆◆◆◆ ◆◆, ◆◆◆◆ ◆◆, . . .

The button controls a test tone so that the tapping pattern produces a pattern of tones. These tones are subjected to a 200 ms time delay and are then directed into one of the patient's earphones. If the patient is able to hear these delayed auditory feedback tones, then his tapping pattern will be disrupted. The tone key is also connected to a chart recorder. The basic procedure is to have the patient keep tapping the required pattern while increasing the hearing level of the DAF tones. At the same time, the audiologist watches the chart recorder for any aberrations in the tapping pattern. The presence of a nonorganic hearing loss is indicated if the tapping pattern is disrupted by DAF tones at levels lower (better) than the patient's admitted thresholds. The main advantage of DFA is that tapping patterns tend to be disrupted by DAF tones that are within 5 to 10 dB of a person's real threshold, which makes it possible to estimate a functional patient's organic hearing levels. However, it is sometimes necessary for the DAF tone to reach a much higher sensation level before it interferes with the tapping pattern (Alberti 1970). The main limitation of DFA is that the patient must be able and willing to produce the tapping pattern and to maintain it over time.

Lombard Reflex Test

The **Lombard reflex** or **effect** is the elevation of vocal effort that occurs when talking in the presence of noise (Lombard 1911). In addition to "talking louder," the Lombard effect also involves several vocal and articulatory changes associated with the increased vocal effort while the noise is present (Junqua 1993). We have all experienced this effect when we try to continue speaking at a noisy party or when a loud airplane or train is passing by. Although many noises can elicit the effect, it has been shown that the Lombard reflex actually depends on the parts of the noise that are within the speech spectrum (Garnier, Henrich, & Dubois 2010; Stowe & Golob 2013).

The Lombard reflex may be used as a test for nonorganic hearing loss on the following basis: A Lombard effect can only be caused by a noise that can be heard. If a noise that is below her voluntary thresholds can induce a patient to raise her speaking level, then her hearing must actually be better than admitted. The **Lombard test** can be accomplished in a variety of ways, but the basic procedure may be described as follows: The patient is asked to read a passage, during which the clinician monitors the level of the patient's speech on the VU meter of the audiometer. Noise is introduced into both of the patient's earphones and its intensity is raised while the audiologist watches the VU meter (and listens) for changes in the patient's

vocal level. An exaggerated hearing loss is suspected if the patient's speech level is raised by a noise that is lower than the patient's admitted thresholds.

Doerfler-Stewart Test

The Doerfler-Stewart (1946) test is based on the notions that a masking noise will cause functional patients to stop repeating spondee words even though the noise level is below the speech level, and interferes with the patient's ability to use a target loudness as a frame of reference for consistent responses. It was originally described as a binaural test that employed sawtooth noise, but it has also been used as a monaural test and with other noises (e.g., speech noise). The procedure involves several SRTs, a noise detection threshold, determining how much noise is needed to interfere with the patient's repetition of spondee words at various levels relative to the SRTs, and calculations among the various measures to decide whether a functional loss is present. Because it relies on this cumbersome procedure just to identify a nonorganic hearing loss as present (which is done more efficiently with many other tests), it is not surprising that the **Doerfler-Stewart test** is rarely if ever used anymore. Those who are interested in this test can find a detailed description and normative information in Hopkinson (1978).

Switching Speech Test

The **switching speech** (or **story**) **test** is an uncommon method for detecting unilateral functional losses. Various descriptions are available (e.g., Watson & Tolan 1949; Calearo 1957), but the basic idea is as follows: A passage, or a series of questions, is presented to the patient with the speech being switched back and forth between the patient's right and left earphones, so each ear gets only part of the information. The presentation levels are above the threshold of the "good" ear and below the admitted threshold of the "bad" ear. A functional loss is revealed by the ensuing confusion and/or how the patient recounts the story or answers the questions. Tests of this type are not recommended because they rely on a very cumbersome approach just to identify a unilateral nonorganic hearing loss, and it is not surprising that they are rarely if ever used.

Physiological Tests

The physiological changes that occur in response to the reception of a sound stimulus reflect the patient's organically based hearing because they occur regardless of whether the patient chooses to volunteer a behavioral response. For this reason, physiological tests are particularly attractive as tests for nonorganic hearing loss. Although physiological tests are said to be objective, one should realize that this objectivity does not extend to the clinician, who can be subject to biases in her interpretation of the physiological results. We will go over only the major physiological approaches to nonorganic hearing loss, but most physiological measurements that have been used to test hearing have also been tried with functional hearing loss.

Electrodermal (Psychogalvanic Skin Response) Audiometry

Electrodermal audiometry (EDA) is the measurement of hearing with the **electrodermal** or **psychogalvanic skin response (PGSR)**, and was employed to confirm the veracity of voluntary thresholds and assess patients with nonorganic hearing loss until the mid-1970s. The PGSR is a change in the electrical resistance of the skin that occurs in response to some stimulus. In EDA, electrodes on the fingertips were used to monitor skin resistance changes in response to hearing a test tone (or speech). Even though sounds can be used to obtain PGSR results, noxious stimuli such as mild electrical shocks are much more effective and reliable. For this reason, the usual EDA procedure involved presenting mild shocks along with tones above the patient's voluntary threshold. These shock-tone pairings enabled the tone itself to reliably elicit a PGSR as a result of classical conditioning. This is the same kind of classical conditioning we all learned about in Psych 101, which caused Pavlov's dogs to salivate whenever they heard a bell that was previously paired with food. The PGSR instrument registered the patient's electrodermal responses on a strip chart recording. Organic hearing thresholds could then be approximated by finding the lowest tone (or speech) levels that resulted in a measurable skin resistance change. In spite of its effectiveness as a tool in the evaluation of nonorganic hearing loss, electrical safety considerations have relegated EDA to the history books. A detailed discussion of this approach may be found in Ventry (1975).

Acoustic Reflex

Acoustic reflex thresholds (ARTs) have been used as a physiological test for functional hearing loss since the 1960s (Feldman 1963; Lamb & Peterson 1967; Alberti 1970). This is not surprising because most audiological evaluations include acoustic reflex testing as a matter of routine, so that applying ARTs to the

assessment of functional impairment comes almost without cost. The other physiological tests mentioned in this chapter do not enjoy this advantage.

A functional impairment is suspected when an ART occurs at or below the patient's hearing threshold, or at an atypically low level even though it exceeds the hearing threshold. How high must an ART be? Recall from Chapter 7 that ARTs depend on the hearing threshold in normal and cochlear-impaired patients, and that there is a range of ARTs that occurs for any given amount of loss. In that chapter we considered ARTs to be atypically high if they exceeded the 90th percentiles. Now we are concerned with atypically low ARTs, and we will use the 10th percentiles as the lower cutoff values for the degree of apparent hearing loss (Gelfand & Piper 1984; Gelfand, Schwander, & Silman 1990; Gelfand 1994). However, the 10th percentiles may be used to identify functional losses only when the voluntary thresholds are *at least 60 dB HL* at the frequency where the ART is tested (Gelfand 1994). Real and feigned losses up to 55 dB HL cannot be distinguished by ARTs because tonal ARTs are essentially the same for hearing thresholds up to roughly 50 to 60 dB HL. **Table 14.2** shows the 10th percentile lower cutoff values for hearing losses ≥ 60 dB HL due to real cochlear impairments at 500, 1000, and 2000 Hz (Gelfand et al 1990).

Table 14.2 Tenth percentile cutoff values in dB HL for acoustic reflex thresholds (ARTs) for hearing losses ≥ 60 dB HL at 500, 1000, and 2000 Hz

Hearing threshold (dB HL)	Frequency		
	500 Hz	1000 Hz	2000 Hz
60	85	85	85
65	90	90	90
70	95	95	90
75	95	95	95
80	100	100	100
85	100	100	110
≥ 90	(10 dB above the hearing threshold)[a]		

[a] An ART that is no more than 5 dB above the hearing threshold is considered to be atypically low for hearing losses ≥ 90 dB HL. This criterion places the lower cutoff value at 10 dB above the hearing threshold assuming that testing is done in 5 dB steps. (Based on Gelfand, Schwander, and Silman [1990].)

The modified bivariate method, which uses the ARTs for both broadband noise (BBN) and tones to identify hearing loss (Chapter 7), has also been proposed as a test for functional impairment (Silman, Gelfand, Piper, Silverman, & VanFrank 1984; Silman 1988). This technique reveals the existence of nonorganic hearing losses in young adults who actually have normal hearing (Silman 1988). However, the modified bivariate cannot be expected to identify functional losses in patients who have a significant degree of underlying organic hearing loss, or those who are ≥ 45 years old. This limitation occurs because the bivariate method depends on the broadband noise ART, which is affected by sensorineural losses and aging.

Gelfand (1994) suggested the following guidelines for interpreting acoustic reflex tests with regard to functional losses. It is assumed that the patient's voluntary thresholds show some degree of significant hearing loss.

1. Reflex thresholds at or below the voluntary threshold for the same tones suggest functional impairments.

2. Modified bivariate results falling within the "normal area" of the bivariate graph (Chapter 7) strongly suggest a nonorganic hearing loss and also that the organic hearing thresholds are more or less within the normal range.

3. Tenth percentiles are appropriate when the voluntary thresholds are at least 60 dB HL at the frequencies used for reflex testing. In this case, a functional loss may be suspected if ARTs fall (a) below the 10th percentiles, and/or (b) up to 5 dB above a voluntary threshold that is ≥ 90 dB HL.

4. Just because the modified bivariate results fall in the "impaired area" of the bivariate graph and the ARTs are at or above the 10th percentiles does not rule out an exaggerated loss.

Auditory Evoked Potentials

The auditory brainstem response (ABR) has been used to identify patients with nonorganic hearing loss as well as to estimate organic hearing sensitivity (Alberti 1970; Sanders & Lazenby 1983; Qiu, Yin, Stucker & Welsh 1998; Balatsouras et al 2003). The major limitations of the ABR in functional hearing loss are due to its reliance on wide-band stimuli such as clicks under routine testing conditions. The effect of high-frequency hearing losses on the ABR can be a complicating factor when assessing nonorganic hearing loss in adults, because they usually have at least some degree of underlying organic hearing loss, particularly in the higher frequencies.

Cortical auditory evoked potentials are also useful in the assessment of functional hearing loss (Alberti 1970; Coles & Mason 1984). A major advantage of cortical potentials is that they make it possible to screen for exaggerated losses and to estimate organic thresholds on a frequency-by-frequency basis. Coles and Mason (1984) suggested that a functional loss is indicated if there is a discrepancy between voluntary thresholds and cortical response findings averaging more than 7.5 dB for three frequencies, or more than 15 dB for a single frequency. Electrocochleography (Spraggs, Burton, & Graham 1994) and middle latency responses (Barrs, Althoff, Krueger, & Olsson 1994) have also been employed as tests for nonorganic hearing loss.

Otoacoustic Emissions

Otoacoustic emissions (OAEs) have great potential as a test for at least some patients with nonorganic hearing loss because they are obliterated by many sensorineural losses. Functional losses have been identified using both transient-evoked and distortion product OAEs (Robinette 1992; Musiek, Bornstein, & Rintelmann 1995; Kvaerner, Engdahl, Aursnes, Arnesen, & Mair 1996; Durrant, Kesterson, & Kamerer 1997; Qiu et al 1998; Lonsbury-Martin, Martin, & Telischi 1999; Balatsouras et al 2003; Saravanappa, Mepham, & Bowdler 2005). It is clear that OAEs will be a very useful tool for identifying exaggerated losses in patients whose hearing is really normal or near normal. However, it should be kept in mind that OAEs are limited in their application as tests for nonorganic hearing losses because the majority of adults with functional impairments also have some degree of underlying organic hearing loss.

■ Some Comments about Counseling in Cases of Nonorganic Hearing Loss

Counseling a patient with a nonorganic hearing loss is a tricky matter. The main goal is to get the patient to elicit valid and reliable responses, if at all possible. In the overwhelming majority of cases, one should *avoid being adversarial, judgmental, or accusatory, and also avoid the use of labels* when counseling a patient who has a nonorganic overlay. Let us be tersely candid to drive home the point: Using words such as "malingering" and "feigning" is like calling the patient a liar or worse, and many patients translate clinical-sounding words such as "functional," "nonorganic," and "psychogenic" into "crazy liar."

Offending the patient is almost always counterproductive. Instead of being confrontational, give the patient as much emotional room as possible so he has the option of changing his responses without losing face. A good initial approach is to simply reinstruct the patient about the tasks, subtly emphasizing the importance of responding no matter how soft the tones are, etc. If a reason is needed, allude to benign miscommunication that was not the patient's fault. The strategic placement of a physiological test sometimes motivates the patient to consider a change in response behavior, especially if the right "spin" is put on the test description ("This test helps us make a diagnosis because it directly tests your hearing nerve"). If all fails (as it often does), the next approach is generally to point out that there are "discrepancies" that make a diagnosis impossible at this time, and to schedule another appointment.

Prudence and discretion are equally important when counseling children with functional losses and their parents. The issue of secondary gain was discussed earlier. It is generally agreed that a normal-hearing child with a nonorganic hearing loss should not be confronted with the issue of his exaggerated thresholds (Veniar & Salston 1983; Bowdler & Rogers 1989; Rintelmann & Schwan 1999). On the contrary, the wise course of action is usually to advise the child that his hearing is normal and to treat him as a normal-hearing child. Supportive psychotherapy has been found beneficial in some children with functional hearing losses (e.g., Veniar & Salston 1983; Bowdler & Rogers 1989; Andaz, Heyworth, & Rowe 1995), although the clinician should be alert to the possibility of more significant emotional problems (e.g., Aplin & Rowson 1986; Brooks & Geoghegan 1992). Hence, psychological referrals should be made when these are appropriate.

Perhaps the most important point to be made in this context is that counseling by a student is not appropriate when nonorganic hearing loss is an issue. New clinicians are equally well advised to involve or at least consult an experienced supervisor whenever these situations arise.

■ Study Questions

1. What is nonorganic (or functional) hearing loss?
2. Describe the signs and behaviors often associated with nonorganic hearing losses.
3. How are nonorganic hearing losses revealed by the relationship between the speech recognition threshold and the pure tone thresholds?
4. Why does the absence of a shadow curve reveal a nonorganic hearing loss in cases of unilateral deafness?
5. How do ascending-descending gap tests reveal nonorganic hearing losses?
6. Describe how nonorganic hearing losses are revealed in standard Bekesy audiometry, the lengthened off-time (LOT) test, and the descending lengthened off-time (DELOT) test.
7. Explain the Stenger effect and how it is used to reveal nonorganic hearing losses with the Stenger test.
8. Describe how delayed feedback audiometry (DFA) reveals the presence of nonorganic hearing losses.
9. Describe how nonorganic hearing losses are identified with acoustic reflex thresholds and auditory evoked potentials.
10. Describe the considerations involved in counseling patients who have demonstrated evidence of nonorganic hearing losses.

References

Alberti PWRM. New tools for old tricks. Ann Otol Rhinol Laryngol 1970;79(4):800–807

Altshuler MW. The Stenger phenomenon. J Commun Dis 1970;3:89–105

Andaz C, Heyworth T, Rowe S. Nonorganic hearing loss in children—a 2-year study. ORL J Otorhinolaryngol Relat Spec 1995;57(1):33–35

Aplin DY, Rowson VJ. Personality and functional hearing loss in children. Br J Clin Psychol 1986;25(Pt 4): 313–314

Aplin DY, Rowson VJ. Psychological characteristics of children with functional hearing loss. Br J Audiol 1990;24(2):77–87

Balatsouras DG, Kaberos A, Korres S, Kandiloros D, Ferekidis E, Economou C. Detection of pseudohypacusis: a prospective, randomized study of the use of otoacoustic emissions. Ear Hear 2003;24(6):518–827

Baran JA, Musiek FE. Evaluation of the adults with hearing complaints and normal audiograms. Hearing Today 1994;6:9–11

Barr B. Psychogenic deafness in school children. Int Audiol 1963;2:125–128

Barrs DM, Althoff LK, Krueger WW, Olsson JE. Work-related, noise-induced hearing loss: evaluation including evoked potential audiometry. Otolaryngol Head Neck Surg 1994;110(2):177–184

Berger K. Nonorganic hearing loss in children. Laryngoscope 1965;75:447–457

Bergman M. The FIT test: monaural threshold finding through binaural fusion. Arch Otolaryngol 1964; 80:440–449

Bowdler DA, Rogers J. The management of pseudohypacusis in school-age children. Clin Otolaryngol Allied Sci 1989;14(3):211–215

Broad RD. Developmental and psychodynamic issues related to cases of childhood functional hearing loss. Child Psychiatry Hum Dev 1980;11(1):49–58

Brooks DN, Geoghegan PM. Non-organic hearing loss in young persons: transient episode or indicator of deep-seated difficulty. Br J Audiol 1992;26(6):347–350

Calearo C. Detection of malingering by periodically switched speech. Laryngoscope 1957;67(2):131–136

Carhart R. Speech audiometry in clinical evaluation. Acta Otolaryngol 1952;41(1–2):18–48

Chaiklin JB. A descending LOT-Bekesy screening test for functional hearing loss. J Speech Hear Disord 1990;55(1):67–74

Chaiklin J, Ventry IM. 1963. Functional hearing loss. In: Jerger J, ed. Modern Developments in Audiology. New York, NY: Academic Press; 76–125

Chaiklin J, Ventry IM. Evaluation of pure-tone audiogram configurations used in identifying adults with functional loss. J Aud Res 1965a;5:212–218

Chaiklin J, Ventry IM. Patient errors during spondee and pure-tone threshold measurement. J Aud Res 1965b;5:219–230

Chaiklin JB, Ventry IM, Barrett LS, Skalbeck GA. Pure-tone threshold patterns observed in functional hearing loss. Laryngoscope 1959;69:1165–1179

Cherry R, Ventry IM. The ascending-descending gap: a tool for identifying a suprathreshold response. J Aud Res 1976;16:281–287

Coles RRA. 1982. Non-organic hearing loss. In: Gibb AG, Smith MFW, eds. Butterworth's International Medical Reviews. London, UK: Butterworth; 150–176

Coles RRA, Mason SM. The results of cortical electric response audiometry in medico-legal investigations. Br J Audiol 1984;18(2):71–78

Coles RRA, Priede VM. Non-organic overlay in noise-induced hearing loss. Proc R Soc Med 1971;64:41–63

Conn M, Ventry IM, Woods RW. Pure-tone average and spondee threshold relationships in simulated hearing loss. J Aud Res 1972;12:234–139

Cooper WA Jr, Stokinger TE, Billings BL. Pure tone delayed auditory feedback: development of criteria of performance deterioration. J Am Audiol Soc 1976;1(5):192–196

Dixon RF, Newby HA. Children with nonorganic hearing problems. AMA Arch Otolaryngol 1959;70:619–623

Doerfler L, Stewart K. Malingering and psychogenic deafness. J Speech Disord 1946;11(3):181–186

Durrant JD, Kesterson RK, Kamerer DB. Evaluation of the nonorganic hearing loss suspect. Am J Otol 1997;18(3):361–367

Feldman AS. Impedance measurements at the eardrum as an aid to diagnosis. J Speech Hear Res 1963;6:315–327

Frank T. Yes-no test for nonorganic hearing loss. Arch Otolaryngol 1976;102(3):162–165

Garnier M, Henrich N, Dubois D. Influence of sound immersion and communicative interaction on the Lombard effect. J Speech Lang Hear Res 2010;53(3):588–608

Gelfand SA. Acoustic reflex threshold tenth percentiles and functional hearing impairment. J Am Acad Audiol 1994;5(1):10–16

Gelfand SA, Piper N. Acoustic reflex thresholds: variability and distribution effects. Ear Hear 1984;5(4):228–234

Gelfand SA, Schwander T, Silman S. Acoustic reflex thresholds in normal and cochlear-impaired ears: effects of no-response rates on 90th percentiles in a large sample. J Speech Hear Disord 1990;55(2):198–205

Gelfand SA, Silman S. Functional hearing loss and its relationship to resolved hearing levels. Ear Hear 1985;6(3):151–158

Gelfand SA, Silman S. Functional components and resolved thresholds in patients with unilateral nonorganic hearing loss. Br J Audiol 1993;27(1):29–34

Gold S, Lubinsky R, Shahar A. Speech discrimination scores at low sensation levels as a possible index of malingering. J Aud Res 1981;21(2):137–141

Goldstein R. Pseudohypacusis. J Speech Hear Disord 1966;31(4):341–352

Hallewell JD, Goetzinger CP, Allen ML, Proud GO. The use of hypnosis in audiologic assessment. Acta Otolaryngol 1966;61(3):205–208

Hanley CN, Tiffany WR. An investigation into the use of electro-mechanically delayed side tone in auditory testing. J Speech Hear Disord 1954;19(3):367–374

Harris DA. A rapid and simple technique for the detection of nonorganic hearing loss. AMA Arch Otolaryngol 1958;68(6):758–760

Hattler KW. The type V Bekesy pattern: the effects of loudness memory. J Speech Hear Res 1968;11(3):567–576

Hattler KW. Lengthened off-time: a self-recording screening device for nonorganicity. J Speech Hear Disord 1970;35(2):113–122

Hattler KW. The development of the LOT-Bekesy Test for nonorganic hearing loss. J Speech Hear Res 1971;14(3):605–617

Hood WH, Campbell RA, Hutton CL. An evaluation of the Bekesy ascending-descending gap. J Speech Hear Res 1964;7:123–132

Hopkinson NT. Comment on "Pseudohypacusis." J Speech Hear Disord 1967;32:293–294

Hopkinson NT. 1973. Functional hearing loss. In: Jerger J, ed. Modern Developments in Audiology, 2nd ed. New York, NY: Academic Press; 175–210

Hopkinson NT. 1978. Speech tests for pseudohypacusis. In: Katz J, ed. Handbook of Clinical Audiology, 2nd ed. Baltimore, MD: Williams & Wilkins; 291–303

Jerger J, Herer G. Unexpected dividend in Bekesy audiometry. J Speech Hear Disord 1961;26:390–391

Junqua JC. The Lombard reflex and its role on human listeners and automatic speech recognizers. J Acoust Soc Am 1993;93(1):510–524

Kerr AG, Gillespie WG, Easton JM. A simple test for malingering. Br J Audiol 1975;9:24–26

Kvaerner KJ, Engdahl B, Aursnes J, Arnesen AR, Mair IWS. Transient-evoked otoacoustic emissions: helpful tool in the detection of pseudohypacusis. Scand Audiol 1996;25(3):173–177

Lamb LE, Peterson JL. Middle ear reflex measurements in pseudohypacusis. J Speech Hear Disord 1967; 32(1):46–51

Lombard E. Le signe de l'elévation de la voix. Ann Maladiers Oreill Larynx Nes Pharynx 1911;37:101–119

Lonsbury-Martin BL, Martin GK, Telischi FF. 1999. Otoacoustic emissions in clinical practice. In: Musiek FE, Rintelmann WF, eds. Contemporary Perspectives in Hearing Assessment. Boston, MA: Allyn & Bacon; 167–196

Lumio JS, Jauhiainen T, Gelhar K. Three cases of functional deafness in the same family. J Laryngol Otol 1969;83(3):299–304

McCanna DL, DeLupa G. A clinical study of twenty-seven children exhibiting functional hearing loss. Lang Speech Hear Serv Sch 1981;12:26–35

Miller AL, Fox MS, Chan G. Pure tone assessments as an aid in detecting suspected non-organic hearing disorders in children. Laryngoscope 1968;78(12):2170–2176

Musiek FE, Bornstein SP, Rintelmann WF. Transient evoked otoacoustic emissions and pseudohypacusis. J Am Acad Audiol 1995;6(4):293–301

Noble W. 1978. Assessment of Impaired Hearing: A Critique and a New Method. New York, NY: Academic Press

Noble W. The conceptual problem of "functional hearing loss." Br J Audiol 1987;21(1):1–3

Pope ML. A FIT solution. J Am Acad Audiol 1998;9(3): 221–226

Pracy JP, Walsh RM, Mepham GA, Bowdler DA. Childhood pseudohypacusis. Int J Pediatr Otorhinolaryngol 1996;37(2):143–149

Qiu WW, Yin SS, Stucker FJ, Welsh LW. Current evaluation of pseudohypacusis: strategies and classification. Ann Otol Rhinol Laryngol 1998;107(8):638–647

Radkowski D, Cleveland S, Friedman EM. Childhood pseudohypacusis in patients with high risk for actual hearing loss. Laryngoscope 1998;108(10):1534–1538

Riedner ED, Efros PL. Nonorganic hearing loss and child abuse: beyond the sound booth. Br J Audiol 1995;29(4):195–197

Rintelmann WF, Carhart R. Loudness tracking by normal hearers via Bekesy audiometer. J Speech Hear Res 1964;7:79–93

Rintelmann W, Harford E. The detection and assessment of pseudohypoacusis among school-age children. J Speech Hear Disord 1963;28:141–152

Rintelmann WF, Harford ER. Type V Bekesy pattern: interpretation and clinical utility. J Speech Hear Res 1967;10(4):733–744

Rintelmann WF, Schwan SA. 1999. Pseudohypacusis. In: Musiek FE, Rintelmann WF, eds. Contemporary Perspectives in Hearing Assessment. Boston, MA: Allyn & Bacon; 415–435

Robinette MS. Clinical observations with transient evoked otoacoustic emissions with adults. Semin Hear 1992;13:23–36

Ross M. The variable intensity pulse count method (VIPCM) for the detection and measurement of the puretone thresholds of children with functional hearing losses. J Speech Hear Disord 1964;29:477–482

Ruhm HB, Cooper WA Jr. Delayed feedback audiometry. J Speech Hear Disord 1964;29:448–455

Sanders JW, Lazenby BB. Auditory brain stem response measurement in the assessment of pseudohypoacusis. Am J Otol 1983;4(4):292–299

Saravanappa N, Mepham GA, Bowdler DA. Diagnostic tools in pseudohypacusis in children. Int J Pediatr Otorhinolaryngol 2005;69(9):1235–1238

Saunders GH, Haggard MP. The clinical assessment of obscure auditory dysfunction–1. Auditory and psychological factors. Ear Hear 1989;10(3):200–208

Schlauch RS, Arnce KD, Olson LM, Sanchez S, Doyle TN. Identification of pseudohypacusis using speech recognition thresholds. Ear Hear 1996;17(3):229–236

Shepherd DC. Non-organic hearing loss and the consistency of behavioral responses. J Speech Hear Res 1965;8:149–163

Silman S. The applicability of the modified bivariate plotting procedure to subjects with functional hearing loss. Scand Audiol 1988;17(2):125–127

Silman S, Gelfand SA, Piper N, Silverman CA, VanFrank L. 1984. Prediction of hearing loss from the acoustic-reflex threshold. In: Silman S, ed. The Acoustic Reflex: Basic Principles and Clinical Applications. Orlando, FL: Academic Press; 187–223

Silman S, Silverman CA. 1991. Auditory Diagnosis: Principles and Applications. San Diego, CA: Academic Press

Spraggs PDR, Burton MJ, Graham JM. Nonorganic hearing loss in cochlear implant candidates. Am J Otol 1994;15(5):652–657

Stowe LM, Golob EJ. Evidence that the Lombard effect is frequency-specific in humans. J Acoust Soc Am 2013;134(1):640–647

Tiffany WR, Hanley CN. Delayed speech feedback as a test for auditory malingering. Science 1952;115(2977): 59–60

Trier TR, Levy R. Social and psychological characteristics of veterans with functional hearing loss. J Aud Res 1965;5:241–256

Veniar FA, Salston RS. An approach to the treatment of pseudohypacusis in children. Am J Dis Child 1983; 137(1):34–36

Ventry IM. A case for psychogenic hearing loss. J Speech Hear Disord 1968;33(1):89–92

Ventry IM. 1975. Conditioned galvanic skin response audiometry. In: Bradford LJ, ed. Physiological Measures of the Audio-Vestibular System. New York, NY: Academic Press; 215–247

Ventry IM, Chaiklin J. The efficiency of audiometric measured used to identify functional loss. J Aud Res 1965; 5:196–211

Watson LA, Tolan T. 1949. Hearing Tests and Hearing Instruments. Baltimore, MD: Williams & Wilkins

15 Audiological Management I

In the grand sense, the terms **audiological (re)habilitation** and **aural (re)habilitation** refer to a wide range of modalities employed by the audiologist to maximize the hearing-impaired patient's ability to live and communicate in a world of sound. Many clinicians use the term **rehabilitation** when working with someone who has an impairment of an already-developed skill, such as an adult with an adventitious hearing loss, and **habilitation** when dealing with an individual who has not yet developed a skill, such as a child with prelingual hearing loss. The modalities of audiological intervention include the use of physical instruments such as hearing aids, cochlear implants, tactile aids, and hearing assistance technologies, as well as therapeutic approaches like patient and family counseling, developing effective communication strategies, and auditory-visual training. To this list must be added referrals to and interactions with other professionals who are involved with the patient's management, such as speech-language pathologists, physicians, psychologists, teachers, etc.

We will cover audiological management in two chapters. This chapter will deal with basic concepts and principles pertaining to hearing aids per se. Our coverage of audiological management will continue in the next chapter, beginning with the clinical use of hearing aids and other instruments, and then moving one to cochlear implants, hearing assistance technology, and intervention approaches.

■ Hearing Aids

It almost goes without saying that the first order of business in the audiological management of a hearing-impaired person must be to increase the intensities of sounds so they become audible. **Hearing aids** are devices that boost sound levels so the patient can hear them. This process is called **amplification**.

Most simply, a hearing aid amplifies sounds just like a megaphone, except the amplified sound is directed right into the listener's ear. It is easiest to think of a hearing aid in terms of its major parts, as shown in **Fig. 15.1**. The hearing aid's **microphone** picks up sounds and converts them into an electrical signal. A device that transforms energy from one form to another is called a **transducer**. Thus, the microphone is an acoustic-to-electrical transducer. Once the sound has been changed into an electrical signal it can be manipulated by electronic circuits. Obviously, the principal manipulation is to boost its intensity, that is, to *amplify* it. This is done by the **amplifier**. The amplified electrical signal is then converted back into sound by an electrical-to-acoustic transducer or loudspeaker. The hearing aid's loudspeaker is called the **receiver**. The amplified sound from the receiver is directed into the patient's ear. Two other components of all hearing aids should be mentioned at this time. One is the **battery**, which provides the power to accomplish all of the hearing aid's functions. The other is the **earmold**, which is the object actually inserted into the patient's ear. In fact, the majority of modern hearing aids are completely contained within the earmold itself. Earmolds are almost always custom-made from an impression taken of the ear.

The sounds picked up by the microphone are called the **input** to the hearing aid and the sounds produced by the receiver are called the **output**. The patient hears the output from the hearing aid. The amount of amplification is called **gain**. Suppose the input is speech at 60 dB SPL and the output is the same speech signal that has been amplified to 95 dB SPL. How much amplification has occurred? The obvious answer is 35 dB because the signal coming out of the instrument is 35 dB higher than the signal that went in. Thus, gain is simply the difference in decibels between the intensity coming out of a hearing aid and the intensity that went in. Numerically,

Fig. 15.1 A simplified hearing aid diagram showing the microphone, amplifier, and receiver. Notice how the output from the receiver is larger than the input into the microphone. The battery is not shown for simplicity.

gain (in dB) equals output (in dB SPL) minus input (in dB SPL). Ten decibels of gain means the output is 10 dB higher than the input, and 0 dB of gain means the input and output are the same. Notice that input and output are given in SPL, but gain is not expressed in SPL. The reason is that the input and output are physical magnitudes, whereas gain refers to the *difference* between them. In fact, 10 dB of gain is simply referred to as "10 dB gain." (The quantitatively oriented student should note that gain is actually the ratio of the intensity of the output to the intensity of the input.) Any hearing aid has a range of gains that it can generate, and the patient has some degree of control over this gain by using a **volume control** (more technically called a **gain control**), just like the volume control of a radio.

The sound level of a hearing aid's output cannot be limitless. The greatest sound magnitude that can be produced by a hearing aid is quite descriptively called its **maximum power output (MPO)** or **output sound pressure level (OSPL)**. We will see later that OSPL is more completely called **OSPL90**, which means how much is coming out of the hearing aid ("O") in decibels of sound pressure level ("SPL") when the input to the hearing aid is a 90 dB SPL signal ("90"). For example, an OSPL of 124 dB means that 124 dB SPL is the strongest sound the hearing aid is capable of producing. In other words, OSPL refers to the output of the hearing aid in dB SPL when the hearing aid is saturated. In fact, OSPL used to be called *saturation sound pressure level (SSPL)*.

To understand what we mean by OSPL, suppose you set a hearing aid to its *highest gain* by turning its volume control all the way up and you also *keep increasing the input*. The output will get bigger and bigger as the input rises, but the output will eventually reach a maximum. Here, the output cannot get any higher no matter how much you raise the input (remember that the volume control is already turned all the way up). At this point we say the hearing aid is *saturated*, or that **saturation** has occurred. This is

analogous to what happens when you keep pouring more and more water into a sponge. It will soak up all the water until some maximum amount is absorbed. At that point we say that the sponge is saturated, meaning that it cannot hold any more water no matter how much more water you pour into it. Similarly, once the hearing aid's maximum power output is reached, its output cannot become any greater than this ceiling no matter how much more the input might increase or the volume control might be turned up. When this happens, the parts of the amplified sound that would have exceeded the ceiling are clipped off, resulting in a distortion of the amplified signal descriptively known as **peak clipping**.

These notions are illustrated by the **input-output (I-O) function** in **Fig. 15.2a**. The diagonal line shows how output increases with input up to a maximum value, where the line becomes horizontal because output no longer rises with increasing input. The diagonal line represents **linear amplification**, and shows that each 10 dB increase of input (on the x-axis) results in a 10 dB increase in the output (on the y-axis). This one-for-one relationship continues until saturation is reached, where output no longer increases with input. In this example, the I-O function becomes flat (saturates) when the output is 110 dB SPL. Parts of the output that would have been above this 110 dB saturation level would be clipped off.

Many hearing aids have **automatic gain control (AGC)** circuits that are usually employed to "slow down" the rate of amplification for louder sounds. Automatic gain control means that output from the hearing aid is changed automatically when the input changes. **Compression** is a kind of AGC where a certain increase in input results in a *smaller* increase the output increase, as shown by the solid line in **Fig. 15.2b**. Here we see that a 10 dB increase in the input level results in *less* than a 10 dB increase in the output level. Notice how compression amplification causes the I-O curve to be *shallower* than it would have been with linear amplification (shown by the dashed line for comparison). As a result, peak clipping is avoided. In addition, compression is used to prevent outputs from becoming strong enough to be uncomfortably loud, which is often desirable for patients who have trouble with loudness recruitment. The amount of compression is expressed by a **compression ratio**, which is simply the relationship of input level changes to output level changes. A compression ratio of 2:1 means that every 2 dB input increase results in an output increase of only 1 dB. Since every 1 dB input increase results in 1 dB output increase with linear amplification, it has a compression ratio of 1:1.

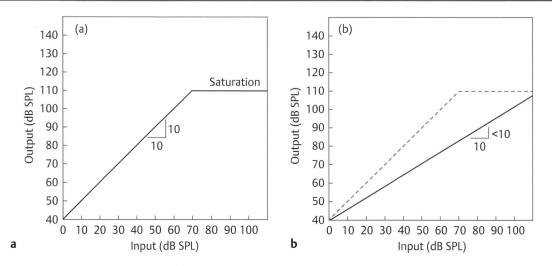

Fig. 15.2 Input-output (I-O) curves showing **(a)** linear amplification with saturation and **(b)** compression amplification. With linear amplification, each 10 dB increase of input (on the x-axis) results in a 10 dB increase in the output (on the y-axis) until saturation is reached, where output no longer increases with input. With compression amplification, a 10 dB increase in the input results in less than a 10 dB increase in output, so the output does not become uncomfortably loud or reach saturation. In frame **b**, notice how compression (solid line) causes the I-O curve to be shallower than it would have been with linear amplification (dashed line shown for comparison).

The student should also be aware of a process called **expansion**, although its applications are beyond the introductory level. Expansion means that the output level rises *faster* than the input level, so that a 10 dB increase of the input results in *more* than a 10 dB increase in the output. In this case, the I-O curve is steeper than it would have been with linear amplification. Analogous to the compression ratio, an **expansion ratio** of 1:2 means that every 1 dB input increase results in an output increase of 2 dB.

Two more commonly encountered hearing aid components are worthy of mention. One of these is the **tone control**. It adds flexibility to the instrument by adjusting the relative levels of the higher and lower frequencies much like the bass and treble on a stereo set.

The **telecoil** is a circuit that allows the hearing aid to pick up magnetic signals generated by many telephone receivers instead of using the microphone. Telecoils are associated with a switch labeled "M/T" or "M/T/MT," allowing the patient to select between using the hearing aid's microphone (**M**) in the normal manner, using the telecoil (**T**) while bypassing the microphone, or in some cases using the microphone and telecoil simultaneously (**MT**). The telecoil allows the patient to hear the telephone signal without interference from noises in the room, and/or to attend to a telephone conversation that would not be possible using the microphone. The MT position might be selected when the patient desires to hear the phone clearly but also needs to hear what is going on around her, or when she needs her hearing aid to monitor her own voice while speaking on the phone.

Types of Hearing Aids

Hearing aids are most broadly classified in terms of whether they are body or ear-level devices, and among the latter, whether they are worn behind the ear, in the ear, or built into eyeglass frames. **Fig. 15.3** shows several examples. Originally, the larger body aids were the most common devices, but smaller and less conspicuous devices now dominate the market (e.g., Strom 2000). One is tempted to conclude that this simply reflects the ability of technological advances to meet patients' desires for hearing aids that are cosmetically acceptable. While the cosmetic issue is real and highly relevant, it is by no means the only reason for the preponderance of small instruments. Technological advances have not only made it possible for modern hearing aids to be smaller, but more importantly modern hearing aids are capable of being genuine high-fidelity devices (Killion 1993). In addition, having a device in the patient's ear means the microphone is picking up sounds as they appear at the patient's ear. This permits the listener to receive a more realistic representation of his acoustic environment, and maximizes the ability to take advantage of binaural cues.

Fig. 15.3 Examples of various types of hearing aids. Behind-the-ear instruments are on the left, in-the-ear instruments are in the middle, and a body hearing aid is on the right. Several coins are shown for size comparison.

Body Hearing Aids

Body hearing aids contain all of their components and controls (except for the receiver and earmold) in a case about the size of a small pocket calculator. A wire leads from the case to the receiver and ear-mold at the patient's ear. The case is usually worn somewhere on the chest. Typical locations are in a chest-level pocket; clipped to a shirt, jacket, or undergarment; or in a specially made harness. Body instruments now account for less than 1% of the hearing aids dispensed in the United States.

Body instruments have always been the most powerful hearing aids, and this continues to be true. Thus, body aids are primarily used for the most severe hearing losses. However, considerable amounts of gain are also available in modern ear-level instruments, so high power is no longer the exclusive domain of the body instrument. Because of their size, body aids have controls and batteries that are larger, more accessible, and easier to manipulate than other types of hearing instruments. This is advantageous for patients with arthritis and other handicapping conditions, as well as for some elderly patients and younger children. An unfortunate dilemma exists because economic considerations make it practical for body aids to be manufactured only as powerful (high-gain) instruments. This is a problem for individuals who need large controls due to manual dexterity or other limitations, as well as low to moderate amounts of gain.

In addition to being big enough to accommodate larger components and batteries, another reason body aids can provide the greatest amounts of gain involves the problem of **acoustic feedback**. This is the whistle or whine produced when the output from the receiver is picked up by the microphone; feedback is a bigger problem when the microphone and receiver are closer together than when they are farther apart. The wide separation between the microphone (on the chest) and receiver (at the ear) with body aids makes feedback less of a problem than it is for ear-level instruments, where the two transducers are very close together.

Body instruments have many limitations, as well. The most obvious problem is cosmetic undesirability, but it is not the only one. Many of the problems are due to the location of the microphone on the torso instead of at ear level. Noise is picked up by the microphone when clothing brushes across the case. The amount and thickness of clothing covering the case can reduce the sound reaching the microphone. (Consider how different one's aided hearing would be with the microphone covered by a sweater and overcoat.) The body itself can adversely affect the intensity and spectrum of the sounds reaching the microphone. These effects are known as the "body shadow" and the "body baffle." Finally, body aids cause sounds to be picked up as though the ears were located on the chest instead of on the sides of the head. This distorts the perception of auditory space and detracts from the perceptual advantages afforded by binaural hearing even if two hearing aids are being used.

Ear-Level Hearing Aids

Ear-level instruments have all of their components in a small package worn in or near the ear, and comprise almost all hearing aids now being dispensed in the United States. They include behind-the-ear, in-the-ear, in-the-canal, and eyeglass instruments. A hearing aid is an ear-level instrument as long as the microphone and receiver are at the patient's ear. This includes currently available or future ear-level units that use a radio signal (or wire) to communicate with signal processing circuits contained in a case that might be kept in one's shirt pocket. In general, the smaller ear-level instruments provide less gain and flexibility than the larger ones, but there is extensive overlap among instrument types. Moreover, the ongoing development of programmable and signal processing hearing aids (see below) continues to cloud the traditional distinctions. Feedback has been limiting factor for ear-level devices, although feedback cancellation technology is available in digital hearing aids (see, e.g., Ross 2006; Johnson, Ricketts, & Hornsby 2007).

Behind-the-ear (BTE) or **post-auricular** instruments have their components contained in a crescent-shaped plastic case that fits behind the auricle. The amplified sound produced by the receiver, which is located in the case of the instrument, is transmitted via a plastic tube to an earmold in the patient's ear. The **receiver-in-the-canal (RIC)** hearing aid is a noteworthy modification of the BTE arrangement in which the receiver is located inside of the patient's ear canal, and is connected to the body of the instrument by a tiny wire. The more powerful models of BTE instruments rival the amounts of gain that could only be provided by body aids in the past, although many patients with very severe and profound losses still require body instruments.

Behind-the-ear hearing aids are preferred for pediatric patients because earmolds must be replaced frequently as infants and children grow, and also because they can be easily coupled with assistive listening devices (AAA 2013; see Chapter 16).

Over the years, BTEs were supplanted by in-the-ear instruments (described below), accounting for slightly less than 20% of the hearing aids dispensed in the United States in 1999. However, the advent of *mini-* or *micro-* BTE hearing aids (of which the RIC is one type) came with a dramatic reversal of the earlier trend, so that BTEs now account for ~ 51% of all instruments dispensed (Kirkwood 2007).

Eyeglass hearing aids have their components built into the temple piece of the patient's glasses. Similar to BTEs, the receiver output goes through a plastic tube to an earmold in the patient's ear. These instruments have various practical problems because they are part of and inseparable from the patient's eyeglasses, and are rarely used anymore.

In-the-ear (ITE) hearing aids have all of their components built into the earmold. In spite of their small size, the technology has progressed to the point that a majority of patients can now be fitted with ITE-type instruments. In-the-ear hearing aids vary widely in size. The largest ones fill the whole concha and extend into the ear canal. Smaller units take up less and less of the concha, and the smallest ones fit completely into the ear canal. The latter group constitutes a category of instruments called **completely-in-the-canal (CIC)** hearing aids. To be considered a CIC instrument, the outermost part of the device must be at least 1 to 2 mm inside of the ear canal entrance. Very tiny CIC instruments are sometimes called **invisible in-the-canal (IIC)** hearing aids. Most CICs also are **deep canal fittings**, meaning that the device extends into the bony part of the canal so its receiver end is within ~ 5 mm of the eardrum. (Actually, a deep canal fitting can be achieved with any kind of hearing aid as long as its earmold extends this deep into the external auditory meatus.) The various types of ITE instruments collectively account for ~ 49% of the hearing aids dispensed in the United States (Kirkwood 2007).

In addition to their obvious cosmetic advantage, CIC and IIC hearing aids also offer several acoustic benefits (e.g., Chasin 1994; Gudmundsen 1994; Mueller 1994). For example: (1) locating the microphone inside the meatus entrance makes it possible to take advantage of pinna and concha effects; (2) compared with shallower ones, deep canal fittings provide more gain and output because the sound is directed into a smaller volume; and (3) they are less likely to make the wearer's own speech sound as if he is talking inside a barrel because the *occlusion effect* is minimized in the bony section of the canal. On the other hand, deep canal fittings also have some potential for negative outcomes (e.g., Branda 2012; Leavitt, Welch, & Thompson 2013). For example, there is the possibility of abrasions of the ear canal and injuries to the eardrum and middle ear structures (especially when deep earmold impressions are being made), as well as the possibility that the enhanced sound amplitudes might cause progression of hearing loss.

Directional Hearing Aids

Hearing aids with directional microphones are called **directional** hearing aids (e.g., Ricketts & Mueller 1999; Valente 2000; Ricketts & Dittberner 2002; Ricketts 2005). **Directional microphones** are designed to be more sensitive to sounds coming from certain directions and less sensitive to sounds coming from other directions. This is in contrast to the more common type of microphone, which is more or less equally sensitive to sounds coming from all directions, or **omnidirectional**. In the directional mode, the hearing aid provides more amplification for sounds coming from the *front* compared with sounds coming from behind the patient. As a result, directional hearing aids provide the patient with an improved signal-to-noise ratio (SNR) in situations where the desired signal is coming from the front and noise is coming mainly from behind. Most patients experience directional benefits; and small albeit significant directional advantages have been found even for patients with severe hearing losses, at least under difficult listening conditions (e.g., Ricketts & Hornsby 2006).

The benefits afforded by directional amplification depend on various factors, such as listening situations. For example, Walden, Surr, Cord, and Dyrlund (2004) found that hearing aid users appear to prefer the directional mode in situations with noisy backgrounds when the signal comes from a nearby source in front of them, but prefer the omnidirectional setting in quiet environments as well as in noisy situations when the signal source is farther away. In addition, the speaker is not always in front of the listener. For example, instruments capable of favoring locations *next to* or *behind* the listener have been shown to be useful when speaking to others in a car (e.g., Wu, Stangl, Bentler, & Stanziola 2013). Directional amplification on a full-time basis is also problematic for children because it reduces their ability to attend to environmental signals and overhear conversations coming from all around them, as well as opportunities for incidental learning (AAA 2013).[1] Thus, patients should be advised to switch between the directional and omnidirectional settings depending on the listening situation, rather than arbitrarily keeping the hearing aid in the directional mode at all times. Signal processing technologies that provide the hearing aid with adaptive directional functions are also available (e.g., Ricketts & Henry 2002; Kuk, Keenan, Lau, & Ludvigsen 2005).

Signal Processing Hearing Aids

Digital hearing aids now account for over 90% of the instruments dispensed in the United States (Kirkwood 2007). In contrast to traditional hearing aids that use standard (analog) electronic circuits to amplify and otherwise adjust the signal, **digital** or **digital signal processing (DSP)** hearing aids use an **analog-to-digital (A/D) converter** to transform the signal entering the microphone into digital form (i.e., a code in which binary numbers represent the sound signal). The instrument then accomplishes all aspects of the amplification process digitally (analogous to how a personal computer handles the activities involved in word processing or computer games). After digital processing, the signal is transformed back into analog form by a **digital-to-analog (D/A) converter**, and is then transduced into amplified sound by a receiver. Digital hearing aids provide a host of signal processing and adaptive functions (in which the hearing aid automatically reacts or adapts to the nature of the signal), such as sophisticated compression schemes, feedback suppression, noise

reduction, switching between directional and omnidirectional modes, and programmable amplification, among others.

Programmable Hearing Aids

Programmable hearing aids are instruments that can be programmed to provide several different kinds of amplification characteristics for use under different kinds of circumstances, such as speech communication in quiet and in the presence of competing noises, listening to music, etc. The wearer can select among the different settings using a switch on the hearing aid itself or with a small remote control device that can be kept in a pocket or handbag.

Bone-conduction Hearing Aids

The hearing aids described so far have been *air-conduction* instruments in which the sound is directed into the ear from a miniature loudspeaker (the receiver) via the normal air-conduction route. **Bone-conduction hearing aids** present amplified sound to the patient using a **bone-conduction vibrator** just like the ones used for bone-conduction audiometry (Chapter 5). The vibrator is typically held in place with a spring headband or built into the temple portion of eyeglasses. Bone-conduction instruments are used only when air-conduction hearing aids are ruled out because of *atresia of the ear canal* or *certain conductive pathologies* like active drainage from the ear, or in situations in which ear disease is activated when an earmold is used.

Surgically Implantable and Bone-Anchored Hearing Aids

Surgically **implantable hearing aids** may be warranted in some patients who have permanent conductive hearing losses, particularly if they cannot use regular hearing aids because of medical considerations such as those mentioned for bone-conduction instruments. Implantable middle ear devices typically attach to the ossicular chain (e.g., Goebel et al 2002; Miller & Sammeth 2002; Spindel 2002; Franz 2007; Traynor & Fredrickson 2007; Bassim & Fayad 2010).

In contrast to the surgically implanted devices, the BAHA bone-anchored hearing aid (**Fig. 15.4**) uses an external bone-conduction device that attaches to a titanium screw implanted in the side of the skull in a manner analogous to dental implants (e.g., Spitzer, Ghossaini, & Wazen 2002; Wazen, Spitzer, Ghossaini, et al 2003; Bosman, Snik, Mylanus, & Cremers 2006, 2009; Pfiffner, Caversaccio, & Kompis 2011; Colquitt,

---

[1] Ching, O'Brien, Dillon, et al (2009) suggested it is probably not necessary to be concerned about a child's ability to hear safety-related and warning signals coming from behind because (1) it is unlikely that the directional hearing aid would reduce the sound coming from behind enough for this to occur, and (2) part of the decrease likely would be counteracted by the hearing aid's compression circuit.

a **Titanium Screw**

b

c

Fig. 15.4 The BAHA bone-anchored hearing aid **(a)** is attached to an implanted titanium screw that protrudes through the skin **(b)**. The BAHA can also be worn using a Softband worn around the head, which is shown here with two instruments **(c)**. (Images provided courtesy of Cochlear Americas. © 2014 Cochlear Americas.)

Loveman, Baguley, et al 2011; Janssen, Hong, Chadha 2012; Bosman, Snik, Hol, & Mylanus 2013). The BAHA instrument can be worn with a headband (Softband; **Fig. 15.4c**) by children too young for implantation, others who cannot have the surgery, and during testing and trial periods by patients who are candidates for the device. Bone-anchored instruments offer several advantages over conventional bone-conduction hearing aids, such as the elimination of feedback, headband pressure, and the instability of vibrator positioning, as well as some improvement in high-frequency response and reduced distortion. The BAHA is also useful as an approach to CROS amplification (see below) in cases of single-sided deafness by picking up sounds on the deaf side and transmit-

ting them to the hearing side via bone-conduction (e.g. Hol et al 2010; Snapp, Fabry, Telischi, Arheart, & Angeli 2010; Wazen et al 2010; Desmet, Bouzegta, Hofkens, et al 2012; Pai, Kelleher, Nunn, et al 2012).

Hearing Aid Configurations

Hearing aids can be worn in one or both ears. **Monaural amplification** means that one hearing aid is being used in one ear, and is illustrated in **Fig. 15.5a**. **Binaural amplification** refers to the use of two separate hearing aids, one in each ear (**Fig. 15.5b**), and provides patients with the benefits of binaural hearing. The hallmark of binaural amplification is the use of two independent instruments, which preserves the acoustical differences between signals picked up separately by the two ears, technically known as **dichotic** inputs.

It is also possible to connect the single output of one hearing aid—almost always a body instrument—to both ears with a wire that is split so it can connect to two receivers, as in **Fig. 15.5c**. This configuration is called a **Y-cord** fitting due to the shape of the wire. Here, the two ears are receiving identical (**diotic**) signals instead of the dichotic stimulation that occurs with two independent instruments. For this reason, Y-cord arrangements constitute **pseudobinaural** (as opposed to true binaural) amplification, and their use is discouraged.

Fig. 15.5 also illustrates two kinds of hearing aid configurations that can be used when the patient must rely on just one ear to hear sounds from both sides of the head. The criteria for these configurations are discussed later, but for now let us assume that one ear is completely deaf. In cases like this, sounds coming from the deaf side reach the good ear at a reduced level due to the acoustical shadow cast by the head. This **head shadow effect** is substantial, especially for the frequencies above 1000 Hz, where it grows with increasing frequency and reaches a size of ~ 15 to 20 dB (Shaw 1974).

The **CROS (contralateral routing of signals)** hearing aid (Harford & Barry 1965) picks up sounds with a microphone placed at one ear and transmits the signal around the head via a wire or a radio signal to a second instrument at the *opposite ear*, which receives the amplified sound (**Fig. 15.5d**). For example, sounds picked up by a microphone at the right ear would be delivered via a receiver in the left ear. This arrangement overcomes the head shadow, allowing the left ear to hear sounds originating from the deaf right side. In addition to hearing sound from the impaired side via the hearing aid, the good ear hears other sounds naturally through a large opening in the earmold. **Transcranial CROS** uses cross-hear-

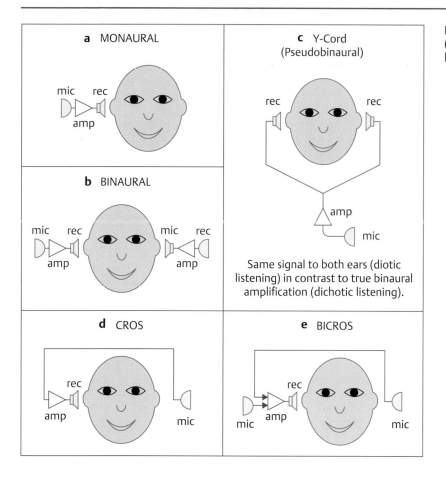

ing to bring sound to the better ear via bone-conduction (e.g., McSpaden & McSpaden 1989; Miller 1989; McSpaden 1990; Chartrand 1991). This can be accomplished with a powerful air-conduction hearing aid (powerCROS), or by using a traditional bone-conduction hearing aid, or, more likely, a BAHA device on the deaf side.

Fig. 15.5e shows a variation of the CROS hearing aid called **BICROS (bilateral CROS)** (Harford 1966). Here, sounds from both sides are picked up by microphones that are located at both ears, and the amplified signals are directed to a single receiver located in just one ear.

Electroacoustic Characteristics of Hearing Aids

Precise terminology is important when dealing with sophisticated devices such as hearing aids. The manner in which hearing aid characteristics are specified is defined in the ANSI S3.22 (2009) standard.[2] In addition to defining terms, the standard also specifies how hearing aid characteristics are to be tested, and gives allowable **tolerances** that tell how closely

a given hearing aid must adhere to the specifications provided by the manufacturer. As a result, we all use the same language, test hearing aids the same way, and know when a hearing aid is operating properly. In addition to audiologists, speech-language pathologists, teachers of the deaf, and others who work with the hearing impaired often need to read hearing aid specifications to understand the functioning (and malfunctioning) of their patient's hearing aids, and must often "translate" this material for others. Parts of this section are a bit technical, but the student will probably find that having some details about the most commonly encountered measurements in an introductory text will serve as a convenient ready reference—if not right away, then surely at some time in the future.

The definitions of a hearing aid's characteristics are closely related to how they are measured. For

---

[2] These measurements are made with pure tone signals. Measurements with a broadband noise signal also may be used when hearing aids have various kinds of adaptive features such as compression, and are addressed in the ANSI S3.42 (2012) standard.

example, we already know that **gain** refers to the amount of amplification or "boost" provided by a hearing aid, defined as the difference between the output level (from the receiver) and the input level (that enters the microphone). Let us see how this is actually done. **Fig. 15.6** shows a conceptualized block diagram of a **hearing aid test system**, and **Fig. 15.7** shows a picture of a commercial system. The hearing aid being tested is located inside a sound-treated test box to minimize the effects of noise in the surrounding room, as shown in **Fig. 15.8**. The test box also contains a loudspeaker that produces test sounds that are picked up by the hearing aid's microphone. The hearing aid's receiver is connected to a **2-cc coupler**, which is a metal cavity with a volume of 2 cc that is designed for testing hearing aids (technically called an **HA1** or **HA2 coupler**, depending on the type being used). There is a measuring microphone at the other end of the coupler that monitors the output of the hearing aid. This arrangement is somewhat reminiscent of that described for earphone calibration in Chapter 4. The measuring microphone leads to instrumentation that analyzes the sounds produced by the hearing aid. In other words, (1) the loudspeaker produces sounds that become the input to the hearing aid; (2) the hearing aid amplifies those

sounds, and its receiver broadcasts its output into the coupler; and (3) the measuring microphone picks up the hearing aid's output in the coupler. The test instrumentation is able to determine what the hearing aid has done to the signal because it controls the loudspeaker (hearing aid input) and also receives the hearing aid's output via the measuring microphone. These measurements can then be viewed on a screen or printed out, usually in the form of a graph. We will review several of the measurements that are made using this kind of a testing system.

Full-on gain means the amount of gain provided by a hearing aid when (1) its volume control is turned up to its highest (hence, full-on) position, and (2) the input signal is 50 dB SPL. As with most measurements done according to this standard, the test range must include the frequencies from at least as low as 200 Hz up to at least 5000 Hz. The hearing aid's output is then measured as a function of frequency over this range.

A convenient summary value called the **high-frequency average (HFA)** is used for most ANSI S3.22 measurements. The HFA is obtained by simply aver-

Fig. 15.6 Artist's conception of the major components of a hearing aid test system.

Fig. 15.7 A typical hearing aid test system.

Fig. 15.8 A hearing aid in the hearing aid test system.

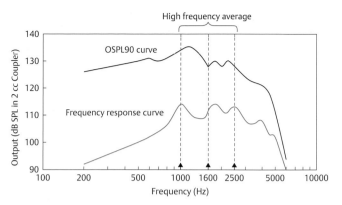

Fig. 15.9 Examples of an OSPL90 curve (above) and a frequency response curve (below) based on ANSI S3.22-2009. The highest point on the OSPL90 curve is called maximum OSPL90. The decibel values of the 1000, 1600, and 2500 Hz points on the OSPL90 curve are averaged to find HFA OSPL90. The average of the three corresponding points on the frequency response curve is 17 dB below HFA OSPL90 at the reference test setting. OSPL90 used to be called SSPL90, and will often be encountered using that terminology.

aging the results obtained at 1000, 1600, and 2500 Hz. The HFA is often provided automatically by commercial hearing aid test systems to make the testing process more convenient and efficient. The HFA full-on gain is simply the average of the amounts of full-on gain obtained at *1000 Hz, 1600 Hz,* and *2500 Hz.* For example, if the full-on gains are 30 dB at 1000 Hz, 34 dB at 1600 Hz, and 36 dB at 2500 Hz, then the HFA full-on gain would be 33 dB. The tolerance for **HFA full-on gain** is ± 5 dB, meaning that a hearing aid's actual HFA full-on gain must be within 5 dB of the value indicated in the manufacturer's specifications. The use of a high-frequency average is sometimes inappropriate, such as when a hearing aid is designed to amplify mainly in the low frequencies. In those cases, the manufacturer may replace the HFA with a **special-purpose average (SPA)** composed of three other frequencies that are appropriate for the hearing aid in question.

Recall that the output sound pressure level represents the maximum output of a hearing aid in dB SPL. Output sound pressure level is determined by turning the hearing aid's volume control to the full-on position and presenting a 90 dB SPL signal from the loudspeaker. This value is called **OSPL90** because we are measuring the OSPL that results from a 90 dB input. Remember that the "90" refers to the 90 dB input, and that the amount of the OSPL90 is the level coming out of the hearing aid (its output). For example, if the 90 dB SPL input causes a hearing aid to produce an output of 129 dB SPL, then the OSPL90 is 129 dB. As for full-on gain, OSPL90 is measured from 200 to 5000 Hz, resulting in an **OSPL90 curve** like the one shown in **Fig. 15.9**. The highest point on the OSPL90

curve is called **maximum OSPL90**, and must be no more than 3 dB higher than the amount shown on the manufacturer's specifications. The **HFA OSPL90** of a hearing aid is obtained by averaging the values of OSPL90 at 1000, 1600, and 2500 Hz. For the OSPL90 curve in the figure, HFA OSPL90 would be (134 + 128 + 128)/3 = 130 dB SPL. The tolerance for HFA OSPL90 is ± 4 dB.

Although OSPL90 and full-on gain tell us the maximum amounts of output and gain provided by a hearing aid, patients rarely set the volume control to the full-on setting. Instead, the patient will actually set the volume control to a lower position, where the amount of gain provided is termed "use gain." Moreover, we do not want the volume control set so high that the peaks of a conversational speech will exceed the hearing aid's maximum output. Conveniently, the volume control position that accomplishes this goal also tends to approximate the setting actually used by the patient. To determine what this setting should be, we must consider the level of conversational speech, which is typically the sound of most interest to the patient. The *average level* of conversational speech is ~ 65 dB SPL (at 1 meter from the talker) and the *peaks* of the speech signal are ~ 12 dB higher. Thus, we need to set the volume control so that the sound coming from the hearing aid will not exceed OSPL90 when the input signal is 65 + 12 = 77 dB SPL. This volume control setting is called the **reference test setting (RTS)** and is formally defined as the *volume control position where the high-frequency average gain (HFAG)* *for a 60 dB SPL input signal is 77 dB below OSPL90* (i.e., where HFAG$_{60}$ = OSPL90 – 77 dB).

How do we find the RTS? We already know HFA OSPL90, which is 130 dB SPL in the above example. Hence, we are looking for the volume control setting that causes an HFAG of 130 – 77 = 53 dB. We begin by turning the hearing aid volume control to some "guesstimated" position, close the test box, and push the button that causes the loudspeaker to present 60 dB SPL test tones. Commercial testing systems can automatically present the three needed tones (1000, 1600, and 2500 Hz) and even calculate the resulting HFAG. We then compare this value to the desired amount (53 dB in our example). If we are off by more than 1.5 dB, then we open the test box, readjust the hearing aid volume control a bit (downward if the result was too high, upward if it was too low), close the box, and press the button to repeat the test. This process continues until we find the volume control setting that gives the desired HFAG (77 dB below HFA-OSPL90 within ± 1.5 dB). This position is the reference test setting, and is used for the remainder of the tests.

The amount of gain provided by a hearing aid when it is at the reference test setting is called its **reference test gain (RTG)**. However, tolerances are not specified for RTG because ANSI S3.22 considers it to be used for information purposes as opposed to a standard for assessing the instrument's performance.

The lower curve in **Fig. 15.9** is the hearing aid's **frequency response curve**, and is obtained by measuring the output as a function of frequency from 200 to 5000 Hz with a 60 dB SPL input (or 50 dB for AGC aids) and the volume control in the reference test setting. Before we can address tolerances for the frequency response curve, an intermediate step is needed so that they will be meaningful. The **frequency range** is determined from the frequency response curve as shown in **Fig. 15.10** by (1) calculating a HFA from the 1000, 1600, and 2500 Hz points on the frequency response curve; (2) measuring down to a point 20 dB below this HFA; and (3) drawing a horizontal line. This horizontal line will intersect the frequency response curve at two points, called the *low-frequency cutoff* (f$_1$) and the *high-frequency cutoff* (f$_2$). The frequency range is the distance between these two points (from f$_1$ to f$_2$), and no tolerances apply to it. The tolerances are different for the lower- and higher-frequency parts (bands) of the curve: (1) ± 4 dB for the lower band, which includes the frequencies from 1.25f$_1$ or 200 Hz (whichever is higher) up to 2000 Hz; and (2) ± 6 dB for the higher band, which includes the frequencies from 2000 Hz up to 0.8f$_2$ or 4000 Hz (whichever is lower).

A **reference test gain curve** can be obtained at the reference test setting by plotting the frequency response curve in terms of *decibels of gain* rather

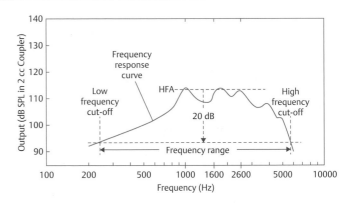

Fig. 15.10 The frequency range is obtained from the frequency response curve, as shown.

than in dB SPL (**Fig. 15.11**), although this is not part of the standard per se. It is usually provided by the hearing aid test system at the touch of a button, and is very useful because it directly shows the amount of amplification provided by the hearing aid (in the 2-cc coupler) on a frequency-by-frequency basis.

The quality of amplification is adversely affected by **distortion** or **noise** produced by the hearing aid. **Harmonic distortion** occurs when the output contains spurious signals at multiples (harmonics) of the input signal. Suppose the input is a 500 Hz tone and the output includes 500, 1000, and 1500 Hz. The 500 Hz signal is the fundamental frequency or first harmonic, and would be the only frequency present in a "perfectly clean" output. The output at 1000 Hz is second harmonic distortion (a spurious signal generated at twice the fundamental, 2 × 500 Hz), and 1500 Hz is third harmonic distortion (3 × 500 Hz). The **percentage of total harmonic distortion (%THD)** may not exceed the manufacturer's specifications by

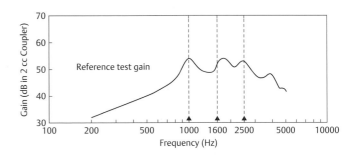

Fig. 15.11 The reference test gain curve shows the frequency response in decibels of gain instead of dB SPL, and represents the amount of amplification provided by the hearing aid (in a 2 cc coupler) on a frequency-by-frequency basis.

more than 3%. It is measured[3] while the hearing aid is at its reference test setting These measurements are done at 500 Hz and 800 Hz using 70 dB SPL input signals, and at 1600 Hz using a 65 dB SPL input.

Equivalent input noise (EIN) is a measure of the noise generated by the hearing aid at the reference test setting based on a comparison of the outputs when there is an input signal and when there is no input signal.[4] A hearing aid's EIN may not exceed the manufacturer's specifications by more than 3 dB.

Several special tests are required for AGC hearing aids. Recall that the input-output function shows how the output of a hearing aid increases as the input level is raised (as in **Fig. 15.2**). With the volume control set to the reference test setting, input-output curves are measured for input levels from 50 to 90 dB SPL in 5dB steps at one or more frequencies (250, 500, 1000, 2000, and/or 4000 Hz). The hearing aid's **input-output function** is compared with the curve in the manufacturer's specifications by lining them up at the point corresponding to the 70 dB input. The output values for the hearing aid must be within ± 5 dB of those in the specifications.

Level changes occur all the time in the real world, such as when a talker suddenly raises his voice to emphasize a point, when a loud drum beat occurs during a musical piece, or when a truck backfires. Instead of acting instantaneously when the input level rises, there will be a delay before the hearing aid's AGC circuit actually reduces the gain in response to the higher level, called **attack time**. Similarly, there will be also be a delay before the gain returns to its original amount after the louder input ends, called **release time**. Attack time is measured by abruptly increasing the input signal from 55 to 90 dB SPL, and measuring how long it takes for the output to stabilize at the level associated with the 90 dB

input (± 3 dB). Release time is measured by abruptly decreasing the input signal from 90 to 55 dB SPL, and measuring how long it takes for the output to stabilize at the level associated with the 55 dB input (± 4 dB). Attack and release times must be within ± 50% or ± 5 ms (whichever is larger) of the manufacturer's specifications.

Telecoil performance is tested by measuring the hearing aid's output in response to a magnetic signal instead of sound. To do this, the hearing aid is switched to the telecoil (T) setting and the volume control is placed in the reference test setting. The hearing aid is placed on a **telephone magnetic field simulator (TMFS)**, which produces the magnetic test signal, and a frequency response curve is obtained. This curve is called a **SPLITS curve** because it shows the *s*ound *p*ressure *l*evel (SPL) as a function of frequency produced by the hearing aid when it is activated by an *i*nduction *t*elephone *s*imulator (ITS). Averaging the values at 1000, 1600, and 2500 Hz gives us the **HFA SPLITS** for the hearing aid, which must be within ± 6 dB of the manufacturer's specifications. Finally, the hearing aid's **simulated telephone sensitivity (STS)** is determined by subtracting reference test gain plus 60 dB (already known from previous measurements) from the HFA SPLITS. The STS gives us an idea of how the hearing aid's gain using the telecoil compares to its normal gain.

Two-cc coupler measurements are excellent for their intended purposes, which involve the reliable determination of hearing aid operating characteristics. However, 2 cc couplers do not replicate the acoustics of the human ear, and the arrangement in the test box certainly does not replicate how sounds are affected by the human head and body. These characteristics are closely replicated by using another kind of coupler called the **Zwislocki ear simulator** (Zwislocki 1971) that is mounted in the ear of a dummy that acoustically mimics the human head and torso, like the **Knowles Electronics Manikin for Acoustic Research (KEMAR)** (Burkhard & Sachs 1975). This type of system is shown in **Fig. 15.12**, and is very useful when it is necessary to make electroacoustic measurements that simulate real-world conditions (ANSI S3.35 2010).

---

[3] For the math-minded student, %THD is found using Method A,

$$\%THD = 100 \sqrt{\frac{\left(p_2^2 + p_4^2 + p_4^2 + \ldots\right)}{p_1^2}}$$

or Method B,

$$\%THD = 100 \sqrt{\left(p_2^2 + p_4^2 + p_4^2 + \ldots\right) / \left(p_1^2 + p_2^2 + p_3^2 + \ldots\right)}$$

where p_1 is the actual pressure (not SPL in dB) of the first harmonic (fundamental), p_2 is the pressure of the second harmonic, etc. The formula $p = 20 \, \mu Pa \times antilog_{10}(dBSPL/20)$ is used to convert dB SPL into pressure (p). Method A must be used whenever %THD exceeds 30%.

[4] For the math-minded, EIN = $HFAG_{50}$ − 50 dB SPL, where $HFAG_{50}$ is the HFA gain obtained with a 50 dB SPL input signal.

Real-Ear Measurements

The measurements described so far tell us how the hearing aid is working as an electroacoustic instrument. But how do we determine whether the hearing aid is actually providing the prescribed amplification performance to a specific, real patient? To do this, actual hearing aid performance must be determined with the hearing aid on the patient herself. The

Fig. 15.12   (a) The KEMAR manikin. (b) A hearing aid being tested on KEMAR. (Photographs courtesy of G.R.A.S. Sound & Vibration A/S.)

nature of these real-ear hearing aid measurements are specified in ANSI standard S3.46 (2013).

The major aspects of a typical real-ear measurement system are shown in **Fig. 15.13**. A sound field loudspeaker is used to present the stimulus sounds, which are picked up by specially placed measurement microphones, to be described momentarily. The core of the system is a computer that controls the loudspeaker and analyzes the sounds monitored by the microphones. The results are displayed on a screen, and can be printed out as desired. Many commercially available systems are programmed to provide a variety of prescription formulas, making it very easy to compare actual hearing aid performance with the prescribed targets.

The key aspect of the real-ear system involves the use of two microphones mounted on the head. One is called the **reference microphone**, which picks up sounds outside the ear, very close to the hearing aid's microphone just before they enter the hearing aid. The other microphone is the **probe microphone**. Even though this microphone is physically located outside the ear, it is connected to a fine pliable **probe tube** that is inserted into the ear canal, with its tip within a few millimeters of the eardrum. The probe tube and microphone (hereafter called the probe

tube) therefore monitor the sound as it is actually received by the eardrum.

Two different kinds of measurements are made with the probe tube system just described. The first measurement is made *without* the hearing aid. The stimulus from the loudspeaker is picked up by both the reference microphone and the probe tube. The reference microphone monitors the signal before it enters the ear canal and the probe tube monitors the signal at the eardrum. The signal will usually be ~ 12 to 17 dB stronger in the 2700 to 5000 Hz range at the eardrum (probe tube) compared with outside the ear (reference microphone). This boost is due to the **ear canal resonance** explained in Chapter 2. The first measurement is called the **real-ear unaided response (REUR)**, and is retained in the memory of the analysis system.

The second measurement is made *with* the hearing aid in the ear. The real-ear system assembly is left in place and the hearing aid is inserted into the patient's ear, being careful not to crimp or displace the probe tube. The probe tube now extends beyond the inside (receiver) end of the hearing aid, so that it monitors the output of the hearing aid that is actually being received by the patient's eardrum. The stimulus signal is then presented from the loudspeaker.

Probe-tube system with unoccluded ear canal

External reference microphone

Stimulus loudspeaker

Ear canal

Eardrum

Probe microphone and probe tube

Real-ear measurement system

Probe-tube system with a hearing aid in place

External reference microphone

Stimulus loudspeaker

Ear canal

Eardrum

Probe microphone and probe
Tube extending beyond hearing aid

Real-ear measurement system

Fig. 15.13 Conceptual representation of real-ear measurements.

The reference microphone monitors the input to the hearing aid, and the probe tube monitors the output of the in-place hearing aid at the eardrum. The difference between them is automatically calculated by the analysis system, and is called the **real-ear aided response (REAR)**.

It would seem that the REAR represents the actual gain provided by the hearing aid. However, let us not forget that a certain amount of gain is provided by the ear canal resonance *without* the hearing aid, represented by the REUR that was previously measured and is being kept in the system's memory. Hence, to arrive at the true gain being provided by the hearing aid, the real-ear system must subtract the unaided response from the aided response. The resulting *true gain* is called the **insertion gain** or **real-ear insertion gain (REIG)**, and the curve showing insertion gain as a function of frequency is the **real-ear insertion response (REIR)**.

We verify whether a hearing aid is providing the patient with the intended amount of amplification by comparing the real-ear insertion gain with the prescribed insertion gain target values based on the prescription method being used. Real-ear measurements are not limited to gain. For example, probe tube measurements also allow us to determine the OSPL90 at the patient's eardrum, which is shown as a function of frequency by the **real-ear saturation response (RESR)**. The phrase *saturation response* here reflects the influence of the term *saturation sound pressure level* (SSPL), which was used before the term was changed to OSPL in the ANSI S3.22 standard. Just as the REIR is compared with prescribed insertion gain target values, the RESR is compared with prescribed target values for OSPL90 at the eardrum. Notice that the patient does not have to do anything except quietly sit still while the measurements are being made. Moreover, we can almost instantly view the results of any number of hearing aid adjustments on the patient. This is a priceless capability when verifying, fine-tuning, or modifying a hearing aid fitting.

The **real-ear to coupler difference (RECD)** is the difference between a real-ear measurement and the equivalent measurement made in a 2-cc coupler (real-ear value minus coupler value). The use of RECDs is especially important when dealing with infants and young children, whose small ears cause them to receive much higher sound levels than an adult fitted with the same hearing aid electroacoustics (e.g., Moodie, Seewald, & Sinclair 1994; Tharpe, Sladen, Huta, & McKinley Rothpletz 2001; Bagatto, Scollie, Seewald, Moodie, & Hoover 2002; AAA 2013).

Functional Gain

The amount of amplification provided by a hearing aid can also be tested behaviorally using **aided thresholds** and/or **functional gain measurements**. Aided thresholds are simply the patient's sound field thresholds while using her hearing aid. Functional gain is simply the difference between the patient's aided and unaided sound field thresholds at each frequency. For example, if an unaided threshold is 55 dB HL and the aided threshold is 30 dB HL, then the functional gain is 55 – 30 = 25 dB. Unfortunately, this approach lacks many of the advantages of real-ear measurements, and also is susceptible to measurement errors and reliability issues (e.g., Hawkins, Montgomery, Prosek, & Walden 1987; Humes & Kirn 1990). These concerns are especially problematic with children, for whom functional gain is not the recommended approach for verifying hearing aid fittings (AAA 2013). However, it is sometimes useful to convert insertion gain measurements into aided thresholds for counseling purposes, such as explaining amplification to the patient.

■ Study Questions

1. Define and explain the following terms with respect to hearing aids: (a) input, (b) output, (c) microphone, (d) receiver, (e) amplifier, (f) telecoil, (g) earmold.

2. Define gain, maximum power output (or output sound pressure level), and saturation.

3. Explain the difference between linear amplification and compression amplification.

4. Define/describe the following types of hearing aids: (a) monaural, (b) binaural, (c) CROS, (d) BICROS, (e) directional, (f) digital, (g) programmable.

5. What are bone-conduction hearing aids and when are they used?

6. What is the high-frequency average (HFA)?

7. Define OSPL90 and how it is determined.

8. Define the reference test setting and how it is determined.

9. What is the frequency response curve of a hearing aid and how is it obtained?

10. Explain the nature of real-ear (probe tube) measurements and why they are used.

References

American Academy of Audiology (AAA). 2013. Clinical Practice Guidelines: Pediatric Amplification. Available at http://www.audiology.org/resources/documentlibrary/Documents/PediatricAmplificationGuidelines.pdf

American National Standards Institute (ANSI). 2009. ANSI S3.22-2009. American National Standard Specification of Hearing Aid Characteristics. New York, NY: ANSI

American National Standards Institute (ANSI). 2010. ANSI S3.35-2010. American National Standard Method of Measurement of Performance Characteristics of Hearing Aids under Simulated Real-Ear Working Conditions. New York, NY: ANSI

American National Standards Institute (ANSI). 2012. ANSI/ASA S3.42-1992 (R2012). American National Standard Testing Hearing Aids with a Broad-Band Noise Signal. New York, NY: ANSI

American National Standards Institute (ANSI). 2013. ANSI/ASA S3.46-2013. Methods of Measurement of Real-Ear Performance Characteristics of Hearing Aids. New York, NY: ANSI

Bagatto M, Scollie S, Seewald R, Moodie K, Hoover B. Real-ear-to-coupler difference (RECD) predictions as a function of age for two coupling procedures. J Am Acad Audiol 2002;13:416–427

Bassim MK, Fayad JN. Implantable middle ear hearing devices: a review. Semin Hear 2010;31(1):28–36

Bosman AJ, Snik AFM, Hol MKS, Mylanus EAM. Evaluation of a new powerful bone-anchored hearing system: a comparison study. J Am Acad Audiol 2013;24(6):505–513

Bosman AJ, Snik AFM, Mylanus EA, Cremers CW. Fitting range of the BAHA Cordelle. Int J Audiol 2006;45(8):429–437

Bosman AJ, Snik FM, Mylanus EA, Cremers WR. Fitting range of the BAHA Intenso. Int J Audiol 2009;48(6):346–352

Branda E. Deep canal fittings: advantages, challenges, and a new approach. Hear Rev 2012;19(4):24–27

Burkhard MD, Sachs RM. Anthropometric manikin for acoustic research. J Acoust Soc Am 1975;58(1):214–222

Chartrand MS. Transcranial or internal CROS fittings: evaluation and validation protocol. Hear J 1991;44:24–28

Chasin M. The acoustic advantages of CIC hearing aids. Hear J 1994;47:13–17

Ching TY, O'Brien A, Dillon H, et al. Directional effects on infants and young children in real life: implications for amplification. J Speech Lang Hear Res 2009;52(5):1241–1254

Colquitt JL, Loveman E, Baguley DM, et al. Bone-anchored hearing aids for people with bilateral hearing impairment: a systematic review. Clin Otolaryngol 2011;36(5):419–441

Desmet J, Bouzegta R, Hofkens A, et al. Clinical need for a BAHA trial in patients with single-sided sensorineural deafness. Analysis of a BAHA database of 196 patients. Eur Arch Otorhinolaryngol 2012;269(3):799–805

Franz D. The middle-ear implant: new solutions for complex challenges. Hear Rev 2007;14(4):42–44

Goebel J, Valente M, Valente M, Enrietto J, Layton KM, Wallace MS. 2002. Fitting strategies for patients with conductive or mixed hearing losses. In: Valente M, ed. Strategies for Selecting and Verifying Hearing Aid Fittings, 2nd ed. New York, NY: Thieme; 272–286

Gudmundsen GI. Fitting CIC hearing aids—some practical pointers. Hear J 1994;47(10):45–47

Harford E. Bilateral CROS: two sided listening with one hearing aid. Arch Otolaryngol 1966;84(4):426–432

Harford E, Barry J. A rehabilitative approach to the problem of unilateral hearing impairment: the contralateral routing of signals (CROS). J Speech Hear Disord 1965;30:121–138

Hawkins DB, Montgomery AA, Prosek RA, Walden BE. Examination of two issues concerning functional gain measurements. J Speech Hear Disord 1987;52(1):56–63

Humes LE, Kirn EU. The reliability of functional gain. J Speech Hear Disord 1990;55(2):193–197

Janssen RM, Hong P, Chadha NK. Bilateral bone-anchored hearing aids for bilateral permanent conductive hearing loss: a systematic review. Otolaryngol Head Neck Surg 2012;147(3):412–422

Johnson EE, Ricketts TA, Hornsby BW. The effect of digital phase cancellation feedback reduction systems on amplified sound quality. J Am Acad Audiol 2007;18(5):404–416

Killion MC. The K-amp hearing aid: an attempt to present high fidelity for persons with impaired hearing. Am J Audiol 1993;2:52–73

Kirkwood DH. Bucking bad economic news, hear aid sales rise by 5.4% on way to record year. Hear J 2007;60(12):11–16

Kuk F, Keenan D, Lau CC, Ludvigsen C. Performance of a fully adaptive directional microphone to signals presented from various azimuths. J Am Acad Audiol 2005;16(6):333–347

Hol MKS, Kunst SJW, Snik AFM, Bosman AJ, Mylanus EAM, Cremers CWRJ. Bone-anchored hearing loss (BAHA) in patients with acquired and congenital unilateral inner ear deafness (BAHA CROS): clinical evaluation of 56 cases. Ann Otol Rhinol Laryngol 2010;119:447–454

Leavitt R, Welch C, Thompson CR. Invisible in-the-canal hearing aids and deep-canal fittings: medical and audiological concerns. Audiol Today 2013;25(4):36–42

McSpaden JB. One approach to a unilateral "dead" ear. Audecibel 1990;39:32–34

McSpaden JB, McSpaden CH. A method for evaluating the efficacy and effectiveness of transcranial CROS fittings. Audecibel 1989;38:10–14

Miller AL. An alternative approach to CROS and bi-CROS hearing aids: an internal CROS. Audecibel 1989;39:20–21

Miller DA, Sammeth CA. 2002. Middle ear implants: an alternative to conventional amplification. In: Valente M, ed. Strategies for Selecting and Verifying Hearing Aid Fittings, 2nd ed. New York, NY: Thieme; 287–310

Moodie KS, Seewald RC, Sinclair ST. Procedure for predicting real-ear hearing aid performance in young children. Am J Audiol 1994;3:23–31

Mueller HG. Small can be good too! Hear J 1994;47:11

Pai I, Kelleher C, Nunn T, et al. Outcome of bone-anchored hearing aids for single-sided deafness: a prospective study. Acta Otolaryngol 2012;132(7):751–755

Pfiffner F, Caversaccio MD, Kompis M. Comparisons of sound processors based on osseointegrated implants in patients with conductive or mixed hearing loss. Otol Neurotol 2011;32(5):728–735

Ricketts TA. Directional hearing aids: then and now. J Rehabil Res Dev 2005;42(4, Suppl 2):133–144

Ricketts T, Dittberner AB. 2002. Directional amplification for improved signal-to-noise ratios: strategies, measurements, and limitations. In: Valente M, ed. Hearing Aids: Standards, Options and Limitations, 2nd ed. New York, NY: Thieme; 274–346

Ricketts T, Henry P. Evaluation of an adaptive, directional-microphone hearing aid. Int J Audiol 2002;41(2): 100–112

Ricketts TA, Hornsby BWY. Directional hearing aid benefit in listeners with severe hearing loss. Int J Audiol 2006;45(3):190–197

Ricketts T, Mueller HG. Making sense of directional microphone hearing aids. Am J Audiol 1999;8(2): 117–127

Ross M. That old familiar squeal: acoustic feedback cancellation systems and open-ear hearing aid fitting. Hear Loss Mag 2006;27(5):20–25

Shaw E. Ear canal pressure generated by a free sound field. J Acoust Soc Am 1974;56:1848–1861

Snapp HA, Fabry DA, Telishi FF, Arheart KL, Angeli SI. A clinical protocol for predicting outcomes with an implantable prosthetic device (BAHA) in patients with single-sided deafness. J Am Acad Audiol 2010;21: 654–662

Spindel JH. Middle ear implantable hearing devices. Am J Audiol 2002;11(2):104–113

Spitzer JB, Ghossaini SN, Wazen JJ. Evolving applications in the use of bone-anchored hearing aids. Am J Audiol 2002;11(2):96–103

Strom KE. The hearing care market at the turn of the 21st century. Hear Rev 2000;7:8–22, 100

Tharpe AM, Sladen D, Huta HM, McKinley Rothpletz A. Practical considerations of real-ear-to-coupler difference measures in infants. Am J Audiol 2001;10(1): 41–49

Traynor RM, Fredrickson JM. (2007). The future is here: the Otologics fully implantable hearing system. http://www.audiologyonline.com/articles/article_detail.asp?article_id=1903. Retrieved Dec. 21, 2007

Valente M. 2000. Use of microphone technology to improve user performance in noise. In: Sandlin R, ed. Textbook of Hearing Aid Amplification: Technical and Clinical Considerations. San Diego, CA: Singular; 247–284

Walden BE, Surr RK, Cord MT, Dyrlund O. Predicting hearing aid microphone preference in everyday listening. J Am Acad Audiol 2004;15(5):365–396

Wazen JJ, Spitzer JB, Ghossaini SN, et al. Transcranial contralateral cochlear stimulation in unilateral deafness. Otolaryngol Head Neck Surg 2003;129(3):248–254

Wazen JJ, Van Ess MJ, Alameda J, Ortega C, Modisett M, Pinsky K. The BAHA system in patients with single-sided deafness and contralateral hearing loss. Otolaryngol Head Neck Surg 2010;142(4):554–559

Wu Y-H, Stangl E, Bentler RA, Stanziola RW. The effect of hearing aid technologies on listening in an automobile. J Am Acad Audiol 2013;24(6):474–485

Zwislocki J. 1971. An Ear-Like Coupler for Earphone Calibration. Lab of Sensory Communication Report LSC-S-9. New York, NY: Syracuse University

16 Audiological Management II

The previous chapter covered the basic concepts and technical considerations involved with hearing aids. We will now continue with our coverage of audiological management with a discussion of the use of hearing aids within the overall framework of audiological management, and will then continue to discuss cochlear implants, hearing assistance technologies, intervention approaches, and tinnitus management.

The primary step in audiological management involves determining the need for amplification, and then providing the patient with it, always staying mindful of the fact that the hearing aid is *part* of the *aural rehabilitation* process, and not an end unto itself. This concept is by no means limited to hearing aids, but applies equally to cochlear implants, hearing assistance technologies, and tinnitus management. In each case, the overall process involves considerations of the patient's *candidacy* for intervention; the *selection* of the instrument; *verification* of its fit, functioning, and ability to provide the prescribed characteristics; and *validation* of the patient's performance; as well as *counseling, monitoring,* and *follow-up.*

■ Candidacy for Audiological Intervention

Who is a candidate for audiological interventions, such as amplification? The consensus of current opinion is that any patient complaining of auditory difficulties in communicative situations should be viewed as a potential candidate for audiological intervention, such as hearing aids or other kinds of assistive devices (e.g., Hawkins, Beck, Bratt, et al 1991). Clearly, the patient should have some degree of hearing loss, and the need for amplification unquestionably rises as the degree of hearing loss worsens. Hence, it is easy to say that a patient with a pure tone average (PTA) or speech recognition threshold (SRT) of 50 dB HL in both ears needs a hearing aid. But let us see what happens when we play the "countdown" game: Is a hearing aid needed at 45 dB? Absolutely. At 40 dB? Yes. At 35 dB? Of course. At 30 dB? Sure. How about 25 dB or 20 dB? Well, uh . . . Notice how we quickly reach a range of losses where we cannot definitively say "yes" or "no." One of the reasons for hedging on the answer is that the overall degree of hearing loss is only one of the many variables to be considered. For example, hearing losses typically increase with frequency, so a patient can have quite a nasty hearing impairment even though the PTA and/or SRT may be just 10 dB (or even zero). Then, of course, there is the issue of unilateral and asymmetrical impairments: Does Mrs. Jones need a hearing aid if her right ear has a 50 dB loss but her left ear is normal? What about Mr. Smith, who has a 60 dB loss in the right ear and a 30 dB loss in the left?

Complicating matters is the distinction between the *need for amplification* due to the extent and impact of the auditory deficit versus how much *benefit the patient experiences* from the hearing aid. When the hearing loss is moderate to severe, unaided speech communication is belabored or impossible (*need*), and this situation improves appreciably albeit not totally when hearing aids are worn (*benefit*). What's more, the improvement is readily appreciated by the patient and by others. However, the need for amplification can be ambiguous in cases considered to be marginal because of a mild, high-frequency, or unilateral loss. Here the degree to which the hearing loss affects speech communication is often subtle, inconsistent, and situational, depending on such factors as speaking level, whether there are background or competing noises, and the communicative demands of the patient's occupational and social interactions.

The benefits of amplification can be similarly subtle and inconsistent in patients with marginal impairments, so that a patient may need a hearing aid but perceive little or no benefit from it. However, little perceived benefit does not mean no benefit. The subtle benefits of amplification often become apparent when the patient forgets to bring his hearing aid to an important meeting or must do without the instrument while it is being repaired. At the opposite extreme, patients with profound losses have the greatest need for hearing aids, but they often receive relatively little benefit in terms of auditory speech reception because their residual auditory capability is often minimal. Again, however, remember that limited benefit for the purpose of hearing speech is not the same as no benefit at all. On the contrary, patients with profound losses benefit considerably from their hearing aids in terms of the ability to hear for alerting, warning, and emergency signals, and as an aid to lipreading.

Clearly, hearing aid candidacy depends on more than auditory status alone, and is particularly affected by the patient's communicative requirements and the need to rely on auditory information. Other motivational factors interact with the hearing loss to induce the patient to see an audiologist, and then to follow the recommendation to obtain hearing aids and to use them. Some of the major factors that appear to motivate patients to obtain a hearing aid for the first time include communication problems at home, in noisy listening situations, in social situations, and at work, as well as encouragement by the spouse (Bender & Mueller 1984). In fact, Palmer, Solodar, Hurley, Byrne, and Williams (2009) showed that self-assessed hearing ability was a strong predictor of whether many patients will actually purchase hearing aids. Just one question is required: "On a scale from 1 to 10, 1 being the worst and 10 being the best, how would you rate your overall hearing ability?" (p. 342). Most patients with ratings of 1 to 5 actually obtained hearing aids and most with ratings of 8 to 10 did not; but instrument purchases were 50-50 for those who rated their hearing ability at 6 or 7.

Acceptance of the hearing impairment itself and of the need for clinical assistance to deal with it also weighs heavily in the patient's decision to obtain amplification. A patient in one of the "marginal" categories is often not willing to accept himself as hearing impaired, let alone so much so that amplification is needed. This is particularly true when the loss has developed slowly and insidiously over a long period of time.

Special candidacy issues come into play with pediatric patients, and it is essential for comprehensive intervention including appropriate amplification to be introduced as soon as possible (e.g., PWG 1996; JCIH 2007, 2013; AAA 2013). It is important to be mindful that infants and children are in the process of developing auditory skills, speech, language, and world knowledge. Thus, the hearing-impaired child is faced with a double challenge because (1) development in these areas relies heavily on auditory input, and (2) she cannot depend on linguistic and world knowledge to make up for missed sounds. At this point, it important to mention a large-sample prospective study by Ching, Dillon, Marnane, et al (2013) because it overcame many of the limitations of prior studies that failed to provide cogent support for early intervention for young children with prelingual hearing loss (see, e.g., Puig, Municio, & Medà 2005; Wolff et al 2010). They found that better speech/language and related performance in prelingually hearing-impaired 3-year-olds was significantly associated with (1) cochlear implants that were turned on at an earlier date, (2) less severe hearing losses, (3) no other disabilities, (4) female gender, and (5) higher maternal education.[1] The significant impact of cochlear implants highlights the efficacy of early intervention with children with severe and profound losses. In fact, delaying cochlear implantation from 10 months to 24 months was associated with a dramatic decrease in performance scores at age 3.

In addition to the considerations already discussed, hearing-impaired infants and children are also candidates for amplification if they have unilateral and/or mild losses, or permanent conductive losses, as well as for a trial period with hearing aids when cochlear implants are being considered and in cases of auditory neuropathy syndrome disorder (see, e.g., GDC 2008; Roush, Frymark, Venediktov, & Wang 2011; AAA 2013).

Functional Assessment Scales

How the patient experiences hearing difficulty as well as a variety of nonauditory factors enter into audiological management, involving a host of social, emotional, occupational, health, and other issues. In addition to addressing hearing disorders in terms of *structure* and *function*, contemporary thinking focuses upon restrictions of *activities* (task performance) and *participation* in day-to-day situations (e.g., WHO 2001; ASHA 2004), and *health-related quality of life* (AAA 2006a,b). In fact, amplification improves one's health-related quality of life by mitigating the social and psychologi-

---

[1] It might seem odd that earlier versus later hearing aid fitting is missing from the list. However, this makes sense when we realize that most of the children with hearing aids had mild or moderate losses, so that they may have been benefiting from auditory stimulation before receiving their aids, and may not have been enrolled in programs working on auditory skill development over time (Ching, Dillon, Marnane, et al 2013).

cal impact of hearing impairment, at least for adult patients (Hnath-Chisolm, Johnson, Danhauer, et al 2007). Because of all of these factors, self-assessment scales play a central feature in assessing the impact of hearing impairment, candidacy for hearing aids and other treatment approaches, and validating the outcomes of audiological management (e.g., ASHA 1998; AAA 2006a, 2011a, 2013).

Functional assessment or **self-assessment scales** and questionnaires are valuable tools for identifying the nature and scope of a patient's communicative and related problems. These measures are also known as **outcome assessment scales** because they are also used for ascertaining the effects of intervention as experienced by the patient. **Table 16.1** shows representative scales typically used with adults and the topics they address, and many of the scales used with infants and children are shown in **Table 16.2**. In addition to describing the direct communicative impact of the hearing loss, many of these instruments also provide insights about its psychological, social, and vocational impact upon the patient. In addition, some instruments assess the impact of a patient's hearing impairment upon the quality of life experienced by the spouse (see, e.g., Scarinci, Worrall, & Hickson 2009; Preminger & Meeks 2012).

Most self-assessment instruments present statements or questions to which the patient must reply along a scale describing how common or true a situation is, how much difficulty or benefit is experienced, or how much he agrees or disagrees with what it says. For example, he might reply on a scale of 1 to 5 (or 1 to 3, 1 to 7, etc.) from "always" to "never," "very little" to "very much," or "completely agree" to "completely disagree."

The information derived from self-assessment scales helps define the kinds of rehabilitative efforts needed by isolating specific problems and difficult environmental situations; it also provides us with a basis for counseling the patient and significant persons in her life. In addition, the outcome of a hearing aid fitting or other aspects of the rehabilitation process can be validated by comparing self-assessment scales administered before and after intervention, as well as over the course of the management program. Some scales ask the patient to indicate several areas of concern or special relevance to his own situation, which become the basis for assessing intervention outcomes. Self-assessment scales are also used in the audiological evaluation process, as well as in hearing screening programs.

Binaural versus Monaural Amplification

The hearing-impaired listener should be provided with usable binaural hearing whenever possible. The desirability of binaural amplification reflects several advantages of binaural hearing compared with monaural hearing (Valente 1982; deJong 1994; Gelfand 2010): Binaural summation results in an advantage over monaural listening corresponding to ~ 3 dB at threshold and ~ 6 dB at suprathreshold levels. Binaural difference limens for both frequency and intensity are smaller (better) than the corresponding values for monaural hearing. Binaural hearing maximizes directional hearing ability (e.g., sound localization) and alleviates the head shadow effect. In addition, binaural listening reduces the adverse effects of noise and reverberation on speech intelligibility in real-world listening conditions.

For practical purposes, this means that binaural amplification is preferred over a monaural hearing aid for most patients with bilateral hearing losses, and many patients with unilateral hearing losses should benefit from the use of a hearing aid in the impaired ear. Binaural amplification clearly is the recommended protocol for children, including bimodal stimulation for children using a cochlear implant in one ear if the opposite has any residual hearing (AAA 2013). The term **bimodal** refers to the use of a cochlear implant in one ear and a hearing aid in the other ear. As one would expect, there are cases where binaural amplification is contraindicated, and these are discussed below.

There is also a compelling negative reason to choose binaural amplification whenever possible. Silman, Gelfand, and Silverman (1984) demonstrated that adults with bilateral sensorineural hearing losses who use monaural hearing aids can develop an **auditory deprivation effect** in which speech recognition scores deteriorate over time in their *unaided* ears even though intelligibility scores remain unchanged in their aided ears. In contrast, binaural hearing aid users do not experience a speech recognition deficit in either ear. This phenomenon has been corroborated by numerous studies in both adults (e.g., Gelfand, Silman, & Ross 1987; Stubblefield & Nye 1989; Silverman & Silman 1990; Silman, Silverman, Emmer, & Gelfand 1992; Hurley 1993, 1999; Gelfand 1995; Silverman, Silman, Emmer, Schoepflin, & Lutolf 2006), and children (Gelfand & Silman 1993). Once a patient has developed an auditory deprivation effect, adding a second hearing aid to the previously unfitted ear may reduce or alleviate the problem in many but not all cases (Silverman & Silman 1990; Silman et al 1992; Hurley 1993; Gelfand 1995). In addition, some patients actually reject a second hearing aid even though the auditory deprivation effect has been reduced or eliminated by its use (e.g., Hurley 1993).

The foregoing discussion demonstrates that binaural hearing aids should be the first consideration for patients with bilateral hearing losses. This conclusion agrees with the consensus of opinion in

Table 16.1 Characteristics of several self-assessment instruments

Scale	Author(s)	Characteristics assessed
Abbreviated Profile of Hearing Aid Performance (AP-HAB)	Cox & Alexander (1995)	Abbreviated version of PHAB addressing ease of communication, reverberation, background noise, aversiveness of sounds.
Attitudes toward Loss of Hearing Questionnaire, v. 2.1 (ATLH)	Saunders, Cienkowski, Forsline, & Fausti (2005)	Hearing loss denial; negative associations; negative coping strategies; manual dexterity and vision; hearing-related esteem.
Client Oriented Scale of Improvement (COSI)	Dillon, James, & Ginis (1997)	Patient nominates up to five specific situations of concern in order of importance, before treatment. Each situation is rated according to (a) how much better/worse and (b) ease of communication, after treatment.
Communication Profile for the Hearing Impaired (CPHI)	Demorest & Erdman (1986)	25 scales addressing communicative performance, importance, environment, strategies, personal adjustment, response biases.
Communication Scale for Older Adults (CSOA)	Kaplan, Bally, Brandt, Busacco, & Pray (1997)	Communication strategies, communication attitudes; for use with non-institutionalized elderly adults.
Expected Consequences of Hearing Aid Ownership (ECHO)	Cox & Alexander (2000)	Patient expectations about hearing aids in terms of (a) acoustical benefits, (b) service and cost, (c) negative features, (d) psychosocial implications.
Glasgow Hearing Aid Benefit Profile (GHABP)	Gatehouse (1999)	Addresses initial disability, handicap, hearing aid usage, hearing aid benefit, residual disability, and satisfaction for each of four situations plus four additional situations nominated by the patient.
Hearing Handicap Inventory for Adults (HHIA)	Newman, Weinstein, Jacobson, & Hug (1991)	Modification of HHIE for use with non-elderly adults.
Hearing Handicap Inventory for Elderly (HHIE)	Ventry & Weinstein (1982)	Social-situational, emotional.
Hearing Impairment Impact—Significant Other Profile (HII-SOP)	Preminger & Meeks (2012)	Impact of hearing loss on *spouse's* quality of life: emotions and relationship, social impact, spouse's communication strategies.
International Outcome Inventory for Hearing Aids (IOI-HA)	Cox & Alexander (2002)	Patient rates hearing aid outcome experience based on daily usage, benefit derived, continuing activity limitations, satisfaction, continuing participation limitations, impact on others, quality of life.
Profile of Hearing Aid Performance (PHAB)	Cox, Gilmore, & Alexander (1991)	Situations involving familiar talkers, ease of communication, reverberation, reduced cues, background noise, aversiveness of sounds, distortion of sounds.
Satisfaction with Amplification in Daily Live (SADL)	Cox & Alexander (1999)	Global (overall) satisfaction with hearing aid, positive effects, service and cost, positive image, negative features.
Self-Assessment of Communication (SAC); Significant Other Assessment of Communication (SOAC)	Schow & Nerbonne (1982)	Communication situations, feelings, opinions about others' views. SOAC completed by familiar other.
Significant Other Scale for Hearing Disability (SOS-HEAR)	Scarinci, Worrall, & Hickson (2009)	Impact of hearing loss on *spouse's* quality of life: communication changes; communicative burden; relationship changes; going out and socializing; emotional reactions; concern for partner.
Speech, Spatial and Qualities of Hearing Scale (SSQ)	Gatehouse & Noble (2004)	Addresses both static and dynamic listening conditions. *Speech hearing* section includes quiet, noise, reverberation, multiple talkers, selective/shifting attention). *Spatial hearing* section includes direction, distance, motion. *Other qualities* section includes sound recognition, segregation, clarity, naturalness, listening effort.

Table 16.2 Examples of functional assessment scales that may be used for outcome assessment in infants and children

Scale	Authors	Age range	Respondent
Auditory Behavior in Everyday Life (ABEL)[a]	Purdy, Farrington, Moran, Chard, & Hodgson (2002)	3–6 years	Parent
Children's Abbreviated Profile of Hearing Aid Benefit (CA-PHAB)[a]	Kopun & Stelmachowicz (1998)	> 6 years	Parent/child
Children's Home Inventory of Listening Difficulties (CHILD)[a]	Anderson & Smaldino (2000)	3–6 years	Parent
Children's Outcome Worksheets (COW)	Williams (2004)	Unspecified	Parent
Classroom Participation Questionnaire (CPQ)	Antia, Sabers, & Stinson (2007)	Grades K–12	Child
Client Oriented Scale of Improvement for Children (COSI-C)[a]	National Acoustics Laboratory (2000)	> 6 years	Child
Developmental Index of Audition and Listening (DIAL)[a]	Palmer & Mormer (1999)	< 3 years	Parent
Early Listening Function (ELF)	Anderson (2002)	≤ 3 years	Parent
Functional Auditory Performance Indicators (FAPI)[a]	Stredler-Brown & DeConde (2003)	< 3 years	Parent
Hearing Performance Inventory for Children (HPIC)[a]	Kessler, Giolas, & Maxon (1990)	> 6 years	Child
Infant-Toddler Meaningful Auditory Integration Scale (IT-MAIS)[a]	Zimmerman-Phillips, Osberger, & Robbins (1998)	< 3 years	Parent
Listening Inventory for Education (LIFE)[a]	Anderson & Smaldino (1998, 1999)	> 6 years	Child/teacher
LittlEARS[a]	Kühn-Inacker, Weichbold, Tsiakpini, Coninx, & D'Haese (2003)	< 3 years	Parent
Meaningful Auditory Integration Scale (MAIS) [a]	Robbins, Renshaw, & Berry (1991)	3–6 years	Parent
Meaningful Use of Speech Scale (MUSS)[a]	Robbins, Svirsky, Osberger, & Pisoni (1998)	3–6 years	Parent
Parents' Evaluation of Aural/Oral Performance of Children (PEACH)[a]	Ching & Hill (2007)	All	Parent
Screening Instrument for Targeting Educational Risk in Pre-School Children (Preschool SIFTER)[a]	Anderson & Matkin (1996)	Age 3–grade K	Teacher
Screening Instrument For Targeting Educational Risk (SIFTER)[a]	Anderson (1989)	Grades K–5	Teacher
Screening Instrument for Targeting Educational Risk in Secondary Students (Secondary SIFTER)	Anderson (2004)	Grades 6–12	Teacher
Self-Evaluation of Listening Function (SELF)[a]	Ching, Hill, & Dillon (2008)	> 6 years	Child
Teachers' Evaluation of Aural/Oral Performance of Children (TEACH)[a]	Ching, Hill, & Dillon (2008)	All	Teacher

[a]Scales included in the AAA (2013) pediatric amplification guidelines. In these cases, the age ranges in this table are consistent with but not necessary identical to those recommended in these guidelines.

the field (e.g., Hawkins et al 1991; PWG 1996; AAA 2013). However, binaural amplification is not always the best overall choice for every patient. For example, Walden and Walden (2005) reported that poorer binaural than monaural performance was reported among patients in the 50- to 90-year-old age range. Moreover, some patients experience a **binaural interference effect**, in which the participation of the more impaired ear (as with binaural hearing aids) results in a deterioration of performance rather than an improvement (Jerger et al 1993). In addition, binaural hearing aids may be rejected by the patient due to any number of reasons that might be perceptual, behavioral, physical, cognitive, emotional, and/or financial.

Candidacy for binaural hearing aids becomes less clear when patients have asymmetrical losses, that is, bilateral impairments that are significantly different between the two ears. The "traditional wisdom" was that preference for binaural hearing aids begins to wane when the two ears have pure tone averages that differ by more than 15 dB and/or speech recognition scores that differ by more than 8%; and binaural amplification is progressively less desirable as the inter-ear difference gets wider. It is reasonable to anticipate that patients with large inter-ear differences probably will not have the same chances of success with binaural hearing aids as their counterparts with more symmetric losses. However, there is no reason to rule out binaural amplification without even a try simply because there is a difference between the ears (e.g., Sandlin & Bongiovanni 2002; AAA 2013). Of course, one should be alert to the possibility of the binaural interference phenomenon when binaural hearing aids are rejected or when binaural performance is poorer than that of the better ear alone.

Open-Canal Fittings

Hearing aid fittings that leave the ear canal unoccluded are often considered for patients with sloping sensorineural hearing losses who have good sensitivity in the low frequencies. The basic approach is to use an open earmold or a vent drilled through the earmold, which facilitates high-frequency amplification without also amplifying the low frequencies. This approach has been used for a long time, and was sometimes referred to as **IROS** ("I" for "ipsilateral") on analogy to CROS, although the term is a misnomer. There has been a major increase in the use of open-canal fittings in which mini-BTE hearing aids are connected to the ear with thin tubing. The benefits of open-canal fittings are often enhanced when used with digital feedback cancellation technology

and directional microphones (see, e.g., Fabry 2006; Mueller & Ricketts 2006; Johnson, Ricketts, & Hornsby 2007).

CROS-Type Fittings

The **CROS** hearing aid was introduced for patients who have one normal ear and one substantially impaired ear that is *unaidable* (Harford & Barry 1965). The impaired ear might be unaidable because it is totally deaf or due to a medical condition that precludes the use of a hearing aid, such as chronic drainage. Even an ear with a reasonable amount of residual hearing sensitivity sometimes proves to be unaidable due to, for example, an extremely low speech recognition score. These patients must rely on one ear, which means that sounds originating from the impaired side will be received at a reduced level due to the head shadow. Depending on the communicative and other demands of their work and social environments, some individuals in this situation can function with little or no difficulty by relying on the remaining normal ear, but others experience a considerable disadvantage and need assistance to hear sounds originating from the impaired side. Imagine, for example, the disadvantage experienced by an executive who cannot hear the people sitting to her left at a business meeting, or a taxi driver with a deaf right ear who cannot hear his passengers.

The "good ear" does not have to be normal for CROS to be used. Instead, CROS can also be used if there is a high-frequency sensorineural hearing loss in the better ear (Harford & Dodds 1966), In fact, it appears that the chances of success with CROS are best when there is a mild to moderate hearing loss above 1500 Hz in the better ear, and are only minimal when it is normal (Valente, Valente, Enrietto, & Layton 2002). This arrangement works for two reasons. First, the open earmold facilitates amplification of the high frequencies without boosting the lows. Second, placing the microphone and receiver in separate ears avoids the acoustic feedback problem that is likely to occur when the microphone and receiver are able to communicate via an open earmold in the same ear. This arrangement minimizes feedback by increasing the distance between the microphone and receiver and taking advantage of the head shadow effect.

Another approach to unilateral hearing loss, often called **transcranial CROS,** involves directing stimuli from the deaf side to the hearing ear via bone-conduction using a conventional bone-conduction hearing aid, a powerful air-conduction hearing aid, or a BAHA device, worn on the deaf side (e.g., Valente et al 2002; Spitzer, et al 2002; Wazen, et al 2003; Hol, Kunst, Snik, & Cremers 2010).

The **BICROS** arrangement is considered when the patient has an unaidable poorer ear for any of the above-mentioned reasons, as well as a hearing loss that can benefit from a hearing aid in the better ear (Harford 1966). It is easiest to think of this arrangement as a regular hearing aid in the better ear, with its own microphone, receiver, and the appropriate kind of earmold (instead of an open CROS-type earmold), plus an additional "off-side" microphone that is located at the unaidable poorer ear on the other side of the head.

Reported outcomes with CROS and BICROS amplification have been rather mixed (e.g., Gelfand 1979; Cashman, Corbin, Riko, & Rossman 1984; Ericson, Svärd, Högset, Devert, & Ekström 1988; Hill, Marcus, Digges, Gillman, & Silverstein 2006; Lin et al 2006; Hol et al 2010; Taylor 2010). However, it is noteworthy that Williams, McArdle, and Chislom (2012) found that user performance and satisfaction improved when previously used BICROS instruments were replaced with newer ones employing state-of-the-art technology.

Prefitting Considerations

The first steps in the process of providing the patient with amplification include patient assessment (see Candidacy for Audiological Intervention, above), obtaining medical clearance, and providing the patient with initial counseling. The purpose of the medical clearance is to meet legal and regulatory requirements and to be sure no medical prob-lems exist that would contraindicate a hearing aid or would create the need for special considerations. Otologic and related pathologies are discussed in Chapter 6. Initial counseling should address such issues as the reasons for amplification and other aural rehabilitation services that might be indicated; the kinds of instrument(s) that are appropriate; the reasons for preferring binaural amplification, if appropriate; and realistic goals and expectations regarding what hearing aids can and cannot do. Other issues often discussed at this point revolve around such practical matters as the costs involved, where the instrument can be purchased, the 30-day trial period, batteries, instrument warrantees, and insurance. The patient, his family, and other pertinent individuals (caregivers, etc.) should have a clear and realistic understanding of these issues so they can be active participants in the audiological management process, of which the hearing aids are an important part (ASHA 1998; AAA 2006a). Earmold impressions might be taken at this point or at a subsequent time, depending on the kinds of instruments being considered and who will be dispensing them. These issues are included in the early phases of both the ASHA (1998) and AAA (2006a) guidelines summarized in **Table 16.3** and **Table 16.4**.

Instrument Selection/Evaluation/Fitting

The process of providing the patient with amplification has been described by various terms over the years, such as *hearing aid evaluation, hearing aid con-*

Table 16.3   Some features of the ASHA (1998) hearing aid guidelines for adults

Stage	Description
Assessment	Determine nature and magnitude of hearing loss. Assess hearing aid/rehabilitation candidacy based on audiometric data, self-assessment protocols, etc. Consider patient's unique circumstances (e.g., physical status, mental status, attitude, motivation, sociological status, communication status).
Treatment planning	Audiologist, patient, and family/caregivers review findings to identify needs, arrive at rehabilitative goals, plan intervention strategies, understand treatment benefits/limitations/costs and how outcomes are assessed.
Selection	Hearing aid(s) selected in terms of electro-acoustic (e.g., frequency gain, OSPL90, input-output function) and other (monaural/binaural; style and size, etc.) characteristics.
Verification	ANSI S3.22 measurements (hearing aid electro-acoustics) and real-ear measurements (e.g., prescriptive targets, performance on patient). Physical and listening checks for physical fit, intermittencies, noisiness, etc. Determine whether audibility, comfort, and tolerance expectations are met.
Orientation	Counseling on hearing aid use and care, realistic expectations, etc.; explore candidacy for hearing assistive technology, audiologic rehabilitation assessment, and further intervention.
Validation	Assess intervention outcomes, reduction of disability, goals addressed using such measures as self-assessment tools, objective or subject's measures of speech perception, other means.

Table 16.4 Some features of the AAA (2006a) Audiological Management Guidelines for Adults

Feature	Description
Assessment and goal setting	Auditory assessment and diagnosis. Self-perception of communication needs using self-assessment instruments. Assess non-auditory needs. Set treatment goals. Determine medical referral/clearance needs.
Technical aspects of treatment	*Hearing aid selection* Make sure hearing aids include specified features and meet quality standards before the fitting appointment. Hearing aid fitting and verification of comfortable fit, prescribed gain, OSPL90, etc., preferably using probe microphone and simulated real ear methods, absence of occlusion effect or feedback problems, consideration of hearing assistive technology.
Orientation	A significant other should be involved if possible. Provide device-related information. Discuss goals, expectations, wearing schedule, adjusting to hearing aid use in various settings, effects of various environments, listening strategies, speechreading, monaural versus binaural amplification, post-fitting issues.
Counseling and follow-up	Provided to new hearing aid users; offered to experienced users. Primary communication partner should be included if possible. Discuss topics pertaining to hearing mechanism, hearing loss and effects including speech in noise, approaches and strategies for minimizing these issues, care and use of hearing aids; possibility of adjustment/acclimatization period before full benefits are apparent; realistic expectation; community resources.
Assessing outcomes	Analogous to validation stage in ASHA (1996). Use of objective measures (e.g., speech recognition tests) and subjective measures (e.g., self-assessment instruments). Determine extent to which goals have been achieved, including effects on communication, activity and participation limitations, and quality-of-life issues.

sultation, *hearing aid selection*, and *hearing aid fitting*. The nature of the fitting process has evolved over the years and continues to do so, and no one method is applicable in all cases, let alone universally accepted. Contemporary approaches implicitly accept a concept that has traditionally been called *selective amplification*. This term originally meant that the amount of gain at each frequency should depend on the degree and configuration of the patient's hearing loss. A more modern definition would say that the hearing aid's electroacoustic characteristics should be chosen or adjusted so that they are most appropriate for the nature of the patient's hearing loss. The selective amplification concept is so ingrained in modern clinical philosophy that the term itself is rarely used anymore. However, the student should be aware that this was not always the case. For example, the influential Harvard (Davis, Stevens, Nichols, et al 1947) and MedResCo (1947) reports concluded that most patients could be optimally fitted with a hearing aid that has a flat or slightly rising frequency response, so that an individualized selection process would be superfluous in all but unusual cases. The

ensuing controversy lasted for decades (see, e.g., Levitt, Pickett, & Houde 1980). As already indicated, individualized hearing aid selection has proven to be the accepted approach, although numerous different methods have been proposed to accomplish this. These methods can be categorized into two broad groups, which we will call the comparative and prescriptive approaches.

Comparative Hearing Aid Evaluations

The traditional **hearing aid evaluation (HAE)** used to involve preselecting several hearing aids that appeared to be appropriate for the patient on the basis of her electroacoustic specifications, and then comparing the patient's performance with each of them using a variety of speech tests presented from loudspeakers. The procedure originally described by Carhart (1946) began with unaided measurements of SRT, the tolerance limit for speech, and a speech recognition score, followed by a series of tests with each of the hearing aids being compared. These tests began by finding the volume control setting where the patient judged speech presented at 40 dB HL to be comfortably loud. This was followed by finding SRTs and tolerance limits at the comfort and full-on gain settings, the signal-to-noise ratio that rendered speech at 50 dB HL barely audible, and speech recognition scores.

The extensive testing involved in the **original Carhart method** quickly led to abbreviated versions, generically known as **comparative hearing aid evaluations** or **modified Carhart methods**. In a typical evaluation, the patient would be tested with each hearing aid to obtain an SRT and speech recognition scores for words presented in quiet and/or against a background of noise. Other methods compared hearing aids based on quality and/or intelligibility judgments (e.g., Punch & Beck 1980; Punch & Parker 1981; Neuman, Levitt, Mills, & Schwander 1987; Cox & McDaniel 1989; Surr & Fabry 1991; Kuk 1994). The hearing aid with the best speech recognition score (or judgment rating) was chosen for the patient. This was often followed by a short trial period with the hearing aid. The patient then purchased an instrument of the same make and model, and would subsequently return to the clinic to determine whether the purchased instrument provided adequate performance.

Comparative HAEs have been abandoned in favor of prescriptive methods, principally because speech recognition tests could not distinguish among hearing aids adequately and reliably. For example, Walden, Schwartz, Williams, Holum-Hardegen, and Crowley (1983) found that the mean difference in speech recognition scores for words presented in noise was only 4.3% among acoustically similar hearing aids. In addition, only 4.5% of the score differences were large enough to be significant on an individual-patient basis.[2] This was the same situation involved in a real-world comparative HAE, where the audiologist preselected several appropriate (hence similar) instruments to compare behaviorally on the patient. In other words, speech recognition scores were unable to distinguish among the instruments being compared. Moreover, the hearing aid with highest speech recognition score was not always the one judged best by a patient after a trial period of actual use.

The comparative HAE approach also had practical limitations: In-the-ear instruments do not lend themselves to comparative assessments because they are custom-ordered. Also, programmable instruments have multiple settings for different listening conditions, so that comparative assessments between instruments are simply unrealistic.

---

[2] The mean difference was only 14.2% even for dissimilar hearing aids, for which fewer than half of the differences were significant on an individual-patient basis.)

Prescriptive Hearing Aid Fitting

Contemporary hearing aid fittings involve **prescriptive methods** in which "formulas" are used to prescribe the amplification characteristics considered to be most appropriate for a patient. The very idea of using formulas to prescribe gain might seem strange. After all, we know from common experience that eyeglasses often restore "20-20" visual acuity. Consequently, it would seem that the amount of gain should be equal to the amount of hearing loss because this would restore 0 dB HL thresholds. This notion would be a great idea except for the fact that it is wrong. Equating gain with the amount of loss invariably results in too much amplification, subjecting the patient to excessive amounts of loudness and distortion, and placing the patient at risk for developing a noise-induced hearing loss. In fact, if we try to give patients too much gain, they often negate the intent by turning down the volume control, and may even reject amplification altogether. If the goal of amplification is not to restore normal hearing, then, alas, what is the goal? The answer is to provide the amount and configuration of gain that maximizes the audibility of conversational speech without making the amplified signal uncomfortably loud. Skinner (1988) described this gain configuration as the one that provides the patient with the best compromise between maximum speech intelligibility and acceptable sound quality.

Hearing aid prescription formulas are really explicitly described sets of rules used to determine the amounts and configurations of gain and output sound pressure level that are most desirable for the patient (the *selection* stage in **Table 16.3** and the *technical aspects* section in **Table 16.4**). The American Academy of Audiology (AAA 2013) stressed the importance of providing *audibility for speech over a wide range of input levels* in the context of fitting infants and young children, but this goal is clearly desirable for older children and adults as well. Depending on which prescriptive method is used, the formula might use the patient's thresholds, comfortable listening levels, and/or loudness discomfort levels as a function of frequency. This information might come from the patient's audiogram, specially administered tests, or a combination of the two. Reviews of this topic and summaries of prescriptive formulas for adults and children are available in several sources (e.g., Skinner 1988; Mueller, Hawkins, & Northern 1992; PWG 1996; Traynor 1997; Valente 2002; Dillon 2012). The student should keep in mind that existing prescriptive approaches are revised and new methods are introduced from time to time, and that different prescriptive methods can recommend different gain configurations for the same patients.

The approaches described by Watson and Knudsen (1940) and by Lybarger (1944) might be considered the prototypes for prescriptive hearing aid fittings. Lybarger's (1944) more widely known *half-gain rule* recommended setting the hearing aid's gain to 50% of the patient's hearing loss at each frequency (except 500 Hz, where 30% gain was used). On the other hand, the method recommended by Watson & Knudsen (1940) essentially involved setting the gain at each frequency so that the speech would approximate the equal-loudness-level curve that was most comfortable for the patient. Since then, many methods have been proposed that prescribe amplification characteristics based on unaided thresholds and/or suprathreshold measures, and also account for a wide range of considerations such as severe to profound hearing loss, conductive components, and the capabilities of modern programmable instruments (e.g., McCandless & Lyregaard 1983; Byrne & Dillon 1986; Libby 1986; Schwartz, Lyregaard, & Lundh 1988; Berger, Hagberg, & Rane 1988; Byrne, Parkinson, & Newall 1990; Killion 1996; Seewald et al 1997; Dillon 1999a,b, 2006; Scollie, Seewald, Cornelisse, et al 2005; Byrne, Dillon, Ching, Katsch, & Keidser 2001; Keidser, Dillon, Dyrlund, Carter, & Hartley 2011; Keidser, Dillon, Carter, & O'Brien 2012; Johnson 2013). Some prescriptive methods attempt to prescribe the gain configuration needed to place the *long-term average speech spectrum* at the listener's MCL or approximately midway between the patient's thresholds and loudness discomfort levels (e.g., Shapiro 1976, 1980; Bragg 1977; Cox 1988; Skinner 1988), or to levels 10 dB below the patient's LDLs for most frequencies. Another protocol uses thresholds and loudness judgments, and attempts to enable the patient to experience soft sound levels as audible and soft, average sound levels as comfortable, and high sound levels as loud but not uncomfortably loud (e.g., Cox 1995; Valente & Van Vliet 1997).

In addition to the desired amount of gain as a function of frequency, it is also important to prescribe OSPL90 values that do not exceed the patient's loudness discomfort levels. Output sound pressure levels can be prescribed based on loudness discomfort level measurements (using, e.g., narrow-band noises or warble tones) or employing various estimating procedures (e.g., Cox 1983, 1985; Hawkins, Walden, Montgomery, & Prosek 1987; PWG 1996; Cox, Alexander, Taylor, & Gray 1997; ASHA 1998; Dillon & Storey 1998; Storey, Dillon, Yeend, & Wigney 1998; Dillon 1999a; Keidser et al 2011, 2012; Johnson 2013).

The prescription may also be viewed in terms of **targets**. For example, the targeted frequency response expresses the amount of gain that we want delivered to the patient's eardrum at each frequency. Similarly, maximum output is also prescribed in terms of target values for OSPL90 at the patient's eardrum. The ideal hearing aid would be the one that actually provides these targeted values. To achieve this goal with BTE and body hearing aids, the clinician selects a stock instrument based on the information provided in the manufacturer's specifications book. For ITE and canal aids, the audiologist places a customized order with the manufacturer, who then fabricates an instrument using electronic and acoustical methods that should provide the prescribed characteristics.

It is important to be aware that hearing aid manufacturers commonly use their own proprietary fitting protocols. However, the preferred practice is for audiologists to use prescriptive targets based on an appropriately chosen, well-documented prescriptive method. This is especially important with children (AAA 2013). Also, programmable hearing aids make it possible to use different prescriptions based on the listening situation. For example, children might switch between hearing aid settings based on the *NAL-NL1* (Byrne et al 2001) and *DSL[i/o]* (Seewald et al 1997) prescriptions depending on whether the listening situation is quiet or noisy (Ching, Scollie, Dillon, et al 2010; Scollie, Ching, Seewald, et al 2010).

Verification

Verification of the hearing aid fitting is carried out to confirm that the instrument actually provides the prescribed amplification characteristics and to adjust these as needed, to ensure that it is working without problems (e.g., distortions, noisiness, intermittencies), and to be sure it fits properly and comfortably. (These issues are included in the section on the *verification* stage in **Table 16.3** and in the *technical aspects* section in **Table 16.4**.)

That the instrument actually meets the intended electroacoustic characteristics selected by the audiologist is **verified** by testing the instrument in a hearing aid test box using the measurements described in the ANSI S3.22 (2009) standard and in place on the patient (in situ) using **real-ear (probe-tube) measurements.** These are essential measurements about the hearing aid itself, but they do not tell us what the instrument is doing for the patient. Hence, we must also test the hearing aid *on the patient* to verify that it is actually providing her with the intended performance. The *preferred method* for verifying hearing aid performance with respect to the patient involves **real-ear** or **probe-tube measurements** (PWG 1996; ASHA 1998; AAA 2006a). **Real-ear to coupler differences** (Chapter 15) should be employed with infants and young children (AAA 2013). It is often necessary for the audiologist to "fine-tune" the hearing aid's characteristics to bring them as close as possible to the targeted values. This is done by making program adjustments for programmable instruments, or by adjusting the hearing aid's internal settings for hearing aids that are not programmable.

Validation (Outcome Assessment)

In addition to verifying the adequacy of the fitting in terms of consistency with the prescribed characteristics, it is also necessary to validate the benefits afforded to the patient using appropriate outcomes instruments like those shown in **Table 16.1** and **Table 16.2** (e.g., Hawkins et al 1991; ASHA 1998; AAA 2006a, 2013), corresponding to the *validation* stage in **Table 16.3** and the *assessing outcomes* section in **Table 16.4**. As the tables show, **validation** or **outcome assessment** may be accomplished in a variety of ways that might employ, for example, speech intelligibility tests, quality and/or intelligibility judgments, paired comparisons, or other assessment tools. Notice that speech intelligibility assessment is now used as one of several ways to validate the adequacy of a hearing aid fitting, whereas it was the criterion measure for selecting among instruments in the traditional HAE approach that was used in the past.

■ Post-Fitting Considerations

There is almost always a 30-day trial period during which the patient may elect to return the hearing aid. Although one should not lose sight of the consumer protection aspects of the trial period, it is probably more important for the audiologist and patient to consider it the time when the *orientation stage* (**Table 16.3**) of the hearing aid fitting process takes place. Consequently, the patient should be urged to return for consultation several times during this period, not just at the end; and it is a very good idea to schedule the first follow-up appointment before the patient leaves. Also, it cannot be overstressed that ongoing follow-ups on a regular basis are especially important with children (AAA 2013).

Once the hearing aid fitting has been judged acceptable, the patient and any significant others (family, parents, etc., depending on the specific circumstances) should be instructed about all aspects of the use and care of the instrument. The patient should know how to insert and remove the instrument, use its controls, clean and maintain it, replace batteries, etc. She should understand the goals of amplification, have realistic expectations for what hearing aids can and cannot do, and know the nature of effective listening strategies. These initial clinical counseling activities should also include the consideration of assistive devices and other aural rehabilitation services.

A word about batteries is in order before proceeding. The patient and others who handle the instruments should also be made aware that hearing aid batteries are to be treated as a dangerous poison. This is not an overstatement. Special attention should be given to battery safety (including the use of tamper-resistant battery compartments) with pediatric patients and others who require special supervision. Batteries should be inaccessible to at least younger children as well as to pets. Even adult patients should be counseled about battery safety and to avoid unsafe practices like using their lips as an extra set of hands while changing batteries. Grandparents and other patients without "baby proof" homes should be counseled about battery safely as well, particularly when children might be visiting.

■ Cochlear Implants

Some hearing losses are so extensive that the patient is unable to derive any appreciable benefit from even the most powerful hearing aids. Other types of sensory aids are needed for these patients. **Cochlear implants** attempt to provide the patient with information about sound by converting it into an electrical current, and then using this electrical signal to directly stimulate any remaining auditory nerve fibers the patient might still have.

Cochlear implants are composed of both internal components that are surgically installed and external devices worn outside the body, as illustrated in **Fig. 16.1**; and examples of contemporary instruments are shown in **Fig. 16.2a–d**. The **external components** include (1) a **microphone** that picks up sound and converts it into an electrical signal, (2) the **speech processor** that analyzes the sound and converts it into a code representing various aspects of the sound, and (3) a **transmitter** that sends the encoded information to the implanted device via an electromagnetic or radiofrequency signal. The **surgically implanted components** include (1) a **receiver** that picks up the signal from the external transmitter and (2) the **electrical stimulator** with its **electrodes** that are inserted into the cochlea. The electrodes send the encoded information to the remaining fibers of the auditory nerve in the form of an electrical signal. In addition, a ground electrode is placed somewhere outside the cochlea, such as in the middle ear. Most contemporary speech processors and microphones are housed in behind-the-ear units like post-auricular hearing aids, which are in turn connected to the external transmitter by a small

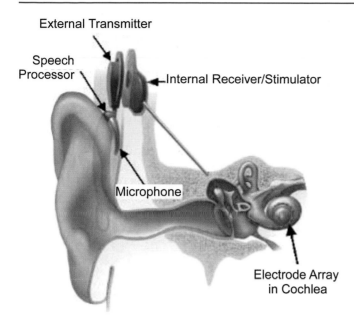

Fig. 16.1 Representation of a cochlear implant in a patient, showing external and implanted components. (Picture courtesy of the National Institutes of Health.)

Fig. 16.2 Examples of cochlear and brainstem implants. (a) Advanced Bionics cochlear implant systems (Neptune freestyle processor at right). (b) MED-EL cochlear implant systems (RONDO self-contained unit at left). (c) Cochlear Americas cochlear implant system. (d) Cochlear Americas hybrid system. (e) MED-EL auditory brainstem implant. (Frame a provided courtesy of Advanced Bionics. Frames b and e provided courtesy of MED-EL. Frames c and d images provided courtesy of Cochlear Americas. © 2014 Cochlear Americas. Used with permission.)

wire, although other arrangements are available. For example, MED-EL's RONDO instrument combines the speech processor and transmitter into one self-contained unit, and the Advanced Bionics Neptune is a "freestyle" speech processor that can be worn in various locations on the head or upper body.

To take advantage of tonotopic organization, cochlear implants have multiple channels to separate the spectrum into frequency bands and multiple electrodes laid out along the cochlea.[3] Depending on the manufacturer, cochlear implants typically have 12 (MED-EL), 16 (Advanced Bionics), or 22 (Cochlear) active electrodes, in addition to ground electrodes. In each case, the electrodes closer to the base of the cochlea represent higher frequencies and those toward the apex represent lower frequencies. In other words, the electrode layout follows the pattern of how frequencies are arranged by place along the cochlea. The cochlear implant's microprocessor analyzes the incoming sound in terms of various

parameters, which are coded into combinations of tiny currents delivered to the electrodes laid out in the cochlea. Various coding strategies are used to represent the speech signal. For example, the patterns of stimulation from the array of electrodes might represent the spectral peaks of the incoming sound, speech features like formants and fricative noises, or the waveform of the incoming signal. Some approaches activate one electrode at a time in rapid succession, whereas other systems activate several electrodes simultaneously. Information about the intensity of a sound is provided by the strength of the current coming from the electrodes.

Cochlear implant technology and clinical applications have been developing rapidly, and this process will continue well into the future. For example, there are ongoing changes in such areas as instrumentation, processing strategies, and candidacy, as well as binaural cochlear implants (combining cochlear implantation with acoustical amplification) and auditory brainstem implants.

Patients can be provided with a combination **of** both electrical and acoustical stimulation in two

---

[3] Early cochlear implants were **single-channel** cochlear implants, exemplified by the 3M/House single-electrode system. This implant treated the sound entering the microphone as a whole, and delivered an electrical signal to the remaining auditory nerve fibers via a single electrode inserted into the scale tympani. The single-channel 3M/House device was discontinued in 1987, and all modern cochlear implants are multiple-channel units.

basic ways, which might be used alone or in various combinations. **Bimodal stimulation** means that the patient is provided with a combination of both electrical and acoustical stimulation. Combined **electric and acoustic stimulation (EAS)** can be accomplished in two basic ways, which might be used alone or in various combinations. One EAS approach is to use a cochlear implant (electrical stimulation) in one ear and a hearing aid (acoustic stimulation) in the other ear, and consequently also provides binaural stimulation. The second bimodal approach involves a **hybrid cochlear implant,** which combines a cochlear implant and a hearing aid in one device that provides both sound and electric stimulation to the same ear. To make this possible, the hybrid device has a shorter electrode array that does not extend as far up the cochlea as regular implants do, which allows the more apical parts of the cochlea to remain intact so that they can respond to sound (e.g., Gantz & Turner 2003, 2004). Overall, the outcomes achieved with binaural and bimodal cochlear implants have been quite successful (e.g., Schafer, Amlani, Seibold, & Shattuck 2007; Wilson & Dorman 2008; Schafer, Amlani, Paiva, Nozari, & Verret 2011)

Auditory brainstem implants deliver the electrical stimulation to the brainstem. The electrode array is arranged on a paddle-shaped silicon holder as shown in **Fig. 16.2e**, and it is usually placed on the cochlear nucleus. Auditory brainstem implants are used when cochlear implants are not possible due to, for example, neurofibromatosis type 2 (NF2) and non-tumor etiologies such as congenital aplasia of the eighth nerve and traumatic injuries. Unlike in Europe, auditory brainstem implants in the United States were limited to adults until clinical trials in children were approved by the Food and Drug Administration in 2013. Early speech perception results with brainstem implants were poor in patients with NF2 compared with those with non-tumor causes, but improved performance in NF2 patients has been reported more recently (e.g., Otto, Brackmann, Hitselberger, Shannon, & Kuchta 2002; Colletti & Shannon 2005; Behr, Müller, Shehata-Dieler, et al 2007; Colletti, Shannon, Carner, Veronese, & Colletti 2009; Skarzyński, Behr, Lorens, Podskarbi-Fayette, & Kochanek 2009; Colletti, Shannon, & Colletti 2012).

Candidacy for Cochlear Implants

A patient's candidacy for a cochlear implant depends on many factors (e.g., Chute & Nevins 2000; ASHA 2004; Waltzman & Roland 2007; AAA 2013). Cochlear implants are currently approved by the Food and Drug Administration (FDA) beginning at 12 months old for children with bilateral profound

sensorineural hearing losses [generally defined as a pure tone average (PTA) ≥ 90 dB HL], and beginning at 18 months of age for those with bilateral severe to profound sensorineural losses (PTA ≥ 70 dB HL). However, cochlear implants can also be used for younger patients and a wider range of losses on an "off-label" basis or in clinical trials; and good results have been obtained for those implanted before 12 months of age (e.g., James & Papsin 2004; Nicholas & Geers 2004; Waltzman 2005; Waltzman & Roland 2005; Lesinski-Schiedat et al 2006; Dettman, Pinder, Briggs, Dowell, & Leigh 2007; Tait, DeRaeve & Nikolopoulos 2007; Ching et al 2013). In addition, children who are candidates for a cochlear implant should be considered for bimodal stimulation (implant in one ear and hearing aid in the other) when there is any residual hearing in the opposite ear (AAA 2013).

Speech perception assessment is a fundamental aspect of cochlear implant use from candidacy decisions through evaluating the effects of intervention. Many speech perception batteries have been developed over the years (e.g., Owens, Kessler, Telleen, & Schubert 1981; Owens, Kessler, Raggio, & Schubert 1985) along with some other selected tests. Other batteries and tests are also available (e.g., Tyler, Preece, & Lowder 1983; Osberger et al 1991; Beiter & Brimacombe 1993; Nilsson, McCaw, & Soli 1996; MSTB 2011), and it is possible to pick and choose among them to formulate the optimum mix for a particular clinical situation.

Speech perception testing for cochlear implants has evolved as the very limited benefits of early single-channel devices have given way to the great potential offered by modern multiple-channel devices and advanced speech processing strategies. To get a flavor for the range of instruments that may be used, we will briefly examine the revised Minimal Auditory Capabilities (MAC) battery, the Monosyllable-Trochee-Spondee test, and the current version of the Minimum Speech Test Battery (MSTB 2011).

The **revised Minimal Auditory Capabilities (MAC) Battery** (Owens et al 1985) exemplified the assessment approaches that were used in the early days of cochlear implantation. As shown in **Table 16.5**, it included 13 auditory-only speech tests arranged in order from easiest to hardest, followed by a visual enhancement test, which also involved lipreading. Several of the tests should be familiar from Chapter 8. Notice that the MAC battery was designed to examine a very wide range of speech perception abilities from simple discriminations among spondee words through open-set monosyllabic speech recognition. In addition, the last test (visual enhancement) was included to ascertain whether the patient's lipreading performance was improved by the addition of auditory cues.

Table 16.5 Description of the subtests of the revised MAC battery[a]

Test name	Description
Spondee Same/Different	Discrimination task in which the patient must indicate whether two spondee words are the same or different.
Four-Choice Spondee	Closed set recognition test in which the patient must identify a spondaic test word from four alternatives.
Noise/Voice	Patient's task must determine whether sounds are noises or the human voice. The stimuli are noises with different spectra and temporal-intensity envelopes (i.e., how intensity varies over time) and sentences spoken by different talkers.
Final Consonants	Closed-set word recognition task in which the patient must identify a monosyllabic test word from four alternatives that have different final consonants (e.g., "rid/rip/rib/ridge").
Accent	Perception of prosody. Four-word phrases are presented in which one word is stressed or accented (e.g., "can you FIX it?"). Patient must select it from four closed-set alternatives.
Everyday Sounds	Open-set task in which the patient must identify familiar sounds (a doorbell, people talking, etc.).
Initial Consonants	Closed-set word recognition task in which the patient must identify a monosyllabic test word from four alternatives that have different initial consonants (e.g., "din/bin/fin/gin").
Question/Statement	Prosody perception task in which the patient must identify phrases as questions (rising inflection) or statements (falling inflection).
Vowels	Closed-set word recognition task in which the patient must identify a monosyllabic test word from four alternatives that have different medial vowels or diphthongs (e.g., "fool/full/fall/foul").
CID Everyday Sentences	Open-set sentence recognition test scored based on key words correctly repeated.
Spondee Recognition	Open-set test in which the patient is asked to repeat each of 25 spondaic words. Half credit is given when one syllable is correct.
Words In Context	Probability-High SPIN sentences are presented. Originally scored based on last word, but scoring was subsequently changed to sentence recognition based on correctly repeated key words. (A key word is considered right as long as its root is correctly identified.)
Monosyllabic Words	Standard monosyllabic word recognition using NU-6 materials.
Visual Enhancement	CID Everyday Sentences (scored by key words) presented (a) visually only (unaided lipreading) and (b) by lipreading plus amplified sound (aided lipreading). Both aided and unaided lipreading are tested to ascertain whether the patient's lipreading performance is enhanced by the auditory cues.

[a]Based on Owens, Kessler, Raggio, and Schubert (1985).

The **Minimum Speech Test Battery (MSTB)** is a contemporary approach for adult cochlear implant patients (MSTB 2011). The MSTB includes the Peterson and Lehiste (1962) CNC word recognition test, given in quiet; the AzBio Sentences (Spahr & Dorman 2004; Spahr, Dorman, Litvak, et al 2012), administered both in quiet and against a background of multi-talker babble; and the Bench-Koval-Bamford Speech-In-Noise (BKB-SIN) test (Etymotic Research 2005). Thus, it provides assessments of the patient's speech perception skills in terms of quiet word recognition, sentence recognition in quiet and noise, and signal-to-noise ratio for sentences. An earlier version of the MSTB (Nilsson, McCaw, & Soli 1996) used the Hearing-in-Noise-Test (HINT) sentences (Nilsson, Soli, & Sullivan 1994); however, they were found to be too easy (Gifford, Shallop, & Peterson 2008) and were thus replaced with the more challenging AzBio sentences. Comparing the MAC battery of the 1980s, which contained several very easy tasks, to the much more demanding focus of the current MSTB illustrates how improved performance with cochlear implants has developed over the years.

When dealing with very limited speech recognition ability, especially in young children, it often becomes important to know whether the patient can at least recognize differences in the temporal or rhythmic patterns of speech. This type of information is provided by the **Monosyllable-Trochee-Spondee (MTS) test** (Erber & Alencewicz 1976), which is often used with cochlear implant batteries or included in them. Recall from Chapter 12 that the MTS uses three kinds of stimulus words that differ with respect to the number of syllables and the stress pattern, including (1) monosyllabic words; (2) spondaic words, which have two equally stressed syllables (e.g., "baseball"); and (3) trochaic words, which have two unequally stressed syllables (e.g., "button"). The test words are presented to the child, who responds by pointing to corresponding pictures. Examining the relationships between the stimulus words and responses reveals whether the child can correctly identify words with different levels of difficulty, and also whether she is able to take advantage of temporal and/or stress patterns in speech.

Typical performance requirements for cochlear implant candidates are (a) ≤ 50% on open-set sentence recognition tests for adults, (b) ≤ 30% on appropriate word recognition tests for children over ~ 24 months of age, and/or (c) a lack of auditory skill development in those too young for speech reception testing (e.g., those up to 24 months old). In the latter case, auditory skill development is assessed using age-appropriate instruments such as the *Infant-Toddler Meaningful Auditory Integration Scale* (IT-MAIS; Zimmerman-Phillips, Robbins, & Osberger 2000) or the *Meaningful Auditory Integration Scale* (MAIS; Robbins, Renshaw, & Berry 1991). Candidates for cochlear implants should typically be receiving only minimal if any benefit from amplification. Implant decisions for infants should include a trial period with hearing aids, if possible (AAA 2013).

Several medical and surgical criteria must be met for cochlear implantation (e.g., Gray 1991; Chute & Nevins 2000; Waltzman & Shapiro 2000). There must be working auditory nerve fibers that can be stimulated by the implant and the existence of the relevant cochlear anatomy. These criteria are met by using high-resolution computerized tomography (CT) scans to rule out such structural abnormalities as cochlear agenesis or dysplagia, or the absence of an auditory nerve. The viability of the remaining auditory nerve fibers can be tested by seeing if an auditory sensation is produced by electrical stimulation of the promontory or round window niche. This procedure involves inserting a needle electrode through the tympanic membrane. The integrity of the existing auditory nerve fibers can also be demonstrated by the presence of low-frequency audiometric thresh-

olds provided they are actually heard as opposed to being tactile responses. In addition to these factors, the patient's general health must be good enough to undergo surgery and general anesthesia.

In addition, the potential complications of cochlear implantation should be discussed with the patient and/or parents. Even though cochlear implant surgery has a relatively low incidence of major complications, they can and do occur (see, e.g., Papsin & Gordon 2007). Bacterial meningitis is a rare but serious potential complication that also needs to be addressed (CDC 2007; FDA 2007). As a result, it has been recommended that (a) children with cochlear implants receive a complete course of meningitis vaccinations, (b) patients and those dealing with them should be able to identify the signs of meningitis so that treatment can be undertaken as early as possible, (c) otitis media be promptly diagnosed and treated, and (d) the prophylactic use of antibiotics be considered during cochlear implant surgery (CDC 2007; FDA 2007).

Realistic expectations play an especially important role in cochlear implant candidacy. The patient and/or parents need to know about the variability of the results and the importance of a strong commitment to training after the device is installed.

After the surgery is completed and healing has occurred, the next step is to program the device for optimal use by the individual patient. The **programming** process is also called **mapping**. Programming involves adjusting the electrical currents produced by the electrodes to yield appropriate thresholds and comfortable listening levels, and allocating frequency bandwidths to the various electrodes. Children often require a period of preprogramming training to teach them the tasks involved in programming the cochlear implant.

Experience with the cochlear implant is essential after it has been installed and programmed. In general, patients should expect to need a minimum of 3 months, and often considerably longer, before they can anticipate reaching the stage where performance levels off (Wilson & Dorman2008). A period of training is highly desirable and often essential; and it can last anywhere from a month or so for adults with adventitious deafness to an extensive and comprehensive long-term intervention program for children with prelingual deafness.

Clinical Outcomes with Cochlear Implants

Let us now look at some of the benefits provided by cochlear implants. Notice that, in general, success with cochlear implants occurs when (1) the onset of the hearing impairment is postlingual rather than prelingual, (2) the duration of deafness is shorter rather than longer, and (3) implantation occurs sooner rather than later.

Although performance varies widely, contemporary cochlear implants provide many adults with *postlingual* deafness considerable speech perception benefits, including open-set recognition performance, which tends to improve with time over the course of about 3 months or so (e.g., Hollow et al 1995; Staller, Menapace, Domico, et al 1997; Geier, Barker, Fisher, & Opie 1999; Rubinstein, Parkinson, Tyler, & Gantz 1999; Waltzman, Cohen, & Roland 1999; Osberger & Fisher 2000; Tyler, Dunn, Witt, & Noble 2007). More or less similar benefits appear to be obtained by elderly patients (e.g., Labadie, Carrasco, Gilmer, & Pillsbury 2000; Francis, Chee, Yeagle, Cheng, & Niparko 2002; Pasanisi, Bacciu, Vincenti, et al 2003; Leung, Wang, Yeagle, et al 2005).

Cochlear implantation is appropriate for children with prelingual hearing impairments as well as those who have postlingual losses (due to, e.g., meningitis). Keeping in mind that performance varies widely, the benefits provided to children by cochlear implants are quite impressive in such areas as speech perception (including open-set speech recognition), speech production, language development, and literacy and academic achievement (e.g., Cohen, Waltzman, Roland, Staller, & Hoffman 1999; Eisenberg, Martinez, Sennaroglu, & Osberger 2000; Geers, Nicholas, Tye-Murray, et al 2000; Meyer & Svirsky 2000; Papsin, Gysin, Picton, Nedzelski, & Harrison 2000; Tyler et al 2000; Teoh, Pisoni, & Miyamoto 2004; Blamey, Sarant, Paatsch, et al 2001; Geers, Nicholas & Sedey 2003; Stacey, Fortnum, Barton, & Summerfield 2006; Geers, Tobey, & Moog 2011). In addition, children and adolescents with cochlear implants provided similar responses to those of their normal-hearing peers on a health-related quality-of-life questionnaire (Loy, Warner-Czyz, Tong, Tobey, & Roland 2010).

The outcomes just described are indeed impressive, and the performance of children with cochlear implants far exceeds what would have been accomplished without them. However, it is essential to reiterate that performance varies widely. It is equally important to realize that although children with cochlear implants often perform similarly to their normal-hearing peers, they still do lag behind them, and that the size of the gap can be on the order of one standard deviation (see, e.g., Geers, Moog, Biedenstein, Brenner, & Hayes 2009; Geers & Hayes 2011; Geers & Sedey 2011; Most, Shina-August, & Meilijon 2010; Ching et al 2013; Guo, Spencer, & Tomblin 2013; Nittrouer, Caldwell, Lowenstein, et al 2013; Nittrouer 2015). Clearly, there is still more to be done.

Performance benefits have been shown to improve with earlier implantation (Fryauf-Bertschy, Tyler, Kelsay, Gantz, & Woodworth 1997; Nicholas & Geers 2004; McConkey Robbins, Koch, Osberger, Zimmerman-Phillips, & Kishon-Rabin 2004; Svirsky, Teoh, & Neuburger 2004; Lesinski-Schiedat et al 2006; Ching et al 2013), the effects of which are enhanced by early identification made possible by universal infant screening programs (Chapter 13) and the trend toward implantation during the first year of life, as noted above. In addition, unlike the leveling off of performance after several months that occurs in adults, children's performance continues to improve with increasing cochlear implant usage over time (e.g., Miyamoto et al 1992; Fryauf-Bertschy et al 1997; Tyler et al 2000).

Until recently, cochlear implants had been placed in just one ear. However, just as we saw that binaural amplification provides advantages over monaural hearing aids, recent studies have shown beneficial outcomes with binaural cochlear implants in both children and adults (e.g., Kühn-Inacker, Shehata-Dieler, Müller, & Helms 2004; Litovsky, Parkinson, Arcaroli, et al 2004; Litovsky, Johnstone, Godar, et al 2006; Verschuur, Lutman, Ramsden, Greenham, & O'Driscoll 2005; Galvin, Mok, & Dowell 2007; Tyler, Dunn, Witt, & Noble 2007). As already pointed out, unilaterally implanted patients should be considered for a hearing aid in the un-implanted ear if it has any residual hearing (AAA 2013).

■ Tactile Aids

Tactile aids are another class of sensory aids for the deaf that use tactile sensations to *substitute* for auditory ones. With tactile aids, sounds are picked up by a microphone, analyzed and encoded by a processor, and then transmitted to the skin using **vibrators (vibrotactile stimulators)** or **electrical (electrotactile** or **electrocutaneous) stimulators**. The stimulators have been worn at various sites, such as the wrist, arm, chest, abdomen, waist, and thighs.

Single-channel tactile devices typically use the incoming speech signal to modulate the vibration, and represent sound amplitude as the strength of the vibration. **Multiple-channel** tactile aids use an array of vibrators laid out on the skin. For example, several stimulators may be arranged in a line, with frequency represented by which vibrators are active, and intensity coded as the strength of the vibration. More complicated representations use a matrix of stimulators in columns and rows, so that the vibratory pattern represents the spectrum of an incoming sound as a graph "drawn" on the skin.

Tactile aids have been studied in some detail (e.g., Sherrick 1984; Hnath-Chisolm & Kishon-Rabin

1988; Cowan et al 1990; Carney et al 1993; Osberger, Maso, & Sam 1993; Weisenberger & Percy 1995; Kishon-Rabin, Boothroyd, & Hanin 1996; Kishon-Rabin, Haras, & Bergman 1997; Sehgal, Kirk, Svirsky, & Miyamoto 1998; Galvin et al 1999; Plant, Gnosspelius, & Levitt 2000; Reed & Delhorne 2003). Although tactile aids are much cheaper than cochlear implants and do not involve surgery, considerable training and practice are needed to make optimal use of the tactual signals. While tactile aids do not enable open-set word recognition for tactual-only stimulation, they do provide the important benefit of lipreading enhancement. In spite of their limitations, one should remember that tactile aids can be desirable for patients who are not candidates for cochlear implants or choose not to have one, and also can be beneficial during the period prior to receiving an implant, for preimplantation training, etc.

■ Room Acoustics

In spite of the benefits provided by their personal hearing aids, hearing-impaired children still have considerable problems communicating in classrooms because of **noise** and **reverberation**. As we will see in the next section, approaches known as hearing assistance technologies are used to minimize these effects and thereby present an optimal signal to each hearing-impaired child (or adult) in the room. Even though we are focusing on the hearing-impaired child trying to listen to the teacher in a classroom, the same issues apply to *all* hearing-impaired persons in *all* noisy and/or reverberant environments, such as theaters, houses of worship, auditoriums, and lecture halls. In fact, hearing assistance technologies are beneficial for a wide range of individuals who may have normal or near normal hearing sensitivity, such as those with auditory processing disorders, developmental disabilities, language and/or learning disorders, and auditory neuropathy spectrum disorder, as well as those operating in their non-native language (e.g., ASHA 2005b; AAA 2007).

Room acoustics have a considerable impact on the effectiveness and quality of communication, and the importance of hearing in all facets of education makes classroom acoustics in particular an area of major concern (e.g., ASHA 2005a,b; Crandell, Smaldino, & Flexer 1997, 2005; Palmer 1997; Rosenberg, Blake-Rahter, Heavner, et al 1999; Crandell & Smaldino 2000; ANSI 2010a,b; Seep et al 2003; Nelson, Soli, & Seltz 2003).

Classroom noise comes from a variety of sources inside and outside the room, with which we are all familiar from common experience. Ambient noise levels vary among public school classrooms, but are typically as high as ~ 60 dB or more (Ross & Giolas 1971; Crandell et al 1997, Rosenberg et al 1999; Crandell & Smaldino 2000; Knecht, Nelson, Whitelaw, & Feth 2002). For example, Knecht et al (2002) found that noise levels in elementary school classrooms ranged from 34.4 to 65.9 dBA; averaging 39.8 dBA in rooms where the heating, ventilation, and air-conditioning (HVAC) systems were off, and 49.7 dBA in rooms where the HVAC systems were on. In addition, Hodgson, Rempel, and Kennedy (1999) found that university classrooms and lecture halls had an average noise level of 44.4 dBA.

Particularly important for speech understanding is the relationship between the levels of the teacher's speech and the noise at the child's ears (or at the microphones of her hearing aids/cochlear implants). Recall that this relationship is a **signal-to-noise ratio (SNR)**. The SNR is often called the **message-to-competition ratio (MCR)** when the noise is a competing speech signal, or the **speech-to-babble ratio (SBR)** when the noise is a babble composed of several voices. Positive SNRs mean that the level of the signal (the speech) is greater than that of the noise, and negative SNRs indicate that the noise is stronger than the speech. For example, a +6 dB SNR means the signal is 6 dB greater than the noise, and a –6 dB SNR means the noise is 6 dB higher than the speech. A 0 dB SNR means the levels of the signal and noise are the same. **Fig. 16.3** illustrates these relationships as well as the manner in which SNR deteriorates with distance from the talker. Notice that the SNR falls from +18 dB immediately in front of the teacher's lips (at 1 foot) to 0 dB at a distance of just 8 feet, and to –6 dB when the child is 16 feet away.

Hearing-impaired persons need higher SNRs than normal individuals to achieve similar levels of performance while listening to speech in noise (Dubno, Dirks, & Morgan 1984; Gelfand, Ross, & Miller 1988). Hearing-impaired children require SNRs of at least +10 to +20 dB for effective classroom performance (Gengel 1971; Finitzo-Hieber & Tillman 1978). Yet typical schoolroom SNRs are often only +1 to +6 dB (Finitzo 1988). In fact, even children who have minimal amounts of sensorineural hearing loss (with pure tone averages between 15 and 30 dB HL) have significantly poorer speech recognition than their normal-hearing counterparts, and the disadvantage becomes greater as the SNR decreases (Crandell 1993), as illustrated in **Fig. 16.4**.

Reverberation is the term used to describe the reflections of sounds from the walls, floors, ceilings, and other hard surfaces in the room. This multiplicity of reflections is perceived as a prolongation of the duration of a sound in a room. It can be heard by sharply clapping one's hands once in a classroom,

Fig. 16.3 Speech level and signal-to-noise ratio (SNR) at various distances from the talker's lips (idealized).

Fig. 16.4 Percent correct speech recognition ability on BKB sentences for children with normal hearing and minimal sensorineural hearing losses (pure tone average 15 to 30 dB HL). (Based on data by Crandell [1993].)

and noticing that the resulting sound lingers after the initial sound. Reverberation is measured in terms of **reverberation time (RT)**, which is the duration of the reflections. Specifically, RT is how long it takes for the reflected sounds to fall to a level that is 60 dB less than the original sound. Typical classroom reverberation times range from ~ 0.2 to roughly 1.3 seconds (Crandell & Smaldino 2000; Knecht et al 2002). Speech recognition is adversely affected by reverberation because the reflections mask the direct sound and also because some speech cues are distorted by their prolongation (Nabelek & Robinette 1978; Gelfand & Silman 1979; Gelfand 2010). Speech perception worsens as reverberation time gets longer and when reverberation is mixed with noise, and the effect is greater for people with hearing loss than it is for those with normal hearing (Gelfand & Hochberg 1976; Finitzo-Hieber & Tillman 1978; Nabelek & Robinette 1978; Yacullo & Hawkins 1987; Crandell & Smaldino 2000). Moreover, it appears that children do not attain adult levels of consonant recognition in noise or reverberation until their early teens, and may not attain adult levels of performance in noise-plus-reverberation until their late teens (Johnson 2000).

The effects of noise and reverberation depend a lot on the distance between the teacher and the child. Let's see why: Under the simplest conditions, sound pressure level drops by 6 dB whenever the distance from the sound source doubles. Suppose the teacher's overall speech level is 78 dB at 1 foot in front of her lips. The speech level will be 72 dB (i.e., 6 dB less) when the distance doubles to 2 feet; then it will drop to 66 dB at 4 feet, 60 dB at 8 feet, and 54 dB at 16 feet. Thus, if the noise level is 60 dB, then the SNR will be 0 dB at a distance of 8 feet and –6 dB at

16 feet from the teacher. The effects of reverberation are also smaller near the teacher's lips and become greater with distance. This is so because the intensity of the original sound is relatively greater than that of the reflections close to the source, whereas the reflections are dominant at some distance away from the source.

The American National Standards for *Acoustical Performance Criteria, Design Requirements, and Guidelines for Schools* (ANSI S12.60-2010 Parts 1 & 2) call for typical classrooms to have a maximum unoccupied noise level of 35 dBA and a maximum reverberation time of 0.6 second. However, the specific criteria depend on factors such as room size, whether there are permanent or relocatable structures, and whether there are core learning spaces (e.g., classrooms) or ancillary ones (e.g., gymnasiums). Some of the key standards that apply to core learning spaces are summarized in **Table 16.6** for permanent classrooms and in **Table 16.7** for relocatable classrooms. Unfortunately, most elementary school classrooms do not appear to meet these guidelines (Knecht et al 2002).

■ Hearing Assistance Technologies

We can now appreciate why a hearing-impaired child experiences so much difficulty listening through her hearing aids in a classroom and other environments. In fact, it is important to stress that the same points presented here in the context of a child in a

Table 16.6 Noise and reverberation requirements for permanent classrooms and other core learning spaces (ANSI S12.60-2010/Part 1)[a]

Noise/reverberation	Requirement	Room size
Background noise	35 dBA or 55 dBC	≤ 20,000 cubic feet (566 m³)
	40 dBA or 60 dBC	> 20,000 cubic feet (566 m³)
Reverberation time	0.6 second	≤ 10,000 cubic feet (283 m³)
	0.7 second	> 10,000 to ≤ 20,000 cubic feet (566 m³)[b]

[a]For rooms that are unoccupied and furnished for these purposes.
[b]No reverberation time requirement for rooms larger than 20,000 cubic feet (566 m³).

classroom actually apply to children and adults alike in all kinds of listening environments, such as theaters, conference rooms, and lecture halls, to name but a few. Hearing aids pick up all sounds present at their microphones, which are located on the child who is sitting in a noisy and reverberant classroom. Thus, the hearing aid delivers a noisy and reverberant signal to the child. The workable solution is to place a microphone close to the teacher's (or other talker's) lips, where her speech is least affected by the acoustics of the room. The signal from this optimally placed microphone can then be amplified and sent directly to receivers in the child's ears. This simple strategy is the basis for a variety of techniques known as **remote microphone hearing assistance technologies** about to be described.

In general, **hearing assistance technologies (HAT)**, also known by terms such as **assistive** or **assistive listening devices**, refer to various kinds of technological approaches (above and beyond hearing aids and cochlear implants) that make the world of sound more accessible. We will concentrate on remote microphone HAT, and will then review some of the other types of devices that are useful for people with hearing losses.

Remote Microphone Hearing Assistance Technologies

Remote microphone hearing assistance technologies are so named because the microphone is not at the patient's ear, but rather is located remotely from the patient at a location close to the teacher's (or other talker's) mouth. The basic components include a microphone near the teacher's mouth, an amplifier with its controls, a mode of transmission from the talker to the listener, and some type of receiver to direct the amplified sound into the listener's ears. To keep the teacher's hands free, most systems use *lapel microphones*, *lavaliere microphones* that hang from a cord around the neck, or *boom microphones* worn

Table 16.7 Noise and reverberation requirements for classrooms and other core learning spaces that can be relocated (ANSI S12.60-2010/Part 2)[a]

Noise/reverberation	Requirement	Room size
Background noise from *exterior* sources	35 dBA	≤ 20,000 cubic feet (566 m³)
Background noise from *interior* sources	41 dBA until 2013 38 dBA as of 2013 35 dBA as of 2017	≤ 20,000 cubic feet (566 m³)
Reverberation time	0.5 second	≤ 10,000 cubic feet (283 m³)
	0.6 second	> 10,000 to ≤ 20,000 cubic feet (566 m³)

[a]For rooms that are unoccupied and furnished for these purposes.

on the head like the ones often used by entertainers and with hands-free telephones. Some systems also include microphones for each child, typically called **environmental microphones**. Environmental microphones permit the children to hear each other, and also allow each child to monitor her own speech. The principal difference among the various types of systems has to do with how the signal from the teacher's microphone is transmitted to the receivers at the children's ears.

At this level, we will review some of the HAT basics. However, as mentioned earlier, it should be stressed that HAT entails an extensive array of clinical considerations and procedures having to do with candidacy, selection, verification, validation, and monitoring. These matters are analogous to those already discussed with hearing aids, but they are not the same. For example, in addition to those with hearing losses, candidates for remote microphone HAT also include individuals with auditory processing disorders, language disorders, learning disabilities, attention deficits, and auditory neuropathy spectrum disorder, as well as those for whom English is not the first language (AAA 2011a). The audiologist also must consider and address a host of issues such as: the type(s) of system(s) to be selected; the clinical and technical considerations and procedures involved in their implementation and use; applicable legal and regulatory matters; and practical issues in the school, home, and community. The interested student will find details addressing these matters for patients from birth to 21 years old in the American Academy of Audiology clinical guidelines for remote microphone for HAT (AAA 2011a,b).[4]

Hard-Wired Systems

The oldest and technologically simplest remote microphone systems involved components that were physically connected by wires. The teacher's microphone was wired to a console containing an amplifier and controls, from which wires went to control boxes and headsets at each of the children's desks. Hard-wired systems can provide high sound levels with good fidelity. They are also relatively low in cost and easy to repair. However, the teacher and students can move no further than the lengths of the cables allow, making them physically restrictive and inflexible.

Although group hard-wired systems are a thing of the past, *personal* systems like the ones shown in **Fig. 16.5** are also available and quite useful. With these devices, the talker speaks into a small, portable microphone/amplifier unit which has a wire that goes to the listener. This cable leads to earphones, or to the patient's hearing via direct audio input or a magnetic inductor. The hard-wired approach is cheaper than personal systems using FM technology, but the wire limits the distance between the talker and listener, and can also be somewhat cumbersome.

Induction Loop Systems

Induction loop classroom amplification systems use a *magnetic signal* to transmit the teacher's speech to the children in the room. The teacher's microphone connects to an amplifier and then to a wire **(induction loop)** that encircles the classroom, as in

Fig. 16.5 Two versions of the Pocketalker personal hardwired system, shown with **(a)** earphones and **(b)** a neck-loop induction coil. (Pictures courtesy of Williams Sound Corp.)

---

[4] These guidelines focus on FM, loop induction, and classroom audio distribution systems. As of this writing, detailed procedures are available for FM systems (AAA 2011a) and classroom audio distribution systems (AAA 2011b). A supplement addressing loop induction systems is currently in preparation.

Induction loop around the room

Fig. 16.6   An induction loop system transmits a magnetic signal to those wearing hearing aids with telecoils or special induction receivers. In the system shown here, the teacher uses a wireless microphone/transmitter that sends an FM radio signal to an amplifier, which is in turn connected to the induction loop around the room.

Fig. 16.6. The induction loop sends a magnetic signal into the room, which is then received by the telecoil of each child's hearing aid. Thus, the child's hearing aid becomes the final amplification device and receiver in induction loop systems (although special induction receivers are also available). This is made possible by switching the hearing aid to its "T" position to receive the signal from the induction loop, or to the "MT" position to hear the teacher via the telecoil and to hear other students and monitor his own speech through the microphone. Although classroom applications have been largely supplanted by FM systems, induction loop systems are widely used in all kinds of business and social environments to provide acoustical access to individuals with hearing losses. Examples include larger areas like conference rooms, meeting halls, and lecture halls, as well as smaller ones like ticket booths, to name but a few. Some of the benefits and limitations of induction loop systems are listed in **Table 16.8**.

FM Systems

Most modern classroom and personal hearing assistive instruments are **FM (frequency modulation) systems**, and a great deal of attention has been given to their use in a wide variety of applications (Ross 1992; Lewis 1994a,b; ASHA 2002; AAA 2007). In an FM system, the talker's voice is picked up by a portable microphone/transmitter and is sent by an FM radio signal to receivers worn by each child using the system. In turn, the FM receiver may lead to earphones, or be connected to

the patient's hearing aid or cochlear implant. The Federal Communications Commission (FCC) designates special radio bandwidths for FM assistive listening systems, which can accommodate up to 10 wide-band or 40 narrow-band channels. Class participation and self-monitoring is made possible by environmental microphones on each receiver. As we saw for hearing aids, speech reception in noise is enhanced when a directional microphone is used with the FM system (Hawkins 1984; Lewis, Crandell, & Kreisman 2004). Clinical guidelines for FM systems are provided by ASHA (2002, 2005a,b) and AAA (2007).

Body-worn FM receivers can deliver the signal to the listener's ears directly using a variety of transducers such as the headphones shown in **Fig. 16.7a**, or they can be connected (coupled) to the hearing aids by induction or direct audio input. One should be aware that the hearing aid's output can be affected by how it is coupled to the FM system (Hawkins & Schum 1985; Thibodeau 1990; Thibodeau & Saucedo 1991).

With induction coupling, the body-worn FM receiver sends a magnetic signal to the hearing aid's telecoil by way of a personally worn inductor, which comes in two general styles. Neck loop inductors **(Fig. 16.7b)** are induction loops worn around the child's neck. Silhouette inductors **(Fig. 16.7c)** house the inductor in a flat case that has the same shape as the hearing aid, and are worn next to the hearing aid itself. Direct audio input **(Fig. 16.7d)** involves a wire that plugs into both the FM receiver and the hearing aid, and requires the hearing aid to be equipped with a direct audio input jack.

Table 16.8 Some advantages and limitations of various remote microphone hearing assistance technologies[a]

System	Advantages	Limitations
Induction loop	– Usable with a wide range of hearing losses – Relative freedom of movement within the room – Takes advantage of individual hearing aids as receivers for system – Relatively low cost to school – Well suited for use in non-school environments such as conference rooms, lecture halls, etc.	– Hearing aids must have telecoils – Hearing aids function differently via telecoil compared with microphone – Broken hearing aid denies child access to group system – Signal varies with location in the room – Signal varies with how telecoil is oriented with respect to the loop – Interference from loops in other rooms (cross-talk) – Interference from other electromagnetic signals – Cannot be used outside of room with induction loop (not portable)
FM	– Usable with a wide range of hearing losses – No cross-talk between rooms because many FM channels available – Environmental microphones for class participation and self-monitoring – Usable outside of building (portable) – Personal hearing aids not needed with self-contained FM system	– Interference from other FM sources – Coupling to hearing may affect performance – Personal systems require a hearing aid – For FM systems built into hearing aids, entire unit unavailable when repairing either component – More complicated maintenance and troubleshooting – Relatively higher relative cost
Infrared	– Convenient for theaters, houses of worship, other public forums – No cross-talk between rooms – Does not require personal hearing aid	– Output levels generally more limited than for FM and induction loop system when used alone – Signals blocked by obstructions between transmitter and receiver – Interference from sunlight prevents outside use (not portable) – No environmental microphones
Sound field amplification	– Advantageous for a wide range of groups – Receiving device not needed – Provides improved signal for everyone in room – Does not stigmatize individuals – Reduces teacher's vocal stress – Easily maintained – Relatively lower cost	– If used all by itself, useful only with relatively milder hearing losses – Loudspeakers must be properly placed and oriented – Cannot be used outside of room if permanently installed (but movable systems are available)

[a]Gilmore and Lederman (1989); Leavitt (1991); Flexer (1992, 1994); Beck, Compton, and Gilmore (1993); Lewis (1994a,b); Compton (2000); Crandell, Smaldino, and Flexer (2005); AAA (2007).

Ear-level FM receivers are either built into a behind-the-ear hearing aid as a self-contained unit, or take the form of a "boot" that snaps onto the bottom of the hearing aid **Fig. 16.7e**), constituting another kind of direct audio input. It is also possible for the hearing aid to receive signals from devices like telephones, personal music players, televisions, etc., via Bluetooth technology using a streaming device. The streamer is worn around the neck as illustrated in **Fig. 16.7f**.

Some of the principal advantages and limitations of FM systems are outlined in **Table 16.8**.

Infrared Systems

With an **infrared system**, the signal from the talker's microphone is sent by an infrared light transmitter to individually worn receivers in the room. The infrared receivers convert the light signal back to sound, which is directed into the wearer's ears. A typical infrared device is shown in **Fig. 16.8**. These systems are rarely used in regular classrooms, but are widely used as assistive devices by hearing-impaired persons in theaters, houses of worship, auditoriums, and other public forums. The system shown in the

Fig. 16.7   An FM amplification system showing a lapel microphone and FM transmitter along with various receiver options. **(a)** A body-worn FM receiver wired to earphones. **(b)** A body-worn FM receiver transmitting the signal to the telecoil in the patient's behind-the-ear (BTE) hearing aid via a neck-loop inductor. **(c)** A body-worn FM receiver sending the signal to the hearing aid telecoil via a silhouette inductor. **(d)** A body-worn FM receiver connected to a BTE hearing aid by direct audio input (DAI). **(e)** A BTE hearing aid directly connected to an attached FM receiver boot. The FM receiver can also be built into the BTE hearing aid itself (not shown). **(f)** A BTE hearing aid/FM receiver being used along with a body-worn streamer device that picks up Bluetooth signals (from telephones, personal music players, televisions, etc.). (Used with permission from Etymotic Research, Inc. and Compton-Conley Consulting.)

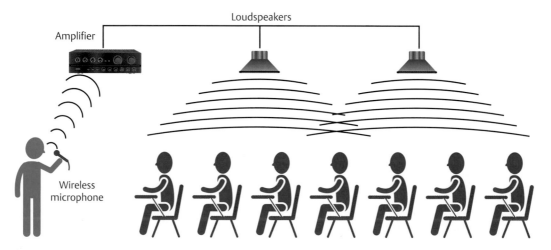

Fig. 16.8   A sound field amplification system sends the speech from the talker's microphone to one or more loudspeakers so that everybody in the room receives an amplified signal and an improved signal-to-noise ratio. In the example shown here, the teacher uses a wireless microphone/transmitter that sends an FM radio signal to an amplifier, which is in turn connected to two appropriately located ceiling-mounted loudspeakers.

figure includes a transmitter for personal use, such as improving the hearing-impaired person's ability to hear television programs. Some of their advantages and limitations are listed in **Table 16.8**.

Classroom Audio Distribution Systems (Sound Field Amplification)

Sound field (or **FM sound field**) **amplification systems** (Crandell & Smaldino 1992; Crandell et al 1997, 2005) differ from the other approaches described because they transmit amplified sound directly into the room (a sound field) rather than to individually worn receivers. Specifically, the signal from the talker's microphone is usually sent to an amplifier by an FM transmitter (although infrared transmission is also available) and is then directed to one or several loudspeakers placed around the room, as shown in **Fig. 16.9**. The idea is to keep the level of the talker's speech ~ 10 dB higher than the ambient noise level all through the room, so that everyone present is provided with an improved signal. Although implementing a sound field amplification system is beyond our scope (see, e.g., Crandell et al 1997, 2005), it should be noted that the proper acoustical analyses need to be done, and that the system cannot be a haphazard modification of a public address (PA) system with a few loudspeakers. For example, sound field amplification may not be appropriate in highly reverberant rooms, and improper loudspeaker arrangements may result in an amplified signal that is inferior to the original one (Leavitt 1991; Flexer 1992, 1994; Rosenberg et al 1999; Crandell et al 2005).

Sound field amplification produces several kinds of benefits for a wide range of individuals (see, e.g., Flexer 1992, 1994; Iglehart 2004; ASHA 2005b; Crandell et al 2005; Dockrell & Shield 2012). Among the advantageous outcomes are improved speech recognition performance, attending skills and academic performance for students, as well as reduced vocal (and other) stress for teachers. Among those who appear to benefit from sound field amplification are (a) children of various ages; (b) children with all kinds of hearing disorders (conductive, sensorineural, minimal, unilateral, fluctuating); (c) cochlear implant users; (d) children with language, articulation, learning and attention disorders, and developmental delays; and (e) children who are not native speakers of English. Several of the benefits and limitations of sound field amplification systems are enumerated in **Table 16.8**. However, one should keep in mind that variations have been reported. For example, Dockrell and Shield (2012) found improvements associated with sound field systems for elementary school children's spoken language comprehension,

Fig. 16.9 An example of an infrared system. The one pictured here is used with a television, and includes both the transmitter (below) and the head-word receiver (cradled on top of the transmitter). (Photography courtesy of Sennheiser electronic GmbH & Co. KG.)

but not for academics, and in classrooms with poorer acoustics (RT ≥ 0.83 s), but not in those with better acoustics (RT ≤ 0.52 s).

Other Assistive Devices

In addition to personal hearing aids, cochlear implants, tactile aids, and group and personal amplification sound enhancement systems, a diverse and growing variety of technologies are available to help meet the communicative requirements of the hearing impaired and deaf. Some devices must be used alone, while others are used in combination with one's hearing aids, speech reading, and sign language interpreters.

Telephone Devices

Hearing aid compatibility has been required for most new telephones since 1991. The simplest systems are telephones that provide amplified signals, often with a volume control. The use of special telephone amplifiers is facilitated by the common use of modular telephone connectors, which are available as special replacement handsets or as in-line amplifiers installed between the telephone and the handset. One should be sure to check for electronic compatibility with the telephone when using replacement handsets and in-line amplifiers. Several telephones specially designed for use by the hearing impaired are also available, as are various portable amplifiers. Portable amplifiers and other instruments can pick up either acoustic or magnetic signals from telephones, or are connected by direct audio input.

Telecommunication devices for the deaf (TDDs) or **text telephones (TTs)** as well as personal computers (PCs) provide telephone access for those who cannot hear amplified speech from the telephone. The TDD is basically a portable terminal that sends and receives typed messages via the telephone. The TDD and telephone are often connected using an acoustic coupler. Communication between people using voice telephones and TDDs (or computers) is made possible by dual-party relay systems, which telephone companies must provide under Public Law 101-336 (the Americans with Disabilities Act). Communication between TDDs and PCs has been somewhat of a problem because TDDs have traditionally used a system called **Baudot code**, whereas PCs use **ASCII code** and also operate at much faster transmission rates. As one might expect, TDDs are now available that can use both formats.

Television and Related Devices

Closed captioning is probably one of the best-known assistive approaches in current use. It involves providing subtitles on a television monitor or movie screen giving the gist of what is being said from moment to moment. Although closed captioning previously necessitated the use of a decoder box, Public Law 101-431 (the Television Decoder Circuitry Act of 1990) mandates that closed caption decoders be built into all new television sets with screens 13 inches in size and larger. **Real-time captioning** involves providing the detailed text of what is being said, and is often desirable for lectures and similar situations.

Alerting and Safety Aides

Many hearing-impaired individuals cannot rely upon the auditory channel to know when the doorbell is ringing, when the alarm clock sounds, or when emergency signals like smoke or burglar alarms go off. For this reason, sound signals like bells, tones, buzzers, and sirens are supplemented or replaced with flashing lights and/or vibrators on all kinds of common devices. In addition, special-purpose devices are also available, such as lights or vibrators that indicate when a call is coming in on a telecommunication device, or when the baby is crying.

Before leaving this section, we must not forget that **hearing dogs** can serve as portable alerting and assistive aides, as well as valued and loved companions, to their severely hearing-impaired or deaf owners. The right of hearing-impaired persons to have and be accompanied by their hearing dogs is protected by several federal laws, such as the *Air Carrier Access Act of 1986* for airlines, the *Americans with Disabilities Act of 1990* for public places, and the *Federal Fair Housing Amendments Act of 1988* for housing.

■ Intervention Approaches and Considerations

Framework for Intervention with Adults

A useful framework for understanding modern approaches to aural rehabilitation for adults is provided by a model described by Goldstein and Stephens (1981). Their *evaluation phase* explores several aspects of the patient's communicative situation as well as interrelated factors: (1) *Communication status* is assessed in terms of all components, such as auditory, visual, language, and manual/gesture skills. (2) *Associated variables* (e.g., psychological, sociological, vocational, and educational) are explored to determine their interactions with the hearing disorder and the need for coordinated efforts with other professionals. (3) *Related conditions* such as the patient's overall mobility, manual dexterity, visual disorders, and the existence of ear pathologies might affect the intervention plan, and are therefore assessed. Consider how factors such as these would change with aging—the differences in approach and supportive counseling that would be appropriate for those who need various degrees of assistance to accomplish their daily activities, and for those who are in nursing facilities. (4) Finally, the patient's *attitude* toward the rehabilitation process is assessed, and is one of the first issues handled during the redemption phase.

The *treatment phase* also addresses several broad areas of redemption: (1) *Psychosocial counseling* is provided, dealing with such factors as explaining the nature of the hearing loss, helping the patient and her family understand its ramifications, and dealing with the patient's attitudes regarding aural rehabilitation. Of course, audiological counseling should not meander into the realm of psychotherapy, the need for which should be handled by appropriate referrals. (2) *Amplification* and other instruments are a major component of the intervention process. These instruments include hearing aids, group amplification devices, and other assistive listening and warning devices. The instruments must be selected and fitted, and must also be adjusted over time. The audiologist also orients and instructs the patient (and often others as well) regarding the use and care of each device, its use in various situations, coordination with other devices, etc. (3) *Communication training* involves learning strategies to improve communicative situations and listening effectiveness, as well as developing skills through auditory-visual training, and other activities. (4) The *overall coordination* phase of the program deals with making use of other professionals and resources that are appropriate in a given case, such as vocational rehabilitation, social work, psychology, medicine, etc.

Auditory and Visual Training

One of our principal goals is to maximize the amount and quality of speech information that the hearing-impaired patient can obtain. This involves (1) providing an optimum acoustical signal with hearing aids or other devices, and (2) training the patient to derive the most information about the spoken message from what he hears and sees by using the acoustical and visual representations of speech to the fullest, and taking advantage of various forms of contextual and linguistic cues. Even though we will be considering some aspects of speechreading and auditory training separately, the student should know from the outset that combined auditory-visual training is usually the preferred treatment mode. Also, virtually all practice exercises can be done in the auditory, visual, or combined audiovisual mode. In fact, it is not uncommon to present exercises in all three modes to demonstrate to the patient the benefits of using all possible communication channels, and to give him practice in doing so. In addition, most techniques are successfully used in both individual and group therapy.

Analytical and Synthetic Techniques

Therapy methods are traditionally divided into analytical and synthetic approaches. **Analytical** exercises concentrate on the recognition of individual sounds and words, and might be thought of as the "micro" approach. In contrast, **synthetic** methods can be conceived of as the "macro" approach because they concentrate upon deriving the meaning of what is being said rather than trying to catch every sound or word. These alternative approaches trace their origins to the classical schools of thought in lipreading instruction. The classical analytical schools were the Mueller-Walle (Bruhn 1920) and Jena (Bunger 1932) methods, and the traditional synthetic schools

of thought were described by Nitchie (1912) and by Kinzie and Kinzie (1931), and are mentioned for historic perspective. Strict adherence to one approach is a thing of the past, and even the traditional schools actually used both analytical and synthetic activities. The terms *analytical* and *synthetic* continue to be employed to describe the two different classes of activities that are used.

Analytic exercises are the most formal. Typical syllable discrimination exercises might involve presenting the patient with two syllables (e.g., "ba-da," or "da-da") and having him indicate whether they are the same or different, or having the patient choose which one of three syllables is different from the other two (e.g., "se-sa-sha"). The same tasks can also be done with words. Recognition drills might involve having the patient identify the presented syllable or word by repeating it, or by choosing it from among several choices. The syllables or words selected depend on the focus of the exercise. In addition, the patient is usually given feedback after each response.

There is an almost unlimited variety of synthetic techniques. These include counseling about effective communicative strategies and group discussion as well as practice exercises per se. One type of exercise involves practice in receiving the main ideas of a sentence, paragraph, or passage-length material. For example, one might first give the patient the key words and/or the general topic of a passage, which is then presented to him. Responses can include anything from answering specific questions to having the patient retell the passage, or to incorporate the main ideas of the passage into a subsequent discussion. Another type of synthetic exercise involves having the patient fill in the gaps in a passage. A useful group therapy exercise involves videotaping a group discussion among several hearing-impaired patients, which is subsequently shown to them. The group can then discuss the communicative styles and strategies used, dealing with such topics as taking advantage of context, listening for main ideas rather than trying to catch every word, the importance of asking for clarification when needed, etc.

Providing the patient (and communication partners) with information and practice in the use of effective communication strategies is an important aspect of the aural rehabilitation process that is appropriate to mention in this context. This may include, for example, **facilitative strategies** that structure the environment and situation to facilitate communication, and **repair strategies** that attempt to recover from communication breakdowns (see, e.g., Tye-Murray 2015). Facilitative strategies include such things as taking steps to maximize the visibility of the talker (e.g., manipulating lighting, viewing angle, and distance) and to minimize noises and competing voices. Repair strategies involve using techniques like repetition, rephrasing, simplifying, or elaborating, and confirmation of what was said.

Continuous-Discourse Tracking

Continuous-discourse tracking (De Filippo & Scott 1978) is a popular therapy technique that provides practice in the use of repair strategies. The clinician orally presents a passage to the patient, who must in turn repeat it back verbatim on an ongoing basis (based on vision, audition, or a combination of the two). Thus, the patient literally tracks what the clinician is saying: the clinician says a phrase, the patient repeats it word for word, the clinician presents the next phrase, the patient says it back exactly, etc. This continues until the patient makes an error. Then the clinician provides the patient with a variety of clues and prompts to help her get the correct word(s). The prompts might include repeating the misperceived word, paraphrasing it, using fill-ins, or any of a host of other tactics to help the patient get the correct word. Tracking performance is assessed in terms of the number of words per minute that can be repeated by the patient.

Adult Auditory-Visual Training Approaches

The traditional approach to auditory training for adults was outlined by Carhart (1960). The goal was to train the patient "to take full advantage of the auditory cues that are still available to him" (p. 381). This involved counseling about the nature of the hearing disorder and listening strategies, reporting on various listening assignments, and formal analytic listening drills. Practice exercises were initially done in quiet, and then under more difficult listening conditions, such as in the presence of noise or reverberation.

Garstecki's (1981) auditory-visual training paradigm involves manipulating the redundancy of the communicative situation in terms of (1) message type, (2) noise type, (3) signal-to-noise ratio, and (4) situational cues. Message type has to do with the content of the speech material, going from low-message-content materials like syllables or individual words to high-content materials like paragraphs or stories. Noise type refers to the kind of acoustical background that is present during the speech. This may be quiet, white noise, one or more competing talkers, etc. The signal-to-noise ratio (SNR) refers to the intensity relationship between the speech signal and the noise being used. It can range from speech that is 12 dB greater than the noise (+12 dB

SNR) down to noise levels that are 6 dB higher than the speech (–6 dB SNR). Situational cues involve the visual or auditory context of the speech material. The types of cues used may be *related* to the message versus *distracting*, or may be *omitted* altogether. Pretests are used to determine the combination of these parameters where the patient is able to achieve a certain percent correct level of performance (the "criterion level"). This becomes the starting point for training. Individual and group practice exercises are designed to help him to perform at successively lower levels of redundancy. Communication strategies such as making predictions from situational and nonverbal cues and optimizing listening situations are also provided.

Computer-based approaches A growing number of computer-based auditory training programs are becoming available. Let's briefly review several of them. The **Seeing and Hearing Speech** (Sensimetrics 2002) program provides practice (and assessment) materials for adult patients in four groups: (1) vowels; (2) consonants; (3) stress, intonation, and length; and (4) everyday communication. The material can be presented in the auditory, visual, or combined auditory-visual mode, and a variety of noise backgrounds may be used.

Sound and Beyond (Cochlear Americas n.d.) includes auditory training materials for adults with severe to profound losses. It includes exercises on pitch discrimination; environmental sound discrimination and identification; discriminating male and female voices; discrimination and identification for vowels and consonants; word discrimination; sentence recognition; and identifying musical instruments and tunes.

Adaptive **Listening and Communication Enhancement** (**LACE**; Sweetow & Sabes 2006) provides auditory training for adults. It includes speech reception exercises in the presence of babble or a competing talker, and for compressed speech; auditory short-term memory and processing speed exercises; and communication strategies. In LACE, the patient receives feedback on his responses, and the approach is adaptive in the sense that exercises increase and decrease in difficulty based on whether the patient's prior responses were correct.

Conversation Made Easy (Tye-Murray 2002) is a computer-based speechreading program that can be used in the vision-only or combined auditory-visual mode; and has versions for adults and teenagers, as well as for children with higher-level and lower-level language skills. It includes speechreading exercises involving (1) analytic exercises with sounds, words, and phrases; (2) unrelated sentence recognition with repair strategies; and (3) contextually related material with both repair and facilitative strategies.

Lipreading (Speechreading) Considerations

Lipreading or **speechreading** involves deriving meaning about what is being said by watching the talker. Although we will use the two terms interchangeably[5], *speechreading* is sometimes considered the preferred term because information is obtained from the visible movements of the articulators, facial expressions, gestures, etc., and not just the lips. Speechreading involves the *visual channel of speech communication*. It is a natural means of communication that we all use to supplement hearing, especially when listening conditions become difficult. It should thus come as no surprise that all people with hearing impairments must rely on speechreading to a greater or lesser extent. In fact, one of the most elegant distinctions between "hearing impairment" and "deafness" is that the primary channel of speech perception is audition for the former and vision for the latter (Ross, Brackett, & Maxon 1982).

Lipreading Tests

Speechreading skills vary widely among individuals, and trying to predict how much a given patient will benefit from lipreading training can be difficult. We can use lipreading tests to gain some insight into a given patient's speechreading ability and the effects of training. Many lipreading tests are available. Two well-known traditional measures are the Utley Lipreading Test (Utley 1946) and the Denver Quick Test of Lipreading Ability (Alpiner 1987). The sentence part of the Utley Test is shown in **Table 16.9**, and it requires the patient to repeat what has been said. The Denver Quick Test includes similar kinds of sentences (e.g., "There is somebody at the door."), and it requires the patient to identify the main idea expressed in each sentence. A more contemporary approach is illustrated by the **Children's Audiovisual Enhancement Test** (**CAVET**; Tye-Murray & Geers 2002), which includes words known to be in the vocabularies of 7- to 9-year-olds who have profound hearing losses. The CAVET is recorded with auditory-only, visual-only, and audiovisual parts, and each section includes both easy- and hard-to-lipread words.

Table 16.9   The Utley Lipreading Test, Form A

1. All right.	17. What did you want?
2. Where have you been?	18. How much do you weigh?
3. I have forgotten.	19. I cannot stand him.
4. I have nothing.	20. She was home last week.
5. That is right.	21. Keep your eye on the ball.
6. Look you.	22. I cannot remember.
7. How have you been?	23. Of course.
8. I don't know if I can.	24. I flew to Washington.
9. How tall are you?	25. You look well.
10. It is awfully cold.	26. The train runs every hour.
11. My folks are home.	27. You had better go slow.
12. How much was it?	28. It says that in the book.
13. Good night.	29. We got home at six o'clock.
14. Where are you going?	30. We drove to the country.
15. Excuse me.	31. How much rain fell?
16. Did you have a good time?	

Factors Affecting Lipreading

One should be aware of the factors that affect speechreading because these become the basis for counseling patients about effective listening strategies and for many practice exercises. Optimal speechreading requires adequate illumination of the talker's face, and the lipreader should try to orient himself so light falls on the talker's face instead of in his own eyes. Other factors that affect speechreading to a greater or lesser extent include the distance between the talker and lipreader, viewing angle, familiarity with the speaker, articulation, speaking rate, facial expressions and gestures, age, feedback between the talker and speechreader, distracting behaviors (e.g., chewing and random gestures), as well as environmental distractions. Unfortunately, our understanding about how some of these factors influence lipreading has been clouded by inconsistent findings across studies. Several these issues are being re-examined using more modern approaches. Speaking rate and viewing angle are two examples. Ijsseldijk (1992) found that different speaking rates and facial views (full face, two-thirds profile, and lips only) did not affect the speechreading performance

---

[5] These terms are not always used interchangeably. Tye-Murray (2015), a leading authority in the field, employs the term *lipreading* to denote the use of vision only and *speechreading* for the combined use of vision and audition.

of 8- to 16-year-olds who had profound hearing losses. Performance was improved by repetition of the material.

Speechreading is also affected by context, situational cues, knowledge of the topic, linguistic factors (e.g., sentence structure and word familiarity), and the redundancy of the message. As one might expect, the speechreader's visual acuity affects lipreading ability, but contrary to common wisdom, lipreading performance is not related to his personality attributes and intelligence (as long as it is not impaired).

Homophonous Sounds and Words Certain speech sounds look the same "on the lips," such as /p/, /b/, and /m/, and therefore cannot be distinguished from one another on the basis of speechreading alone. Such sounds are called **homophonous sounds** or **homophemes**. Similarly, words that look the same are called **homophonous words** (e.g., "pat," "bat," and "mat"). Therefore, the speechreader can only distinguish among sounds that belong to different homophonous groups, but cannot be expected to distinguish between sounds within the same group. Such visually distinguishable groups of sounds are called **visemes** (Fisher 1968). Owens and Blazek (1985) found sets of homophonous sound groups that were in good agreement with visually identifiable articulatory movements described by Jeffers and Barley (1971). These are shown in **Table 16.10**. The existence of homophonous sounds and words brings home the point that lipreading cannot independently serve as a replacement for hearing, and one must learn to make use of linguistic and contextual constraints as well as the redundancy of the message.

Using Both Hearing and Vision Speech perception is improved by the use of hearing plus speechreading, compared with either audition or vision alone (Walden, Prosek & Worthington 1974; Erber 1975;

MacLeod & Summerfield 1987). It is easy to understand why this occurs. It is not always possible to determine what is being said from either audition or vision alone because (1) speechreading does not give enough information for adequate speech understanding all by itself, and (2) sound cues may be inaudible or distorted due to adverse listening conditions or a hearing impairment. Combined hearing and speechreading provides the person with complementary cues, so that the total amount of information becomes sufficient to perceive what is being said. For example, place of articulation cues (e.g., "pile" versus "tile") that might be misheard because of a hearing loss can be filled in by speechreading, and voicing distinctions (e.g., "bad" versus "pad") that are not visible can often be filled in by hearing.

We want hearing-impaired patients to use both hearing and lipreading whenever possible, but many people think of lipreading as an "alternative" to hearing, or are reluctant for whatever reason to both look and listen. It is therefore important to make the patient aware that almost everybody benefits from the *combined* use of speechreading and audition, including those with profound hearing losses who must use powerful hearing aids or cochlear implants to receive even a modicum of auditory input. Telling this to the patient is often not enough. A simple and effective demonstration involves giving the patient a speech recognition "test" by hearing alone (with your mouth covered), by speechreading alone (with no sound), and then by hearing plus speechreading. The speech level used should be reasonably difficult for the patient so that there is room to show how the scores improve when audition and vision are combined. This exercise can usually be done sitting face to face in a regular room (unless it is done as part of a formal assessment) with whatever kind of speech material is appropriate to demonstrate the intended effect. It is often useful for this type of exercise to be worked into individual and group practice sessions.

Effectiveness of Formal Training Exercises

There is no question that formal training procedures are essential and beneficial for hearing-impaired children. On the other hand, the ability of formal auditory training and lipreading instruction to improve the speech recognition ability of adults with adventitious hearing losses is another issue.

A systematic review by Sweetow and Palmer (2005) suggested that individualized synthetic auditory training leads to improved use of active listening strategies among adults. Rubinstein and Boothroyd (1987) found that auditory training using either synthetic

Table 16.10 Visemes[a] and their associated articulatory movements[b]

Visemes	Articulatory movements
p, b, m	Lips together
f, v	Lower lip to upper teeth
θ, ð	Tongue between teeth
w, r	Puckered lips
tʃ, dʒ, ʃ, ʒ	Lips forward
t, d, s, k, n, g, l	Teeth approximated

[a] Owens and Blazek (1985).
[b] Jeffers and Barley (1971).

techniques alone or a combination of synthetic and analytic methods yielded a significant improvement in speech recognition performance on the probability-high SPIN test (HI-SPIN) but not on the probability-low SPIN test (LO-SPIN). Recall from Chapter 8 that each test word on the SPIN is at the end of a sentence. The HI-SPIN sentences provide contextual cues for the test words, but the LO-SPIN sentences do not provide any contextual cues about the test words. Thus, Rubinstein and Boothroyd's results suggest that auditory training improves the listener's ability to take advantage of the context. In addition, a systematic review by Hawkins (2005) found that group counseling provides benefits in terms of perceived handicap and quality of life, and might also enhance effective communication strategies and hearing aid usage. Similar group therapy benefits were subsequently reported by Hickson, Worrall, and Scarinci (2007).

In contrast, Sweetow and Palmer's (2005) systematic review also indicated that the effects of analytic training were unclear, and that there was some but very limited evidence supporting the efficacy of individualized auditory training. However, it is important to realize that these conclusions were based on the outcomes of just six studies that met the rigorous requirements for inclusion in the 2005 systematic review. More importantly, the effectiveness of individual auditory training has been supported by the outcomes of subsequent investigations, which took advantage of computer-assisted training protocols (Burk, Humes, Amos, & Strauser 2006; Sweetow & Sabes 2006; Burke & Humes 2007, 2008; Henderson Sabes & Sweetow 2007; Olson, Preminger, & Shinn 2013). Thus, individual aural rehabilitation therapy does seem to be an efficacious management approach that can be made available to adults with hearing impairment.

Speech Production Management

Speech conservation efforts are sometimes needed because speech production occasionally deteriorates in adults who develop hearing losses. Aberrations of final consonants, sibilants, and vocal loudness or quality are among the reported speech production problems of these patients (Calvert & Silverman 1975). The incidence of these problems is exceedingly variable, and it is affected by the degree and configuration of the hearing loss, among other, less clear factors. In fact, significant amounts of speech deterioration in cases of adult-onset deafness have been reported to occur by some (Cowie, Douglas-Cowie, & Kerr 1983) but not by others (Goehl & Kaufman 1984). In addition, speech deterioration effects due to adult-onset hearing losses tend to develop gradu-

ally over time. Cases of clinically significant speech deterioration have been rare (but not absent) in the author's experience, and the dearth of coverage on this topic in current aural rehabilitation textbooks seems to confirm this. (Jackson (1982) is still one of the few available discussions of the topic, and includes clinically applicable material.) Even though these effects are relatively uncommon, we must be alert to their development so that the appropriate intervention can be undertaken.

Intervention Considerations for Infants and Children

Our goal from the very beginning of the intervention process is to provide the hearing-impaired child with the best possible access to auditory stimuli, optimize her auditory perceptual skills, and integrate these into her overall communicative, cognitive, educational, and psychosocial development. Thus, the **early intervention (EI)** process for the hearing-impaired child is very much a comprehensive undertaking. A set of recommended goals and a framework for coordinated EI services for hearing-impaired children through age 3 and their families has been formulated by the Joint Committee on Infant Hearing (2013), and is readily available on the Internet.

Recall from Chapter 13 that early identification is linked to early intervention, and is a primary goal in the audiological management of children with all kinds and degrees of hearing impairments. Even relatively small amounts of hearing loss can have numerous adverse effects (e.g., Bess, Dodd-Murphy, & Parker 1998), and *early identification* linked with *early intervention* produces impressive benefits (Yoshinaga-Itano, Sedey, Coulter, & Mehl 1998; Yoshinaga-Itano 1999). For example, language performance is significantly better in children whose hearing losses are identified before 6 months of age compared with those identified after 6 months old (Yoshinaga-Itano et al 1998). Thus, the goal is screening by 1 month of age, diagnosis by 3 months, and instituting an EI program by 6 months (JCIH 2007). In fact, current guidelines call for children who are deaf or hard of hearing to be referred for EI services within 2 days of the audiological diagnosis, followed by the completion of an *individualized family service plan (IFSP)* inside of 45 days (JCIH 2013). It is important to remember that evaluation and planning do not end with the onset of intervention, but regular monitoring of the child's audiological status and progress is an ongoing aspect of the program. For example, comprehensive and monitoring of the child's progress has been recommended at least every 6 months up to age 3, and every year from then on (JCIH 2013).

Audiological rehabilitation for the very young hearing-impaired child begins with an at-home focus, with most of the earliest activities performed by parents or other caregivers in consultation with the audiologist and other professionals. The intervention environment expands as the child enters preschool, elementary school, and then higher grades, where increasingly greater roles are taken on by professionals.

Carhart's (1960) auditory training approach for children stresses the development of sound awareness, gross sound discriminations, and discriminations among speech sounds. The first goal is for the child to become aware that sounds exist, attend to them, and associate them with objects and activities in her environment. This involves surrounding the child with the sounds of everyday life and associating them with the objects and activities that produce them. Work on sound discrimination begins with gross distinctions between sounds that are very different, and then proceeds to finer distinctions. Typical noisemakers used for these activities include drums, horns, toys, or other objects that produce reasonably distinctive sounds that are within the child's aided audible range. Work on speech sound discriminations also starts with more gross discriminations (e.g., between vowels and consonants) and then moving on to finer ones (e.g., place differences between consonants).

Current intervention programs for hearing-impaired infants and young children are exemplified by the SKI-HI, SPICE, Erber, and DASL approaches. These and other resources are listed in Appendix N. In the **SKI-HI program** (Watkins & Clark 1993; Watkins 2004), activities are designed to address a series of 11 major classes of auditory/speech/language skills that are arranged into four overlapping developmental phases. Phase I includes (1) attending to sound and (2) early vocalization skills. Phase II involves (3) recognizing sounds, (4) locating sound sources, and (5) vocalizing with inflections. The skills in Phase III include (6) locating sounds that are at some distance as well as at levels above and below the child, and (7) the production of several vowels and consonants. Phase IV is concerned with the discrimination and comprehension of (8) environmental sounds; (9) vocal sounds, words, and phases; and (10) distinct speech sounds; as well as (11) the imitation and/or meaningful production of speech. The SKI-HI program itself is a well-known example of early intervention approaches in which the professional clinician guides parents, family members, and other caregivers so that they can provide the child with a comprehensive at-home program of auditory, speech, and language stimulation.

Speech Perception Instructional Curriculum and Evaluation (SPICE) is an audiovisual training curriculum developed at the Central Institute for the Deaf (Moog, Biedenstein, & Davidson 1995). The materials in the SPICE program might be used with hearing-impaired children between about 3 and 12 years old; and includes four levels, beginning with (1) detection (e.g., speech awareness) and progressing to (2) suprasegmentals (dealing with speech distinctions relying on intonation, stress, and duration), (3) vowels and consonants, and finally (4) connected speech.

Erber (1982) stresses that auditory training should be incorporated into the child's overall communicative activities and school program. In his auditory training approach, the child's auditory skills are viewed in terms of a model that takes into account both the speech stimulus and the response task. The *speech stimulus* involves the characteristics and complexity of the speech material that the child must perceive, and may involve any of six levels: (1) *speech elements*, (2) *syllables*, (3) *words*, (4) *phrases*, (5) *sentences*, and (6) *connected discourse*. The *response task* involves the kind of perceptual activity that is involved in responding to the speech signal. These include four general categories: (1) *detection*, (2) *discrimination*, (3) *identification*, and (4) *comprehension*.

Auditory activities can be viewed in terms of any combination of these six speech materials and four response tasks. The child's auditory skills are assessed in terms of Erber's model with the **Glendonald Auditory Screening Procedure (GASP)**. The GASP includes three combinations of these stimuli and response tasks: (1) detection of speech elements, (2) word identification, and (3) sentence comprehension.

Auditory training activities in Erber's approach may involve any of three general styles, including (1) practice on specific tasks, (2) a moderately structured method, and (3) a natural conversational method. Practice on specific tasks is the most structured approach. It focuses on a specific listening skill, and involves structured activities in which the teacher determines the speech stimuli and the range of responses to be used by the child. A moderately structured activity might use material selected from recent class work in a multiple-choice identification task, followed by comprehension tasks or basic speech development activities, procedures, and comprehension tasks. The natural conversational approach is the most flexible method, in which auditory training activities are integrated into the context of the current classroom activity. The approach is *adaptive* in the sense that the nature of the child's responses for one activity influences the nature of the subsequent activity.

The **Developmental Approach to Successful Listening II (DASL-II)** program, developed by Stout and Windle (1992), also uses a sequential approach to auditory training in which a child's auditory capabilities are addressed in terms of sound awareness, phonetic listening, and auditory comprehension. Similar to the program described by Erber, DASL-II employs an auditory skills test to determine the child's level of auditory performance so that she can be placed properly in the intervention program.

Sanders (1993) presents a comprehensive intervention approach for hearing-impaired children. Several of its aspects are mentioned to give the student a flavor for the approach, although these points do not even begin to the scratch the surface. Sanders's intervention procedures for younger preschool children are directed toward the development of auditory behavior in the child, and are analogous to but more comprehensive than what Carhart (1960) described as developing sound awareness and discriminations. The major areas of concentration include (1) parent/caregiver education, (2) stimulating the use of hearing, (3) optimization of the child's auditory environment, and (4) developing auditory discrimination and recognition.

Intervention approaches for older preschool children realize the place of the preschool educational environment as a supplement to at-home activities, and highlight the importance of learning through active experiences. Structured communication training is introduced. This includes (1) the use of language that is appropriate for the child's developmental level, (2) maximizing redundancy to optimize the child's understanding of relationships and the ability to make accurate predictions about what is being said, and (3) techniques to encourage the development of auditory-visual perceptions.

The intervention process for the hearing-impaired school-age child is multifaceted. A major issue to be faced is the choice of the type of school placement, which is discussed below. Several of the audiologist's responsibilities at this level include providing information to the classroom teacher about issues such as the manner in which hearing loss affects communication, the use and care of hearing aids and other amplification and assistive devices, preferential seating to optimize the hearing-impaired child's auditory-visual reception of classroom activities, etc. Auditory-visual training and language enrichment are integrated into the overall academic program.

Speech Production Assessment and Training

The speech production characteristics of children with hearing impairments have been described for those who have mild-to-moderate losses (Markides 1970, 1983; Elfenbein, Hardin-Jones, & Davis 1994) and severe hearing impairments (McDermott & Jones 1984), as well as for those with profound losses who are typically described as deaf (Hudgins & Numbers 1942; Smith 1975). Speech production problems are observed among children with all levels of loss; however, speech does not generally become significantly unintelligible until the loss is worse than roughly 70 dB HL (Jensema, Karchmer, & Trybus 1978), beyond which it becomes less intelligible as the person's hearing loss and speech reception capabilities become worse (Boothroyd 1984, 1985). It is therefore not surprising that speech production considerations are a major issue in the habilitation and education of hearing-impaired and deaf children. Details of speech production evaluation and training for hearing-impaired and deaf children are generally within the province of speech-language pathologists and educators of the deaf. However, the interested student will find excellent coverage in several well-known texts on the subject (Vorce 1974; Calvert & Silverman 1975; Hochberg, Levitt, & Osberger 1983; Ling 2002).

Educational Options and Approaches

The legal requirement for providing comprehensive educational and related services to hearing-impaired and deaf children is well established. Children with hearing impairments are included among those with a wide range of handicaps covered under the Individuals with Disabilities Education Act of 1975, better known as Public Law (PL) 92-142. For our purposes, PL 94-142 (along with its extensions under PL 99-457) mandates (1) the least restrictive, individually appropriate free public education for hearing-impaired children from 3 to 21 years old, (2) provision of the full range of intervention modalities involved in aural rehabilitation, and (3) empowerment of parents with significant input into the child's educational plan.

Educational Placement Options

Potential educational placements for hearing-impaired children fall along a continuum from attending conventional classes in a regular school (**inclusion** or complete **mainstreaming**) to being enrolled in a residential school for the deaf. Complete mainstreaming is considered to be the least restrictive environment and the residential school represents the most restrictive one. The options between these extremes (going from less to more restrictive) include mainstreaming with various modifications of the environment (e.g., an FM system) and/or some adjustments in the requirements (e.g., modified assignments or tests), or with a modified curriculum; attending a classroom that has both a regular teacher and a teacher for the hearing impaired (co-enrollment); attending regular classes but spending part of the time getting individualized assistance in a resource room or with an itinerant specialist teacher or therapist; being enrolled in a self-contained classroom for the hearing impaired inside the regular school building; and attending a day school for the deaf. There is evidence to suggest that overall academic performance is best when high-quality services are provided in less restrictive settings (Ross, Brackett, & Maxon 1982).

What constitutes the optimal educational placement for a given hearing-impaired child can be a vexing question. The factors to be considered go beyond the degree of hearing loss, and include such issues as the kinds of special services needed by the child, the presence of other handicaps, maximization of the child's psychosocial development, family considerations, geographical limitations, and viewpoints about educational approaches for the hearing impaired.

Communicative Approaches

Several communication approaches and techniques are available for use by the hearing impaired and deaf. Because the means of communication cannot be separated from the overall habilitation and education of this population, the choice of which communication method will be used is a central issue in the education of the hearing impaired and deaf. Audiologists have a responsibility to inform parents about the approaches available for their children. However, we must remember that we share this responsibility with other professionals such as educators of the deaf and speech-language pathologists, and that the final placement decision rests with the child's parents. In fact, even though the JCIH (2013) guidelines highlight the importance of *listening and spoken language*, they make it clear that *language* means "all spoken and signed languages" (p. e1325); thus, families may choose American Sign Language (ASL) as the preferred communication mode, and services in these cases should be provided by people who are fully competent in ASL.

Spoken Language: Oral/Aural Approach

Candidly stated, there is no question that spoken language is the means of communication naturally developed by normal individuals, and is employed by the overwhelming preponderance of people throughout the world. These points provide the basic argument for teaching the hearing impaired to employ spoken language as their principal means of communication as well. This viewpoint has been implied throughout the current discussion. Educational approaches that use spoken language as the primary and often exclusive means of communication are said to employ the **oral/aural method**.

It is unlikely that anyone would disagree with this point of view provided we are discussing children whose residual auditory capabilities are sufficient for hearing to be the principal channel for receiving language. However, the oral/aural method becomes an issue of heated controversy when we are dealing with deaf children, for whom the visual channel effectively becomes their natural, primary channel for receiving linguistic information. Of course, cochlear implants make it possible for many deaf children to become oral/aural communicators and learners. Also, Geers and colleagues (Geers, Brenner, Nicholas, et al 2002; Geers 2002; Geers, Nicholas, & Sedey 2003) found that children with cochlear implants accrue greater speech, language, and reading performance benefits with the oral/aural approach compared with manual ones.

Of course, vision will remain the principal communication channel when cochlear implants are either not chosen or not successful. In these cases, the primary arguments against oral/aural education are that (1) these children learn visually oriented or manual systems as their natural, primary means of communication; and (2) the manual method is the preferred system within the deaf community. This line of reasoning leads to the use of the manual and total communication methods in the education of deaf children.

Manual Systems

American Sign Language (ASL) developed as the manual language of the deaf community. It is not a "translation" of the English language into a set of equivalent signs, but is rather a language unto itself with its own lexicon and grammatical rules. This concept can be difficult for hearing individuals to understand even if they have learned to speak a foreign language like Spanish or German, either of which is a spoken language. In contrast to *spoken* languages, which are suited to transmission via sound (acoustic spectra that change with time), ASL is a manual system suited to the visual channel. Thus, ASL uses *spatial* dimensions (hand shakes, movements, and locations and orientations relative to the signer's body) over time. Signed English (Bornstein 1974) is similar in many ways to ASL, with modifications intended for use by younger children, such as the addition of signed pronouns, helping verbs, and syntactic markers. A variety of other signing systems have been developed over the years that have attempted to represent the spoken language manually; however, these have not received the wide acceptance enjoyed by ASL.

Fingerspelling involves hand positions and motions corresponding to the conventional 26 letters of the alphabet. Words are spelled out with letters in order. Fingerspelling is employed by users of both oral/aural and manual systems.

Cued speech (Cornett 1967) is a visual system used to supplement lipreading. It uses a total of 12 hand postures and positions produced by the talker while speaking to help the speechreader distinguish between homophonous sounds.

Total Communication

Total communication encourages the combined use of both speech and/or sign language in whatever combination fosters the child's best language development (Jordan, Gustason, & Rosen 1979). This approach has replaced oralism as the principal means of communication in most educational institutions for the hearing impaired.

The relative advantages of oral versus total communication programs for the speech communication abilities of profoundly hearing-impaired children have always been controversial. Studies comparing the effects of these two types of settings have yielded conflicting results. One reason for the inconsistencies involves comparisons among elementary school children whose communicative skills are still being developed. Geers and Moog (1992) improved our understanding of this issue by comparing two large, well-matched groups of teenagers with profound hearing impairments who were educated in either oral versus total communication programs since they were in preschool. They found that speech perception, speech production, and oral communication skills were significantly better for the subjects who were educated in oral programs.

Todoma

Todoma is a manual system employed by individuals who are both deaf and blind. In the Todoma method, the "listener" feels the talker's face and neck. Reed

and colleagues (1985) found that speech reception by Todoma relies principally on the feel of lip and jaw movements, laryngeal vibration, and oral air flow, and secondarily on the feel of muscle tension and nasal air flow.

Audiological Management of Tinnitus and Hyperacusis

Tinnitus is the perception of sounds having no external stimulus, and it may occur with or without hearing loss. The assessment of tinnitus is a multidisciplinary endeavor. Medical assessment of the tinnitus patient is an important step to identify and address a variety of disorders requiring medical and/or surgical treatment, ranging from impacted cerumen to acoustic neuroma, Meniere's disease, and vascular tumors (e.g., Perry & Gantz 2000; Levine 2001; Wackym & Friedland 2004). Our discussion here assumes that these issues already have been ruled out or addressed, so that we are able to concentrate on the tinnitus per se.

In addition to the regular audiological evaluation and case history, the assessment of patients with problematic tinnitus involves (a) psychoacoustic measurements of the tinnitus (its pitch, loudness, quality, and duration, and how it is affected by sound stimulation); (b) loudness discomfort levels; (c) electrophysiological measurements such as auditory brainstem responses and otoacoustic emissions; and (d) self-assessment inventories and in-depth interviews (see, e.g., Henry, Zaugg, & Schechter 2005c).

Tinnitus self-assessment inventories are used in both evaluation and outcome assessment. They are analogous to the hearing impairment scales discussed in Chapter 13 and earlier in this text, but they concentrate upon the experience and impact of tinnitus and hyperacusis on the patient's life, dealing with issues like annoyance, sleep interference, emotional stress, anxiety, and other psychological issues, as well as how it might otherwise interfere with one's day-to-day activities (Newman, Sandridge, & Jacobson 2014). As examples, see the *Iowa Tinnitus Handicap Questionnaire* (Kuk, Tyler, Russell, & Jordan 1990), shown in **Table 16.11**, and the *Iowa Tinnitus Activities Questionnaire* (Tyler et al 2006), in **Table 16.12**. Some other well-known examples include the *Tinnitus Effects Questionnaire* (Hallam, Jakes, & Hinchcliffe 1988), the *Tinnitus Reaction Questionnaire* (Wilson, Henry, Bowen, & Haralambous 1991), and the *Tinnitus Handicap Inventory* (Newman, Jacobson, & Spitzer 1996). Three additions to these tools are particularly interesting and useful: The *Tinnitus and Hearing Aid Survey* (Henry, Zaugg, Myers, & Kendall 2010; Henry, Griest, Zaugg, et al 2015) helps distinguish between

Table 16.11 Iowa Tinnitus Handicap Questionnaire[a]

INSTRUCTIONS: This questionnaire has 27 questions. Please indicate 0 that you strongly disagree (up to) 100 that you strongly agree. Please do not skip any questions.

1. I am unable to follow conversation during meetings because of tinnitus.
2. Tinnitus creates family problems.
3. I think I have a healthy outlook on tinnitus.
4. I feel uneasy in social situations because of tinnitus.
5. I have trouble falling asleep at night because of tinnitus.
6. Tinnitus contributes to a feeling of general ill health.
7. Tinnitus interferes with my ability to tell where sounds are coming from.
8. I have support from my friends regarding my tinnitus.
9. I am unable to relax because of tinnitus.
10. I do not enjoy life because of tinnitus.
11. My tinnitus has gotten worse over the years.
12. I cannot concentrate because of tinnitus.
13. Tinnitus makes me feel tired.
14. Tinnitus causes me to feel depressed.
15. The general public does not know about the devastating nature of tinnitus.
16. Tinnitus causes me to avoid noisy situations.
17. Tinnitus interferes with my speech understanding when talking with someone in a noisy room.
18. I find it difficult to explain what tinnitus is to others.
19. I complain more because of tinnitus.
20. Tinnitus makes me feel annoyed.
21. Tinnitus makes me feel insecure.
22. Tinnitus interferes with my speech understanding when listening to the television.
23. Tinnitus affects the quality of my relationships.
24. Tinnitus has caused a reduction in my speech understanding ability.
25. Tinnitus causes stress.
26. Tinnitus makes me feel anxious.
27. I feel frustrated frequently because of tinnitus.

Raw %

Factor 1

Factor 2

Factor 3

TOTAL

Scoring:
Factor 1—Social, Emotional, and Behavior Tinnitus Effects:
(add responses to 5, 6, 9, 10, 12, 13, 14, 18, 19, 20, 21, 23, 25, 26, 27)
= _____/15 = _____%

Factor 2—Tinnitus and Hearing:
(add responses to 1, 2, 4, 7, 16, 17, 22, 24)
= _____/8 = _____%

Factor 3—Outlook on Tinnitus:
(add responses to 11, and 15, plus [100 − response to 3] plus [100 − response to 8])
= _____/4 = _____%

TOTAL
[(Factor 1 × 15/27) + (Factor 2 × 8/27) + (Factor 3 × 4/27)]
= _____%

[a]Source: Kuk, Tyler, Russell, and Jordan (1990) and UITC (2011), which includes a scoring template. Used with permission of the University of Iowa Tinnitus Clinic.

Table 16.12 Iowa Tinnitus Activities Questionnaire[a]

INSTRUCTIONS: This questionnaire has 20 questions. Please indicate 0 that you strongly disagree (up to) 100 that you strongly agree. Please do not skip any questions.

1. My tinnitus is annoying.
2. My tinnitus masks some speech sounds.
3. When there are lots of things happening at once, my tinnitus interferes with my ability to attend to the most important thing.
4. My emotional peace is one of the worst effects of my tinnitus.
5. I have difficulty getting to sleep at night because of my tinnitus.
6. The effects of tinnitus on my hearing are worse than the effects of my hearing loss.
7. I feel like my tinnitus makes it difficult for me to concentrate on some tasks.
8. I am depressed because of my tinnitus.
9. My tinnitus, not my hearing loss, interferes with my appreciation of music and songs.
10. I am anxious because of my tinnitus.
11. I have difficulty focusing my attention on some important tasks because of tinnitus.
12. I just wish my tinnitus would go away. It is so frustrating.
13. The difficulty I have sleeping is one of the worst effects of my tinnitus.
14. In addition to my hearing loss, my tinnitus interferes with my understanding of speech.
15. My inability to think about something undisturbed is one of the worst effects of my tinnitus.
16. I am tired during the day because my tinnitus has disrupted my sleep.
17. One of the worst things about my tinnitus is its effect on my speech understanding, over and above any effect of my hearing loss.
18. I lie awake at night because of my tinnitus.
19. I have trouble concentrating while I am reading in a quiet room because of tinnitus.
20. When I wake up in the night, my tinnitus makes it difficult to get back to sleep.

Raw %
Concentration
Emotional Well Being
Hearing
Sleep
TOTAL

Scoring:
Concentration: (add responses to 3, 7, 11, 15, and 19) = _____/5 = _____%
Emotional: (add responses to 1, 4, 8, 10, and 12) = _____/5 = _____%
Hearing: (add responses to 2, 6, 9, 14, and 17) = _____/5 = _____%
Sleep: (add responses to 5, 13, 16, 18, and 20) = _____/5 = _____%

TOTAL:
[Concentration % + Emotional % + Hearing % + Sleep %]/4 = _____%

[a]Source: Tyler et al (2006) and UITC (2011), which includes a scoring template. Used with permission of the University of Iowa Tinnitus Clinic.

problems due to hearing loss and tinnitus, and is a useful screening tool for identifying who is an appropriate patient for tinnitus intervention. The *Self-Efficacy for Tinnitus Management Questionnaire* (Smith & Fagelson 2011) focuses on patients' confidence in their ability to manage their tinnitus and its effects. The third inventory is the *Tinnitus Functional Index* (Meikle, Henry, Griest, et al 2012), which not only enables audiologists to effectively scale the severity of tinnitus, but also is precise enough to identify changes resulting from intervention.

Although we are concentrating on tinnitus, the student should be aware that as many as ~ 45% of patients with tinnitus also complain of **hyperacusis**, or intolerance for loud sounds (Henry, Dennis & Schechter 2005a), and that these related complaints are typically treated together. In fact, one of the major components in assessing patients for tinnitus retraining therapy (discussed below) involves assigning them to diagnostic/treatment categories based on the difficulties they experience with tinnitus and sound tolerance (e.g., Jastreboff & Jastreboff 2000; Henry, Jastreboff, Jastreboff, Schechter, & Fausti 2002). The common features of hyperacusis treatment involve *avoiding overprotection* of the ears from sound exposure and the evasion of sounds in one's environment, *enhancing* the patient's *acoustical environment*, and a gradual process of *progressive desensitization* to sound using wearable sound generators and other means of enriching the patient's acoustical environment (Henry, Zaugg, & Schechter 2005c,d).

To date, most treatments to alleviate tinnitus itself, including various forms of medical and surgical intervention, have been largely unsuccessful (see, e.g., Langguth & Elgoyhen 2012), and invasive treatments are best avoided (Folmer, Theodoroff, Martin, & Shi 2014). Thus, instead of trying to alleviate the tinnitus, most contemporary intervention approaches attempt to remove or reduce its impact upon and objectionableness to the patient. Even though prior reviews suggested that tinnitus management techniques lacked adequate supporting evidence (e.g., Dobie 1999, 2004), the accumulating literature now provides us with several efficacious approaches and combinations of approaches (e.g., Henry et al 2005a,b,c,d; Henry, Schechter, Zaugg, et al 2006; Tyler 2006; Davis, Paki, & Hanley 2007; Bauer & Brozoski 2011; Cima, Maes, Joore, et al 2012; Newman & Sandridge 2012; Shekhawat, Searchfield, & Stinear 2013). Let us mention a few of the best-established approaches.

Sound therapy involves using various kinds of sounds to provide relief from tinnitus by such mechanisms as masking and habituation. It is often effective when used in association with various counseling approaches, but it is not yet clear whether sound therapy provides a reliably effective treatment all by itself (Hoare, Searchfield, El Refaie, & Henry 2014). **Tinnitus masking** is the traditional form of sound therapy for tinnitus, and is illustrated in **Fig. 16.10a**. Tinnitus masking seeks to provide immediate relief from disturbing tinnitus by rendering it inaudible (complete masking) or at least less audible (partial masking) by furnishing a more acceptable noise (e.g., Vernon & Meikle 2000; Schechter & Henry 2002). This is typically done by having the patient wear ear-level (a) noise generators (tinnitus maskers), (b) hearing aids to amplify sounds from the environment for those who also have hearing loss, as well as (c) combination devices that incorporate the hearing aid and noise generator in the same instrument (e.g., Shekhawat et al 2013; Hoare et al 2014). Supplemental sound sources such as CD players, radios, bedside masking devices, etc. may also be recommended to provide relief when the patient is not wearing the ear-level device. Other sound therapy approaches are discussed below.

Tinnitus retraining therapy (TRT) is an approach that combines directive counseling and sound therapy, based on a **neurophysiological model** of tinnitus (e.g., Jastreboff 1990; Jastreboff & Hazell 1993, 2004; Hazell 1999; Jastreboff & Jastreboff 2000). We normally habituate to unimportant background sounds, so we typically are unaware of, say, air-conditioner noise or a ticking clock. However, we tend not to habituate to sounds that carry important meanings (like footsteps behind us on a dark street or the noise of an approaching truck), which elicit primitive survival reactions mediated by the limbic and autonomic nervous systems. According to the neurophysiological model, tinnitus becomes problematic when it is linked by classical conditioning to fears and negative associations that evoke such responses (e.g., worries that the tinnitus is a symptom of a brain tumor or impending deafness). What develops is a vicious cycle in which the tinnitus evokes emotional and annoyance reactions, which, in turn, further focus the patient's attention on the tinnitus.

In TRT, a program of **directive counseling** supported by informative illustrations and examples is used to "demystify" the tinnitus, breaking down its negative associations over time (typically a 1- to 2-year period). Thus, the patient is retrained to respond to the tinnitus as a neutral stimulus, to which we can then habituate. Effective counseling can often be accomplished in group sessions (Henry, Loovis, Montero, et al 2007). **Sound therapy** in TRT involves the use of wearable ear-level noise generators that provide the patient with a backdrop of relatively low-level ongoing sound stimulation, which reduces the contrast between the tinnitus and background sounds (**Fig. 16.10b**). This makes the tinnitus less distinctive, thereby facilitating its **habituation**. A comparison of TRT with tinnitus masking plus counseling revealed that both approaches provided significant benefits, but TRT yielded greater improvements, especially for patients with more severe tinnitus problems (Henry et al 2006). A study comparing TRT and general counseling similarly found that while improvements were achieved with both approaches, TRT yielded greater benefits (Bauer & Brozoski 2011).

A different kind of sound therapy to achieve tinnitus habituation is employed by **neuromonics tinnitus treatment** (**NTT**; Davis, Wilde, & Steed 2001, 2002a,b; Davis 2005; Davis et al 2007). Here, the sound therapy stimulus is wide-band relaxing music that is spectrally adjusted to account for the patient's hearing loss, and is presented binaurally using a personal stimulating device similar to an MP3 player. The sound therapy is self-administered in daily sessions of 2 or more hours. Music is used because it promotes desensitization to the tinnitus by (a) eliciting *relaxation responses* and (b) producing *intermittent* masking of the tinnitus due to its increasing and decreasing levels over time. **Fig. 16.10c** illustrates how tinnitus is made intermittently audible and inaudible by the peaks and troughs of the music.

The NTT approach involves about 6 months of sound therapy along with educational and supportive counseling. The music stimulus may be used throughout the therapy regimen, or a staged protocol might be used. In the staged approach, the music is combined with masking noise during the earlier phases of treatment, after which only the music stimulus is used. Combining the music with masking noise completely covers the tinnitus because the troughs in the music are filled with the noise. Davis et al (2007) reported similar outcomes for the two approaches, with 91% of their subjects realizing clinically significant improvements in tinnitus disturbance after 6 months of treatment. Newman and Sandridge (2012) found that 6 months of treatment produced significant and similar amounts of improvement for patients receiving NTT and for those using noise generators.

Audiologic tinnitus management (ATM) involves an in-depth assessment phase followed by an ongoing treatment protocol for tinnitus and/ or hyperacusis (Henry et al 2005c,d). The treatment approach initially involves structured informational counseling and, if indicated, the fitting of wearable sound therapy devices (sound generators, hearing aids, combination devices). This is followed on an

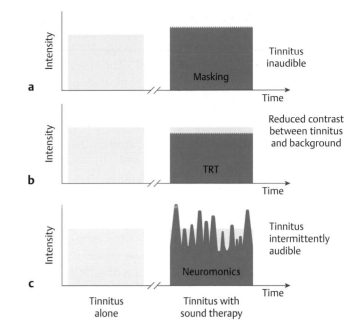

Fig. 16.10 (a–c) Artist's conceptualizations of different tinnitus sound therapy approaches. Blush represents tinnitus; green represents the sound therapy stimulus.

ongoing basis by structured informational counseling, monitoring the use of the wearable devices, augmentative sound sources (e.g., wearable CD players, table-top sound sources), and outcome assessment using questionnaires and interviews. Repeated testing of loudness discomfort levels is also done for hyperacusis patients. Because many patients with less severe tinnitus problems do not require ongoing management, ATM also includes a short-term counseling program. In fact, its authors described a "progressive intervention approach" involving five levels of intervention (Henry et al 2005b). The first level uses telephone *screening* to identify those requiring intervention and answer basic concerns, and level 2 provides *informational counseling* on a group basis. The third level involves a *tinnitus intake assessment*, which includes individual educational counseling and identifies patients requiring *ongoing treatment* (level 4). Level 5 involves *extended treatment* beyond 1 or 2 years of ongoing treatment. Referrals for psychological management are considered at every level, particularly for those requiring extended treatment.

Various *counseling techniques* have been employed for tinnitus management. Andersson and Lyttkens (1999) found that psychological approaches are effective in reducing annoyance caused by tinnitus (although not its loudness). **Cognitive-behavioral therapy (CBT)** is the principal and perhaps the most efficacious counseling approach for tinnitus management (e.g., Sweetow 2000; Andersson 2001, 2002; Henry & Wilson 2001; Cima et al 2012; Cima, Andersson, Schmidt, & Henry 2014). Analogous to similar techniques for pain management, CBT for tinnitus concentrates on (a) addressing the patient's thoughts and beliefs about the tinnitus using cognitive structuring approaches; and (b) modifying maladaptive reactions using techniques like applied relaxation, increased physical activity, positive imagery, distraction, and sleep management. While CBT is generally associated with psychotherapists, it can be used for tinnitus treatment by appropriately trained audiologists; and positive outcomes have also been reported for a CBT protocol administered in the form of an Internet-based self-help protocol (Kaldo-Sandström, Larsen, & Andersson 2004). The patient is also counseled about the availability of sound therapy, although it is not directly involved in CBT itself. A large-scale study by Cima et al (2012) found that a combined CBT-TBT approach by audiologists, psychologists, and others was significantly more effective than the "usual care" (which involved informational counseling, tinnitus maskers, hearing aids, and counseling by a social worker in more difficult cases).

■ Study Questions

1. Explain the considerations involved in the use of monaural versus binaural amplification.

2. Under what conditions would we consider the use of CROS and BICROS hearing aids?

3. What are prescriptive hearing aid fitting methods and how are they used?

4. Describe what is involved in the (a) verification and (b) validation of a hearing aid fitting.

5. Describe the components of cochlear implants, and explain how they provide patients with auditory stimulation.

6. Explain the considerations for cochlear implant candidacy for children and adults.

7. Explain (a) how noise, reverberation, and distance affect the speech signal reaching a hearing aid user, and (b) how these problems are addressed with FM systems, induction systems, and sound field amplification.

8. Explain the nature of analytical and synthetic activities in auditory-visual training for the hearing impaired.

9. Describe the characteristics of some contemporary intervention approaches for young children with hearing impairment.

10. Describe the techniques used in contemporary tinnitus management approaches.

References

Alpiner JG. 1987. Evaluation of adult communication function. In: Alpiner JG, McCarthy PA, eds. Rehabilitative Audiology: Children and Adults. Baltimore, MD: Williams & Wilkins; 44–114

American Academy of Audiology (AAA). 2006a. Guidelines for the Audiologic Management of Adult Hearing Impairment. Available at http://www.audiology.org/publications/documents/positions/Adultrehab/

American Academy of Audiology (AAA). Health-related quality of life benefits of amplification in adults. Audiol Today 2006b;18(5):28–31

American Academy of Audiology (AAA). 2007. AAA Clinical Practice Guidelines: Remote Microphone Hearing Assistance Technologies for Children and Youth Birth–21 Years (DRAFT 11.13.07). Available at http://www.audiology.org/NR/rdonlyres/0A8B687B-FEFA-4F4A-A9EC-67B0CE64D414/0/FINALHATGuidelines-Draft111307.pdf

American Academy of Audiology (AAA). 2011a. Clinical Practice Guidelines: Remote Microphone Hearing Assistance Technologies for Children and Youth Birth–21 Years and Supplement A (April 2011). Available at http://www.audiology.org/resources/documentlibrary/Documents/HAT_Guidelines_Supplement_A.pdf

American Academy of Audiology (AAA). 2011b. Clinical Practice Guidelines: Remote Microphone Hearing Assistance Technologies for Children and Youth Birth–21 Years. Supplement B: Classroom Audio Distribution Systems—Selection and Verification (July 2011). Available at http://www.audiology.org/resources/documentlibrary/Documents/20110926_HAT_GuidelinesSupp_B.pdf

American Academy of Audiology (AAA). 2013. Clinical Practice Guidelines: Pediatric Amplification. Available at http://www.audiology.org/resources/documentlibrary/Documents/PediatricAmplificationGuidelines.pdf

American National Standards Institute (ANSI). 2009. ANSI S3.22-2009. American National Standard Specification of Hearing Aid Characteristics. New York, NY: ANSI

American National Standards Institute (ANSI). 2010a. S12.60-2010/Part 1. Acoustical Performance Criteria, Design Requirements, and Guidelines for Schools, Part 1: Permanent Schools. New York, NY: ANSI

American National Standards Institute (ANSI). 2010b. S12.60-2010/Part 2. Acoustical Performance Criteria, Design Requirements, and Guidelines for Schools, Part 2: Relocatable Classroom Factors. New York, NY: ANSI

American Speech-Language-Hearing Association (ASHA). Guidelines for hearing aid fitting for adults. Am J Audiol 1998;7:5–13

American Speech-Language-Hearing Association (ASHA). 2002. Guidelines for Fitting and Monitoring FM Systems. Available at www.asha.org/policy

American Speech-Language-Hearing Association (ASHA). 2004. Technical report: Cochlear implants. Supplement 24. Available at http://www.asha.org/NR/rdonlyres/215CC9B8-6831-494F-83ED-E02A6832A8A9/0/24402_1.pdf

American Speech-Language-Hearing Association (ASHA). 2005a. Acoustics in Educational Settings: Technical Report. Available at http://www.asha.org/members/deskref-journals/deskref/default

American Speech-Language-Hearing Association (ASHA). 2005b. Guidelines for Addressing Acoustics in Educational Settings. Available at http://www.asha.org/members/deskref-journals/deskref/default

American Speech-Language-Hearing Association. (ASHA). 2006. Preferred Practice Patterns for the Profession of Audiology. Available at www.asha.org

Anderson K. 1989. Screening Instrument for Targeting Educational Risk (SIFTER). Austin, TX: Pro-Ed

Anderson K. 2002. ELF—Early Listening Function. Available at http://www.cms-kids.com/home/resources/es_policy_0113/Attachments/6_SHINE_elf_questionnaire.pdf

Anderson K. 2004. Screening Instrument for Targeting Educational Risk in Secondary Students (Secondary SIFTER). Available at http://csd.cbcs.usf.edu/_assets/docs/clinic_forms/SIFTER_for_each_teacher.pdf

Anderson K, Matkin N. 1996. Screening Instrument for Targeting Educational Risk in Pre-School Children (Age 3–Kindergarten) (Pre-School SIFTER). Tampa, FL: Educational Audiology Association

Anderson K, Smaldino J. 1998. Listening Inventories for Education (L.I.F.E.). Tampa, FL: Educational Audiology Association

Anderson K, Smaldino J. Listening inventories for education: a classroom measurement tool. Hear J 1999;52:74–76

Anderson K, Smaldino J. 2000. Children's home inventory of listening difficulties (CHILD). Available at http://depts.washington.edu/isei/ptrl/upload/com_child_questionnaire_gb-2.pdf

Andersson G. The role of psychology in managing tinnitus: a cognitive behavioral approach. Semin Hear 2001;22:65–76

Andersson G. Psychological aspects of tinnitus and the application of cognitive-behavioral therapy. Clin Psychol Rev 2002;22(7):977–990

Andersson G, Lyttkens L. A meta-analytic review of psychological treatments for tinnitus. Br J Audiol 1999; 33(4):201–210

Antia SD, Sabers DL, Stinson MS. Validity and reliability of the classroom participation questionnaire with deaf and hard of hearing students in public schools. J Deaf Stud Deaf Educ 2007;12(2):158–171

Bauer CA, Brozoski TJ. Effect of tinnitus retraining therapy on the loudness and annoyance of tinnitus: a controlled trial. Ear Hear 2011;32(2):145–155

Beck L, Compton C, Gilmore R, et al. Telecoils: past, present and future. Hear Instr 1993;44:22–27,40

Behr R, Müller J, Shehata-Dieler W, et al. The high rate CIS auditory brainstem implant for restoration of hearing in NF-2 patients. Skull Base 2007;17(2):91–107

Beiter AL, Brimacombe JA. 1993. Cochlear implants. In: Alpiner JG, McCarthy PA, eds. Rehabilitative Audiology in Children and Adults, 2nd ed. Baltimore, MD: Williams & Wilkins; 417–440

Bender D, Mueller HG. 1984. Factors influencing the decision to obtain amplification. Paper presented at American Speech-Language-Hearing Association Convention. San Francisco, CA.

Berger KW, Hagberg EN, Rane RL. 1988. Prescription of Hearing Aids: Rationale, Procedure, and Results. Kent, OH: Herald

Bess FH, Dodd-Murphy J, Parker RA. Children with minimal sensorineural hearing loss: prevalence, educational performance, and functional status. Ear Hear 1998;19(5):339–354

Blamey PJ, Sarant JZ, Paatsch LE, et al. Relationships among speech perception, production, language, hearing loss, and age in children with impaired hearing. J Speech Lang Hear Res 2001;44(2):264–285

Boothroyd A. Auditory perception of speech contrasts by subjects with sensorineural hearing loss. J Speech Hear Res 1984;27(1):134–144

Boothroyd A. 1985. Residual Hearing and the Problem of Carry-over in the Speech of the Deaf. ASHA report no. 15, 8–14

Bornstein H. Signed English: a manual approach to English language development. J Speech Hear Disord 1974;39(3):330–343

Bragg VC. Toward a more objective hearing aid fitting procedure. Hear Instr 1977;28:6–9

Bruhn M. 1920. The Mueller-Walle Method of Lipreading for the Deaf. Lynn, MA: Nichols

Bunger A. 1932. Speech Reading—Jena Method. Danville: Interstate

Burk MH, Humes LE. Effects of training on speech recognition performance in noise using lexically hard words. J Speech Lang Hear Res 2007;50(1):25–40

Burk MH, Humes LE. Effects of long-term training on aided speech-recognition performance in noise in older adults. J Speech Lang Hear Res 2008;51(3):759–771

Burk MH, Humes LE, Amos NE, Strauser LE. Effect of training on word-recognition performance in noise for young normal-hearing and older hearing-impaired listeners. Ear Hear 2006;27(3):263–278

Byrne D, Dillon H. The National Acoustic Laboratories' (NAL) new procedure for selecting the gain and frequency response of a hearing aid. Ear Hear 1986;7(4): 257–265

Byrne D, Dillon H, Ching T, Katsch R, Keidser G. NAL-NL1 procedure for fitting nonlinear hearing aids: characteristics and comparisons with other procedures. J Am Acad Audiol 2001;12(1):37–51

Byrne D, Parkinson A, Newall P. Hearing aid gain and frequency response requirements for the severely/profoundly hearing impaired. Ear Hear 1990;11(1):40–49

Calvert DR, Silverman SR. 1975. Speech and Deafness. Washington, DC: Alexander Graham Bell Association for the Deaf

Carhart R. Tests for selection of hearing aids. Laryngoscope 1946;56(12):780–794

Carhart R. 1960. Auditory training. In Davis H, Silverman SR (Eds.): Hearing and Deafness. New York, NY: Holt, Rinehart & Winston; 368–386

Carney AE, Osberger MJ, Carney E, Robbins AM, Renshaw J, Miyamoto RT. A comparison of speech discrimination with cochlear implants and tactile aids. J Acoust Soc Am 1993;94(4):2036–2049

Cashman M, Corbin H, Riko K, Rossman R. Effect of recent hearing aid improvements on management of the hearing impaired. J Otolaryngol 1984;13(4):227–231

Centers for Disease Control and Prevention (CDC). 2007. Use of Meningitis Vaccine in Persons with Cochlear Implants (June 4, 2007). Available at http://www.cdc.gov/vaccines/vpd-vac/mening/cochlear/dis-cochlear-hcp.htm

Ching TY, Dillon H, Marnane V, et al. Outcomes of early- and late-identified children at 3 years of age: findings from a prospective population-based study. Ear Hear 2013;34(5):535–552

Ching TYC, Hill M. The Parents' Evaluation of Aural/Oral Performance of Children (PEACH) scale: normative data. J Am Acad Audiol 2007;18(3):220–235

Ching TYC, Hill M, Dillon H. Effect of variations in hearing-aid frequency response on real-life functional performance of children with severe or profound hearing loss. Int J Audiol 2008;47(8):461–475

Ching TYC, Scollie SD, Dillon H, et al. Evaluation of the NAL-NL1 and the DSL v.4.1 prescriptions for children: paired-comparison intelligibility judgments and functional performance ratings. Int J Audiol 2010;49(Suppl 1):S35–S48

Chute PM, Nevins ME. 2000. Cochlear implants in children. In: Roeser RJ, Valente M, Hosford-Hill H, eds. Audiology: Treatment. New York, NY: Thieme Medical Publishers; 511–535

Cima RFF, Andersson G, Schmidt CJ, Henry JA. Cognitive-behavioral treatments for tinnitus: a review of the literature. J Am Acad Audiol 2014;25(1):29–61

Cima RFF, Maes IH, Joore MA, et al. Specialised treatment based on cognitive behaviour therapy versus usual care for tinnitus: a randomised controlled trial. Lancet 2012;379(9830):1951–1959

Cochlear Americas. N.d. Sound and Beyond. Available at www.cochlearamericas.com

Cohen NL, Waltzman SB, Roland JT Jr, Staller SJ, Hoffman RA. Early results using the nucleus CI24M in children. Am J Otol 1999;20(2):198–204

Colletti V, Shannon RV. Open set speech perception with auditory brainstem implant? Laryngoscope 2005;115(11):1974–1978

Colletti V, Shannon RV, Carner M, Veronese S, Colletti L. Progress in restoration of hearing with the auditory brainstem implant. Prog Brain Res 2009;175:333–345

Colletti L, Shannon R, Colletti V. Auditory brainstem implants for neurofibromatosis type 2. Curr Opin Otolaryngol Head Neck Surg 2012;20(5):353–357

Compton CL. 2000. Assistive technology for the enhancement of receptive communication. In: Alpiner JG, McCarthy PA, eds. Rehabilitative Audiology: Children and Adults, 3rd ed. Baltimore, MD: Lippincott Williams & Wilkins; 501–555

Cornett R. Cued speech. Am Ann Deaf 1967;112:3–13

Cowan RS, Blamey PJ, Galvin KL, Sarant JZ, Alcántara JI, Clark GM. Perception of sentences, words, and speech features by profoundly hearing-impaired children using a multichannel electrotactile speech processor. J Acoust Soc Am 1990;88(3):1374–1384

Cowie R, Douglas-Cowie E, Kerr AG. A study of speech deterioration in profound post-lingually deafened adults. J Laryngol Otol 1983;96:101–112

Cox RM. Using ULCL measures to find frequency-gain and SSPL90. Hear Instr 1983;34:17–21

Cox RM. A structured approach to hearing aid selection. Ear Hear 1985;6(5):226–239

Cox RM. The MSUv3 hearing instrument prescription procedure. Hear Instr 1988;39:6–10

Cox RM. Using loudness data for hearing aid selection: The IHAFF approach. Hear J 1995;47:39–42

Cox RM, Alexander GC. The abbreviated profile of hearing aid benefit. Ear Hear 1995;16(2):176–186

Cox RM, Alexander GC. Measuring satisfaction with amplification in daily life: the SADL scale. Ear Hear 1999;20(4):306–320

Cox RM, Alexander GC. Expectations about hearing aids and their relationship to fitting outcome. J Am Acad Audiol 2000;11(7):368–382

Cox RM, Alexander GC. The International Outcome Inventory for Hearing Aids (IOI-HA):psychometric properties of the English version. Int J Audiol 2002;41:30–35

Cox RM, Alexander GC, Taylor IM, Gray GA. The contour test of loudness perception. Ear Hear 1997;18(5):388–400

Cox RM, Gilmore C, Alexander GC. Comparison of two questionnaires for patient-assessed hearing aid benefit. J Am Acad Audiol 1991;2(3):134–145

Cox RM, McDaniel DM. Development of the Speech Intelligibility Rating (SIR) test for hearing aid comparisons. J Speech Hear Res 1989;32(2):347–352

Crandell CC. Speech recognition in noise by children with minimal degrees of sensorineural hearing loss. Ear Hear 1993;14(3):210–216

Crandell CC, Smaldino JJ. Sound-field amplification in the classroom. Am J Audiol 1992;1:16–18

Crandell CC, Smaldino JJ. 2000. Room acoustics for listeners with normal-hearing and hearing impairment. In: Roeser RJ, Valente M, Hosford-Dunn H, eds. Audiology: Treatment. New York, NY: Thieme; 601–637

Crandell CC, Smaldino JJ, Flexer C. A suggested protocol for implementing sound-field FM technology in the educational setting. J Educ Audiol 1997;5:13–21

Crandell CC, Smaldino JJ, Flexer C. 2005. Sound-Field FM Amplification: Applications to Speech Perception and Classroom Acoustics, 2nd ed. San Diego, CA: Singular

Davis H, Stevens SS, Nichols RH, et al. 1947. Hearing Aids: An Experimental Study of Design Objectives. Cambridge, MA: Harvard University Press

Davis PB. 2005. Music and the acoustic desensitization protocol. In: Tyler R, ed. Tinnitus Treatments. New York, NY: Thieme; 146–160

Davis PB, Paki B, Hanley PJ. Neuromonics Tinnitus Treatment: third clinical trial. Ear Hear 2007;28(2): 242–259

Davis PB, Wilde RA, Steed L. Relative effects of acoustic stimulation and counseling in the tinnitus rehabilitation process. Aust N Z J Audiol 2001;23:84–85

Davis PB, Wilde RA, Steed L. 2002a. Trials of tinnitus desensitisation music: Neurophysiology-influenced rehabilitation. Seventh International Tinnitus Seminar. Perth: University of Western Australia; 74–80

Davis PB, Wilde RA, Steed L. 2002b. A habituation-based rehabilitation technique using the acoustic desensitisation protocol. Seventh International Tinnitus Seminar. Perth: University of Western Australia; 188–191

De Filippo CL, Scott BL. A method for training and evaluating the reception of ongoing speech. J Acoust Soc Am 1978;63(4):1186–1192

deJong R. 1994. Selecting and verifying hearing aid fittings for symmetrical hearing loss. In: Valente M, ed. Strategies for Selecting and Verifying Hearing Aid Fittings. New York, NY: Thieme; 180–206

Demorest ME, Erdman SA. Scale composition and item analysis of the Communication Profile for the Hearing Impaired. J Speech Hear Res 1986;29(4):515–535

Dettman SJ, Pinder D, Briggs RJS, Dowell RC, Leigh JR. Communication development in children who receive the cochlear implant younger than 12 months: risks versus benefits. Ear Hear 2007;28(2, Suppl):11S–18S

Dillon H. NAL-NL1: a new procedure for fitting non-linear hearing aids. Hear Instr 1999a;52:10–16

Dillon H. Using the NAL-NL1 prescriptive procedure with advanced hearing instruments. Hear Rev 1999b;6:8–20

Dillon H. What's new from NAL in hearing aid prescriptions? Hear J 2006;5(10):10–16

Dillon H. 2012. Hearing Aids, 2nd ed. Sydney: Boomerang Press

Dillon H, James A, Ginis J. Client Oriented Scale of Improvement (COSI) and its relationship to several other measures of benefit and satisfaction provided by hearing aids. J Am Acad Audiol 1997;8(1):27–43

Dillon H, Storey L. The National Acoustic Laboratories' procedure for selecting the saturation sound pressure level of hearing aids: theoretical derivation. Ear Hear 1998;19(4):255–266

Dobie RA. A review of randomized clinical trials in tinnitus. Laryngoscope 1999;109(8):1202–1211

Dobie RA. 2004. Clinical trials and drug therapy for tinnitus. In: Snow JB, ed. Tinnitus: Theory and Management. Hamilton, Ontario: BC Decker; 266–277

Dockrell JE, Shield B. The impact of sound-field systems on learning and attention in elementary school classrooms. J Speech Lang Hear Res 2012;55(4): 1163–1176

Dorman MF, Gifford RH. Combining acoustic and electric stimulation in the service of speech recognition. Int J Audiol 2010;49(12):912–919

Dubno JR, Dirks DD, Morgan DE. Effects of age and mild hearing loss on speech recognition in noise. J Acoust Soc Am 1984;76(1):87–96

Dunn CC, Perreau A, Gantz B, Tyler RS. Benefits of localization and speech perception with multiple noise sources in listeners with a short-electrode cochlear implant. J Am Acad Audiol 2010;21(1):44–51

Dunn CC, Tyler RS, Oakley S, Gantz BJ, Noble W. Comparison of speech recognition and localization performance in bilateral and unilateral cochlear implant users matched on duration of deafness and age at implantation. Ear Hear 2008;29(3):352–359

Eisenberg LS, Martinez AS, Sennaroglu G, Osberger MJ. Establishing new criteria in selecting children for a cochlear implant: performance of "platinum" hearing aid users. Ann Otol Rhinol Laryngol Suppl 2000;185: 30–33

Elfenbein JL, Hardin-Jones MA, Davis JM. Oral communication skills of children who are hard of hearing. J Speech Hear Res 1994;37(1):216–226

Erber NP. Auditory-visual perception of speech. J Speech Hear Disord 1975;40(4):481–492

Erber NP. 1982. Auditory Training. Washington, DC: AG Bell Association for the Deaf

Erber NP, Alencewicz CM. Audiologic evaluation of deaf children. J Speech Hear Disord 1976;41(2):256–267

Ericson H, Svärd I, Högset O, Devert G, Ekström L. Contralateral routing of signals in unilateral hearing impairment. A better method of fitting. Scand Audiol 1988;17(2):111–116

Etymotic Research. Bench-Koval-Bamford Speech-In-Noise (BKB-SIN) Test 2005;3:••• Elk Grove Village, IL: Etymotic Research

Fabry DA. Facts vs myths: the "skinny" on slim-tube open fittings. Hear Rev 2006;13(5):20–25

Finitzo T. 1988. Classroom acoustics. In: Roeser RJ, Downs MP, eds. Auditory Disorders in School Children, 2nd ed. New York, NY: Thieme; 221–233

Finitzo-Hieber T, Tillman TW. Room acoustics effects on monosyllabic word discrimination ability for normal and hearing-impaired children. J Speech Hear Res 1978;21(3):440–458

Fisher CG. Confusions among visually perceived consonants. J Speech Hear Res 1968;11(4):796–804

Flexer C. 1992. FM classroom public address systems. In: Ross M, ed. FM Auditory Training Systems: Characteristics, Selection and Use. Timonium, MD: York Press; 189–210

Flexer C. 1994. Facilitating Hearing and Listening in Young Children. San Diego, CA: Singular

Folmer RL, Theodoroff SM, Martin WH, Shi Y. Experimental, controversial, and futuristic treatments for chronic tinnitus. J Am Acad Audiol 2014;25(1):106–125

Food and Drug Administration (FDA). 2007. FDA Public Health Notification: Importance of Vaccination in Cochlear Implant Recipient (Oct. 10, 2007). Available at http://www.fda.gov/cdrh/safety/101007-cochlear.html

Francis HW, Chee N, Yeagle J, Cheng A, Niparko JK. Impact of cochlear implants on the functional health status of older adults. Laryngoscope 2002;112(8 Pt 1): 1482–1488

Fryauf-Bertschy H, Tyler RS, Kelsay DM, Gantz BJ, Woodworth GG. Cochlear implant use by prelingually deafened children: the influences of age at implant and length of device use. J Speech Lang Hear Res 1997; 40(1):183–199

Galvin KL, Mavrias G, Moore A, Cowan RSC, Blamey PJ, Clark GM. A comparison of Tactaid II+ and Tactaid 7 use by adults with a profound hearing impairment. Ear Hear 1999;20(6):471–482

Galvin KL, Mok M, Dowell RC. Perceptual benefit and functional outcomes for children using sequential bilateral cochlear implants. Ear Hear 2007;28(4):470–482

Gantz BJ, Turner CW. Combining acoustic and electrical hearing. Laryngoscope 2003;113(10):1726–1730

Gantz BJ, Turner C. Combining acoustic and electrical speech processing: Iowa/Nucleus hybrid implant. Acta Otolaryngol 2004;124(4):344–347

Garstecki DC. Auditory-visual training program for hearing-impaired adults. J Acad Rehab Audiol 1981; 14:223–238

Gatehouse S. Glasgow hearing aid benefit profile: derivation and validation of a client-centered outcome measure for hearing aid services. J Am Acad Audiol 1999;10:80–103

Gatehouse S, Noble W. The Speech, Spatial and Qualities of Hearing Scale (SSQ). Int J Audiol 2004;43(2): 85–99

Geers AE. Factors affecting the development of speech, language, and literacy in children with early cochlear implantation. Lang Speech Hear Svcs Schools 2002;33:172–183

Geers A, Brenner C, Nicholas J, Uchanski R, Tye-Murray N, Tobey E. Rehabilitation factors contributing to implant benefit in children. Ann Otol Rhinol Laryngol Suppl 2002;189:127–130

Geers AE, Hayes H. Reading, writing, and phonological processing skills of adolescents with 10 or more years of cochlear implant experience. Ear Hear 2011;32(1, Suppl):49S–59S

Geers AE, Moog JS. Speech perception and production skills of students with impaired hearing from oral and total communication education settings. J Speech Hear Res 1992;35(6):1384–1393

Geers AE, Moog JS, Biedenstein J, Brenner C, Hayes H. Spoken language scores of children using cochlear implants compared to hearing age-mates at school entry. J Deaf Stud Deaf Educ 2009;14(3):371–385

Geers AE, Nicholas JG, Sedey AL. Language skills of children with early cochlear implantation. Ear Hear 2003;24(1, Suppl):46S–58S

Geers AE, Nicholas J, Tye-Murray N, et al. Effects of communication mode on skills of long-term cochlear implant users. Ann Otol Rhinol Laryngol Suppl 2000;185: 89–92

Geers AE, Sedey AL. Language and verbal reasoning skills in adolescents with 10 or more years of cochlear implant experience. Ear Hear 2011;32(1, Suppl):39S–48S

Geers AE, Tobey EA, Moog JS, Eds. 2011. Long term outcomes of cochlear implantation in early childhood. Ear Hear 32;(Suppl. 1):1S–92S.

Geier L, Barker M, Fisher L, Opie J. The effect of long-term deafness on speech recognition in postlingually deafened adult CLARION cochlear implant users. Ann Otol Rhinol Laryngol Suppl 1999;177(Suppl. 177):80–83

Gelfand SA. Usage of CROS hearing aids by unilaterally deaf patients. Arch Otolaryngol 1979;105(6):328–332

Gelfand SA. Long-term recovery and no recovery from the auditory deprivation effect with binaural amplification: six cases. J Am Acad Audiol 1995;6(2):141–149

Gelfand SA. 2010. Hearing: An Introduction to Psychological and Physiological Acoustics, 5th ed. London, UK: Informa Healthcare

Gelfand SA, Hochberg I. Binaural and monaural speech discrimination under reverberation. Audiology 1976;15(1):72–84

Gelfand SA, Ross L, Miller S. Sentence reception in noise from one versus two sources: effects of aging and hearing loss. J Acoust Soc Am 1988;83(1):248–256

Gelfand SA, Silman S. Effects of small room reverberation upon the recognition of some consonant features. J Acoust Soc Am 1979;66:22–29

Gelfand SA, Silman S. Apparent auditory deprivation in children: implications of monaural versus binaural amplification. J Am Acad Audiol 1993;4(5):313–318

Gelfand SA, Silman S, Ross L. Long-term effects of monaural, binaural and no amplification in subjects with bilateral hearing loss. Scand Audiol 1987;16(4):201–207

Gengel R. Acceptable speech-to-noise ratios for aided speech discrimination by the hearing impaired. J Aud Res 1971;11:219–222

Gifford RH, Shallop JK, Peterson AM. Speech recognition materials and ceiling effects: considerations for cochlear implant programs. Audiol Neurotol 2008; 13(3):193–205

Gilmore R, Lederman N. Induction loop assistive listening systems: back to the future? Hear Instr 1989;40:14–20

Goehl H, Kaufman DK. Do the effects of adventitious deafness include disordered speech? J Speech Hear Disord 1984;49(1):58–64

Goldstein DP, Stephens SDG. Audiological rehabilitation: management model I. Audiology 1981;20(5): 432–452

Gray RF. 1991. Cochlear implants: the medical criteria for patient selection. In: H Cooper, ed. Cochlear Implants: A Practical Guide. London, UK: Whurr; 146–154

Guidelines Development Conference (GDC). 2008. Guidelines for Identification and Management of Infants and Young Children with Auditory Neuropathy Spectrum Disorder. Como, Italy. Monograph available at http://www.childrenscolorado.org/pdf/ANSD%20Monograph%20Bill%20Daniels%20Center%20for%20Childrens%20Hearing.pdf

Guo L-Y, Spencer LJ, Tomblin JB. Acquisition of tense marking in English-speaking children with cochlear implants: a longitudinal study. J Deaf Stud Deaf Educ 2013;18(2):187–205

Hallam RS, Jakes SC, Hinchcliffe R. Cognitive variables in tinnitus annoyance. Br J Clin Psychol 1988;27(Pt 3): 213–222

Harford E. Bilateral CROS: two-sided listening with one hearing aid. Arch Otolaryngol 1966;84(4):426–432

Harford E, Barry J. A rehabilitative approach to the problem of unilateral hearing impairment: the contralateral routing of signals (CROS). J Speech Hear Disord 1965;30:121–138

Harford E, Dodds E. The clinical application of CROS: a hearing aid for unilateral deafness. Arch Otolaryngol 1966;83(5):455–464

Hawkins DB. Comparisons of speech recognition in noise by mildly-to-moderately hearing-impaired children using hearing aids and FM systems. J Speech Hear Disord 1984;49(4):409–418

Hawkins DB. Effectiveness of counseling-based adult group aural rehabilitation programs: a systematic review of the evidence. J Am Acad Audiol 2005;16(7):485–493

Hawkins DB, Beck LB, Bratt GW, Fabry DA, Mueller HC, Stelmachowicz PB. The Vanderbilt/Department of Veterans Affairs 1990 conference consensus statement: recommended components of a hearing aid selection procedure for adults. Audiol Today 1991;3:16–18

Hawkins DB, Schum DJ. Some effects of FM-system coupling on hearing aid characteristics. J Speech Hear Disord 1985;50(2):132–141

Hawkins DB, Walden BE, Montgomery A, Prosek RA. Description and validation of an LDL procedure designed to select SSPL90. Ear Hear 1987;8(3):162–169

Hazell JWP. 1999. The TRT method in practice. Proceedings of Sixth International Tinnitus Seminar. London, UK: Tinnitus and Hyperacusis Centre; 92–98

Helms J, Müller J, Schön F, et al. Comparison of the TEMPO+ ear-level speech processor and the CIS PRO+ body-worn processor in adult MED-EL cochlear implant users. ORL J Otorhinolaryngol Relat Spec 2001;63(1, Spec):31–40

Henderson Sabes J, Sweetow RW. Variables predicting outcomes on listening and communication enhancement (LACE) training. Int J Audiol 2007;46(7):374–383

Henry JA, Dennis KC, Schechter MA. General review of tinnitus: prevalence, mechanisms, effects, and management. J Speech Lang Hear Res 2005a;48(5):1204–1235

Henry JA, Griest S, Zaugg TL, et al. Tinnitus and hearing survey: a screening tool to differentiate bothersome tinnitus from hearing difficulties. Am J Audiol 2015;24(1):66–77

Henry JA, Jastreboff MM, Jastreboff PJ, Schechter MA, Fausti SA. Assessment of patients for treatment with tinnitus retraining therapy. J Am Acad Audiol 2002;13(10):523–544

Henry JA, Loovis C, Montero M, et al. Randomized clinical trial: group counseling based on tinnitus retraining therapy. J Rehabil Res Dev 2007;44(1):21–32

Henry JA, Schechter MA, Loovis CL, Zaugg TL, Kaelin C, Montero M. Clinical management of tinnitus using a "progressive intervention" approach. J Rehabil Res Dev 2005b;42(4, Suppl 2):95–116

Henry JA, Schechter MA, Zaugg TL, et al. Outcomes of clinical trial: tinnitus masking versus tinnitus retraining therapy. J Am Acad Audiol 2006;17(2):104–132

Henry JA, Zaugg TL, Myers PM, Kendall CJ. 2010. Progressive Tinnitus Management: Clinical Handbook for Audiologists. San Diego: Plural. Also available online at: http://www.ncrar.research.va.gov/Education/Documents/TinnitusDocuments/Index.asp

Henry JA, Zaugg TL, Schechter MA. Clinical guide for audiologic tinnitus management I: Assessment. Am J Audiol 2005c;14(1):21–48

Henry JA, Zaugg TL, Schechter MA. Clinical guide for audiologic tinnitus management II: Treatment. Am J Audiol 2005d;14(1):49–70

Henry JL, Wilson PH. 2001. The Psychological Management of Chronic Tinnitus. Needham Heights, MA: Allyn & Bacon

Hickson L, Worrall L, Scarinci N. A randomized controlled trial evaluating the active communication education program for older people with hearing impairment. Ear Hear 2007;28(2):212–230

Hill SL III, Marcus A, Digges ENB, Gillman N, Silverstein H. Assessment of patient satisfaction with various configurations of digital CROS and BICROS hearing aids. Ear Nose Throat J 2006;85(7):427–430, 442

Hnath-Chisolm T, Johnson CE, Danhauer JL, et al. A systematic review of health-related quality of life and hearing aids: final report of the American Academy of Audiology Task Force On the Health-Related Quality of Life Benefits of Amplification in Adults. J Am Acad Audiol 2007;18(2):151–183

Hnath-Chisolm T, Kishon-Rabin L. Tactile presentation of voice fundamental frequency as an aid to the perception of speech pattern contrasts. Ear Hear 1988;9(6):329–334

Hoare DJ, Searchfield GD, El Refaie A, Henry JA. Sound therapy for tinnitus management: practicable options. J Am Acad Audiol 2014;25(1):62–75

Hochberg I, Levitt H, Osberger MJ. 1983. Speech of the Hearing Impaired: Research, Training, and Personal Preparation. Baltimore, MD: University Park Press

Hodgson M, Rempel R, Kennedy S. Measurement and prediction of typical speech and background noise levels in university classrooms during lectures. J Acoust Soc Am 1999;105:226–233

Hol MKS, Kunst SJW, Snik AFM, Cremers CWRJ. Pilot study on the effectiveness of the conventional CROS, the transcranial CROS and the BAHA transcranial CROS in adults with unilateral inner ear deafness. Eur Arch Otorhinolaryngol 2010;267(6):889–896

Hollow RD, Dowell RC, Cowan RSC, Skok MC, Pyman BC, Clark GM. Continuing improvements in speech processing for adult cochlear implant patients. Ann Otol Rhinol Laryngol Suppl 1995;166(Suppl.):292–294

Hudgins CF, Numbers F. An investigation of the intelligibility of the speech of the deaf. Genet Psychol Monogr 1942;25:289–392

Hurley RM. Monaural hearing aid effect: case presentations. J Am Acad Audiol 1993;4(5):285–294, discussion 295

Hurley RM. Onset of auditory deprivation. J Am Acad Audiol 1999;10(10):529–534

Iglehart F. Speech perception by students with cochlear implants using sound-field systems in classrooms. Am J Audiol 2004;13(1):62–72

Ijsseldijk FJ. Speechreading performance under different conditions of video image, repetition, and speech rate. J Speech Hear Res 1992;35(2):466–471

Incerti PV, Ching TY, Cowan R. A systematic review of electric-acoustic stimulation: device fitting ranges, outcomes, and clinical fitting practices. Trends Amplif 2013;17(1):3–26

Jackson PL. 1982. Techniques for speech conservation. In: Hull R, ed. Rehabilitative Audiology. New York, NY: Grune & Stratton; 129–152

James AL, Papsin BC. Cochlear implant surgery at 12 months of age or younger. Laryngoscope 2004;114(12):2191–2195

Jastreboff PJ. Phantom auditory perception (tinnitus): mechanisms of generation and perception. Neurosci Res 1990;8(4):221–254

Jastreboff PJ, Hazell JW. A neurophysiological approach to tinnitus: clinical implications. Br J Audiol 1993;27(1):7–17

Jastreboff PJ, Hazell JWP. 2004. Tinnitus Retraining Therapy: Implementing the Tinnitus Retraining Model. New York, NY: Cambridge University Press

Jastreboff PJ, Jastreboff MM. Tinnitus Retraining Therapy (TRT) as a method for treatment of tinnitus and hyperacusis patients. J Am Acad Audiol 2000;11(3):162–177

Jeffers J, Barley M. 1971. Speechreading. Springfield, IL: CC Thomas

Jensema CJ, Karchmer MA, Trybus R. 1978. The Rated Intelligibility of Hearing-Impaired Children: Basic Relationships. Washington, DC: Gallaudet College

Jerger J, Silman S, Lew HL, Chmiel R. Case studies in binaural interference: converging evidence from behavioral and electrophysiologic measures. J Am Acad Audiol 1993;4(2):122–131

Johnson CE. Children's phoneme identification in reverberation and noise. J Speech Lang Hear Res 2000;43(1):144–157

Johnson EE. Prescriptive amplification recommendations for hearing losses with a conductive component and their impact on the required maximum power output: an update with accompanying clinical explanation. J Am Acad Audiol 2013;24(6):452–460

Johnson EE, Ricketts TA, Hornsby BW. The effect of digital phase cancellation feedback reduction systems on amplified sound quality. J Am Acad Audiol 2007;18(5):404–416

Joint Committee on Infant Hearing (JCIH), American Academy of Pediatrics. Year 2007 position statement: Principles and guidelines for early hearing detection and intervention programs. Pediatrics 2007;120(4):898–921

Joint Committee on Infant Hearing (JCIH), American Academy of Pediatrics. Supplement to the JCIH 2007 position statement: principles and guidelines for early intervention after confirmation that a child is deaf or hard of hearing. Pediatrics 2013;131(4):e1324–e1349

Jordan IK, Gustason G, Rosen R. An update on communication trends at programs for the deaf. Am Ann Deaf 1979;124(3):350–357

Kaldo-Sandström V, Larsen HC, Andersson G. Internet-based cognitive-behavioral self-help treatment of tinnitus: clinical effectiveness and predictors of outcome. Am J Audiol 2004;13(2):185–192

Kaplan H, Bally S, Brandt F, Busacco D, Pray J. Communication scale for older adults (CSOA). J Am Acad Audiol 1997;8(3):203–217

Keidser G, Dillon H, Carter L, O'Brien A. NAL-NL2 empirical adjustments. Trends Amplif 2012;16(4):211–223

Keidser G, Dillon H, Dyrlund O, Carter L, Hartley D. The NAL-NL2 prescription procedure. Audiol Res 2011;1(e24):88–90

Kessler AR, Giolas TG, Maxon AB. 1990. The Hearing Performance Inventory for Children (HPIC): reliability and validity. Presented at convention of American Speech-Language-Hearing Association, Seattle, WA

Killion MC. 1996. Talking hair cells: what they have to say about hearing aids. In: Berlin CI, ed. Hair Cells and Hearing Aids. San Diego, CA: Singular

Kinzie C, Kinzie R. 1931. Lipreading for the Deafened Adult. Chicago, IL: Winston

Kishon-Rabin L, Boothroyd A, Hanin L. Speechreading enhancement: a comparison of spatial-tactile display of voice fundamental frequency (F0) with auditory F0. J Acoust Soc Am 1996;100(1):593–602

Kishon-Rabin L, Haras N, Bergman M. Multisensory speech perception of young children with profound hearing loss. J Speech Lang Hear Res 1997;40(5):1135–1150

Knecht HA, Nelson PB, Whitelaw GM, Feth LL. Background noise levels and reverberation times in unoccupied classrooms: predictions and measurements. Am J Audiol 2002;11(2):65–71

Kopun JG, Stelmachowicz PG. Perceived communication difficulties of children with hearing loss. Am J Audiol 1998;7:30–38

Kühn-Inacker H, Shehata-Dieler W, Müller J, Helms J. Bilateral cochlear implants: a way to optimize auditory perception abilities in deaf children? Int J Pediatr Otorhinolaryngol 2004;68(10):1257–1266

Kühn-Inacker H, Weichbold V, Tsiakpini L, Coninx F, D'Haese P. 2003. LittlEARS Auditory Questionnaire: Parents Questionnaire to Assess Auditory Behavior. Innsbruck, Austria: MED-EL

Kuk FK. A screening procedure for modified simplex in frequency-gain response selection. Ear Hear 1994;15(1):62–70

Kuk FK, Tyler RS, Russell D, Jordan H. The psychometric properties of a tinnitus handicap questionnaire. Ear Hear 1990;11(6):434–445

Labadie RF, Carrasco VN, Gilmer CH, Pillsbury HC III. Cochlear implant performance in senior citizens. Otolaryngol Head Neck Surg 2000;123(4):419–424

Langguth B, Elgoyhen AB. Current pharmacological treatments for tinnitus. Expert Opin Pharmacother 2012;13(17):2495–2509

Leavitt R. Group amplification systems for students with hearing impairment. Semin Hear 1991;12:380–387

Lesinski-Schiedat A, Illg A, Warnecke A, Heermann R, Bertram B, Lenarz T. Kochleaimplantation bei Kindern im 1. Lebensjahr: Vorläufige Ergebnisse [Paediatric cochlear implantation in the first year of life: preliminary results]. HNO 2006;54(7):565–572

Leung J, Wang N-Y, Yeagle JD, et al. Predictive models for cochlear implantation in elderly candidates. Arch Otolaryngol Head Neck Surg 2005;131(12):1049–1054

Levine RA. Diagnostic issues in tinnitus: a neuro-otological perspective. Semin Hear 2001;22:23–36

Levitt H, Picket/t JM, Houde RA. 1980. Sensory Aids for the Hearing Impaired. New York, NY: IEEE Press

Levitt H, Sullivan JA, Neuman AC, Rubin-Spitz JA. Experiments with a programmable master hearing aid. J Rehabil Res Dev 1987;24(4):29–54

Lewis DE. Assistive devices for classroom listening. Am J Audiol 1994a;3:58–69

Lewis DE. Assistive devices for classroom listening: FM systems. Am J Audiol 1994b;3:70–83

Lewis MS, Crandell CC, Kreisman NV. Effects of frequency modulation (FM) transmitter microphone directivity on speech perception in noise. Am J Audiol 2004;13(1):16–22

Libby, 1986. The 1/3–2/3 insertion gain hearing aid selection guide. Hear Instr 37:27–28

Lin LM, Bowditch S, Anderson MJ, May B, Cox KM, Niparko JK. Amplification in the rehabilitation of unilateral deafness: speech in noise and directional hearing effects with bone-anchored hearing and contralateral routing of signal amplification. Otol Neurotol 2006;27(2):172–182

Ling D. 2002. Speech and the Hearing-Impaired Child: Theory and Practice, 2nd ed. Washington, DC: Alexander Graham Bell Association for the Deaf

Litovsky RY, Parkinson A, Arcaroli J, et al. Bilateral cochlear implants in adults and children. Arch Otolaryngol Head Neck Surg 2004;130(5):648–655

Litovsky RY, Johnstone PM, Godar S, et al. Bilateral cochlear implants in children: localization acuity measured with minimum audible angle. Ear Hear 2006;27(1):43–59

Loy B, Warner-Czyz AD, Tong L, Tobey EA, Roland PS. The children speak: an examination of the quality of life of pediatric cochlear implant users. Otolaryngol Head Neck Surg 2010;142(2):247–253

Lybarger SF. 1944. U.S. Patent application SN 543, 278

MacLeod A, Summerfield Q. Quantifying the contribution of vision to speech perception in noise. Br J Audiol 1987;21(2):131–141

Markides A. The speech of deaf and partially-hearing children with special reference to factors affecting intelligibility. Br J Disord Commun 1970;5(2):126–140

Markides A. 1983. The Speech of Hearing-Impaired Children. Dover, NH: Manchester University Press

McCandless GA, Lyregaard PE. Prescription of gain/output (POGO) for hearing aids. Hear Instr 1983;34:16–21

McConkey Robbins A, Koch DB, Osberger MJ, Zimmerman-Phillips S, Kishon-Rabin L. Effect of age at cochlear implantation on auditory skill development in infants and toddlers. Arch Otolaryngol Head Neck Surg 2004;130(5):570–574

McDermott R, Jones T. Articulation characteristics and listeners' judgments of the speech of children with severe hearing loss. Lang Speech Hear Serv Sch 1984; 15:110–126

Medical Research Council (MedResCo). 1947. Hearing Aids and Audiometers. Report of the Committee on Electro-Acoustics. Special Report 261. London, UK: His Majesty's Stationery Office

Meikle MB, Henry JA, Griest SE, et al. The tinnitus functional index: development of a new clinical measure for chronic, intrusive tinnitus. Ear Hear 2012;33(2): 153–176

Meyer TA, Svirsky MA. Speech perception by children with the Clarion (CIS) or nucleus 22 (SPEAK) cochlear implant or hearing aids. Ann Otol Rhinol Laryngol Suppl 2000;185:49–51

Minimum Speech Test Battery (MSTB) for Adult Cochlear Implant Users (MSTB). 2011. Manual available at http://www.auditorypotential.com/MSTBfiles/MSTB-Manual2011-06-20%20.pdf

Miyamoto RT, Osberger MJ, Robbins AM, Myres WA, Kessler K, Pope ML. Longitudinal evaluation of communication skills of children with single- or multichannel cochlear implants. Am J Otol 1992;13(3):215–222

Moog J, Biedenstein J, Davidson L. 1995. Speech Perception Instructional Curriculum and Evaluation (SPICE). St. Louis: Central Institute for the Deaf.

Most T, Shina-August E, Meilijson S. Pragmatic abilities of children with hearing loss using cochlear implants or hearing aids compared to hearing children. J Deaf Stud Deaf Educ 2010;15:422–437.

Mueller HG, Hawkins DB, Northern JL. 1992. Probe Microphone Measurements: Hearing Aid Selection and Assessment. San Diego, CA: Singular

Mueller HG, Ricketts TA. Open-canal fittings: ten take-home tips. Hear J 2006;59(11):24–39

Nábělek AK, Robinette L. Reverberation as a parameter in clinical testing. Audiology 1978;17(3):239–259

National Acoustics Laboratory (NAL). 2000. Outcome Measures. New South Wales, Australia: NAL. Available at http://www.nal.gov.au/outcome-measures_tab_cosi.shtml

Nelson PB, Soli SD, Seltz A. 2003. Classroom Acoustics II: Acoustical Barriers to Learning. Melville, NY: Acoustical Society of America

Neuman AC, Levitt H, Mills R, Schwander T. An evaluation of three adaptive hearing aid selection strategies. J Acoust Soc Am 1987;82(6):1967–1976

Newman CW, Jacobson GP, Spitzer JB. Development of the Tinnitus Handicap Inventory. Arch Otolaryngol Head Neck Surg 1996;122(2):143–148

Newman CW, Sandridge SA. A comparison of benefit and economic value between two sound therapy tinnitus management options. J Am Acad Audiol 2012; 23(2):126–138

Newman CW, Sandridge SA, Jacobson GP. Assessing outcomes of tinnitus intervention. J Am Acad Audiol 2014; 25(1):76–105

Newman CW, Weinstein BE, Jacobson GP, Hug GA. Test-retest reliability of the hearing handicap inventory for adults. Ear Hear 1991;12(5):355–357

Nicholas JG, Geers AE. Effect of age of cochlear implantation on receptive and expressive spoken language in 3-year-old deaf children. Int Congr Ser 2004;1273:340–343

Nilsson M, McCaw V, Soli S. 1996. Minimum Speech Test Battery for Adult Cochlear Implant Users: User Manual. Los Angeles, CA: House Ear Institute

Nilsson M, Soli SD, Sullivan JA. Development of the Hearing in Noise Test for the measurement of speech reception thresholds in quiet and in noise. J Acoust Soc Am 1994;95(2):1085–1099

Nitchie E. 1912. Lipreading: Principles and Practice. New York, NY: Stokes

Nittrouer S. (2015). After the implant. Asha Leader 2015; 20(3):46–48

Nittrouer S, Caldwell A, Lowenstein JH, Tarr E, Holloman C. Emergent literacy in kindgergarteners with cochlear implants. Ear Hear 2013;33:683–697

Olson AD, Preminger JE, Shinn JB. The effect of LACE DVD training in new and experienced hearing aid users. J Am Acad Audiol 2013;24(3):214–230

Osberger MJ, Fisher L. New directions in speech processing: patient performance with simultaneous analog stimulation. Ann Otol Rhinol Laryngol Suppl 2000;185:70–73

Osberger MJ, Maso M, Sam LK. Speech intelligibility of children with cochlear implants, tactile aids, or hearing aids. J Speech Hear Res 1993;36(1):186–203

Osberger MJ, Miyamoto RT, Zimmerman-Phillips S, et al. Independent evaluation of the speech perception abilities of children with the Nucleus 22-channel cochlear implant system. Ear Hear 1991;12(4, Suppl):66S–80S

Otto SR, Brackmann DE, Hitselberger WE, Shannon RV, Kuchta J. Multichannel auditory brainstem implant: update on performance in 61 patients. J Neurosurg 2002;96(6):1063–1071

Owens E, Blazek B. Visemes observed by hearing-impaired and normal-hearing adult viewers. J Speech Hear Res 1985;28(3):381–393

Owens E, Kessler DK, Raggio MW, Schubert ED. Analysis and revision of the minimal auditory capabilities (MAC) battery. Ear Hear 1985;6(6):280–290

Owens E, Kessler DK, Telleen CC, Schubert ED. 1981. The minimum auditory capabilities (MAC) battery. Hear Aid J 1981;34(9):10, 32, 34

Palmer CV. Hearing and listening in a typical classroom. Lang Speech Hear Serv Sch 1997;28:213–218

Palmer CV, Mormer E. Goals and expectations of the hearing aid fitting. Trends Amplif 1999;4(2):61–71

Palmer CV, Solodar HS, Hurley WR, Byrne DC, Williams KO. Self-perception of hearing ability as a strong predictor of hearing aid purchase. J Am Acad Audiol 2009;20(6):341–347

Papsin BC, Gordon KA. Cochlear implants for children with severe-to-profound hearing loss. N Engl J Med 2007;357(23):2380–2387

Papsin BC, Gysin C, Picton N, Nedzelski J, Harrison RV. Speech perception outcome measures in prelingually deaf children up to four years after cochlear implantation. Ann Otol Rhinol Laryngol Suppl 2000;185:38–42

Pasanisi E, Bacciu A, Vincenti V, et al. Speech recognition in elderly cochlear implant recipients. Clin Otolaryngol Allied Sci 2003;28(2):154–157

Pediatric Working Group of the Conference on Amplification for Children with Auditory Deficits (PWG). 1996. Amplification for infants and children with hearing loss. Am J Audiol 5:53–68

Perry PB, Gantz BJ. 2000. Medical and surgical evaluation and management of tinnitus. In: Tyler RS, ed. Tinnitus Handbook. San Diego, CA: Singular; 221–241

Peterson GE, Lehiste I. Revised CNC lists for auditory tests. J Speech Hear Disord 1962;27:62–70

Plant G, Gnosspelius J, Levitt H. The use of tactile supplements in lipreading Swedish and English: a single-subject study. J Speech Lang Hear Res 2000;43(1):172–183

Preminger JE, Meeks S. The Hearing Impairment Impact–Significant Other Profile (HII-SOP): a tool to measure hearing loss-related quality of life in spouses of people with hearing loss. J Am Acad Audiol 2012;23(10):807–823

Public Law 101-431. Television Decoder Circuitry Act of 1990. 47 USC §§303(u); 330(b)

Puig T, Municio A, Medà C. Universal neonatal hearing screening versus selective screening as part of the management of childhood deafness. Cochrane Database Syst Rev 2005; (2):CD003731 http://www.ncbi.nlm.nih.gov/pubmed/15846679

Punch JL, Beck EL. Low-frequency response of hearing aids and judgments of aided speech quality. J Speech Hear Disord 1980;45(3):325–335

Punch JL, Parker CA. Pairwise listener preferences in hearing aid evaluation. J Speech Hear Res 1981;24(3):366–374

Purdy SC, Farrington DR, Moran CA, Chard LL, Hodgson SA. A parental questionnaire to evaluate children's Auditory Behavior in Everyday Life (ABEL). Am J Audiol 2002;11(2):72–82

Reed CM, Delhorne LA. The reception of environmental sounds through wearable tactual aids. Ear Hear 2003;24(6):528–538

Reed CM, Rabinowitz WM, Durlach NI, Braida LD, Conway-Fithian S, Schultz MC. Research on the Tadoma method of speech communication. J Acoust Soc Am 1985;77(1):247–257

Robbins AM, Renshaw JJ, Berry SW. Evaluating meaningful auditory integration in profoundly hearing-impaired children. Am J Otol 1991;12(Suppl):144–150

Robbins AM, Svirsky M, Osberger MJ, Pisoni DB. 1998. Beyond the audiogram: the role of functional assessments. In: Bess F, ed. Children with Hearing Impairment: Contemporary Trends. Nashville, TN: Vanderbilt Bill Wilkerson Center Press; 105–124

Rosenberg GG, Blake-Rahter P, Heavner J, et al. Improving classroom acoustics (ICA): a three-year FM soundfield classroom amplification study. J Educ Audiol 1999;7:8–28

Ross M, ed. 1992. FM Auditory Training Systems: Characteristics, Selection and Use. Timonium, MD: York Press

Ross M, Brackett D, Maxon AM. 1982. Hard of Hearing Children in Regular Schools. Englewood Cliffs, NJ: Prentice-Hall

Ross M, Giolas TG. Effect of three classroom listening conditions on speech intelligibility. Am Ann Deaf 1971;116(6):580–584

Roush P, Frymark T, Venediktov R, Wang B. Audiologic management of auditory neuropathy spectrum disorder in children: a systematic review of the literature. Am J Audiol 2011;20(2):159–170

Rubinstein A, Boothroyd A. Effect of two approaches to auditory training on speech recognition by hearing-impaired adults. J Speech Hear Res 1987;30(2):153–160

Rubinstein JT, Parkinson WS, Tyler RS, Gantz BJ. Residual speech recognition and cochlear implant performance: effects of implantation criteria. Am J Otol 1999;20(4):445–452

Sanders DA. 1993. Management of Hearing Handicap: Infants to Elderly. Englewood Cliffs, NJ: Prentice-Hall

Sandlin RE. Bongiovanni R. 2002 Fitting binaural amplification to asymmetrical hearing loss. In: Valente M, ed. Strategies for Selecting and Verifying Hearing Aid Fittings, 2nd ed. New York, NY: Thieme; 221–252

Saunders GH, Cienkowski KM, Forsline A, Fausti S. Normative data for the Attitudes towards Loss of Hearing Questionnaire. J Am Acad Audiol 2005;16(9):637–652

Scarinci N, Worrall L, Hickson L. The effect of hearing impairment in older people on the spouse: development and psychometric testing of the Significant Other Scale for Hearing Disability (SOS-HEAR). Int J Audiol 2009;48(10):671–683

Schafer EC, Amlani AM, Paiva D, Nozari L, Verret S. A meta-analysis to compare speech recognition in noise with bilateral cochlear implants and bimodal stimulation. Int J Audiol 2011;50(12):871–880

Schafer EC, Amlani AM, Seibold A, Shattuck PL. A meta-analytic comparison of binaural benefits between bilateral cochlear implants and bimodal stimulation. J Am Acad Audiol 2007;18(9):760–776

Schechter MA, Henry JA. Assessment and treatment of tinnitus patients using a "masking approach.". J Am Acad Audiol 2002;13(10):545–558

Schow RL, Nerbonne MA. Communication screening profile: use with elderly clients. Ear Hear 1982;3(3):135–147

Schwartz D, Lyregaard PE, Lundh P. Hearing aid selection for severe-to-profound hearing losses. Hear J 1988;4:13–17

Scollie S, Seewald R, Cornelisse L, et al. The Desired Sensation Level multistage input/output algorithm. Trends Amplif 2005;9(4):159–197

Scollie S, Ching TYC, Seewald R, et al. Evaluation of the NAL-NL1 and DSL v4.1 prescriptions for children: preference in real world use. Int J Audiol 2010;49(Suppl 1):S49–S63

Seep B, Glosemeyer R, Hulce E, Linn M, Aytar P, Coffeen R. 2003. Classroom Acoustics I: A Resource for Creating Learning Environments with Desirable Listening Conditions (Revised). Melville, NY: Acoustical Society of America

Seewald RC, Cornelisse LE, Ramji KV, Sinclair ST, Moodie KS, Jamieson DG. 1997. DSL 4.1 for Windows: Software Implementation of the Desired Sensation Level [DSL(i/o)] Method for Fitting Linear Gain and Wide Dynamic Range Compression Hearing Instruments. London: University of Western Ontario

Sehgal ST, Kirk KI, Svirsky M, Miyamoto RT. The effects of processor strategy on the speech perception performance of pediatric nucleus multichannel cochlear implant users. Ear Hear 1998;19(2):149–161

Sensimetrics. (2002). Seeing and Hearing Speech: Lessons in Lipreading and Listening. Available at www.seeing-speech.com.

Shapiro I. Hearing aid fitting by prescription. Audiology 1976;15(2):163–173

Shapiro I. Comparison of three hearing aid prescription procedures. Ear Hear 1980;1(4):211–214

Shekhawat GS, Searchfield GD, Stinear CM. Role of hearing AIDS in tinnitus intervention: a scoping review. J Am Acad Audiol 2013;24(8):747–762

Sherrick CE. Basic and applied research in tactile aids for deaf people: progress and prospects. J Acoust Soc Am 1984;75:1325–1342

Silman S, Gelfand SA, Silverman CA. Late-onset auditory deprivation: effects of monaural versus binaural hearing aids. J Acoust Soc Am 1984;76(5):1357–1362

Silman S, Silverman CA, Emmer MB, Gelfand SA. Adult-onset auditory deprivation. J Am Acad Audiol 1992;3(6):390–396

Silverman CA, Silman S, Emmer MB, Schoepflin JR, Lutolf JJ. Auditory deprivation in adults with asymmetric, sensorineural hearing impairment. J Am Acad Audiol 2006;17(10):747–762

Silverman CA, Silman S. Apparent auditory deprivation from monaural amplification and recovery with binaural amplification: two case studies. J Am Acad Audiol 1990;1(4):175–180

Skarzyński H, Behr R, Lorens A, Podskarbi-Fayette R, Kochanek K. Bilateral electric stimulation from auditory brainstem implants in a patient with neurofibromatosis type 2. Med Sci Monit 2009;15(6):CS100–CS104

Skinner MW. 1988. Hearing Aid Evaluation. Englewood Cliffs, NJ: Prentice-Hall

Smith CR. Residual hearing and speech production in deaf children. J Speech Hear Res 1975;18(4):795–811

Smith SL, Fagelson M. Development of the self-efficacy for tinnitus management questionnaire. J Am Acad Audiol 2011;22(7):424–440

Spahr AJ, Dorman MF. Performance of subjects fit with the Advanced Bionics CII and Nucleus 3G cochlear implant devices. Arch Otolaryngol Head Neck Surg 2004;130(5):624–628

Spahr AJ, Dorman MF, Litvak LM, et al. Development and validation of the AzBio sentence lists. Ear Hear 2012;33(1):112–117

Spitzer JB, Ghossaini SN, Wazen JJ. Evolving applications in the use of bone-anchored hearing aids. Am J Audiol 2002;11(2):96–103

Stacey PC, Fortnum HM, Barton GR, Summerfield AQ. Hearing-impaired children in the United Kingdom, I: Auditory performance, communication skills, educational achievements, quality of life, and cochlear implantation. Ear Hear 2006;27(2):161–186

Staller S, Menapace C, Domico E, et al. Speech perception abilities of adult and pediatric Nucleus implant recipients using the Spectral Peak (SPEAK) coding strategy. Otolaryngol Head Neck Surg 1997;117(3 Pt 1):236–242

Storey L, Dillon H, Yeend I, Wigney D. The National Acoustic Laboratories' procedure for selecting the saturation sound pressure level of hearing aids: experimental validation. Ear Hear 1998;19(4):267–279

Stout G, Windle J. 1992. Developmental Approach to Successful Listening II. Englewood, CO: Resource Point

Stredler-Brown A, DeConde JC. (2003). Functional Auditory Performance Indicators: An Integrated Approach to Auditory Development. Boulder, CO: Marion Downs National Center

Stubblefield J, Nye C. Aided and unaided time-related differences in word discrimination. Hear Instr 1989;40:38–45

Surr RK, Fabry DA. Comparison of three hearing aid fittings using the Speech Intelligibility Rating (SIR) Test. Ear Hear 1991;12(1):32–38

Svirsky MA, Teoh SW, Neuburger H. Development of language and speech perception in congenitally, profoundly deaf children as a function of age at cochlear implantation. Audiol Neurootol 2004;9(4):224–233

Sweetow R, Palmer CV. Efficacy of individual auditory training in adults: a systematic review of the evidence. J Am Acad Audiol 2005;16(7):494–504

Sweetow RW, Sabes JH. The need for and development of an adaptive Listening and Communication Enhancement (LACE) program. J Am Acad Audiol 2006;17(8):538–558

Sweetow RW. 2000. Cognitive-behavior modification. In: Tyler RS, ed. Handbook of Tinnitus. San Diego, CA: Singular; 297–311

Tait M, De Raeve L, Nikolopoulos TP. Deaf children with cochlear implants before the age of 1 year: comparison of preverbal communication with normally hearing children. Int J Pediatr Otorhinolaryngol 2007;71(10):1605–1611

Taylor B. Contralateral routing of the signal amplification strategies. Semin Hear 2010;31:378–392

Teoh S, Pisoni D, Miyamoto R. Cochlear implantation in adults with prelingual deafness. Part I. Clinical results. Laryngoscope 2004;114:1536–1540

Thibodeau LM, Saucedo KA. Consistency of electroacoustic characteristics across components of FM systems. J Speech Hear Res 1991;34(3):628–635

Thibodeau L. Electroacoustic performance of direct-input hearing aids with FM amplification systems. Lang Speech Hear Svcs Schools 1990;21:49–56

Traynor RM. 1997. Prescriptive procedures. In: Tobin H, ed. Practical Hearing Aid Selection and Fitting. Washington, DC: U.S. Department of Veterans Affairs; 59–74

Tye-Murray N. 2002. Conversation Made Easy: Speechreading and Conversation Strategies Training for Children with Hearing Loss. St. Louis, MO: Central Institute for the Deaf

Tye-Murray N. 2015. Foundations of Aural Rehabilitation: Children, Adults, and Their Family Members, 4th ed. Stamford, CT: Centage Learning

Tye-Murray N, Geers A. 2002. The Children's Audiovisual Enhancement Test (CAVET). St. Louis, MO: Central Institute for the Deaf

Tyler RS, ed. 2006. Tinnitus Treatments: Clinical Protocols. New York, NY: Thieme

Tyler RS, Dunn CC, Witt SA, Noble WG. Speech perception and localization with adults with bilateral sequential cochlear implants. Ear Hear 2007;28(2, Suppl):86S–90S

Tyler RS, Gehringer AK, Noble W, Dunn CC, Witt SA, Bardia A. 2006. Tinnitus activities treatment. In: Tyler RS, ed. Tinnitus Treatment: Clinical Protocols. New York, NY: Thieme Medical Publishers; 116–132

Tyler RS, Preece JP, Lowder MW. 1983. The Iowa Cochlear-Implant Test Battery. Iowa City, IA: Department of Otolaryngology—Head and Neck Surgery, University of Iowa

Tyler RS, Teagle HFB, Kelsay DMR, Gantz BJ, Woodworth GG, Parkinson AJ. Speech perception by prelingually deaf children after six years of Cochlear implant use: effects of age at implantation. Ann Otol Rhinol Laryngol Suppl 2000;185:82–84

University of Iowa Tinnitus Clinic (UITC). 2011. Tinnitus questionnaires. Available at: http://www.uihealthcare.org/Tinnitus/

Utley J. A test of lip reading ability. J Speech Disord 1946;11:109–116

Valente M. Binaural amplification. Audiol J Cont Ed 1982;7:79–93

Valente M, ed. 2002. Strategies for Selecting and Verifying Hearing Aid Fittings, 2nd ed. New York, NY: Thieme

Valente M, Valente M(aureen), Enrietto J, Layton KM. 2002. Fitting strategies for patients with unilateral hearing loss. In: Valente M, ed. Strategies for Selecting and Verifying Hearing Aid Fittings, 2nd ed. New York, NY: Thieme; 253–271

Valente M, Van Vliet D. The Independent Hearing Aid Fitting Forum (IHAFF) protocol. Trends Amplif 1997;2:6–35

Ventry IM, Weinstein BE. Identification of elderly people with hearing problems. Ear Hear 1982;3:128–134

Vernon JA, Meikle MB. 2000. Tinnitus masking. In: Tyler RS, ed. Handbook of Tinnitus. San Diego, CA: Singular; 313–356

Verschuur CA, Lutman ME, Ramsden R, Greenham P, O'Driscoll M. Auditory localization abilities in bilateral cochlear implant recipients. Otol Neurotol 2005;26(5):965–971

Vorce E. 1974. Teaching Speech to Deaf Children. Washington, DC: Alexander Graham Bell Association for the Deaf

Wackym PA, Friedland DR. 2004. Otologic Evaluation. In: Snow JB, ed. Tinnitus: Theory and Management. Hamilton, Ontario: BC Decker; 205–219

Walden BE, Prosek RA, Worthington DW. Predicting audiovisual consonant recognition performance of hearing-impaired adults. J Speech Hear Res 1974;17(2):270–278

Walden BE, Schwartz DM, Williams DL, Holum-Hardegen LL, Crowley JM. Test of the assumptions underlying comparative hearing aid evaluations. J Speech Hear Disord 1983;48(3):264–273

Walden TC, Walden BE. Unilateral versus bilateral amplification for adults with impaired hearing. J Am Acad Audiol 2005;16(8):574–584

Waltzman SB. Expanding patient criteria for cochlear implantation. Audiol Today 2005;17(5):20–21

Waltzman SB, Cohen NL, Roland JT Jr. A comparison of the growth of open-set speech perception between the nucleus 22 and nucleus 24 cochlear implant systems. Am J Otol 1999;20(4):435–441

Waltzman SB, Roland JT Jr. Cochlear implantation in children younger than 12 months. Pediatrics 2005;116(4):e487–e493

Waltzman SB, Roland JT, eds. 2007. Cochlear Implants, 2nd ed. New York, NY: Thieme Medical Publishers

Waltzman SB, Shapiro WH. 2000. Cochlear implants in adults. In: Roeser RJ, Valente M, Hosford-Hill H, eds. Audiology: Treatment; 537–546

Watkins S, Clark T. 1993. SKI-HI Resource Manual: Family-Centered Home-Based Programming for Infants, Toddlers, and Pre-School Aged Children with Hearing Impairment. Logan: Hope

Watkins S, ed. 2004. The SKI-HI Curriculum: Family-Centered Programming for Infants and Young Children with Hearing Loss. Logan: Hope

Watson NA, Knudsen VO. Selective amplification in hearing aids. J Acoust Soc Am 1940;11:406–419

Wazen JJ, Spitzer JB, Ghossaini SN, et al. Transcranial contralateral cochlear stimulation in unilateral deafness. Otolaryngol Head Neck Surg 2003;129(3):248–254

Weisenberger JM, Percy ME. The transmission of phoneme-level information by multichannel tactile speech perception aids. Ear Hear 1995;16(4):392–406

Williams CN. 2004. COW—Designed with children in mind. Hear J 57(3):68. Worksheets available at http://www.oticon.com/~asset/cache.ashx?id=10833&type=14&format=web

Williams VA, McArdle RA, Chisolm TH. Subjective and objective outcomes from new BICROS technology in a veteran sample. J Am Acad Audiol 2012;23(10):789–806

Wilson BS, Dorman MF. Cochlear implants: current designs and future possibilities. J Rehabil Res Dev 2008;45(5):695–730

Wilson PH, Henry J, Bowen M, Haralambous G. Tinnitus reaction questionnaire: psychometric properties of a measure of distress associated with tinnitus. J Speech Hear Res 1991;34(1):197–201

Wolff R, Hommerich J, Riemsma R, Antes G, Lange S, Kleijnen J. Hearing screening in newborns: systematic review of accuracy, effectiveness, and effects of interventions after screening. Arch Dis Child 2010;95(2):130–135

World Health Organization (WHO). 2001. International Classification of Functioning, Disability, and Health. Geneva: World Health Organization. Available at http://www.who.int/classifications/icf/en/

Yacullo WS, Hawkins DB. Speech recognition in noise and reverberation by school-age children. Audiology 1987;26(4):235–246

Yoshinaga-Itano C. Early identification: an opportunity and challenge for audiology. Semin Hear 1999;20:317–331

Yoshinaga-Itano C, Sedey AL, Coulter DK, Mehl AL. Language of early- and later-identified children with hearing loss. Pediatrics 1998;102(5):1161–1171

Zimmerman-Phillips S, Osberger MJ, Robbins AM. 1998. Infant-Toddler: Meaningful Auditory Integration Scale (IT-MAIS). In: Eastabrooks W, ed. Cochlear Implants for Kids. Washington DC: AG Bell Association for the Deaf

Zimmerman-Phillips S, Robbins AM, Osberger MJ. Assessing cochlear implant benefit in very young children. Ann Otol Rhinol Laryngol Suppl 2000;185(Suppl 185):42–43

17 Effects of Noise and Hearing Conservation

This chapter is concerned with the branch of audiology that deals with the effects and ramifications of excessive sound exposure. Terms like *noise exposure* and *sound exposure* will be used interchangeably in this context because we are dealing with issues involving too much sound. The topics that will be addressed here include the effects of noise on hearing ability and speech communication, its non-auditory effects, occupational noise exposure and industrial hearing conservation, and the related issue of workers' compensation for noise-induced hearing losses. We will begin by expanding on several concepts about how noises are described and measured, which is often part of audiological practice and is also prerequisite to understanding the effects of noise exposure.

■ Noise Levels and Their Measurement

We are already familiar with the concepts involved in describing the magnitude and spectral content of a sound in terms of its overall sound pressure level (SPL), octave-band levels, and weighted (A, B, C) sound levels. It is also important to characterize noise exposures in terms of their *temporal characteristics* (Hamernik & Hsueh 1991; Ward 1991). Noise exposures are considered **continuous** if they remain above the level of "effective quiet" (the level below which a noise is too soft to cause a threshold shift). Noises that are not continuous may be considered (1) **interrupted** if they are on for relatively long periods of time (hours) above the level of effective quiet; (2) **intermittent** if the noise exposure is split up by short breaks (e.g., a few seconds to an hour) of quiet or effective quiet; or (3) **time-varying** if the noise stays above effective quiet but its level varies over time. **Transient noises** produced by the sudden release of

energy (e.g., gunshots) are called **impulse** noises, and often exceed 140 dB SPL. On the other hand, **impact** noises are transients caused by impacts between objects (e.g., hammering on metal) and are usually less than 140 dB SPL. Special sound level meters with extremely fast response characteristics are needed to measure transient noises accurately.

Most noise events last for some period of time, from a few seconds to many hours. Also, the levels of the noise will usually vary during this period, often considerably. It is desirable to integrate these noise levels into a single number that summarizes the overall level of the exposure "averaged" over its duration, called its **equivalent level** (L_{eq}). However, it is important to remember that decibels are logarithmic values, so that combining a series of sound level measurements into L_{eq} cannot be done by using their simple arithmetic average. Instead, L_{eq} is obtained using a method analogous to the one described in Chapter 1 for combining octave-band levels into overall SPL or dBA. The curious student will find the appropriate formulas and descriptions of their use in Berger, Royster, Royster, Driscol, and Layne (2000). In practice, L_{eq} values are often obtained directly using an integrating sound level meter or a dosimeter (described below). Special types of L_{eq} are used for compliance with occupational hearing conservation regulations (e.g., OSHA, 1983). The equivalent level for a 24-hour period of exposure is often expressed as $L_{eq}(24)$. When annoyance is an issue, the **day-night level** (DNL or L_{dn}) is used to describe the equivalent noise level for a 24-hour period in a way that assigns a penalty to nighttime noises because these are considered more objectionable. This is done by adding 10 dB to all noise levels that occur between the hours of 10 pm and 7 am. **Community noise equivalent level** (CNEL) is a variation of the DNL concept that adds a 5 dB penalty for evening noises and a 10 dB penalty for nighttime noises. All-day equivalent levels do not adequately represent objectionable single noise events like aircraft fly-overs, so a supplemental measurement is often necessary to characterize them. These single incidents can be expressed in terms of an equivalent 1-second exposure called **sound exposure level (SEL)**. There are also other approaches to identify the interference or annoyance capability of noises. For example, the spectrum of a noise can be compared with **noise criterion (NC) curves**, including **balanced noise criterion (NCB) curves,** which also consider the effects of vibration and audible rattles (Beranek 1957, 1989).

Noise Level Surveys

Noise surveys (or **sound surveys**) are systematic measurements of the sound levels in an industrial setting, or in other environments like the neighborhoods in the vicinity of an airport. Noise surveys are done for several reasons:

1. To identify locations where individuals (typically employees) are exposed to noise levels that exceed a certain criterion. This criterion is usually a **time-weighted average (TWA)** of ≥ 85 dBA because this value is the level specified by federal occupational hearing conservation regulations (OSHA 1983). The time-weighted average is a special kind of equivalent level normalized to an 8-hour workday.

2. To identify which employees are being exposed to noise levels of ≥ 85 dBA TWA or some other level of interest.

3. To ascertain which noise sources may require engineering controls, and to provide engineers with the information they need to determine what kinds of noise control methods are best suited to the problem at hand.

4. To determine how much attenuation must be provided by the hearing protection devices (e.g., earplugs and earmuffs) used by noise-exposed employees.

5. In addition, the information provided by noise surveys can also be used to identify and help alleviate problems pertaining to the audibility of emergency warning signals and the effectiveness of speech communication in the workplace.

Levels in dBA are usually needed for determining employee noise exposures. Octave-band levels are needed to evaluate the nature of the noise in detail, for engineering purposes such as determining appropriate noise control techniques, and for assessing hearing protectors. Noise levels in dBC are also needed for assessing hearing protectors, especially

when octave-band levels are not available. Environmental noise surveys often use other measurements to concentrate on annoyance factors around airports, major highways, and other non-occupational noise sources.

The noise level measurements obtained in various locations can be used to develop **noise level maps**. Noise maps are diagrams that depict noise levels as contour lines superimposed on the floor plan of the area that was surveyed. The contours on a noise map show which areas have similar noise levels, just as contours on a geographical map show regions with similar elevations above sea level. An example of a noise level contour map is shown in **Fig. 17.1**. Maps of this type make it easier to identify noise sources and employees who are being exposed to unacceptable noise levels, and to communicate this information to others. In addition to area measurements, it is usually necessary to measure representative personal exposures (1) because noise levels often vary with location; (2) because many employees move around among work locations that have different noise levels, and/or in and out of noise exposure areas; and (3) to account for times when employees may be away from high-noise locations, such as lunch and rest breaks. Similar noise contour maps are made around airports and other environmental noise sources.

Sound Level Meters

The principal noise measurement tools are sound level meters and noise dosimeters. Recall from Chapter 1 that the **sound level meter (SLM)** is the basic instrument for measuring the magnitude of sound.

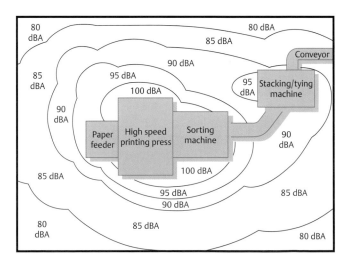

Fig. 17.1 A typical noise contour map.

The SLM can be used to measure overall sound pressure level at its linear setting; weighted sound levels in dBA, dBB, and dBC; as well as octave- and third-octave-band levels with the appropriate filters. The characteristics of the A-, B-, and C-weightings and the octave-band were summarized in **Fig. 1.23** and **Table 1.7** of Chapter 1. In this section we will expand on some of the fundamental aspects of sound measurement, and apply this information to noise measurement.

Sound level meters are classified as types 0, 1, 2, and S (ANSI-S1.4 2006a). The most precise sound level meters with the most restricted tolerances are **Type 0** or laboratory standard models. These instruments have the most exacting tolerances, which require them to be correct within ± 0.7 dB from 100 to 4000 Hz. Type 0 SLMs are used for exacting calibration and reference purposes under laboratory conditions, but are not required for noise level analyses. **Type 1** or **precision** SLMs are intended for precise sound level measurements in the laboratory and in the field, and have tolerances of ± 1 dB from 50 to 4000 Hz. **General-purpose** or **type 2** SLMs are field measurement instruments with tolerances as narrow as ± 1.5 dB from 100 Hz to 1250 Hz, and are the ones required to meet the noise level compliance standards of the Occupational Safety and Health Administration (OSHA) and other regulatory agencies. The student can get an appreciation for the tolerance differences among the three classes of SLMs from the samples listed in **Table 17.1**. One can also find "survey" (formerly type 3) SLMs, but they are not appropriate for our use. **Special-purpose (type S)** SLMs have a limited number of selected functions intended for a particular application rather than all of the features of the type 0, 1, and 2 meters.

It takes a certain amount of time for a meter to respond to an abrupt increase in sound level. Response time is expressed as a **time constant**, which is how long it takes the meter to reach 63% of its eventual maximum reading. Sound level meters have "slow" and "fast" response speeds that date back to the early days of their development, and are specified for use in many noise measurements by various federal and state laws and regulations. In particular, OSHA requires most noise measurements to be made at the slow speed. The **slow** speed has a time constant of 1 second. This sluggish response has the effect of averaging out sound level fluctuations, making the meter easier to read; but it also makes the slow speed inappropriate for estimating sound level variability over time. With a time constant of 0.125 second, the **fast** speed is better suited for assessing the variability of a sound, but the fluctuating meter readings make it more difficult to determine an overall level. However, even the fast response is far too slow for measuring

Table 17.1 Tolerance limits (maximum allowable measurement errors) at selected frequencies for type 0, 1, and 2 sound level meters [ANSI-S1.4, 1983 (R2006)]

Frequency (Hz)	Tolerances in dB for		
	Type 0	Type 1	Type 2
31.5	± 1	± 1.5	± 3
63	± 1	± 1	± 2
125	± 0.7	± 1	± 1.5
250	± 0.7	± 1	± 1.5
500	± 0.7	± 1	± 1.5
1000	± 0.7	± 1	± 1.5
2000	± 0.7	± 1	± 2
3150	± 0.7	± 1	± 2.5
4000	± 0.7	± 1	± 3
6300	− 1.5 to + 1	− 2 to + 1.5	± 4.5
8000	− 2 to + 1	− 3 to + 1.5	± 5

transient noises like impulses and impacts. A **true peak** or **instantaneous** response setting is needed to measure these kinds of sounds. At their true peak settings, type 0 SLMs must be able to respond to pulses as short as 50 *micro*seconds, and type 1 and 2 meters must be able to respond to 100-microsecond pulses. It is important to be aware that the **impulse** setting on SLMs, which has a 35-*milli*second rising time constant and a 1.5-second decay time, is not appropriate for measuring impulse sounds, in spite of its name.

Dosimeters

Noise dosimeters are sound measurement devices that are used to record the amount of sound exposure that accumulates over the course of an entire workday. An example is shown in **Fig. 17.2**. A dosimeter may be thought of as a sound level meter that has been modified to simplify and automate the process of taking noise exposure measurements over a period of time, making noise exposure monitoring a very practical activity. **Personal** noise exposure measurements are obtained by having an employee wear the dosimeter over the course of the workday. In this case, the dosimeter is typically carried

Fig. 17.2 An example of a noise dosimeter commonly used for industrial noise exposure measurements. (Courtesy of Quest Technologies, Inc.)

on the employee's belt with its microphone located on top of his shoulder, or perhaps elsewhere on the body. The effect of where the microphone is worn depends on the nature of the acoustical situation, with small measurement differences in reverberant environments and large differences when noises are directional (Byrne & Reeves 2008). **Area** sound exposure measurements may be obtained by placing the dosimeter at an appropriate location in the work environment. Most dosimeters have a very large dynamic range, which means they are able to integrate a wide range of intensity levels into the exposure measurements. To comply with federal regulations (OSHA 1983), dosimeters usually include all sound levels ≥ 80 dB in the noise measurements, whereas those below this *floor* or lower threshold are often omitted. (Other floors are also available but are not appropriate for compliance with noise exposure regulations.) The overall, accumulated noise exposure for the workday is generally given in terms of a noise dose (analogous to a radiation dose) and/or the equivalent time-weighted average in dBA for an 8-hour exposure. In addition, modern dosimeters can make measurements in both dBA and dBC using all kinds of meter responses (slow, fast, instantaneous, etc.), providing various kinds of accumulated exposure levels, and providing a profile showing a detailed noise exposure history for the period that was monitored.

The Noise Spectrum

Spectral information is not provided by the overall noise level measurements obtained with the linear setting of an SLM, or with its A, B, and C weighting networks. However, a general idea about the spectral content of a noise can sometimes be obtained by comparing the sound levels measured with the linear and A-weighted settings of the sound level meter. This is possible because the overall SPL provided by the linear setting treats all frequencies equally, whereas the low frequencies are de-emphasized by the A-weighting network. In effect, a noise level reading in dB SPL includes the lows, whereas dBA "ignores" the lows. For this reason, a difference between the two levels implies that the noise contains low-frequency energy "seen" by the dB SPL reading but "ignored" by the dBA reading. On the other hand, similar levels in dB SPL and dBA imply that the noise does not have much energy in the low frequencies. This kind of comparison can also be made between noise levels in dBA and dBC because the C-weighting network largely approximates the linear response.

The spectrum of a noise can be determined by **octave-band analysis**, and an even finer picture of the spectrum of a noise from a **third-octave-band analysis**. These measurements can be done with a sound level meter that has octave- or third-octave filters, or with a self-contained instrument often called an octave-band analyzer (or third-octave-band analyzer). **Fig. 17.3** shows an example of an octave-band analysis using the noise present in a hypothetical

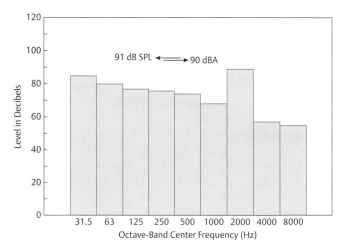

Fig. 17.3 Octave-band levels of the noise in a hypothetical industrial environment with an overall noise level corresponding to 91 dB SPL and 90 dBA. Notice the noise has a low-frequency emphasis as well as the dominant 89 dB peak in the 2000 Hz octave-band.

industrial environment. Notice that the amplitude of this noise is generally greater in the lower frequencies except for a pronounced peak in the 2000 Hz octave-band. This peak happens to be associated with the operation of a particular machine in the plant. These spectral characteristics cannot be ascertained from the overall noise level measurements, which were 90 dBA and 91 dB SPL. The dBA and dB SPL values are very close because of the dominance of the peak in the 2000 Hz octave-band. Another approach is to use a **spectrum analyzer** that determines the spectrum by performing a Fourier analysis on the sound electronically using a process called **fast Fourier transformation (FFT)**.

■ Effects of Noise

Effects of Noise on Hearing

Noise-Induced Hearing Loss

The effect of noise exposure on hearing sensitivity is expressed in terms of threshold shift. A **temporary threshold shift (TTS)** is a temporary change in hearing sensitivity that occurs following an exposure to high sound levels, and is a phenomenon that we have all experienced. The basic concept of a TTS is very simple. Suppose someone's threshold is 5 dB HL, and she is exposed to a relatively intense noise for a period of time. Retesting her hearing after the noise stops reveals her threshold has changed (shifted) to 21 dB HL, and retesting a few hours later shows her threshold has eventually returned to 5 dB HL. Her threshold shift soon after the noise ended is 21 – 5 = 16 dB (the difference between the pre- and post-exposure thresholds), and it is a temporary threshold shift because her threshold eventually returned to its pre-exposure value. If her threshold never returned to its pre-exposure value, then it would have been a **permanent threshold shift (PTS)**, also known as a **noise-induced permanent threshold shift (NIPTS)** or a **noise-induced hearing loss (NIHL)**.[1]

Temporary and permanent threshold shifts have been studied in great detail and involve many factors (Miller 1974; Clark 1991a; Hamernik, Ahroon, & Hsueh 1991; Melnick 1991; Ward 1991; Kujawa & Liberman 2009). The nature of noise-induced damage to the auditory system was discussed in Chap-

ter 6. In general, higher-frequency noise exposures cause larger threshold shifts than do equally intense lower-frequency exposures. In addition, the greatest amount of TTS tends to occur at a frequency that is about one half octave higher than the offending band of noise. However, not all sounds affect hearing sensitivity. The term **equivalent quiet** (or **effective quiet**) describes the intensity below which sound exposures do not cause a TTS. The weakest sound pressure levels that cause a TTS are ~ 75 to 80 dB for broadband noise, and decrease with frequency from 77 dB for the 250 Hz octave-band to 65 dB for the 4000 Hz octave-band. Thus, we are interested in the duration and intensity of exposures that are above equivalent quiet. In any case, it is stressed that noise-induced threshold shifts are very *variable* across individuals.

Temporary threshold shift is usually measured 2 minutes after a noise is turned off because its value is unstable before that point, and it is thus called **TTS$_2$**. The three functions in **Fig. 17.4** illustrate how TTS$_2$ is affected by the duration and intensity of a noise exposure. We will assume that all three exposures are above equivalent quiet, and that the TTS$_2$ is being measured at the frequency most affected by our hypothetical band of noise. All three functions show that TTS$_2$ increases as the duration of the exposure gets progressively longer. As we would expect, more TTS$_2$ is produced by higher noise levels than by softer ones for any particular exposure duration. The rate at which TTS$_2$ grows with duration is essentially

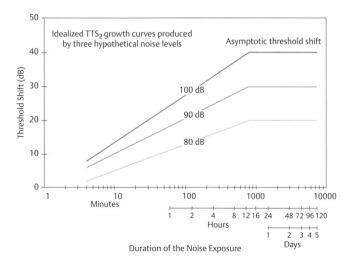

Fig. 17.4 Idealized curves showing the growth of TTS$_2$ at some frequency due to increasing durations of exposure to a narrow-band noise at three different hypothetical levels above equivalent quite (80, 90, and 100 dB). Duration is shown on a logarithmic scale. A maximum amount of ATS (asymptotic threshold shift) is eventually reached for each noise level.

---

[1] Although we are focusing on threshold shifts per se, one should be aware of findings in mice showing that noise exposure can cause permanent auditory neuron degeneration even when the TTS has been completely resolved (Kujawa & Liberman 2009).

linear when plotted on a logarithmic scale. However, TTS_2 grows faster as the intensity of the noise increases, that is, the lines get steeper going from 80 dB to 90 dB to 100 dB. The linear increase continues for durations up to ~ 8 to 16 hours. The functions then level off to become asymptotic (shown by the horizontal line segments), indicating that TTS_2 does not increase any more no matter how much longer the noise is kept on. In other words, the horizontal lines show the biggest TTS_2 that a particular noise is capable of producing regardless of its duration. This maximum amount of TTS_2 is called the **asymptotic threshold shift (ATS)**.

The threshold shift produced by a noise exposure is largest when it is first measured (i.e., TTS_2), and then decreases with the passage of time since the noise ended. This process is called **recovery** and is illustrated in **Fig. 17.5**. Notice that the time scale is logarithmic, as it was in the prior figure. As a rule, *complete* linear recovery is expected to occur within ~ 16 hours after the noise ends, provided TTS_2 is less than roughly 40 dB *and* it was caused by a continuous noise exposure lasting no more than 8 to 12 hours (shown by the lowest function in the figure). Otherwise, the recovery will be *delayed* (e.g., if the noise was intermittent, more than 8 to 12 hours in duration, and/or there is more TTS_2). The middle curve in the figure is an example of delayed recovery that eventually becomes complete after 2 days. However, once the amount of TTS_2 gets into the vicinity of ~ 40 dB, there is a likelihood that recovery may be *incomplete* as well as delayed. The top curve in the figure shows an example. Here, what started out as

a 40 dB TTS ends up as a 15 dB PTS—an irreversible noise-induced hearing loss.

Even though the PTS is usually smaller than the original size of the TTS, it is possible for the PTS to be as large as the TTS. However, it cannot be any larger. Recall that TTS increases with the duration of a noise until the asymptotic threshold shift is reached. This means that there is a maximum amount of TTS (i.e., ATS) that can be caused by a particular noise at a given intensity, no matter how long it lasts. Consequently, the biggest PTS that can be caused by that noise is limited to the ATS. Keep in mind, however, that the TTS caused by a noise exposure is often superimposed upon a pre-existing sensorineural loss. For example, a TTS of 15 dB experienced by a patient who started out with a loss of 30 dB HL would bring his threshold to 45 dB HL.

Occupational noise exposure The early use of terms like *boilermakers' disease* to describe deafness among industrial workers highlights the fact that occupational noise exposure has been recognized as a major cause of hearing loss for a very long time. Industrial noises vary widely in intensity, spectrum, and time course. We can get a sense of the intensities involved from the partial list in **Table 17.2**, based on studies analyzed by Passchier-Vermeer (1974) and Rösler (1994). Overall, somewhere between 36 and 71% of manufacturing employees have daily workplace exposures of 90 dBA or more (Royster & Royster 1990b).

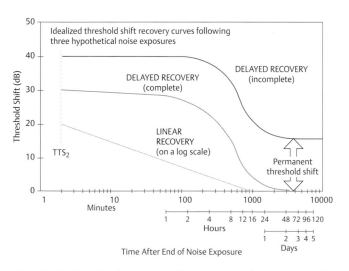

Fig. 17.5 Idealized recovery from noise-induced threshold shift with time after the exposure has ended. Duration is on a logarithmic scale. Notice the largest threshold shift never recovered completely, leaving a permanent threshold shift.

Table 17.2 Some examples of various occupational noise level intensities[a]

Noise type	Example(s) of reported levels
Miscellaneous industrial	88–104 dB SPL; 80–103 dBA
Weaving machines	102 dB SPL
Boiler shop	91 dBA
Riveting	113 dB SPL
Shipyard caulking	111.5 dB SPL
Drop forging	
Background	109 dB SPL
Drop hammer	126.5 peak SPL
Mining industry trucks	102–120 dB SPL
Mining equipment	96–114 dB SPL
Military weapons	168–188 peak SPL

[a]Derived from Passchier-Vermeer (1974) and Rösler (1994).

Numerous studies have reported the noise-induced hearing losses experienced by workers in many industries. Based on an analysis of eight well-documented studies, Passchier-Vermeer (1974) reported that (1) occupational NIHL at 4000 Hz increases rapidly for ~ 10 years, at which time it is similar to the amount of TTS associated with an 8-hour exposure to a similar noise, and (2) the continued development of NIPTS at 4000 Hz slows down or plateaus thereafter. On the other hand, NIHL at 2000 Hz develops slowly for the first 10 years, after which the loss at 2000 Hz increases progressively with time. The general pattern of development of occupational NIHL is illustrated in **Fig. 17.6**. Here, we see the median NIHLs of female workers who were exposed to noise levels of 99 to 102 dB SPL for durations of 1 to 52 years in the jute weaving industry (Taylor, Pearson, Mair, & Burns 1965). As a group, their hearing losses started as a 4000 Hz notch, and became deeper and wider as the workers were exposed to more years of noise. It is important to remember that these are median audiograms, and that Taylor et al (1965) reported a great deal of variability among individuals.

Rösler (1994) compared the long-term development of NIHL in 11 studies representing a wide variety of different kinds and levels of occupationally related noises. **Fig. 17.7** summarizes the mean (or median) audiograms after (a) 5 to 10 and (b) ≥ 25 years of exposure, and shows presbycusis curves for comparison. Notice the similarity among the configurations after ≥ 25 years of exposure in spite of the widely variant kinds of noises. The "outliers" in **Fig. 17.7b** are the two groups of firearms users. Finnish regular army personnel developed their maximum average losses within the first 5 to 10 years,

and are the least affected in **Fig. 17.7b**. On the other hand, Eskimos who hunted without hearing protectors at least weekly since childhood had thresholds that continued to deteriorate throughout a period of ~ 45 years, and are the most affected in **Fig. 17.7b**.

Nonoccupational noise exposure Industrial noise exposures are not the only origin of NIHL. Hearing loss is also caused by *environmental, recreational,* and other *nonoccupational* noise exposures, and is sometimes called **sociocusis**. This is not surprising when we realize that many sounds encountered in daily life and leisure activities produce noise levels that approach and often far exceed 90 dBA. Some examples are shown in **Fig. 17.8**. Recreational impulse noises have been reported to reach peak SPLs of 160 to 170+ dB for rifles and shotguns

Fig. 17.7 Mean (or median) audiograms after **(a)** 5 to 10 years and **(b)** 25 to 40+ years from 11 studies involving different kinds of occupational noises. For reference and comparison purposes, the open circles labeled "30 years" in **a** and "50 and 60 years" in **b** are due to age alone, based on ISO-1999 (1990). (Adapted from Rösler [1994], with permission of *Scandinavian Audiology.*)

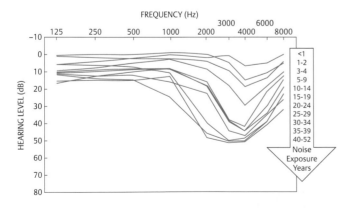

Fig. 17.6 Median audiograms of female weavers exposed to 99 to 102 dB SPL noises for 1 to 52 work years. (Based on Taylor, Pearson, Mair, and Burns [1965]).

Fig. 17.8 Examples of typical sources of environmental noise and their approximate maximum levels in dBA. (Based on data reported by the EPA [1974] and Clark and Bohne [1984].)

(Odess 1972; Davis, Fortnum, Coles, Haggard, & Lutman 1985). A 0.22-caliber rifle generates a peak level of 137 or 140 dBA[2] at the shooter's ears (Rasmussen, Flamme, Stewart, Meinke, & Lankford 2009), and a toy cap pistol can produce ~ 140 dB (Suter 1992a). Rifles and shotguns can cause an asymmetrical loss that is poorer in the left ear, which usually faces the muzzle. Unfortunately, a majority of hunters do not wear hearing protectors or do so sporadically, even when using shotguns and high-power rifles (e.g., Stewart, Foley, Lehman, & Gerlach 2011).

Music is probably the most common source of recreational sound exposure. Rock music averages 103.4 dBA (Clark 1991b), and some car stereo systems have been "clocked" at 140 dB SPL (Suter 1992a).[3] However, **personal listening devices (PLDs)** or **portable music/media players (PMPs)** like iPods and other MP3 players as well as iPhones and other smart phones are the most ubiquitous sources of music-related sound exposure[4] (for reviews, see, e.g., Fligor 2009; Punch, Elfenbein, & James 2011; Rawool 2012).

It is known that PLDs can generate sound levels that are considered to be capable of producing hearing loss (e.g., Fligor & Cox 2004; Portnuff & Fligor 2006; Keith, Michaud, & Chiu 2008), usually defined

as an exposure to ≥ 85 dBA for 8 hours or its equivalent. Whether listeners actually do use their PLDs at harmful levels is a different question. Although the use of MP3 players and other PLDs varies among listeners and across studies, it appears that adolescents and young adults typically listen to their PLDs at less than harmful levels, although volume controls are often turned up when there is background noise and in various situations such as listening to favorite songs (e.g., Airo, Pekkarinen, & Olkinuora 1996; Williams 2005; Fligor & Ives 2006a,b; Ahmed, Fallah, Garrido, et al 2007; Torre 2008; Portnuff, Fligor, & Arehart 2009; Epstein, Marozeau, & Cleveland 2010; McNeill, Keith, Feder, Konkle, & Michaud 2010; Hoover & Krishnamurti 2010; Hoenig 2010; Keith, Michaud, Feder, et al 2011; Punch et al 2011; Danhauer, Johnson, Dunne, et al 2012).

Potentially damaging listening levels have also been reported (e.g., Ahmed, et al 2007; Farina 2008; Vogel, Verschuure, van der Ploeg, Brug, & Raat 2009; Snowden & Zapala 2010; Levey, Levey, & Fligor 2011). For example, Levey et al (2011) found that ~ 58% of the college students in their study used levels equivalent to > 85 dBA for an 8-hour exposure, and Snowden and Zapala (2010) found that the overall use of unsafe levels was 63% among the middle school students they studied. Of particular concern, Snowden and Zapala (2010) reported that many middle schoolers simultaneously listened to the same iPod in pairs, with each using one of the two earphones. This "sharing" practice encouraged them to turn up the volume to make up for the loss of binaural summation when listening monaurally as opposed to binaurally. As a result, the use of unsafe levels went up from 53% when listening with both

---

[2] The level depended on meter characteristics: 137 dB in fast mode and 140 dB in impulse mode.

[3] Interestingly, Florentine, Hunter, Robinson, Ballou, & Buus (1998) found that ~ 9% of the subjects they studied had maladaptive patterns of listening to loud music suggestive of those associated with substance abuse.

[4] The forerunners of the devices such as the once-common Sony Walkman, cassette players and CD players are also PLDs.

earphones to 65% with each child listening to just one receiver.

The sound levels actually produced by MP3 players vary widely depending on the individual's preferred listening level and other influences such as the nature of the listening environment (e.g., background noise) and the type of earphone being used (earbud, supra-aural, insert). Listeners turn up their volume controls to overcome background noise and distracting sounds, which of course increases the potential for harmful sound levels (e.g., Airo et al 1996; Ahmed et al 2007; Hodgetts, Rieger, & Szarko 2007; Atienza, Bhagwan, Kramer, et al 2008; Danhauer, Johnson, Byrd, et al 2009; Hoenig 2010; Danhauer et al 2012). In addition, the physical level of the sound produced at a given volume control setting is affected by the type of earphone (e.g., Fligor & Ives 2006a,b; Portnuff & Fligor 2006; Atienza et al 2008; Keith et al 2008; Rabinowitz 2010). Here is why. Recall that the same sound causes a higher pressure in a smaller volume than in a larger one. As a result, the more deeply placed insert receivers produce greater sound levels than the more shallowly placed receivers like "earbuds," which, in turn, tend to produce higher levels than supra-aural earphones worn over the ears (e.g., Portnuff & Fligor 2006; Atienza et al 2008; Keith et al 2008). As a result, the potential for producing harmful sound levels is greatest for insert receivers. On the other hand, insert receivers attenuate outside noises better than earbuds and supra-aurals, so that insert users turn up their volume controls to overcome background noise less than those using other kinds of earphones (e.g., Atienza et al 2008; Hoenig 2010; Punch et al 2011).

The student has probably noticed that the discussion did not address the question of whether PLDs actually *cause* hearing loss. Perhaps the best available answer is provided by the following very carefully worded statement based on a systematic review by Punch et al (2011):

> "The literature does *not* provide a consensus view regarding a *causative relationship* between PLD use and hearing loss, although many investigators have concluded that PLDs, especially as used by many teenagers and young adults, *present a substantial risk* of hearing loss *or are a probable contributing factor* to hearing loss over the lifespan" (Punch et al 2011, p. 70, emphasis added).

All things considered, it appears wise to limit PLD usage to reasonable levels and durations, as well as to provide hearing health information in schools and the media (e.g., Ahmed et al 2007; Fligor 2009; Punch et al 2011; Danhauer et al 2012). A review of the evidence to date led Fligor (2009) to suggest that listeners

should restrict their PLD use to ≤ 80% of the maximum volume setting and ≤ 90 minutes per day. Since this limit applies to the standard equipment receivers that come with the PLD (typically earbuds), lower volume settings and shorter listening durations would apply when insert receivers are used. Interested students will find an informative set of suggestions for providing hearing health information and messages in the article by Punch and colleagues (2011).

In light of this discussion, one might expect that the prevalence of hearing loss would be getting worse over time. There have been several pessimistic reports, but the most troubling findings were reported by Shargorodsky, Curhan, Curhan, and Eavey (2010; see also Chapter 13). They compared the hearing loss statistics in the 2005–2006 National Health and Nutrition Examination Survey (NHANES)[5] to those in the 1988-1994 survey. According to their analysis, the prevalence of hearing loss among American 12- to 19-year-olds rose from 14.9 to 19.5% overall and from 12.8 to 15.4% for the high frequencies between the two surveys.

However, subsequent analyses of the same NHANES data showed that the prevalence of high-frequency hearing loss among adolescents actually did not increase between 1988–1994 and 2005–2006 (Henderson, Testa, & Hartnick 2011; Schlauch & Carney 2011, 2012; Schlauch 2013). The more optimistic outcomes were revealed by controlling for confounding variables, such as any signs of conductive disorders, threshold shifts affecting both the low and high frequencies as opposed to just the highs, and important calibration and reliability issues. After analyzing the 2005–2006 survey data with these rigorous controls, Schlauch and Carney (2012) showed that the prevalence of high-frequency hearing loss among adolescents actually approximated only 7.4 to 7.9%. Other findings also suggested that the prevalence of high-frequency hearing loss has not been increasing among adolescents and young adults, at least to date (Augustsson & Engstrand 2006; Rabinowitz, Slade, Galusha, Dixon-Ernst, & Cullen 2006). Moreover, the overall hearing loss among American adults may well be improving over time, as well. For example, median adult thresholds improved between 1959–1962 and 1999–2004 (Hoffman, Dobie, Ko, Themann, & Murphy 2010); and the prevalence of hearing loss ≥ 25 dB HL dropped from 27.9 to 19.1% between 1971–1973 and 1999–2004 for those without diabetes (Cheng et al 2009).

The reasons for these improving trends are not completely clear, but, if real, they probably reflect several potential influences (see, e.g., Cruickshanks,

---

[5] These surveys are available from the Centers for Disease Control and Prevention at http://www.cdc.gov/nchs/nhanes.htm.

Nondahl, Tweed, et al 2010; Hoffman et al 2010; Punch et al 2011; Zhan, Cruickshanks, Klein, et al 2011; Schlauch & Carney 2012; Schlauch 2013). Some of the possibilities might include benefits derived from improved public awareness of noise effects, as well as overall health improvements related to factors like nutrition, supplements, health habits, and medical conditions and care. It is clear, however, that we must not become complacent about the effects of noise exposure, especially in light of ever-increasing opportunities for occupational, environmental, and recreational noise exposure for almost all age groups.

Individual susceptibility and interactions with other factors Individual susceptibility to NIHL varies widely and is affected by several factors (Boettcher, Henderson, Gratton, Danielson, & Byrne 1987; Henderson, Subramaniam, & Boettcher 1993). At first glance, it would seem wise to use *temporary threshold shifts* as the test for susceptibility to NIHL because they precede permanent threshold shifts, and the amount of TTS after an 8-hour workday seems to be similar to the amount of PTS after 10 years of occupational exposure on a group basis. However, the correlation between TTS and PTS is too ambiguous for TTS results to be used as a test of one's susceptibility to NIHL, especially when intermittent exposures and impulse noises are involved. The use of TTS testing is also unattractive because of litigation fears.

The effect of noise exposure is exacerbated by *vibration*, but vibration alone does not produce a hearing loss. Susceptibility is also affected by the effectiveness of the *acoustic reflex* and possibly by the *efferent auditory system*. Susceptibility is also affected by *noise exposure history*: repeated intermittent noise exposures produced progressively smaller hearing losses in laboratory animals over time (Clark, Bohne, & Boettcher 1987; Subramaniam, Campo, & Henderson 1991a,b). Does a prior noise exposure affect susceptibility to future exposures? This question has been addressed by measuring threshold shifts in laboratory animals that were subjected to (1) a *prior* (initial) noise exposure (2) followed by a *recovery period*, and (3) then subjected to a *subsequent* noise exposure (Canlon, Borg, & Flock 1988; Campo, Subramaniam, & Henderson 1991; Subramaniam, Henderson, Campo, & Spongr 1992). Subsequent low-frequency exposures produced smaller threshold shifts after a low-frequency prior exposure; but susceptibility to a subsequent high-frequency noise was made worse by prior exposures (with low- or high-frequency noises).

Susceptibility to NIHL is increased by *nonauditory factors* as well, including *ototoxic drugs* (aminoglycosides and cis-platinum, possibly and less so for salicylates) and *industrial and environmental toxins* (e.g., solvents, carbon monoxide). Other factors have been identified, but they account for a very small part of the variability, often with inconclusive or equivocal results. These include the following, with the more susceptible groups identified in parentheses: *age* (very young and the elderly), *gender* (males), *eye color* (blue), and *smoking* (smokers).

Damage Risk Criteria and Noise Exposure Standards

There are probably two closely related key questions that concern people about noise exposure and hearing loss: First, what are the chances of getting a hearing loss from being exposed to some noise for some period of time? Second, how much noise exposure is acceptable before it becomes damaging to hearing? These questions are addressed by **damage risk criteria (DRC)**, which are standards or guidelines that pertain to the hazards of noise exposure. However, this apparently straightforward issue actually involves many interrelated questions, the answers to which are complicated, not necessarily understood, and often controversial. Some questions deal with the noise and predicting its effects: How should noise be quantified for the purpose of assessing damage risk, and how should we handle different kinds of noises (continuous, impulsive, intermittent, and time varying)? Are there valid and reliable "predictors" of NIHL, and if so, what are they and how are they related to hearing loss? Other questions deal with the amount of NIHL and how many people are affected: How much hearing loss is acceptable or at least tolerable, and at which frequency(ies)? Since people vary in susceptibility, what is the acceptable/tolerable percentage of the population that should be "allowed" to develop more than the acceptable/tolerable amount of NIHL? Still other questions pertain to distinguishing between different sources of hearing impairment: Can we separate NIPTS from other sources of hearing impairment (e.g., pure presbycusis and disease), and if so, how? Can we distinguish between the effects of *occupational* noise exposure and *nonoccupational* causes of hearing loss, including nonoccupational noise exposures? The latter is an important issue because we are usually concerned with industrial exposures. For this reason, we often use the term *industrial noise-induced permanent threshold shift* to refer to the part of a hearing loss actually attributable to industrial (or other occupational) noise exposures. These questions should be kept in mind when dealing with the effects of noise exposure in general, and particularly when dealing with hearing conservation programs and assessing hearing handicap for compensation purposes.

One approach to damage risk criteria is to protect just about everybody from just about any degree of NIHL. This notion is illustrated by the "Levels Document" issued by the Environmental Protection Agency (EPA, 1974), which suggested that NIPTS could be limited to less than 5 dB at 4000 Hz in 96% of the population by limiting noise exposures to 75 dB $L_{eq}(8)$ or 70 dB $L_{eq}(24)$ over a 40-year period. Changing the criterion to 77 dB $L_{eq}(24)$ would protect 50% of the population.

The Committee on Hearing and Bioacoustics and Biomechanics (CHABA) published damage risk criteria intended to limit the amount of industrial NIPTS to 10 dB at ≤ 1000 Hz, 15 dB at 2000 Hz, and 20 dB at ≥ 3000 Hz among 50% of workers who are exposed to steady or intermittent noises for 10 years (Kryter, Ward, Miller, & Eldredge 1966). The CHABA DRC was based on the amount of TTS_2 that occurs after an 8-hour noise exposure, and relied on the notion that this value seems to correspond to the amount of NIPTS that is present after 10 years of occupational exposure. However, it has never been proven that TTS validly predicts NIPTS, and this notion has several serious problems (e.g., Melnick 1991; Ward 1991). Damage risk criteria for impulsive noises using similar criteria were introduced by Coles, Garinther, Hodge, and Rice (1968). The CHABA damage risk criteria required noises to be measured in third-octave or octave-bands, and expressed maximum exposure levels for durations up to 8 hours per day. The maximum allowable octave-band levels for an 8-hour exposure were ~ 85 dB for frequencies ≥ 1000 Hz but were higher for lower frequencies, because they cause smaller threshold shifts than do equally intense higher-frequency exposures. The allowable noise levels also became higher as the duration of the exposure decreased below 8 hours, because the amount of threshold shift is related to exposure duration. Botsford (1967) developed equivalent values that make it possible to apply the CHABA damage risk criteria to noises measured in dBA instead of octave-band levels.

Several well-known approaches and estimates of the risks for developing a hearing loss due to occupational noise exposure have been developed over the years (e.g., NIOSH 1972, 1998; EPA 1973; ISO 2013, ANSI 2006b; Prince, Stayner, Smith, & Gilbert 1997). The NIOSH (1972) risk criteria were based on linear fit to the data collected in the 1968–1972 NIOSH Occupational Noise and Hearing Survey (Lempert & Henderson 1973), which was reanalyzed using a best-fitting nonlinear model by Prince et al (1997), also known as the NIOSH-1997 model. [The 1968–1972 survey provides valuable data that are still used today because it pre-dated regulations requiring the use of hearing protectors (see below), the use of which makes it hard to determine actual exposure levels from modern noise surveys.] The criteria for

material impairment used by Prince et al (1997) involved an average hearing loss in both ears of more than 25 dB for certain combinations of frequencies: (a) 500, 1000, and 2000 Hz; (b) 1000, 2000, and 3000 Hz; and (c) 1000, 2000, 3000, and 4000 Hz. The latter is similar to the criterion recommended by ASHA (1981), discussed later in this chapter.[6] In addition, the National Institute for Occupational Safety and Health (NIOSH, 1998) has adopted a binaural average loss exceeding 25 dB HL for the 1000 to 4000 Hz average as its criterion for material hearing impairment.

The International Standards Organization ISO-1999 standard (2013) considers the hearing loss of noise-exposed people to be due to the combination of an age-related component and NIPTS, which are almost additive.[7] Formulas are used to predict the effects of noise exposure levels (from 85 to 100 dBA) and durations (up to 40 years) at each frequency for different percentiles of the population (e.g., the 10% with the most loss, the 10% with the least loss, medians, etc.). This approach has been adopted in the ANSI S3.44 standard (2006b). In effect, NIPTS is determined by comparing the thresholds of a noise-exposed group to a comparable unexposed group of the same age. These standards provide two sets of age-related hearing level distributions. One is based on a population *highly screened* to be free of ear disease and noise exposure (representing more or less "pure" presbycusis), and the other is from an essentially *unscreened general population*.

To estimate the risks to hearing attributable to a certain amount of occupational noise exposure, we need to compare the percentage of people exposed to that noise who get material amounts of hearing impairment to the percentage of unexposed people of the same age who also get a material hearing impairment. Obviously, the risk estimate will depend on the *criterion* used to determine when a *material hearing impairment* begins. In other words, **excess risk** for occupational hearing impairment is simply the percentage of exposed people with material impairments minus the percentage of unexposed people with material impairments. **Fig. 17.9** shows the amount of

---

[6] Prince et al (1997) weighted the 1000–4000 Hz average based on the articulation index (see below) as opposed to ASHA's (1981) simple 1000–4000 Hz average; however, the two variations yielded similar risk estimate outcomes.

[7] Specifically, the total hearing loss in dB due to age and NIPTS combined (TOTAL) is related to the hearing loss due to age (AGE) and the NIPTS according to the formula TOTAL = AGE + NIPTS − (AGE × NIPTS)/120. Subtracting the term (AGE × NIPTS)/120 prevents the total loss from becoming impossibly large and also causes the combined effects of age and noise to be somewhat less than additive.

excess risk of hearing impairment due to 40 years of occupational noise exposures of 80, 85, and 90 dBA (8-hour TWA) estimated by several of the methods just described. It is clear that excess risk becomes readily apparent by the time occupational noise exposure levels reach 85 dBA even though the actual percentages estimated by the various methods and pure tone combinations differ. Notice, too, the higher excessive risk estimates for NIOSH than for ISO. The higher excess risk estimates for NIOSH may be due to differences at the lower frequencies that were not due to noise between the exposed and control groups (Dobie 2007). Clearly, it is important to remember that the estimated risk of NIHL is affected by which reference population is used (see, e.g., Prince et al 2003).

OSHA noise exposure criteria Noise exposure standards are particularly effectual when they carry the weight of law. Numerous examples are found in state and local ordinances and in military regulations, but the most influential are federal labor regulations found in the Walsh-Healey noise standard and OSHA Hearing Conservation Amendment (HCA) (DOL 1969; OSHA 1983). These noise exposure limits are shown in **Table 17.3** (first and second columns), where we see that the maximum noise exposure limit is 90 dBA for 8 hours. In addition, impulse or impact noises are not supposed to exceed 140 dB peak SPL. If the noise level exceeds 90 dBA, then the exposure duration must be reduced by one half for each 5 dB increase. In other words, the maximum exposures are 8 hours at 90 dBA, 4 hours at 95 dBA, 2 hours at 100 dBA, down to one-quarter hour at 115 dBA. However, the noise level is not permitted to exceed 115 dBA even for durations shorter than one-quarter hour. This trade-off of 5 dB per doubling of time is called the **5 dB trading rule** or **exchange rate**, and is based on the premise that sounds that produce equal amounts of TTS are equally hazardous. This is the same **equal-TTS** principle discussed previously for the CHABA damage risk criteria. The major alternative approach is to reduce the intensity by 3 dB for each doubling of duration (the **3 dB trading rule** or **exchange rate**), which is employed by the military, the EPA, and many foreign countries. The 3 dB trading rule is based on the **equal-energy** concept that considers equal amounts of noise energy to be equally hazardous, and is more strongly supported by scientific evidence than the 5 dB rule (e.g., Suter 1992b; NIOSH 1998).

The maximum allowable noise exposure is known as the **permissible exposure level (PEL)** and is considered to be one full dose of noise. Using the OSHA (1983) criteria, a person has received **one dose** (or a **100% dose**) of noise regardless of whether he was exposed to 90 dBA for 8 hours or 105 dBA for 1 hour. This is the same kind of terminology that is used for

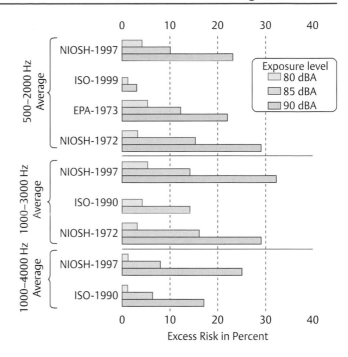

Fig. 17.9 Excess risk of material hearing impairment (binaural average > 25 dB HL) using various approaches and pure tone averages expected to result from 40 years of occupational noise exposures of 80, 85, and 90 dBA (8 hours TWA) among 60-year-old workers. The approach labeled "NIOSH-1997" refers to Prince et al (1997). (Based on NIOSH [1998].)

exposures to radiation or noxious chemicals: a full day's dose is a full dose whether it accumulates over 8 hours or just a few minutes. Because of the 90 dB PEL and the 5 dB trading rule, an 8-hour exposure to 85 dBA would be a half dose (50% dose) and an 8-hour exposure to 80 dBA would be a quarter dose (25% dose). Similarly, an 8-hour exposure to 95 dBA would be a 200% dose or two doses. Hence, we can also express a noise exposure in terms of an *equivalent 8-hour exposure*, that is, its 8-hour TWA. Equivalent values of noise level exposures in terms of TWA and dosage are shown in **Fig. 17.10**.[8] Using the plot labeled "OSHA (1983)," we see that the following are examples of equivalent noise exposures:

90 dBA TWA and *1 dose* and a *100% dose (the PEL)*
95 dBA TWA and *2 doses* and a *200% dose*
100 dBA TWA and *4 doses* and a *400% dose*
105 dBA TWA and *8 doses* and an *800% dose*
120 dBA TWA and *70 doses* and a *6000% dose*

---

[8] For reference purposes, the relationship between TWA in dBA and noise dose in percent (D) can be calculated as follows: TWA = $16.61 \times \log(D/100) + 90$ for OSHA (1983) purposes, and TWA = $10 \times \log(D/100) + 85$ according to the NIOSH (1998) criteria..

Table 17.3　Maximum permissible noise exposures according to the OSHA (1983) regulations and NIOSH (1998) recommendations

Maximum exposure level in dBA	Maximum exposure duration	
	OSHA (1983) regulations[a]	NIOSH (1998) recommendations
85[b]		8 hours
88		4 hours
90[c]	8 hours	2 hours 31 minute
92	6 hours	1 hour 35 minutes
95	4 hours	47 minutes 37 seconds
97	3 hours	30 minutes
100	2 hours	15 minutes
102	1 hour 30 minutes	9 minutes 27 seconds
105	1 hour	4 minutes 43 seconds
110	30 minutes	1 minute 29 seconds
115	15 minutes or less	28 seconds

[a]From OSHA (1983), Table G-16, which also indicates: "When the daily noise exposure is composed of two or more periods of noise exposure of different levels, their combined effect should be considered, rather than the individual effect of each. If the sum of the following fractions: $C_1/T_1 + C_2/T_2 + ... + C_n/T_n$ exceeds unity [i.e., 1], then the mixed exposure should be considered to exceed the limit value. C_n indicates the total time of exposure at a specified noise level, and T_n indicates the total time of exposure permitted at that level."

[b]OSHA (1983) PEL for an 8-hour TWA exposure.

[c]NIOSH (1998) REL for an 8-hour TWA exposure.

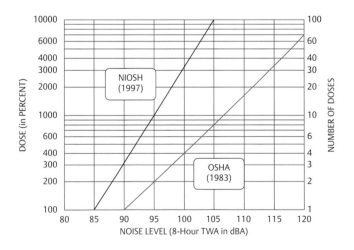

Fig. 17.10　Noise exposure in terms 8-hour TWA in dBA and noise dose (shown in percent on the left axis and as the number of doses on the right axis) according to OSHA (1983) regulations compared with recommendations by NIOSH (1998; see text).

Noises that have been measured in terms of octave-band levels need to be converted into 0 dBA so that allowable exposures can be determined for them. The methods used to convert octave-band levels into overall level in dBA were described in Chapter 1. However, a simplified approach for compliance with the OSHA noise standard can be achieved by using the conversion chart shown in **Fig. 17.11**. The procedure involves plotting the octave-band levels of the noise on the chart, and then comparing them to the conversion curves. The highest curve that is crossed by any part of the noise spectrum constitutes the *equivalent* noise level in dBA. This value in dBA can then be used to assign noise exposure limits according to the first and second columns of **Table 17.3** for OSHA purposes.

NIOSH noise exposure criteria We are very interested in the OSHA HCA because it continues to be the dominant force in occupational hearing conservation in most industries as the legally enforceable federal regulation. However, the National Institute

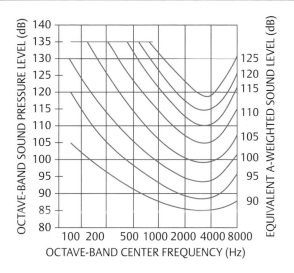

Fig. 17.11 Curves for converting octave-band levels into equivalent A-weighted sound level (based on OSHA, 1983, Figure G-9). Octave-band sound levels measured for a noise are plotted on this graph (using the left axis). The highest contour penetrated by the noise spectrum constitutes the equivalent noise level in dBA (using the right axis).

of Occupational Safety and Health (NIOSH 1998) developed revised criteria and recommendations for occupational hearing conservation programs that have considerable efficacy because they reflect the preponderance of scientific evidence. With regard to noise exposure limits, NIOSH called for (1) replacing the PEL of 90 dBA TWA with a **recommended exposure level (REL)** of 85 dBA TWA, (2) changing the exchange rate from the 5 dB rule to the 3 dB (equal energy) rule, and (3) setting a ceiling exposure of 140 dBA regardless of the type of the noise.

The 85 dBA REL and 3 dB exchange rate used by NIOSH result in different and more protective exposure values than those used by OSHA, which is seen clearly by comparing the two sets of maximum exposure durations in **Table 17.3**. For example, notice that a 90-dBA exposure is permissible for 8 hours by OSHA but for only 2½ hours by NIOSH, and that OSHA permits a 2-hour exposure to 100 dBA compared with only 15 minutes according the NIOSH recommendations. Noise exposure dosages are also considerably different according to the two sets of criteria. Referring to the plot labeled "NIOSH (1998)" in **Fig. 17.10**, we see that a TWA of 85 dBA corresponds to one dose or a 100% dose according to NIOSH; OSHA's 90 dBA PEL is considered to be two doses or a 200% dose, and 105 dBA constitutes 100 doses or a 10,000% dose. Although the graph only goes up to a 10,000% dose, a 120 dBA TWA exposure would correspond to about a 316,000% dose (roughly 316 doses).

Other Effects of Noise

The effects of noise exposure are not limited to hearing impairment. We often experience many of the noises that we encounter as being disturbing in a way that goes beyond being too loud. Traffic and construction noise, airplane flyovers, sirens, squeaky floor boards, the screech of fingernails drawn across a blackboard, and a neighbor's loud music are but a few examples. These sounds may be unwanted for one or more reasons. For example, sounds might be unwanted because they interfere with one's work, leisure activities, rest, or sleep; interfere with speech communication; are distracting or startling; or convey a disturbing meaning.

Noisiness and Annoyance

Kryter (1985) distinguishes between two types of unwanted sounds, described as perceived noisiness and annoyance. **Perceived noisiness** (or just **noisiness**) is the "unwantedness" of a sound that is not unexpected or surprising, does not cause pain or provoke fear, and has nothing to do with the meaning of the sound. The same physical factors that make a sound louder also make it noisier, but noisiness is also affected by the time course of a sound. For example, increasing the duration of a sound beyond a second does not make it louder but does make it noisier. Also, a sound that builds up over time is noisier than a sound that dies down over the same amount of time (e.g., an approaching train is noisier than a departing train). The magnitude of perceived noisiness can be quantified in **noys** (analogous to loudness in sones), and equally objectionable sounds can be expressed in units of **PNdB (perceived noise decibels)** (analogous to *loudness level* in *phons*). If one sound is twice as noisy as another, then it will be 10 PNdB higher and it will have double the number of noys.

In contrast to perceived noisiness, **annoyance** is the "objectionability" of a sound, which that involves the novelty, meaning, or emotional implications of the sound, as well as its physical characteristics. It has been suggested that noise levels would have to be ≤ 45 dB DNL in homes, hospitals, and schools, and ≤ 55 dB outdoors to meet the goal of avoiding all interference and annoyance by noise (EPA 1974). The amount of annoyance increases with increasing noise levels (e.g., Kryter 1985) and also appears to be related to the source of the noise. For example, Miedema and Vos (1998) found that annoyance due to transportation noises is related to the mode of transportation, with the percentage of highly annoyed individuals being the greatest for aircraft noise, followed by road traffic noise, and then by railroad noise. Stansfeld, Berglund, Clark, et al (2005) found that annoyance is also related to both aircraft and traffic noise among 9- to 11-year-old school children, again with the stronger relationship for airplane noise. Moreover, annoyance is greater for combined railroad and traffic noise than for either type alone (Ohrström et al 2007).

Fields (1993) found that residential noise annoyance is affected by the amount of isolation from noise at home, fear of danger from the noise sources, beliefs about noise prevention, general noise sensitivity, concern about the non-noise consequences of the noise source, and beliefs about the importance of the noise source. However, annoyance was not substantially affected by ambient noise levels, the number of hours spent at home, or a variety of demographic variables (e.g., age, sex, socioeconomic status). Fields (1998) also found that the annoyance resulting from a particular noise source (e.g., aircraft) is little if at all affected by the amount of ambient noise produced by other noise sources (e.g., road traffic). Miedema and Vos (1999) found that fears relating to the noise source and self-assessed noise sensitivity had a large effect on transportation noise annoyance, but that most demographic factors had small effects on annoyance. In contrast to Fields's (1993) finding that annoyance was not related to age, Miedema and Vos also found that younger and older adults were less annoyed by transportation noise than were those in the roughly 30- to 50-year-old range. Van Gerven, Vos, Van Boxtel, Janssen, & Miedema (2009) similarly found that middle-aged adults experienced more annoyance from environmental noises than younger and older people.

Another source of annoyance has come with the advent of wind turbines (windmills) to generate electricity. These noises are principally produced by the rotating blades interacting with the wind, and involve largely whooshing sounds with considerable low-frequency and vibration energy, and that modulate in amplitude (see, e.g., Rogers, Manwell, & Wright 2006; Punch, James, & Pabst 2010). In addition to annoyance per se, wind turbine noise has been associated with sleep disturbances, and a variety of stress-related and physiological complaints sometimes called "wind turbine syndrome" (Pedersen & Persson Waye 2007; Pierpont 2009; Pedersen 2011).

A series of studies in the Netherlands found that a larger percentage of people are annoyed by turbine noise than by other industrial noises, and that it becomes annoying to a larger percentage of people at lower sound levels (e.g., Pedersen & Waye 2004; Pedersen & Larsman 2008; Pedersen, van den Berg, Bakker, & Bouma 2009; Janssen, Vos, Eisses, & Pedersen 2011). On the other hand, these studies also found that annoyance from wind turbines is affected by various individual characteristics and situational factors, especially the visibility of the wind farm from one's home and whether any economic benefits are derived from them.

Leventhall and colleagues (Colby, Dobie, Leventhall, et al 2009; Leventhall 2013) suggested that the literature to date does not provide evidence that wind turbines produce direct auditory or vibratory effects that are harmful. However, it is important to realize that these findings were based on A-weighted levels, which de-emphasize the low frequencies and have been shown to be inappropriate when dealing with the low-frequency vibrations involved in wind turbine noise (Salt & Lichtenhan 2014). In fact, compelling evidence summarized by Salt and Lichtenhan (2014) revealed the physiological mechanisms that can account for many of the characteristics of "wind turbine syndrome." As the student has probably surmised, these issues are by no means settled, the effects of wind turbines on people are still being studied and ardently debated (see, e.g., Leventhall 2013; Schomer 2013; Timmerman 2013; Salt & Lichtenhan 2014).

Speech Communication Interference

Interference with speech communication is one of the most important and pervasive problems caused by noise. The adverse effects of noise on speech communication are experienced in many ways: masking of the speech signal may render it completely inaudible, or it may be audible but limited in intelligibility; speaker effort must be increased; listening becomes laborious and stressful; there is an increased need for repetition, clarification, and confirmation of the message; reliance on visual cues becomes increasingly important; message content may have to be adjusted or limited; distances between the talker and listener must be reduced; and errors and confusion abound.

How does a particular noise affect speech communication in a given environment? The most direct answer comes from giving subjects speech intelligibility tests for various kinds of materials (words, sentences, etc.) in each situation, but this approach is unrealistic. The practical solution is to make acoustical measurements of the noise, and then to predict how it should affect communication based on known relationships between noise and speech intelligibility. We will briefly outline the principal methods.

Articulation index/speech intelligibility index The **articulation index (AI)** is a method for predicting speech intelligibility from the audibility of speech signals, originated by French and

Steinberg (1947). Audibility depends on how well the speech signal can be heard above the listener's threshold and any noise that is present.

Some background information is needed to understand the AI. French and Steinberg measured speech intelligibility when subjects were provided with only part of the frequency range. One set of experiments involved **high-pass filtering**, which means that the frequencies above a certain cutoff frequency were "passed" and the frequencies below the cutoff were "rejected" or not passed. For example, if the cutoff frequency is 800 Hz, then the subjects could hear the frequencies above 800 Hz (the "pass band") but could not hear the frequencies below 800 Hz (the "reject band"). This was done for many different cutoff frequencies, and the results are shown by the curve marked "high pass" in **Fig. 17.12**. Intelligibility is close to 100% when the high-pass cutoff is 200 Hz, at point **a**, because the subjects can hear all of the frequencies above 200 Hz and are only denied the small range below it. Performance falls as the cutoff moves upward in frequency, and is only ~ 5% at point **b**, where the high-frequency cutoff is 5000 Hz. This happens because high-pass filtering at 5000 Hz is the same as removing the wide range of important frequencies below 5000 Hz. The same measurements were done with **low-pass filtering**, and these results are shown by the curve marked "low pass." Notice that intelligibility is very good (~ 95%) for low-pass filtering at 5000 Hz, at point **c**, because the subjects can hear all of the frequencies up to 5000 Hz. However, intelligibility drops to near zero for the 200 Hz cutoff, at point **d**, because the subjects can hear only the frequencies up to 200 Hz but cannot hear anything higher than 200 Hz (because passing the lows is the same as rejecting the highs). Notice that the two curves *intersect* at ~ 1900 Hz (where the score happens to be 68%). This means that the frequencies above 1900 Hz provide as much information about speech intelligibility as the frequencies below 1900 Hz. The frequency range of speech has been divided into two ranges or bandwidths (≤ 1900 Hz and ≥ 1900 Hz), each of which makes the same contribution to speech intelligibility. If the frequencies above and below 1900 Hz contribute equally, why do they intersect at 68% instead of at 50%? The answer is that the speech signal contains **redundant** information. Incidentally, 1900 Hz and 68% are not magical values; the curves will intersect at different locations depending on the nature of the speech material being tested.

It is also possible to divide the frequency range into 20 bands, each of which makes an equal contribution to speech intelligibility. French and Steinberg (1947) did this very thing to develop the original version of the articulation index. Specifically, the AI is composed of 20 contiguous bands found to be equally important for speech understanding. Hence, each band contributes 5% to intelligibility (20 bands × 5% = 100%). The AI is expressed as a decimal value between 0 and 1.0, where 1.0 is the same as 100% (20 bands × 0.05 = 1.0). Each band is counted according to the audibility of the speech signal it contains. We are concerned with the effects of noise on speech communication, so we will assume that the sounds are well above threshold, and concentrate on the signal-to-noise ratio (SNR) in each band. (Recall that the signal ratio is the number of decibels for the signal minus the number of decibels for the noise.) A 30 dB range of SNR is considered, where a SNR of +18 dB gets "full credit" for the band (0.05), down to –12 dB, which gets no credit for that band (0.0). In effect, each decibel of SNR counts for 1/30 of the band's 0.05 value. This SNR is used to determine how much of the band's 0.05 value will be counted. The resulting 20 values (one from each band) are added to arrive at the AI, which will range from 0 to 1.0. The original AI has been modified to use standard third-octave and octave-bands, adjustments in the importance attached to each band, etc., which led to the development of a new standard for a **speech intelligibility index (SII)**, as well as for use with the hearing impaired (e.g., Kryter 1962; Pavlovic, Studebaker, & Sherbecoe 1986; Pavlovic 1987, 1991; ANSI 2012a).

The AI can be used to predict the intelligibility of various kinds of speech material, some examples of which are illustrated in **Fig. 17.13**. For example, an AI of 0.5 corresponds to intelligibility scores of

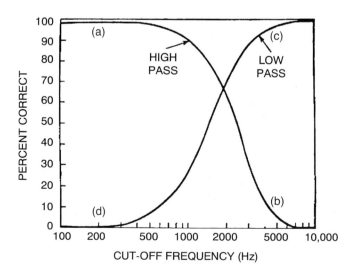

Fig. 17.12 Percent correct identification of syllables as a function of high- and low-pass filtering. Points labeled a, b, c, and d refer to the text. (Adapted from French and Steinberg (1947), with permission of the *Journal of the Acoustical Society of America*.)

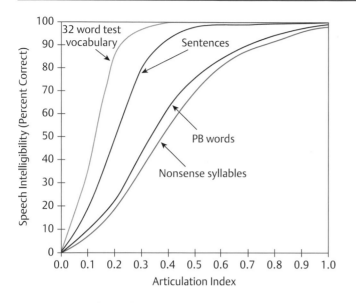

Fig. 17.13 Relationship between the articulation index and percent correct speech intelligibility for various materials. (Based on Kryter [1962, 1985].)

roughly 70% for nonsense syllables, 75% for monosyllabic (PB) words, 97% for sentences, and 100% when the test vocabulary is limited to only 32 words. As a rule of thumb, the conditions for speech communication are (1) probably satisfactory when the AI is above 0.6, (2) unsatisfactory when the AI is under 0.3, and (3) sufficiently suspicious to warrant intelligibility testing (if possible) when the AI is between 0.3 and 0.6 (Beranek 1954/1986). Notice in **Fig. 17.13** that an AI of 0.3 corresponds to word intelligibility of roughly 45% and sentence scores of ~ 80%, whereas performance reaches ~ 85% for words and ~ 98% for sentences when the AI is 0.6.

Speech interference level The **speech interference level (SIL)** (Beranek 1954/1986) is a simplified variation of the articulation index that identifies how much noise will just permit communication to take place. The SIL is provided for various distances between the talker and listener, and for different amounts of vocal effort from normal conversational speech to shouting. **Fig. 17.14** shows SIL values developed by Beranek (1954/1986). It shows, for example, that (1) normal conversational speech can just take place at a distance of 12 feet provided the noise (i.e., the SIL) is 43 dB, but at no more than 4 feet if the SIL is 53 dB; (2) an SIL of 61 dB will allow communication to take place for raised speech level at 3 feet, very loud speech at 6 feet, and shouting at 12 feet; and (3) an SIL of 71 dB limits the distance to 4 feet when shouting, 2 feet for very loud speech, 1 foot for raised speech, and just 6 inches for normal speech.

The SIL itself is obtained by simply averaging the noise levels in three or four bands. The original SIL used the 600 to 1200 Hz, 1200 to 2400 Hz, and 2400 to 4800 Hz bands, and included the 300 to 600 Hz band in the average if its level was > 10 dB more than in the 600 to 1200 Hz band. Many modifications of the SIL have been developed using the *preferred* octave-bands centered at 500, 1000, 2000, and 4000 Hz (called **PSIL** for this reason), as well as measurements in dBA and dBC (e.g., Webster 1969, 1978; ANSI 1997; Lazarus 1987).

Speech transmission index The **speech transmission index (STI)** (Steeneken & Houtgast 1983; Anderson & Kalb 1987) is another method for estimating speech communication efficiency from acoustical measurements. It extends the AI concept to account for the effects of all kinds of distortions, including those that occur over time, like reverberation. **Reverberation** refers to multiple echoes from reflective surfaces in a room that continue for a period of time after the original sound has ended. Some degree of reverberation adds "liveness" to a room, but substantial reverberation is a very common problem that causes speech intelligibility to deteriorate. The STI uses a sophisticated method of physical analysis called the **modulation transfer function (MTF)** to determine how a test signal is affected by noise and distortion in the octave-bands from 125 to 8000 Hz. The MTF results are converted to a transmission index for each band. The bands are weighted according to their importance for speech communi-

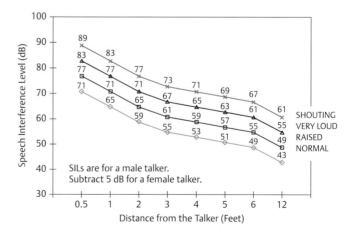

Fig. 17.14 The speech interference levels (SILs) at which word intelligibility is barely reliable at distances of ½ foot to 12 feet away from the talker in an environment without reflections, for various levels of vocal effort (normal, raised, very loud, shouting). Subtract 5 dB for a female talker. Add 5 dB for sentences or if a limited vocabulary is used. (Based on data by Beranek [1954/1986].)

cation (as for the AI) and are then combined to produce the STI, which ranges from 0 to 100% (or 0 to 1.0). The higher the STI, the better are the conditions for speech communication. The curves in **Fig. 17.15** show how speech recognition is related to the STI.

A simple and efficient method for making STI measurements is provided by the **rapid speech transmission index (RASTI)** (IEC 1987), which can be accomplished using instrumentation made for this purpose (e.g., Bruel & Kjaer 1985). The equipment includes a loudspeaker placed in the location of a talker and a microphone placed where the listener would be. The loudspeaker presents a test signal into the room being evaluated, and the sound picked up by the microphone reflects how the original test signal has been affected by the noise and other acoustical characteristics in the room. The results are expressed as RASTI values from 0 to 1.0, which can be used to indicate relative speech intelligibility—for example, ≤ 0.29, bad; 0.3 to 0.44, poor; 0.45 to 0.59, fair; 0.6 to 0.74, good; ≥ 0.75, excellent (Orfield 1987).

Other Effects of Noise

The student should be aware that noise can affect other aspects of life besides hearing and speech communication. It has been known for some time that exposure to noise can have wide-reaching negative effects on many aspects of physical and mental health and performance (e.g., Cohen 1977; Miller 1974; Cohen & Weinstein 1981; Kryter 1985; Suter 1992a; HCN 1996; de Kluizenaar, Janssen, van Lenthe, Miedema, & Mackenbach 2009; Pedersen 2011). These include (1) sleep interference; (2) stress and anxiety reactions; (3) startle responses and reflexive muscle reactions; (4) changes in heart rate, breathing pattern, gastrointestinal motility, pupillary size, and digestive secretions; (5) nervous system arousal; (6) constriction and flow reduction in peripheral blood vessels; (7) vestibular disturbances with very intense sounds; (8) negative impact on the performance of cognitive and sensorimotor tasks due to arousal, distraction, startle responses, and increased fatigue after completion of tasks; (9) increased incidences of cardiovascular, vestibular, and ear-nose-throat disorders; (10) a slight effect on prematurity and reduced birth weight; (11) possible effects on immune responses suggested by noise-related changes in the concentrations of some blood components; and (12) evidence of relatively poorer school performance.

Several recent studies expanded upon what we know about the effects of noise upon health risks and decrements in school-related performance. For example, occupational noise among auto workers has been shown to be related to elevated blood pressure and heart rates (Lusk, Hagerty, Gillespie, & Caruso 2002; Lusk, Gillespie, Hagerty, & Ziemba 2004), as well as increased risks of cardiovascular disease (Virkkunen, Kauppinen, & Tenkanen 2005; Willich, Wegscheider, Stallmann, & Keil 2006). Two studies reported that high levels of noise exposure over years may increase the risks for developing acoustic neuromas (Preston-Martin, Thomas, Wright, & Henderson 1989; Edwards, Schwartzbaum, Lönn, Ahlbom, & Feychting 2006); however, it has been argued that their findings are not conclusive due to methodological issues (Patel 2006). With respect to school-related performance, a large-sample study of elementary school children in three countries demonstrated performance on reading comprehension and recognition memory tasks was adversely affected by aircraft noise, although not by traffic noise (Stansfeld et al 2005). In this context, it is interesting to recall from earlier in this chapter that these children reported greater annoyance from aircraft noise than from traffic noise.

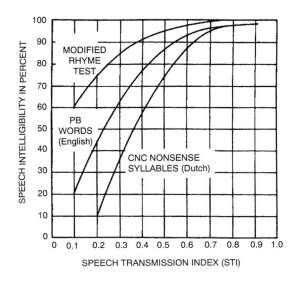

Fig. 17.15 The relationship between the speech transmission index and speech recognition scores for PB-50 words (English), the Modified Rhyme Test (MRT, estimated), and Dutch CVC nonsense syllables. (Adapted from Anderson and Kalb [1987], with permission of the *Journal of the Acoustical Society of America.*)

■ Occupational Hearing Conservation

The requirements of occupational hearing conservation programs are largely defined by compliance with federal regulations known as the **Hearing Con-**

servation **Amendment (HCA)** (OSHA 1983).[9] The current HCA is the culmination of a series of laws and regulations beginning with noise exposure regulations instituted in 1969 under the authority of the Walsh-Healey Public Contracts Act of 1935 (DOL 1969). Subsequently, the Williams-Steiger Occupational Safety and Health Act of 1970 established OSHA under the Department of Labor. In turn, OSHA amended the Walsh-Healey noise standard by developing the original version of the HCA in 1971. After a long and bumpy evolution (see, e.g., Suter 1984; Suter & von Gierke 1987; OSHA 2002), the HCA was published in 1983 (OSHA 1983) and the final rule for reporting and recording hearing loss was published in 2002 (OSHA 1983, 2002).

The HCA requires that a **hearing conservation program** must be implemented for all employees who are exposed to noise levels of 85 dBA TWA, or a 50% dose (recall that the PEL is 90 dBA TWA or a 100% dose). A time-weighted average of 85 dBA (or a 50% dose) is often called the **action level** for this reason, although we will see that some aspects of the program are triggered when exposures achieve 90 dBA TWA. The OSHA-mandated hearing conservation program involves five major components: monitoring of noise levels; audiometric testing; hearing protectors (ear plugs or muffs that reduce the sound levels reaching the eardrum); a training program; and record keeping. Invaluable information and guidance pertaining to the details of hearing conservation programs may be found in several readily available sources (e.g., Berger et al 2000; NIOSH 1990, 1996, 1998; Royster & Royster 1990a; Suter 1993; Rawool 2012; and the OSHA Web site[10]).

Before proceeding, the student should be aware that although the OSHA HCA is the federally mandated program, other approaches have also been recommended. For example, NIOSH (1998) proposed that all components of the hearing conservation program should be triggered at 85 dBA TWA, as well as the use of less strict criteria for deciding when workplace noise has caused a significant change in an employee's hearing, among other differences from the OSHA rules.

Monitoring of Noise Levels

The Hearing Conservation Amendment requires noise level monitoring to be done whenever there is information suggesting that employees might be exposed to noise levels ≥ 85 dBA TWA. All continuous, intermittent, and impulsive noises between 80 and 130 dB are integrated into the noise exposure measurements. Representative personal noise exposure sampling is done when area-wide monitoring is not appropriate, such as when the employees move around a lot, or when there are variations in sound level within the area in question. All affected employees must be notified that they are being exposed to noise levels ≥ 85 dBA TWA. Noise level monitoring must be repeated whenever changes occur that might cause (1) additional employees to be exposed to ≥ 85 dBA TWA, or (2) the employees' hearing protectors no longer to be providing adequate attenuation.

Audiometric Testing

The audiometric testing component of the program includes a baseline audiogram, annual audiograms, certain retests, and referrals. Air-conduction audiograms are done for each ear for at least *500, 1000, 2000, 3000, 4000,* and *6000 Hz,* using a manual, self-recording, or microprocessor-controlled (computerized) audiometer. These tests may be performed by an audiologist, a physician, or a technician who is certified by the Council of Accreditation in Occupational Hearing Conservation (CAOHC) or who has demonstrated satisfactory competence. Technicians who operate microprocessor-based audiometers do not have to be certified. All technicians must be responsible to an audiologist or a physician. The term *physician* is used here even though the HCA actually says "an otolaryngologist or physician" because all otolaryngologists are physicians. Confusing wording is also found in the HCA with regard to technicians who may operate manual versus microprocessor-controlled audiometers. The fact that technicians can be certified by CAOHC or have "satisfactorily demonstrated competence" effectively negates any distinction between a certified and an uncertified technician.

Employees must have a **baseline audiogram** within the first 6 months of exposure to noise levels ≥ 85 dBA TWA. Future audiograms will be compared with the baseline audiogram to determine if there has been any deterioration of hearing that may have been caused by occupational noise exposure. To minimize the effects of TTS on the baseline audiogram, employees must be without workplace noise exposure for at least 14 hours before testing, and must be advised to avoid nonoccupational noise exposures during this period as well. However, hearing protectors may be used as a substitute for being away from workplace noise during the 14 hours before testing. A special exception to the 6-month time limit for

---

[9] Although we are focusing on OSHA, the student should be aware that other hearing conservation programs also exist, such as those for the mining industry (MSHA 1999) and for the military (DOD 2004).

[10] The OSHA Web site is located at www.osha.gov.

baseline audiograms is allowed if the audiometric services are provided by a mobile testing van that comes to the workplace. Mobile testing vans are often used when on-site testing facilities are not available. In these cases, the time limit for the baseline audiogram is extended to a full year, but hearing protectors must be used after the first 6 months.

Annual monitoring audiograms are done for each employee exposed to noise levels ≥ 85 dBA TWA. The annual audiogram is compared with the baseline audiogram to determine if there has been a **standard threshold shift (STS)** in either or both ears. A standard threshold shift is simply a change for the worse in threshold with an *average of 10 dB or more averaged across 2000, 3000, and 4000 Hz*. OSHA (2002) requires the recording and reporting of standard threshold shifts resulting in a total hearing loss of 25 dB HL. An **age correction** may be made when determining if there has been a STS, which essentially reduces the size of the threshold shift by an amount that is attributed to presbycusis. **Table 17.4** shows the age correction values that may be used for this purpose, and illustrates the procedure prescribed by the HCA. A retest may be done within 30 days if there has been a standard threshold shift, in which case the retest may be used as the annual audiogram. Comparisons between annual and baseline audiograms may be done by a technician. However, decisions about whether a STS is work-related, reviews of problem cases, and determinations about the need for further evaluation must be done by a physician or "other licensed health care professional" (audiologist).

An **exit audiogram** should be obtained when an employee is no longer exposed to potentially hazardous noise levels or leaves the employer.

Follow-up and Referral Procedures

An employee who has sustained a standard threshold shift must be advised of this within 21 days. Unless a physician determines that the standard threshold shift was unrelated to occupational noise exposure, the employee must be provided with hearing protectors and be *required* to use them, or be refitted with new ones that provide greater attenuation if he is already using hearing protectors. *Referrals* for audiological and/or otological evaluations are made if more testing is needed or if there is suspicion of ear pathology related to the use of hearing protectors. Employees must also be *informed* about any suspicion of ear diseases that are not related to hearing protector use. Just as an employee must be told about the presence of a standard threshold shift, he must also be informed if subsequent tests show that the standard threshold shift is not consistent. In that

case, he may choose to stop using hearing protectors provided his noise exposures are less than 90 dBA TWA. The annual audiogram becomes a **revised baseline audiogram** for future comparisons if the audiologist or physician judges that (1) there is a persistent standard threshold shift or (2) the thresholds on the annual audiogram are better (lower) than those on the baseline.

Audiometer Calibration and Testing Environment

Audiometers used in the occupational hearing conservation program are required to be calibrated to ANSI specifications (see **Table 4.1** in Chapter 4) for at least the frequencies between 500 and 6000 Hz. A *biological calibration* using a person who has known thresholds as well as a listening check for distortion and spurious noises must be accomplished daily before any testing is done. An *acoustical calibration* is required at least annually, and an *exhaustive calibration* must be done at least once every 2 years. In addition, the HCA calls for an acoustical calibration to be done whenever the biological calibration is off by ≥ 10 dB, and for an exhaustive calibration whenever there is a deviation of ≥ 15 dB on an acoustical calibration.

The HCA permits the audiometric test room to have ambient noise octave-band levels that are substantially higher than the maximum ambient noise levels specified by the ANSI S3.1 (2008a) standard for audiometric environments, as shown in **Table 17.5**. The serious implication of this discrepancy is that a test room can meet the HCA requirements for audiometric testing without really being quiet enough for thresholds to be obtained down to 0 dB HL. This can be a source of error and variability that should be avoided by using test rooms that come as close as possible to meeting the ANSI standard for audiometric test environments whenever feasible. Moreover, testing in rooms meeting the ANSI standard was recommended by NIOSH (1998).[11]

Hearing Protectors

The employer must *provide* a reasonable choice of adequate hearing protectors free of charge to all employees who are exposed to noise levels of

---

[11] NIOSH (1998) actually refers to a previous version of the ANSI 3.1 standard published in 1991, but presumably would have referred to ANSI S3.1 1999 (R2008) if it had been published in 1999 or later.

Table 17.4 Age correction values for males and females (according to OSHA 1983, Tables F-1 and F-2)[a]

Frequency (Hz):	Males					Females				
Age (years)	1000	2000	3000	4000	6000	1000	2000	3000	4000	6000
20 or younger	5	3	4	5	8	7	4	3	3	6
21	5	3	4	5	8	7	4	4	3	6
22	5	3	4	5	8	7	4	4	4	6
23	5	3	4	6	9	7	5	4	4	7
24	5	3	5	6	9	7	5	4	4	7
25	5	3	5	7	10	8	5	4	4	7
26	5	4	5	7	10	8	5	5	4	8
27	5	4	6	7	11	8	5	5	5	8
28	6	4	6	8	11	8	5	5	5	8
29	6	4	6	8	12	8	5	5	5	9
30	6	4	6	9	12	8	6	5	5	9
31	6	4	7	9	13	8	6	6	5	9
32	6	5	7	10	14	9	6	6	6	10
33	6	5	7	10	14	9	6	6	6	10
34	6	5	8	11	15	9	6	6	6	10
35	7	5	8	11	15	9	6	7	7	11
36	7	5	9	12	16	9	7	7	7	11
37	7	6	9	12	17	9	7	7	7	12
38	7	6	9	13	17	10	7	7	7	12
39	7	6	10	14	18	10	7	8	8	12
40	7	6	10	14	19	10	7	8	8	13
41	7	6	10	14	20	10	8	8	8	13
42	8	7	11	16	20	10	8	9	9	13
43	8	7	12	16	21	11	8	9	9	14
44	8	7	12	17	22	11	8	9	9	14

≥ 85 dBA TWA, and replace them as necessary. The employer is also responsible for the proper initial fitting of hearing protectors, providing employees with training in their use and care, and supervising their correct use. There are three classes of employees who not only must be provided with ear protectors but also are required to actually use them. They include all employees exposed to levels exceeding the PEL of 90 dBA TWA, and employees exposed at ≥ 85 dBA TWA who (1) are waiting longer than 6 months for a baseline audiogram under the exception for mobile test vans or (2) have experienced a standard threshold shift. Here, again, the onus for compliance is

upon the employer. Hearing protectors are discussed in more detail below.

Efforts to reduce noise exposure have concentrated on the use of hearing protectors. However, the Walsh-Healey regulation actually states that when employees are exposed to noise levels above the PEL "feasible *administrative or engineering controls shall be utilized*" (emphasis added). If engineering and/or administrative controls fail to reduce sound levels within the levels of Table G-16 of OSHA (1983) (i.e., the PELs identified in the first and second columns of **Table 17.3**), then "personal protective equipment shall be provided and used to reduce sound levels

Frequency (Hz):	Males					Females				
Age (years)	1000	2000	3000	4000	6000	1000	2000	3000	4000	6000
45	8	7	13	18	23	11	8	10	10	15
46	8	8	13	19	24	11	9	10	10	15
47	8	8	14	19	24	11	9	10	11	16
48	9	8	14	20	25	12	9	11	11	16
49	9	9	15	21	26	12	9	11	11	16
50	9	9	16	22	27	12	10	11	12	17
51	9	9	16	23	28	12	10	12	12	17
52	9	10	17	24	29	12	10	12	13	18
53	9	10	18	25	30	13	10	13	13	18
54	10	10	18	26	31	13	11	13	14	19
55	10	11	19	27	32	13	11	14	14	19
56	10	11	20	28	34	13	11	14	15	20
57	10	11	21	29	35	13	11	15	15	20
58	10	12	22	31	36	14	12	15	16	21
59	11	12	22	32	37	14	12	16	16	21
60 or older	11	13	23	33	38	14	12	16	17	22

[a]*Example of how to use age correction values:* Using 4000 Hz as an example, suppose the threshold on the annual audiogram is 20 dB at age 32, and the threshold on the baseline audiogram was 5 dB at age 20. The uncorrected threshold shift would be

$$20 \text{ dB (annual)} - 5 \text{ dB (baseline)} = 15 \text{ dB (threshold shift)}$$

Now, find the age correction values that apply to the baseline and annual audiograms. Find the difference between these age correction values. For males at 4000 Hz, these values are 10dB at age 32 and 5 dB at age 20, and the difference between them is

$$10 \text{ dB (at age 32)} - 5 \text{ dB (at age 20)} = 5 \text{ dB (age correction)}$$

This difference becomes the age correction. It is subtracted from the uncorrected threshold shift to find the age-corrected threshold shift. In our example, this is

$$15 \text{ dB (uncorrected)} - 5 \text{ dB (correction)} = 10 \text{ dB (age corrected)}$$

The age-corrected threshold shift is then used to find the (now age-corrected) standard threshold shift.

within the levels of the table" (OSHA 1983, 29 CFR 1910.95(b)(1)). It is important to be aware that the HCA did *not* supersede or replace these requirements of the original regulations.

Training Program

Employers are responsible for providing an annual training program for employees exposed to ≥85 dBA TWA and ensuring they participate in the program. The training program is required to address at least three topics: (1) the effects of noise on hearing; (2)

hearing protectors, including their purpose, advantages and disadvantages of different types, and their selection, fitting, use, and care; and (3) the purposes of and procedures involved in audiometric testing.

Although annual training sessions are required, it would be foolish to believe that the effectiveness of any hearing conservation program can be maintained by a passively supported meeting once a year, no matter how impressive the talker, demonstrations, and videotapes might be. Several sessions spread over the year can be helpful, especially if they are interactive and relatively short. All kinds of educational and training materials are available,

Table 17.5 Comparison between the octave-band levels (in dB) of ambient noise in an audiometric test room allowed by the Hearing Conservation Amendment (OSHA, 1983) and those specified for ears-covered testing by the ANSI S3.1-1999 (R2008) Standard

Center frequency (Hz)	OSHA (1983) (dB)	ANSI S3.1-1999 (R2008) (dB)	Discrepancy (dB)
500	40	21	19
1000	40	26	14
2000	47	34	13
4000	57	37	20
8000	62	37	25

including motivational posters that not only prompt employees to wear their hearing protectors, but also remind them how to do so properly. Motivational approaches run the gamut from simple praise to innovative reward systems, but also include disciplinary personnel actions. The importance of active support by management, including supervisors and foremen, cannot be over-stressed, so that employees are aware that the hearing conservation program is treated as a mutually beneficial commitment that is enthusiastically encouraged and actively enforced.

Record Keeping

Employers are required to keep records on noise exposure measurements, audiometric test results, and the background levels in the test rooms. In addition to the employee's name, job classification, test dates, and results, each audiometric test record is also required to show the examiner's name, the date of the audiometer's most recent acoustic or exhaustive calibration, and the date of the employee's last noise exposure assessment. Noise exposure measurements have to be retained for 2 years and audiometric records are kept for the entire duration of employment for each employee. Moreover, a standard threshold shift of $\geq$ 10 dB resulting in a total hearing loss of $\geq$ 25 dB must be recorded and reported to OSHA.

Employees (or their representatives) must be allowed to observe the measurements and to have access to the noise standard and related information, training materials, and records.

Program Effectiveness

The effectiveness of a hearing conservation program might be addressed in many different ways, each providing different kinds of information. For example, one might determine how many standard threshold shifts have occurred, or perhaps track the degree of employee compliance for ear protection use or for keeping appointments for hearing tests or training sessions. However, the contemporary method is a statistical approach called **audiometric database analysis (ADBA)** (e.g., Royster & Royster 1999, 2000; ANSI S12.13 TR-2002 [R2010]). The basic concept of ADBA is to monitor the effectiveness of a hearing conservation program by evaluating audiometric findings on a group basis. This approach makes it possible to identify undesirable trends that can be alleviated by program-wide changes in policies and procedures. Instead of comparing threshold shifts between audiograms, audiometric database analysis looks at the *variability* between sequential pairs of audiograms (e.g., between the first and second annual audiograms, the second and third, etc.). This variability is compared with criterion ranges to determine whether it is acceptable, marginal, or unacceptable. Marginally or unacceptably high variability indicates the possibility that a problem exists that needs to be addressed. For example, the hearing conservation program may be failing to provide an adequate degree of protection from on-the-job noise exposure. This might be due to poor utilization of hearing protectors, the need for engineering and/or administrative controls, deficiencies in the educational program or motivation, etc. However, other factors may also account for the variability. The most likely ones involve deficiencies in the audiometric testing program, and often have to do with inadequate audiometer calibration, acoustical test environments, and test methods.

■ Controlling Noise and Noise Exposure

Administrative Controls

Administrative controls involve modifications of scheduling and other policies that effectively reduce employees' exposures to excessive noise levels. For example, instead of having one group of employees working an 8-hour shift in a high-noise area exceeding the PEL, two smaller groups could be rotated between work assignments in high-noise and low-noise areas so their TWA exposures are all below the PEL. However, approaches of this type are rarely used because they present untenable practical problems for the employer and are often just as objectionable to employees and labor unions.

Engineering Controls

Numerous engineering approaches can be used to control noise exposure by reducing noise at its *source* and/or by modifying its transmission path to or at the *receiver* (i.e., the listener). Many of the major considerations have been reviewed by Erdreich (1999) and Driscoll and Royster (2000), and a clearly illustrated outline of noise control methods may be found in Bruel and Kjaer (1986). One approach that addresses the noise source is the *replacement* of noisier equipment, processes, and materials with quieter ones. Several examples include the replacement of gear drives with belt drives, compressed-air-driven (pneumatic) tools with electric ones, riveting with welding or bolts, and steel wheels and gears with rubber or plastic ones. Another approach involves *modifications* of the sound sources. For example, industrial processes that involve impacts on vibrating surfaces can be made less noisy by reducing the driving force. This can be accomplished by decreasing the speed of repetitive impacts, keeping the equipment well balanced, and placing a vibration isolator (e.g., a rubber lining) at the point of impact. Vibratory responses can be reduced by adding damping materials, or by adding stiffness or mass to change the resonance of the vibrating surface. The amount of noise radiated by a vibrating surface can be diminished by reducing its area, which can be accomplished by decreasing

its overall size or by adding perforations. Noises produced by flowing fluids or a turbulent stream of air (e.g., air ejection systems and high-pressure vents) can be abated by reducing the speed of fluid flow and the amount of turbulence. Mufflers and wrapping with sound-absorbing materials are also used.

Modifying the acoustical path may be accomplished by placing enclosures around the offending equipment, using shields or barriers between the source and the listener, using acoustically lined ducts and mufflers, and sometimes by providing sound-isolating control rooms for workers (i.e., an enclosure around the listener). In effect, hearing protectors modify the acoustical path at its far end by obstructing the transmission of noise just before it is picked up by the ear. Noise levels are also reduced by using acoustically absorptive materials on room surfaces (ceilings, walls, etc.), which is particularly important in reverberant environments. Active noise control methods have also been developed that use advanced signal processing methods to produce a sound that cancels all or part of the original noise (e.g., Nelson & Elliot 1992; Ericksson 1996; Kuo & Morgan 1996).

Towne (1994) has provided advice about noise considerations when choosing a place to live, including practical applications of noise control principles in the home. A few examples are quite instructive: Floors should be carpeted except in the kitchen, where a resilient mat should separate vinyl or linoleum floor coverings from the subflooring, especially in multistory dwellings. The entrance door should have a heavy, solid core with minimal spaces around its perimeter, and a rubber bumper to reduce noise when slammed. Similarly, sliding doors should have rubber wheels and resilient bumpers.

Hearing Protectors

Hearing protection devices (HPDs) include a variety of ear plugs and muffs used to reduce the amount of sound reaching the wearer's ears (Berger 2000).[12,13] Hearing protectors are generally categorized as ear muffs, ear plugs, and canal caps or semiaural plugs. **Ear muffs** are rigid plastic cups or shells with soft plastic cushions that completely enclose the ears

---

[12] NIOSH maintains an online compendium of HPDs at http://www.cdc.gov/niosh/topics/noise/hpcomp.html

[13] We will limit our discussion to "passive" HPDs, but the student should be aware that there are also active HPDs, which use electronic techniques to reduce the amount of sound entering the ear (see, e.g., Gauger 2002).

(**Fig. 17.16a**). The shells are filled with sound-attenuating material and the cushions are filled with foam or liquid so they fit snugly against the sides of the head, sealing off the sound path to the ears. The cups are held firmly against the head by a spring headband. The effectiveness of ear muffs is reduced by ~ 5 dB when eyeglasses are worn (Royster, Berger, & Merry 1996). Ear muffs are also available in combination with hard hats for use in jobs where head protection is also needed (**Fig. 17.16b**).

Ear plugs are inserted snugly into the ear canals (**Fig. 17.17**). *Premolded* plugs are made of flexible plastic, silicone, or similar materials that have one or more flanges that provide a snug fit when placed into the ear canal. They usually come in several sizes, although some premolded plugs are made with several tapered flanges so that "one size fits all." *Formable* or *user-molded* plugs are made of pliable materials that conform to the size and shape of the ear canal when they are inserted. The most common materials are expandable polymer foam, silicon putty, wax-impregnated cotton, and fiberglass down or "wool." The latter type of material should be encapsulated within a plastic membrane to protect the ear canal from direct contact with the fiberglass. The expandable foam material is compressed by rolling it between the fingers before being inserted into the ear canal. After being inserted, the foam expands and snugly seals the ear canal. Inserting balls of untreated absorbent cotton (the type commonly sold in health and beauty aid stores) into the ears provides little if any attenuation and should not be used for hearing protection. *Custom-molded* ear plugs can also be made from ear impressions like those used to make hearing aid earmolds and swim molds. In spite of the fact that they are custom-made, the amount of attenuation provided by individually molded ear plugs varies widely.

a

b

Fig. 17.16 Examples of **(a)** ear muffs used for hearing protection and **(b)** ear muffs in combination with a hard hat. (Courtesy of 3M Company, St. Paul, Minnesota.)

Fig. 17.17 Examples of ear plugs used for hearing protection. Formable plugs are shown above and preformed plugs are shown below. (Courtesy of 3M Company, St. Paul, Minnesota.)

Semi-aural hearing protectors are modified ear plugs held in place by a lightweight plastic headband (**Fig. 17.18**). The *canal cap* variety of semi-aural devices covers the entrance to the ear canal and generally provides less attenuation than *pod-type* tips, which insert part of the way into the ear canal. Semi-aurals are easily and conveniently put on and taken off, but they provide the least amount of attenuation among the different types of HPDs. For these reasons, they are best suited for individuals who need hearing protection for short-duration, intermittent exposures.

Compared with ear plugs, ear muffs generally provide somewhat more attenuation, except for the expandable foam plugs; are well suited for situations where HPDs must be put on and removed frequently; provide somewhat more consistent amounts of attenuation in actual field use; are more comfortable in cold environments; and can be easier to fit regardless of head size or shape. Ear muffs are also quite noticeable, so their use is easier to monitor. Ear muffs have several disadvantages as well. For example, headband pressure causes discomfort, particularly with longer durations of use; they are uncomfortable and promote perspiration in hot environments; and they can be problematic when the user is also wearing protective glasses and other kinds of safety devices. Although ear muffs interfere with the use of regular hard hats, this problem can be alleviated by using hard hats with built-in muffs.

Fig. 17.18 Examples of semi-aural hearing protectors: **(a)** canal cap type; **(b)** pod type. (Courtesy of 3M Company, St. Paul, Minnesota.)

In contrast to muffs, ear plugs are more comfortable when they are being worn for longer periods of time, are somewhat less expensive at least on an individual-unit basis, and do not interfere with the use of safety goggles, hard hats, or other safety gear. With the noteworthy exception of the expandable foam variety, most types of ear plugs provide somewhat less attenuation than ear muffs. The amount of attenuation actually provided by ear plugs depends on how deeply and securely they are inserted. (Using both muffs and plugs together typically provides roughly 5 to 10 dB more attenuation than either one alone.) Ear plugs are more difficult to put on than muffs, and, once inserted, many plugs often work themselves loose over the course of the workday, especially when there is jaw movement associated with talking and chewing. Cleanliness becomes an important issue when plugs must be reinserted during the day, especially with dirty hands and in work environments where there is a lot of dust, metal shavings, or other splintering materials. Because they are less visible than muffs, it can be a bit harder to monitor employee compliance with plugs. While it is true that plugs are easier to lose than muffs, they are also available with strings that minimize loss and are certainly less trouble to carry.

Many HPD users are concerned that hearing protectors might interfere with the ability to hear speech. In addition, industrial employees are equally concerned about the ability to hear warning signals and potentially important changes in equipment sounds, and musicians are concerned about interference with the accurate perception of music. In general, it appears that HPDs do not interfere with the speech reception of normal-hearing persons (and may even improve it) as long as the noise levels exceed ~ 85 dBA; but speech interference is a problem in low and moderate noise levels and in quiet (e.g., Berger 2000). Speech intelligibility is adversely affected by HPDs when the wearer has a sensorineural hearing loss or is not a fluent speaker of the language (e.g., Abel, Alberti, Haythornthwaite, & Riko 1982; Abel, Alberti, & Riko 1980; Bauman & Marston 1986). The degree to which HPDs interfere with the reception of desired signals is reduced by using special kinds of HPDs that use acoustical (passive) and/or electronic (active) methods that adjust the amount of attenuation depending on the noise level (such as in military battlefield situations), or so that its frequency response is similar to that of an unoccluded ear (e.g., Maxwell, Williams, Robertson, & Thomas 1987; Killion, DeVilbiss, & Stewart 1988; Berger 1991; Bockstael, De Coensel, Botteldooren, et al 2011; Norin, Emanuel, & Letowski 2011). Earmuffs equipped with amplifiers and volume controls have been found to provide noise protection as well as improved speech reception for hearing-impaired HPD users (Dolan & O'Loughlin 2005).

Determining the Effectiveness of Hearing Protectors

The effectiveness of an HPD is determined by how much attenuation it provides, which can be measured in several ways (Berger 1986; Berger, Franks, & Lindgren 1996; ANSI 2008b; Berger, Voix, Kieper, & Le Cocq 2011). The two principal techniques are **real ear attenuation at threshold (REAT)**, which is a behavioral method, and the **microphone in real ear (MIRE)** approach, which involves physical measurements. In the REAT method, thresholds are obtained for the same ear with and without an HPD. The amount of attenuation provided by the HPD is the difference between the two thresholds. For example, if a subject's threshold is 10 dB with the ear open and 33 dB with an ear plug, then the ear plug has provided 33 – 10 = 23 dB of attenuation. The MIRE approach uses a tiny probe microphone located inside of the ear behind the HPD and another microphone located outside of the hearing protector. Test sounds are thus monitored on both sides of the hearing protector, and the amount of attenuation is the difference between the sound levels picked up inside and outside of the HPD. It appears that the amount of attenuation measured for an HPD is slightly larger when it is based on MIRE compared with REAT measurements (Casali, Mauney, & Burks 1995).

The Environmental Protection Agency (EPA 1979) requires HPDs to be labeled according to the amount of attenuation they provide, expressed in terms of octave-band levels or a **noise reduction rating (NRR)**. The NRR combines the attenuation in each of the octave-bands into a single number. The NRR is the difference between the overall noise level of the "unprotected" exposure in dBC and the noise level under the HPD (the "protected" exposure) in dBA, along with a 3 dB adjustment for "spectral variations," or

$$NRR = dBC_{unprotected} - dBA_{protected} - 3\ dB$$

The attenuation values are obtained by testing a group of subjects in the laboratory, and would typically be expressed in the form of a mean. However, the *average* amount of attenuation theoretically represents the protection provided to only *half* the population who would be using a particular kind of HPD. For this reason, two standard deviations are subtracted from the mean amount of attenuation found in the laboratory, so that the NRR theoretically represents the attenuation that would be afforded to ~ 98% of the population who use that hearing protector. The **single number rating (SNR)** (ISO 1994) is a similar system for describing HPD attenuation, and

tends to estimate attenuation values that are ~ 3 dB larger than the NRR.

Recall that the purpose of a hearing protector is to reduce an employee's effective exposure to noise down to an acceptable maximum level. The amount of noise exposure experienced by a worker while using a particular HPD (the "protected" exposure) in dBA is estimated by subtracting the NRR on the manufacturer's label from the noise level in dBC, or

$$dBA_{protected} = dBC_{unprotected} - NRR$$

This is one of the reasons noise levels are often measured in both dBA and dBC, even though damage risk and compliance are usually viewed in terms of just dBA. (Remember that all of these values are really time-weighted averages.) If the dBC levels are not known, OSHA permits HPD effectiveness to be based on unprotected noise levels in dBA, but the NRR is reduced by 7 dB:

$$dBA_{protected} = dBC_{unprotected} - \left[NRR - 7 \right]$$

Comparisons of laboratory versus field data and studies have shown that HPDs provide substantially less attenuation in actual (field) use compared with the laboratory-based NRRs on their labels (Berger 1993, Berger, Franks, & Lindgren 1996; Royster et al 1996; Berger, Franks, Behar, et al 1998). This point is revealed in **Fig. 17.19**, which summarizes the findings of many studies that compared the attenuation provided by various kinds of HPDs in the laboratory (as labeled on the HPD package) and in the field (Berger 1993; Berger et al 1996).[14] The graph suggests that most ear plugs can be expected to provide most wearers with at least 5 to 10 dB of attenuation in actual use compared with 10 to 15 dB for expandable foam plugs and ear muffs. This is not a problem because more than 90% of noise-exposed workers need only 10 dB of attenuation to bring their exposures down to acceptable levels (Royster 1995).

Issues like these led authorities to suggest replacing the NRR with a **subject-fit noise reduction rating [NRR(SF)** Royster 1995; Royster et al 1996; Berger

---

[14] The NRRs in the graph apply to 98% of the laboratory population and 84% of the field population because the mean attenuation is reduced by two standard deviations in the laboratory and one standard deviation in the field data to keep the values realistic. Thus, the amounts of attenuation shown in the figure apply to ~ 98% of laboratory subjects and 84% of HPD wearers in the field, which is less than the average (mean) amount of attenuation that would occur in both situations.

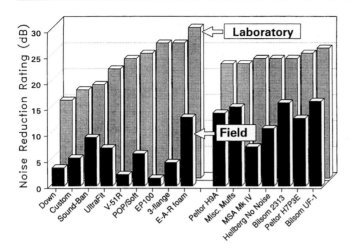

Fig. 17.19 Noise reduction ratings for various kinds of hearing protectors in the laboratory (as labeled) versus in actual use in the field. The group on the left are ear plugs and the group on the right are ear muffs. (© 1993, 3M. All rights reserved. From Berger EH. 1993. The Naked Truth about NRRs. E-A-RLog 20. Indianapolis, IN: 3M. Used with permission by author and 3M.)

1999; ANSI 2008b). The NRR(SF) is determined by subtracting one standard deviation from the mean attenuation values obtained when *naive subjects insert their own HPDs according to the manufacturer's instructions* (hence, "subject-fit"). Hence, the NRR(SF) would better approximate the actual attenuation expected for 84% of actual users in the field. The validity of the subject-fit method was established by Berger et al (1998). NIOSH (1998) proposed reducing **(derating)** the NRRs on the manufacturers' labels by 25% for ear muffs, 50% for formable ear plugs, and 70% for other types of ear plugs until HPDs are tested and labeled using the subject-fit approach. These recommendations were based on comparisons between NRRs and actual attenuation values for various kinds of HPDs (e.g., Berger et al 1996), and are superior to the single 50% derating for all HPDs, used by OSHA inspectors for quite some time.

Instead of using a single NRR number, the ANSI S12.6 (2008b) standard describes the HPD attenuation as a *range* between two values, say 19 dB and 29 dB. The lower number (19 dB in our example) is the amount of protection expected to be obtained by 80% (i.e., most) of trained HPD users, and is called the **Noise Level Reduction Statistic (NRS)** for the 80th percentile, or **NRS$_{80}$**. The higher value (29 dB in our example) is the greater amount of protection expected for the small number of highly proficient and motivated users whose HPDs are meticulously inserted and carefully maintained. It is called the **NRS** for the 20th percentile, or just **NRS$_{20}$**. Laboratory

results and a database of representative industrial noises are used to provide NRS$_{A80}$ and NRS$_{A20}$ values for use with noise levels measured in dBA.[15]

The noise level in dBA experienced by the person wearing the HPD is the **effective A-weighted sound pressure level**, which we have been calling the "protected exposure." This effective or protected exposure is estimated by subtracting the NRS$_A$ for the HPD being used from the noise level in dBA. For the typical HPD wearer, we use the smaller amount of protection represented by NRS$_{A80}$:

$$dBA_{protected} = dBA_{unprotected} - NRS_{A80}$$

For the highly motivated and skillful HPD wearer, we use the greater amount of protection represented by NRS$_{A20}$:

$$dBA_{protected} = dBA_{unprotected} - NRS_{A20}$$

Notice that we *do not subtract* 7 dB from the NRS when the original noise exposure is measured in dBA, as we did when using the NRR.

■ Occupational Hearing Loss and Workers' Compensation

People who have sustained occupational hearing losses may be entitled to payments under workers' compensation programs, although the details vary widely among states and other kinds of jurisdictions. In addition, the terms **impairment**, **handicap**, and **disability**, which are used almost interchangeably in daily clinical discourse, actually have different meanings that become important when employment-related compensation issues are involved. The generally accepted definitions of these terms are as follows (AMA 1979, p. 2055, emphasis added):

Impairment: A change for the worse in either structure or function, *outside the range of normal.*

Handicap: The disadvantage imposed by an impairment *sufficient to affect a person's efficiency* in activities of daily living. Handicap implies a *material* impairment.

Disability: An actual or presumed inability to remain *employed at full wages.*

---

[15] NRS$_{G80}$ and NRS$_{G20}$ are used with a graphical method requiring noises to be measured in dBC (NRS$_{G80}$ and NRS$_{G20}$), and a third and more complicated approach uses octave-bands [see ANSI/ASA S12.68-2007 (R2012)]).

Notice that any deviation from the normal range can be an impairment, but an impairment is not considered to be a handicap unless it interferes materially with the ability to engage in daily activities. Finally, a handicap is not a disability until it affects compensable employment. These distinctions are very important because hearing impairments are often handicapping but are infrequently disabling according to these definitions. In fact, it was not until a 1948 New York court decision that hearing impairments became compensable in spite of the fact that they might not cause lost wages. On the other hand, the Maryland courts took the opposite point of view in 1961, and it took legislative action in 1967 to make occupational hearing impairments compensable regardless of disability in that state.

The amounts of compensation awarded for hearing loss and the duration of the payments vary from jurisdiction to jurisdiction, as do waiting periods, corrections for age (presbycusis),[16] prior losses, etc. In general, there is some maximum amount of compensation, and a proportion of these maximum compensation benefits will be awarded depending on the percentage of the hearing impairment. The arduous task of determining the occupational hearing loss compensation practices from state to state was addressed by ASHA (1992) and Dobie and Megerson (2000), whose findings are summarized in **Table 17.6**.

Compensation methods or **formulas** are used to convert the degree of hearing loss into a *percentage* of impairment for these purposes. Before reviewing the major compensation formulas, it is worthwhile mentioning that they reflect economic, social, and political considerations as much as clinical judgments about the extent to which a hearing loss is handicapping.

Several characteristics are common to just about all of the compensation formulas in current use. Only certain frequencies are considered by each formula, and the amount of hearing loss is averaged across these frequencies separately for each ear. There is a certain minimum amount of hearing loss that must be present before a loss is potentially compensable. (This notion is the same as the criterion for what constitutes a material hearing impairment when estimating the risks of noise exposure.) This border is called the **low fence**, and it constitutes a 0% impairment. If the low fence is 25 dB, then only the part of a hearing loss above 25 dB would be considered

in determining the amount of impairment. There is also a **high fence**, which constitutes a 100% impairment. If the high fence is 92 dB, then any loss of 92 dB or more would count as a 100% impairment. The range of decibels between the low fence and the high fence corresponds to the range of impairments from 0% to 100%. In our example, this range is 92 − 25 = 67 dB wide, so each decibel of hearing loss above 25 dB contributes 1.5% toward the percentage of impairment. These principles are illustrated on the left side of **Fig. 17.20**.

After averaging the losses for the appropriate frequencies in a given ear, this average loss is compared with the low and high fences. In **Fig. 17.20**, the average loss in case A is 23 dB. This value is less than the 25 dB low fence, so this ear has a 0% impairment. Case B has an average loss of 33 dB, which is above the low fence and under the high fence. Only the decibels above the low fence count toward the percentage of impairment, which is 33 − 25 = 8 dB. Because each decibel above the low fence counts for 1.5%, the impairment for this ear is 8 × 1.5% = 12%. Case C has an average loss of 97 dB, which is automatically considered a 100% impairment because it exceeds the 92 dB high fence.

The patient's final (binaural) percentage of impairment is arrived at by combining the percentages of impairment for the two ears, but this is done in a special way that gives the better ear substantially more weight than the poorer ear. The better ear in this context means the ear with a lower percentage of impairment. The procedure is to average the percentages of impairments of the two ears in a way that reflects the greater weighting of the better ear, and is easily understood by considering an example. Suppose that the impairments were found to be 12% for the right ear and 29% for the left ear, and that the better ear must be counted 5 times more than the poorer ear. Here, the better ear would be multiplied by 5, and this product would be added to the poorer ear:

$$(12\% \times 5) + 29\% = 60\% + 29\% = 89\%$$

Notice that this sum of 89% is the result of adding six values, five from the better ear and one from the poorer ear. Hence, the average value is found by dividing the sum by 6:

$$89\% \div 6 = 14.8\%$$

Consequently, this patient's overall or binaural impairment is 14.8%, which would normally be rounded to 15%. The procedural principles just illustrated are essentially the same for all of the compen-

---

[16] The **allocation** of part of an individual patient's hearing loss to age and part of it to noise exposure is a topic with considerable legal ramifications. Dobie (1993, 1996) proposed an approach to doing this, although it is not without controversy (Lipscomb 1999).

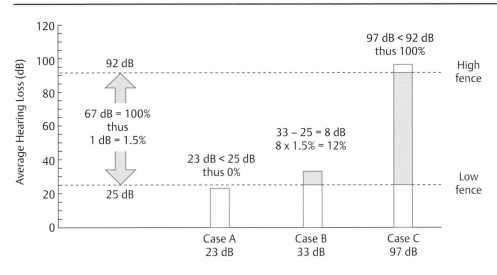

Fig. 17.20 Illustrative examples of the low fence, high fence, and percentage of impairment for each decibel of hearing loss above the low fence (see text).

sation formulas in current use. We will review some of the better-known and more interesting formulas. A reasonably complete listing of the available hearing loss compensation formulas is given in **Table 17.7**.

Early Methods

One occasionally comes across references to the early compensation formulas developed by Fletcher (1929) and the American Medical Association (AMA 1942, 1947) even though they are no longer used. The Fletcher method is often called the *point-eight rule* because it converted a range of losses from 0 dB to 128 dB into percentages, so each decibel is worth 0.8%. The early AMA approaches applied value weightings to the amount of hearing loss at each frequency considered, and the 1947 version is also known as the Fowler-Sabine method.

AAOO 1959/1971 Method

The best-known compensation formulas are those developed by the American Academy of Otolaryngology—Head and Neck Surgery (AAO), formerly known as the American Academy of Ophthalmology and Otolaryngology (AAOO), and the AMA. The AAOO introduced a compensation formula in 1959 that was updated in 1971 for use with the current ANSI standards for audiometers. This method involves the average of 500, 1000, and 2000 Hz; a low fence of 25 dB HL and a high fence of 92 dB HL; 1.5% per decibel; and counting the better ear five times more than the poorer ear. It was proposed that these criteria reflect the ability to hear and repeat sentences, which was in turn supposed to reveal "correct hearing for everyday speech," although this contention was not sup-

ported with research evidence. The appropriateness of the 1959/1971 AAOO formula as a measure of impairment is questionable because it ignores the frequencies above 2000 Hz that are important for everyday speech understanding, sentence reception in quiet is a poor representation of real-life speech recognition ability, and a 25 dB low fence based on the 500 to 2000 Hz average is unfairly high. Suter (1985) demonstrated that the AAOO formula fails to reflect the actual speech recognition problems of hearing-impaired subjects.

AAO-AMA 1979 Method

The formula subsequently recommended by the AAO and the AMA addressed the issues just described by changing the frequencies that are averaged to include 500, 1000, 2000, and 3000 Hz (AMA 1979). The fences, better-ear weighting, and percentage per decibel are the same as in the earlier formula. As a result, the 1979 AAO-AMA method accounts for the high-frequency nature of many occupational losses, at least to the extent that 3000 Hz is involved in the hearing loss. The 1979 AAO-AMA method is widely used, as suggested in **Table 17.6**. Kryter (1998) suggested modifying the 1979 AAO-AMA method by reducing the low fence to 15 dB and the high fence to 75 dB, adjusting the values for presbycusis, and changing the better-ear weighting to 3 instead of 5.

NIOSH and CHABA Methods

Similar to the AAO-AMA method, the **1972 NIOSH formula** uses the same fences, percentages per decibel, and five-times weighting for the better ear. However, it applies these criteria to the average of

Table 17.6   Workers' compensation methods for hearing loss by state[a]

State	Method	Presbycusis considered?	Tinnitus considered?	Prior loss considered?
Alabama	Medical evidence	No	Yes with hrng. impt.	Yes
Alaska	AAO-1979	No	Yes with hrng. impt.	Yes
Arizona	AAO-1979/med. ev.	No	Yes with hrng. impt.	Yes
Arkansas	AAO-1979	Possibly	Possibly	Yes
California	AAO-1979	No	Yes	Yes
Colorado	AAO-1979/med. ev.	Yes	Yes	No
Connecticut	Medical evidence	Possibly	Yes	Yes
Delaware	AAO-1979/med. ev.	No	No	No
Florida	AAO-1979/med. ev.	No	Yes with hrng. impt.	Possibly
Georgia	AAOO-1959 (1971)	No	No	Yes
Hawaii	AAOO-1959 (1971)/ med. ev.	No	Yes	No
Idaho	AAO-1979/med. ev.	No	No	Yes
Illinois	Illinois formula	No	Yes	Yes
Indiana	Medical evidence	Yes	Yes	Yes
Iowa	AAO-1979	Yes	Yes	Yes
Kansas	AAO-1979	Yes	Yes with hrng. impt.	Yes
Kentucky	AAO-1979/med. ev.	No	No	No
Louisiana	AAO-1979/med. ev.	No	Yes with hrng. impt.	Yes
Maine	AAOO-1959 (1971)	Yes	Yes with hrng. impt	Yes
Maryland	AAOO-1959 (1971)	Possibly	Possibly	Yes
Massachusetts	Medical evidence	Yes	Yes	Yes
Michigan	(Medical expenses and wage loss for hearing loss injury)			
Minnesota	AAO-1979	No	No	Yes
Mississippi	Medical evidence	No	Yes	No
Missouri	AAOO-1959 (1971)	Yes	Yes	No
Montana	AAOO-1959 (1971)	Yes	No	No
Nebraska	AAO-1979/med. ev.	No	Possibly	Yes
Nevada	AAO-1979	Possibly	Yes	Yes
New Hampshire	AAO-1979/med. ev.	No	Yes	Yes
New Jersey	New Jersey formula	No	Yes	Yes
New Mexico	AAO-1979/med. ev.	No	Yes	Yes
New York	AAO-1979	No	No	Yes
North Carolina	AAO-1979	No	No	Yes
North Dakota	AAO-1979	Possibly	Yes with hrng. impt.	Yes
Ohio	AAO-1979/med. ev.	No	No	No
Oklahoma	AAO-1979	No	Yes	Yes
Oregon	Oregon formula	Yes	Yes	Yes
Pennsylvania	Medical evidence	No	No	Yes
Rhode Island	AAO-1979	No	No	Yes
South Carolina	AAO-1979	Yes	No	Yes
South Dakota	AAO-1979	Yes	No	Yes

State	Method	Presbycusis considered?	Tinnitus considered?	Prior loss considered?
Tennessee	AAO-1979/med. ev.	Yes	Yes with hrng. impt.	Yes
Texas	AAO-1979	No	No	Yes
Utah	AAO-1979	Yes	No	Yes
Vermont	AAO-1979/med. ev.	No	Yes with hrng. impt.	No
Virginia	AAO-1979	No	No	Yes
Washington	AAO-1979	No	Yes with hrng. impt.	Yes
Washington, D.C.	AAO-1979	Possibly	Possibly	Possibly
West Virginia	AAO-1979	Yes	No	Yes
Wisconsin	Wisconsin formula	No	No	Yes
Wyoming	AAO-1979/med. ev.	No	No	Yes

[a]Based on compilations reported by ASHA (1992) and Dobie and Megerson (2000).

1000, 2000, and 3000 Hz, making it one of the most generous compensation formulas. The **1975 CHABA formula** also uses a 1000, 2000, and 3000 Hz average, but its low fence is raised to 35 dB, and a four-times better-ear weighting is used. The low fence is elevated so that compensation awards are the same as they would be using the 500, 1000, and 2000 Hz average with a 25-dB low fence.

ASHA 1981 Method

The method proposed by a task force of the American Speech-Language-Hearing Association (ASHA, 1981) is based on notions consistent with the following revised definitions of hearing impairment, handicap, and disability (ASHA 1981, p. 297, emphasis added):

Hearing impairment: a deviation or change for the worse in either auditory structure or auditory function, *usually outside the range of normal.*

Hearing handicap: the disadvantage imposed by a hearing impairment on a person's communicative performance in the *activities of daily living.*

Hearing disability: the determination of a financial reward for the actual or presumed loss of ability to perform *activities of daily living.*

These definitions focus on the nature of auditory disorders, how they are experienced by the patient with a hearing loss, and how they interfere with communication. Consequently, it is not surprising to find that they diverge in several ways from the more general notions embodied in the AMA definitions described earlier: Changes for the worse do not always have to be outside the normal range to constitute an impairment. A handicap does not necessarily imply a material degree of impairment. Compensable disability is tied to activities of daily living rather than to lost income. In light of these considerations, the ASHA method involves the average of 1000, 2000, 3000, and 4000 Hz; a 25 dB low fence; a 75 dB high fence; 2% per decibel; and a five-times weighting for the better ear. There is growing support for the 1000–4000 Hz average (Phaneuf, Hétu, & Hanley 1985; Prince et al 1997; NIOSH 1998), and it has been adopted with a 25 dB low fence as the criterion for material hearing impairment by NIOSH (1998). Of course, the ASHA method provides larger estimates of compensable impairment than the other formulas, and has not been adopted for compensation purposed by any jurisdictions to the author's knowledge.

VA Method

An interesting approach for determining the percentage of impairment for compensation purposes is used by the Department of Veterans Affairs. In

Table 17.7 Major characteristics of various methods ("formulas") used for determining the percentage of hearing impairment for workers' compensation

Method ("formula")	Frequencies averaged (Hz)	Low fence (dB)	High fence (dB)	Percent per dB	Better-ear weighting
AAOO 1959/1971	500, 1000, 2000	25	92	1.5	× 5
AAO/AMA 1979	500, 1000, 2000, 3000	25	92	1.5	× 5
NIOSH 1972	1000, 2000, 3000	25	92	1.5	× 5
CHABA 1975	1000, 2000, 3000	35	92	1.75	× 4
ASHA	1000, 2000, 3000, 4000	25	75	2.0	× 5
Illinois	1000, 2000, 2000	30	85	1.82	(Computed monaurally)
New Jersey	1000, 2000, 3000	30	97	1.7	× 5
Oregon	500, 1000, 2000, 3000, 4000, 6000	25	92	1.5	× 7
Wisconsin	500, 1000, 2000, 3000	30	92	1.6	× 4

Table 17.8a Numerical hearing impairment categories used by the Department of Veterans Affairs for each ear according to the average hearing loss at 1000, 2000, 3000, and 4000 Hz combined with the speech recognition score

Speech recognition score in percent	Average pure tone loss in decibels								
	0–41	42–49	50–57	58–65	66–73	74–81	82–89	90–97	98+
92–100	I	I	I	II	II	II	III	III	IV
84–90	II	II	II	III	III	III	IV	IV	IV
76–82	III	III	IV	IV	IV	V	V	V	V
68–74	IV	IV	V	V	VI	VI	VII	VII	VII
60–66	V	V	VI	VI	VII	VII	VIII	VIII	VIII
52–58	VI	VI	VII	VII	VIII	VIII	VIII	VIII	IX
44–50	VII	VII	VIII	VIII	VIII	IX	IX	IX	X
36–42	VIII	VIII	VIII	IX	IX	IX	X	X	X
0–34	IX	X	XI	XI	XI	XI	XI	XI	XI

Adapted from *Federal Register*, 52, 222, 44120, Tables VI and VIa.

Table 17.8b Categories based on just the pure tone average (under special circumstances, e.g., unreliable speech recognition due to foreign accent)

	Average pure tone loss in decibels									
	0–41	42–48	49–55	56–62	63–69	70–76	77–83	84–90	91–97	98–104	105+
Numeric designation of hearing impairment	I	II	II	IV	V	VI	VII	VIII	IX	X	XI

Adapted from *Federal Register*, 52, 222, 44120, Tables VI and VIa.

this method, each ear is categorized into one of 11 categories (I to XI) based on both its speech recognition score and the average pure tone hearing loss for 1000, 2000, 3000, and 4000 Hz. These categories are shown in **Table 17.8**. For example, if one of a patient's ears has an average loss of 59 dB and a speech recognition score of 58%, it would be placed into category VII. If his other ear has an average loss of 39 dB and a speech recognition score of 74%, then it would be placed into category IV. The percentage of impairment is then obtained using **Table 17.9**. Notice that the better ear is more heavily weighted than the poorer ear, analogous to what we have seen in the formula methods. The patient in our example has a better ear in category IV and a poorer ear in category VII. According to **Table 17.9**, he would have a 20% hearing impairment for compensation purposes.

■ Study Questions

1. What is a noise dosimeter and how is it used?
2. Define the terms *temporary threshold shift, effective quiet, asymptotic threshold shift,* and *permanent threshold shift.*
3. Explain the meaning of excess risk with respect to occupational noise-induced hearing loss.
4. What is the time-weighted average (TWA) and how is it related to noise dose?
5. Explain the concepts of perceived noisiness and annoyance.
6. Describe the articulation index (AI) or speech intelligibility index (SII).
7. Describe the major features of the hearing conservation program mandated by the Hearing Conservation Amendment.
8. Describe the major types of hearing protection devices.
9. How do we determine and describe the effectiveness of hearing protection devices?
10. What factors are involved in determining the percentage of hearing impairment for workers' compensation purposes?

Table 17.9 Percentage of hearing impairment used by the Department of Veterans Affairs, based on the numerical categories of each ear obtained from **Table 17.8**

Better ear	XI	X	IX	VIII	VII	VI	V	IV	III	II	I
XI	100										
X	90	80									
IX	80	70	60								
VIII	70	60	50	50							
VII	60	60	50	40	40						
VI	50	50	40	40	30	30					
V	40	40	40	30	30	20	20				
IV	30	30	30	20	20	20	10	10			
III	20	20	20	20	20	10	10	10	0		
II	10	10	10	10	10	10	10	0	0	0	
I	10	10	0	0	0	0	0	0	0	0	0
	XI	X	IX	VIII	VII	VI	V	IV	III	II	I
	Poorer ear										

Adapted from *Federal Register*, 52, 222, 44121, Table 7.

References

Abel SM, Alberti PW, Haythornthwaite C, Riko K. Speech intelligibility in noise: effects of fluency and hearing protector type. J Acoust Soc Am 1982;71(3):708–715

Abel SM, Alberti PW, Riko K. Speech intelligibility in noise with ear protectors. J Otolaryngol 1980;9(3):256–265

Ahmed S, Fallah S, Garrido B, et al. Use of portable audio devices by university students. Can Acoust 2007;35:35–52

Airo E, Pekkarinen J, Olkinuora P. Listening to music with headphones: an assessment of noise exposure. Acustica 1996;82:885–894

American Medical Association (AMA). Council on Physical Therapy. Tentative standard procedure for evaluating the percentage loss of hearing in medicolegal cases. J Am Med Assn 1942;119:1108–1109

American Medical Association (AMA). Council on Physical Medicine. Tentative standard procedure for evaluating the percentage loss of hearing in medicolegal cases. J Am Med Assoc 1947;133(6):396–397

American Medical Association (AMA). Guide for the evaluation of hearing handicap. JAMA 1979;241(19):2055–2059

American National Standards Institute (ANSI). 1997. ANSI S3.14-1977 (R1997): American National Standard for Rating Noise with Respect to Speech Interference. New York, NY: ANSI

American National Standards Institute (ANSI). 2006a. ANSI S1.4-1983 (R2006). American National Standard Specification for Sound Level Meters. New York, NY: ANSI

American National Standards Institute (ANSI). 2006b. ANSI S3.44-1996 (R2006): American National Standard Determination of Occupational Noise Exposure and Estimation of Noise-Induced Hearing Impairment. New York, NY: ANSI

American National Standards Institute (ANSI). 2008a. ANSI S3.1-1999 (R2008): Maximum Permissible Ambient Noise Levels for Audiometric Test Rooms. New York, NY: ANSI

American National Standards Institute (ANSI). 2008b. ANSI S12.6-2008: American National Standard Methods for Measuring Real-Ear Attenuation of Hearing Protectors. New York, NY: ANSI

American National Standards Institute (ANSI). 2010. ANSI S12.13 TR-2002 (R2010): Technical Report: Evaluating the Effectiveness of Hearing Conservation Programs. New York, NY: ANSI

American National Standards Institute (ANSI). 2012a. ANSI S3.5-1997 (R2012): American National Standard Methods for Calculation of the Speech Intelligibility Index. New York, NY: ANSI

American National Standards Institute (ANSI). 2012b. ANSI/ASA S12.68-2007 (R2012): American National Standard Methods of Estimating A-Weighted Sound Pressure Levels When Hearing Protectors Are Worn. New York, NY: ANSI

American Speech-Language-Hearing Association (ASHA). On the definition of hearing handicap. ASHA 1981;23(4):293–297

American Speech-Language-Hearing Association (ASHA). Ad Hoc Committee on Worker's Compensation. A survey of states' workers' compensation practices for occupational hearing loss. ASHA Suppl 1992;34(8):2–8

Anderson BW, Kalb JT. English verification of the STI method for estimating speech intelligibility of a communication channel. J Acoust Soc Am 1987;81:1982–1985

Atienza H, Bhagwan S, Kramer A, et al. 2008. Preferred MP3 listening levels: earphones and environments. Poster presented at annual conference of American Academy of Audiology, Charlotte, NC

Augustsson I, Engstrand I. Hearing ability according to screening at conscription; comparison with earlier reports and with previous screening results for individuals without known ear disease. Int J Pediatr Otorhinolaryngol 2006;70(5):909–913

Bauman KS, Marston LE. Effects of hearing protection on speech intelligibility in noise. Sound Vibrat 1986;20:12–14

Beranek LL. 1954/1986. Acoustics. New York, NY: Acoustical Society of America

Beranek LL. Revised criteria for noise control in buildings. Noise Control 1957;3:19–27

Beranek LL. Balanced noise-criterion (NCB) curves. J Acoust Soc Am 1989;86:650–664

Berger EH. Methods of measuring the attenuation of hearing protection devices. J Acoust Soc Am 1986;79(6):1655–1687

Berger EH. Flat-response, moderate-attenuation, and level-dependent HPDs: how they work, and what they can do for you. Spectrum 1991;8(Suppl 1):17

Berger EH. 1993. The Naked Truth about NRRs. E-A-RLog 20. Indianapolis, IN: 3M

Berger EH. So, how do you want your NRRs: Realistic or sunny-side up? Hear Rev 1999;6:68–72

Berger EH. 2000. Hearing protection devices. In: Berger EH, Royster LH, Royster JD, Driscol, DP, Layne M, eds. The Noise Manual, 5th ed. Fairfax, VA: American Industrial Hygiene Association; 379–454

Berger EH, Franks JR, Behar A, et al. Development of a new standard laboratory protocol for estimating the field attenuation of hearing protection devices. Part III. The validity of using subject-fit data. J Acoust Soc Am 1998;103(2):665–672

Berger EH, Franks JR, Lindgren F. 1996. International review of field studies of hearing protector attenuation. In: Axelsson A, Borchgrevink H, Hamernick RP, Hellstrom P, Henderson D, Salvi RJ, eds. Scientific Basis of Noise-Induced Hearing Loss. New York, NY: Thieme; 361–377

Berger EH, Royster LH, Royster JD, Driscol DP, Layne M, eds. 2000. The Noise Manual, 5th ed. Fairfax, VA: American Industrial Hygiene Association

Berger EH, Voix J, Kieper RW, Le Cocq C. Development and validation of a field microphone-in-real-ear approach for measuring hearing protector attenuation. Noise Health 2011;13(51):163–175

Bockstael A, De Coensel B, Botteldooren D, et al. Speech recognition in noise with active and passive hearing protectors: a comparative study. J Acoust Soc Am 2011;129(6):3702–3715

Boettcher FA, Henderson D, Gratton MA, Danielson RW, Byrne CD. Synergistic interactions of noise and other ototraumatic agents. Ear Hear 1987;8(4):192–212.

Botsford JH. Simple method for identifying acceptable noise exposures. J Acoust Soc Am 1967;42(4):810–819

Bruel & Kjaer. 1985. The Modulation Transfer Function in Room Acoustics. RASTI: A Tool for Evaluating Auditoria. Technical review no. 3-1985. MA: Bruel & Kjaer

Bruel & Kjaer. 1986. Noise Control: Principles and Practice. MA: Bruel & Kjaer

Byrne DC, Reeves ER. Analysis of nonstandard noise dosimeter microphone positions. J Occup Environ Hyg 2008;5(3):197–209

Campo P, Subramaniam M, Henderson D. The effect of "conditioning" exposures on hearing loss from traumatic exposure. Hear Res 1991;55(2):195–200

Canlon B, Borg E, Flock A. Protection against noise trauma by pre-exposure to a low level acoustic stimulus. Hear Res 1988;34(2):197–200

Casali JG, Mauney DW, Burks JA. Physical vs. psychophysical measurements of hearing protector attenuation—a.k.a. MIRE vs. REAT. Sound Vibrat 1995;29:20–27

Cheng YJ, Gregg EW, Saaddine JB, Imperatore G, Zhang X, Albright AL. Three decade change in the prevalence of hearing impairment and its association with diabetes in the United States. Prev Med 2009;49(5):360–364

Clark WW. Recent studies of temporary threshold shift (TTS) and permanent threshold shift (PTS) in animals. J Acoust Soc Am 1991a;90(1):155–163

Clark WW. Noise exposure from leisure activities: a review. J Acoust Soc Am 1991b;90(1):175–181

Clark WW, Bohne BA. The effects of noise on hearing and the ear. Med Times 1984;122:17–22

Clark WW, Bohne BA, Boettcher FA. Effect of periodic rest on hearing loss and cochlear damage following exposure to noise. J Acoust Soc Am 1987;82(4):1253–1264

Cohen A. 1977. Extraauditory effects of noise on behavior and health. In: Lee DK, Falk HL, Murphy SD, Geiger SR, eds. Handbook of Physiology: Reactions to Environmental Agents, sec. 9. Baltimore, MD: Williams & Wilkins

Cohen S, Weinstein N. Nonauditory effects of noise on behavior and health. J Soc Issues 1981;37:36–70

Colby WD, Dobie R, Leventhall G, et al. 2009. Wind Turbine Sound and Health Effects: An Expert Panel Review. Available at http://www.canwea.ca/pdf/talkwind/Wind_Turbine_Sound_and_Health_Effects.pdf

Coles RRA, Garinther GR, Hodge DC, Rice CG. Hazardous exposure to impulse noise. J Acoust Soc Am 1968;43(2):336–343

Cruickshanks KJ, Nondahl DM, Tweed TS, et al. Education, occupation, noise exposure history and the 10-yr cumulative incidence of hearing impairment in older adults. Hear Res 2010;264(1-2):3–9

Danhauer JL, Johnson CE, Byrd A, et al. Survey of college students on iPod use and hearing health. J Am Acad Audiol 2009;20(1):5–27, quiz 83–84

Danhauer JL, Johnson CE, Dunne AF, et al. Survey of high school students' perceptions about their iPod use, knowledge of hearing health, and need for education. Lang Speech Hear Serv Sch 2012;43(1):14–35

Davis AC, Fortnum HM, Coles RRA, Haggard MP, Lutman ME. 1985. Damage to Hearing from Leisure Noise: A Review of the Literature. MRC Inst. Hear Res. Nottingham, UK: University of Nottingham

de Kluizenaar Y, Janssen SA, van Lenthe FJ, Miedema HME, Mackenbach JP. Long-term road traffic noise exposure is associated with an increase in morning tiredness. J Acoust Soc Am 2009;126(2):626–633

Department of Defense (DOD). 2004. DoD Hearing Conservation Program (HCP). Department of Defense Instruction No. 6055.12 (March 5, 2004). Available at http://www.dtic.mil/whs/directives/corres/pdf/605512p.pdf

Department of Labor (DOL). Occupational noise exposure. Fed Regist 1969;34:7946–7949

Dobie RA. 1993. Medico-Legal Evaluation of Hearing Loss. New York, NY: Van Nostrand Reinhold

Dobie RA. 1996. Estimation of occupational contribution to hearing handicap. In: Axelsson A, Borchgrevink H, Hamernick RP, Hellstrom P, Henderson D, Salvi RJ, eds. Scientific Basis of Noise-Induced Hearing Loss. New York, NY: Thieme; 415–422

Dobie RA. Noise-induced permanent threshold shifts in the occupational noise and hearing survey: an explanation for elevated risk estimates. Ear Hear 2007;28(4):580–591

Dobie RA, Megerson SC. 2000. Workers' compensation. In: Berger EH, Royster LH, Royster JD, Driscol, DP, Layne M, eds. The Noise Manual, 5th ed. Fairfax, VA: American Industrial Hygiene Association; 689–710

Dolan TG, O'Loughlin D. Amplified earmuffs: impact on speech intelligibility in industrial noise for listeners with hearing loss. Am J Audiol 2005;14(1):80–85

Driscoll DP, Royster LH. 2000. Noise control engineering. In: Berger EH, Royster LH, Royster JD, Driscol, DP, Layne M, eds. The Noise Manual, 5th ed. Fairfax, VA: American Industrial Hygiene Association; 279–378

Edwards CG, Schwartzbaum JA, Lönn S, Ahlbom A, Feychting M. Exposure to loud noise and risk of acoustic neuroma. Am J Epidemiol 2006;163(4):327–333

Environmental Protection Agency (EPA). 1973. Public Health and Welfare Criteria for Noise (EPA 550/9-73-002). Washington, DC: EPA

Environmental Protection Agency (EPA). 1974. Information on Levels of Environmental Noise Requisite to Protect Public Health and Welfare with an Adequate Margin of Safety (EPA 550/9-74-004). Washington, DC: EPA

Environmental Protection Agency (EPA). Noise labeling requirements for hearing protectors. Fed Regist 1979;190:56139–56147

Epstein M, Marozeau J, Cleveland S. Listening habits of iPod users. J Speech Lang Hear Res 2010;53(6):1472–1477

Erdreich J. Engineering controls for noise abatement. Hear Rev 1999;6:42–46s

Ericksson LJ. Active sound and vibration control: a technology in transition. Noise Control Eng J 1996;44:1–9

Farina A. Assessment of hearing damage when listening to music through a personal digital audio player. Paper presented at Acoustics '08, Paris. J Acoust Soc Am 2008;123:3458 (Abstr.)

Fields JM. Effect of personal and situational variables on noise annoyance in residential areas. J Acoust Soc Am 1993;93:2753–2763

Fields JM. Reactions to environmental noise in an ambient noise context in residential areas. J Acoust Soc Am 1998;104:2245–2260

Fletcher H. 1929. Speech and Hearing. New York, NY: Van Nostrand

Fligor BJ. Risk for noise-induced hearing loss from use of portable media players: a summary of evidence through 2008. Perspect Audiol 2009;5:10–20

Fligor BJ, Cox LC. Output levels of commercially available portable compact disc players and the potential risk to hearing. Ear Hear 2004;25(6):513–527

Fligor BJ, Ives TE. 2006a. Does earphone type affect risk for recreational noise-induced hearing loss? Paper presented at Noise-Induced Hearing Loss in Children Conference. Cincinnati, OH

Fligor BJ, Ives T. 2006b. Does earphone type affect risk for recreational noise-induced hearing loss? Paper presented at Conference: Noise-Induced Hearing Loss in Children at Work & Play. Oct. 19–20, 2006, Covington, KY

Florentine M, Hunter W, Robinson M, Ballou M, Buus S. On the behavioral characteristics of loud-music listening. Ear Hear 1998;19(6):420–428

French NR, Steinberg GC. Factors governing the intelligibility of speech sounds. J Acoust Soc Am 1947;19:90–119

Gauger D. Active noise reduction (ANR) and hearing protection: where it's appropriate and why. Spectrum 2002;19(Suppl 1):20–21

Hamernik RP, Ahroon WA, Hsueh KD. The energy spectrum of an impulse: its relation to hearing loss. J Acoust Soc Am 1991;90(1):197–204

Hamernik RP, Hsueh KD. Impulse noise: some definitions, physical acoustics and other considerations. J Acoust Soc Am 1991;90(1):189–196

Health Council of the Netherlands (HCN). 1996. Effects of noise on health: Chapter 3 of a report on noise and health prepared by a Committee of the Health Council of the Netherlands. Reproduced in Noise/News Intl 4(3):137–150

Henderson D, Subramaniam M, Boettcher FA. Individual susceptibility to noise-induced hearing loss: an old topic revisited. Ear Hear 1993;14(3):152–168

Henderson E, Testa MA, Hartnick C. Prevalence of noise-induced hearing-threshold shifts and hearing loss among US youths. Pediatrics 2011;127(1):e39–e46

Hodgetts WE, Rieger JM, Szarko RA. The effects of listening environment and earphone style on preferred listening levels of normal hearing adults using an MP3 player. Ear Hear 2007;28(3):290–297

Hoenig DR. 2010. Preferred Listening Levels of Normal Hearing Individuals Who Listen to Their IPod While Riding the New York City Subway System. Unpublished AuD Capstone Thesis. New York, NY: City University of New York

Hoffman HJ, Dobie RA, Ko C-W, Themann CL, Murphy WJ. Americans hear as well or better today compared with 40 years ago: hearing threshold levels in the unscreened adult population of the United States, 1959–1962 and 1999–2004. Ear Hear 2010;31(6):725–734

Hoover A, Krishnamurti S. Survey of college students' MP3 listening: habits, safety issues, attitudes, and education. Am J Audiol 2010;19(1):73–83

International Electrotechnical Commission (IEC). 1987. Publ. 268: Sound System Equipment Part 16: Report on the RASTI Method for Objective Rating of Speech Intelligibility in Auditoria

International Standards Organization (ISO). 1994. Acoustics—Hearing Protectors, Part 2: Estimation of Effective A-Weighted Sound Pressure Levels When Hearing Protectors Are Worn (ISO-4869-2). Geneva: ISO

International Standards Organization (ISO). 2013. Acoustics—Estimation of Noise-Induced Hearing Loss (ISO-1999). Geneva: ISO

Janssen SA, Vos H, Eisses AR, Pedersen E. A comparison between exposure-response relationships for wind turbine annoyance and annoyance due to other noise sources. J Acoust Soc Am 2011;130(6):3746–3753

Keith SE, Michaud DS, Chiu V. Evaluating the maximum playback sound levels from portable digital audio players. J Acoust Soc Am 2008;123(6):4227–4237

Keith SE, Michaud DS, Feder K, et al. MP3 player listening sound pressure levels among 10 to 17 year old students. J Acoust Soc Am 2011;130(5):2756–2764

Killion M, DeVilbiss E, Stewart J. An earplug with uniform 15-dB attenuation. Hear J 1988;41(5):14–17

Kryter KD. Methods for the calculation and use of the articulation index. J Acoust Soc Am 1962;34:1689–1697

Kryter KD. 1985. The Effects of Noise on Man, 2nd ed. Orlando, FL: Academic Press

Kryter KD. Evaluation of hearing handicap. J Am Acad Audiol 1998;9:141–146

Kryter KD, Ward WD, Miller JD, Eldredge DH. Hazardous exposure to intermittent and steady-state noise. J Acoust Soc Am 1966;39(3):451–464

Kujawa SG, Liberman MC. Adding insult to injury: cochlear nerve degeneration after "temporary" noise-induced hearing loss. J Neurosci 2009;29(45):14077–14085

Kuo SM, Morgan DR. 1996. Active Noise Control Systems. Hoboken, NJ: Wiley

Lazarus H. Prediction of verbal communication in noise: a development of generalized SIL curves and the quality of communication, Part 2. Appl Acoust 1987;20:245–261

Lempert BL, Henderson TL. 1973. Occupational Noise and Hearing 1968 to 1972: A NIOSH Study. Cincinnati, OH: NIOSH

Leventhall G. Concerns about infrasound from wind turbines. Acoustics Today 2013;9(3):30–38

Levey S, Levey T, Fligor BJ. Noise exposure estimates of urban MP3 player users. J Speech Lang Hear Res 2011;54(1):263–277

Lipscomb DM. Allocation among causes of hearing loss: the concept, its pros and cons. Hear Rev 1999;6(9):48–64

Lusk SL, Gillespie B, Hagerty BM, Ziemba RA. Acute effects of noise on blood pressure and heart rate. Arch Environ Health 2004;59(8):392–399

Lusk SL, Hagerty BM, Gillespie B, Caruso CC. Chronic effects of workplace noise on blood pressure and heart rate. Arch Environ Health 2002;57(4):273–281

Maxwell DW, Williams CE, Robertson RM, Thomas GB. Performance characteristics of active hearing protection devices. Sound Vibrat 1987;21(5):14–18

McNeill K, Keith SE, Feder K, Konkle ATM, Michaud DS. MP3 player listening habits of 17 to 23 year old university students. J Acoust Soc Am 2010;128(2):646–653

Melnick W. Human temporary threshold shift (TTS) and damage risk. J Acoust Soc Am 1991;90(1):147–154

Miedema HME, Vos H. Demographic and attitudinal factors that modify annoyance from transportation noise. J Acoust Soc Am 1999;105:3336–3344

Miedema HME, Vos H. Exposure-response relationships for transportation noise. J Acoust Soc Am 1998;104(6):3432–3445

Miller JD. Effects of noise on people. J Acoust Soc Am 1974;56(3):729–764

Mine Safety and Health Administration (MSHA). Health standards for occupational noise exposure. Final rule. 30 CFR Part 62. Fed Regist 1999;64:49548–49634, 49636–49637

National Institute for Occupational Safety and Health (NIOSH). 1972. Criteria for a Recommended Standard: Occupational Exposure to Noise. Publication No. HSM 73-11001. Cincinnati, OH: NIOSH

National Institute for Occupational Safety and Health (NIOSH). 1990. A Practical Guide to Effective Hearing Conservation Programs in the Workplace. Publication No. 90-120. Cincinnati, OH: NIOSH

National Institute for Occupational Safety and Health (NIOSH). 1996. Preventing Occupational Hearing Loss—A Practical Guide. Publication No. 96-110. Cincinnati, OH: NIOSH

National Institute for Occupational Safety and Health (NIOSH). 1998. Criteria for a Recommended Standard: Occupational Noise Exposure—Revised Criteria 1998. Publication No. 98-126. Cincinnati, OH: NIOSH

Nelson PA, Elliot SJ. 1992. Active Control of Sound. London, UK: Academic

Norin JA, Emanuel DC, Letowski TR. Speech intelligibility and passive, level-dependent earplugs. Ear Hear 2011;32(5):642–649

Occupational Safety and Health Administration (OSHA). 1983. §1910.95 Occupational noise exposure. March 8, 1983/Rules and regulations. Fed. Reg., 48:46:9776–9785

Occupational Safety and Health Administration (OSHA). 2002. §1904.10 Occupational injury and illness recording and reporting requirements. July 1, 2002/ Rules and regulations. Fed. Reg., 67:126:44037–44048

Odess JS. Acoustic trauma of sportsman hunter due to gun firing. Laryngoscope 1972;82(11):1971–1989

Ohrström E, Barregård L, Andersson E, Skånberg A, Svensson H, Angerheim P. Annoyance due to single and combined sound exposure from railway and road traffic. J Acoust Soc Am 2007;122(5):2642–2652

Orfield SJ. The RASTI method of testing relative intelligibility. Sound Vibrat 1987;21(12):20–22

Passchier-Vermeer W. Hearing loss due to continuous exposure to steady-state broad-band noise. J Acoust Soc Am 1974;56(5):1585–1593

Patel D. Exposure to loud noise and risk of acoustic neuroma. Occup Med (Lond) 2006;56(7):514

Pavlovic CV. Derivation of primary parameters and procedures for use in speech intelligibility predictions. J Acoust Soc Am 1987;82(2):413–422

Pavlovic CV. Speech recognition and five articulation indexes. Hear Instr 1991;42(9):20–23

Pavlovic CV, Studebaker GA, Sherbecoe RL. An articulation index based procedure for predicting the speech recognition performance of hearing-impaired individuals. J Acoust Soc Am 1986;80(1):50–57

Pedersen E. Health aspects associated with wind turbine noise—Results from three field studies. Noise Control Eng J 2011;59(1):47–53

Pedersen E, Larsman P. The impact of visual factors on noise annoyance among people living in the vicinity of wind turbines. J Environ Psychol 2008;28:379–389

Pedersen E, Persson Waye K. Wind turbine noise, annoyance and self-reported health and well-being in different living environments. Occup Environ Med 2007; 64(7):480–486

Pedersen E, van den Berg F, Bakker R, Bouma J. Response to noise from modern wind farms in the Netherlands. J Acoust Soc Am 2009;126(2):634–643

Pedersen E, Waye KP. Perception and annoyance due to wind turbine noise—a dose-response relationship. J Acoust Soc Am 2004;116(6):3460–3470

Phaneuf R, Hétu R, Hanley JA. A Bayesian approach for predicting judged hearing disability. Am J Ind Med 1985;7(4):343–352

Pierpont N. 2009. Wind-Turbine Syndrome: A Report on a Natural Experiment. Santa Fe, NM: K-Selected Books

Portnuff CDF, Fligor BJ. 2006. Sound output levels of the iPod and other MP3 players: is there potential risk to hearing? Paper presented at Conference: Noise-Induced Hearing Loss in Children at Work & Play. Oct. 19–20, 2006, Covington, KY

Portnuff C, Fligor B, Arehart K. 2009. Teenage use of portable listening devices: a hazard to hearing? Presentation at annual conference of National Hearing Conservation Association, Atlanta, GA.

Preston-Martin S, Thomas DC, Wright WE, Henderson BE. Noise trauma in the aetiology of acoustic neuromas in men in Los Angeles County, 1978–1985. Br J Cancer 1989;59(5):783–786

Prince MM, Gilbert SJ, Smith RJ, Stayner LT. Evaluation of the risk of noise-induced hearing loss among unscreened male industrial workers. J Acoust Soc Am 2003;113(2):871–880

Prince MM, Stayner LT, Smith RJ, Gilbert SJ. A re-examination of risk estimates from the NIOSH occupational noise and hearing survey (ONHS). J Acoust Soc Am 1997;101(2):950–963

Punch JL, Elfenbein JL, James RR. Targeting hearing health messages for users of personal listening devices. Am J Audiol 2011;20(1):69–82

Punch J, James R, Pabst D. Wind-turbine noise: what audiologists should know. Audiol Today 2010;22(4):20–31

Rabinowitz PM. Hearing loss and personal music players. BMJ 2010;340:c1261

Rabinowitz PM, Slade MD, Galusha D, Dixon-Ernst C, Cullen MR. Trends in the prevalence of hearing loss among young adults entering an industrial workforce 1985 to 2004. Ear Hear 2006;27(4):369–375

Rasmussen P, Flamme G, Stewart M, Meinke D, Lankford J. Measuring recreational firearm noise. Sound Vibrat 2009;43(8):14–18

Rawool VW. 2012. Hearing Conservation: In Occupational, Recreational, Educational, and Home Settings. New York, NY: Thieme Medical Publishers

Rogers AL, Manwell JF, Wright S. 2006. Wind turbine acoustic noise. Available at http://www.minutemanwind.com/pdf/Understanding%20Wind%20Turbine%20Acoustic%20Noise.pdf

Rösler G. Progression of hearing loss caused by occupational noise. Scand Audiol 1994;23(1):13–37

Royster JD, Berger EH, Merry CJ, et al. Development of a new laboratory standard protocol for estimating the field attenuation of hearing protection devices. Part I. Research of working group 11, Accredited Standards Committee S12, Noise. J Acoust Soc Am 1996;99:1506–1526

Royster JD, Royster LH. 1990a. Hearing Conservation Programs: Guidelines for Success. Chelsea, MI: Lewis

Royster JD, Royster LH. How can we evaluate the effectiveness of occupational hearing conservation programs? Hear Rev 1999;6(9):28–34

Royster JD, Royster LH. 2000. Evaluating hearing conservation program effectiveness. In: Berger EH, Royster LH, Royster JD, Driscol, DP, Layne M, eds. The Noise Manual, 5th ed. Fairfax, VA: American Industrial Hygiene Association; 517–548

Royster LH. Recommendations for the labeling of hearing protectors. Sound Vibrat 1995;29(7):16–19

Royster LH, Royster JD. Employment related exposure to noise and its effect on hearing. Hear Instr 1990b;41(10):17–18

Salt AN, Lichtenhan JT. How does wind turbine noise affect people? Acoustics Today 2014;10(1):20–28

Schlauch RS. Noise-induced hearing loss in teenagers. Acoustics Today 2013;9(4):14–18

Schlauch RS, Carney E. Are false-positive rates leading to an overestimation of noise-induced hearing loss? J Speech Lang Hear Res 2011;54(2):679–692

Schlauch RS, Carney E. The challenge of detecting minimal hearing loss in audiometric surveys. Am J Audiol 2012;21(1):106–119

Schomer PD. Comments on recently published article, "Concerns about infrasound from wind turbines." Acoustics Today 2013;9(4):7–9

Shargorodsky J, Curhan SG, Curhan GC, Eavey R. Change in prevalence of hearing loss in US adolescents. JAMA 2010;304(7):772–778

Snowden CK, Zapala DA. Do middle school students set safe volume levels for routine iPod use? A comparison of monaural versus binaural listening trends. Audiol Today 2010;22(4):53–59

Stansfeld SA, Berglund B, Clark C, et al; RANCH study team. Aircraft and road traffic noise and children's cognition and health: a cross-national study. Lancet 2005;365(9475):1942–1949

Steeneken HJM, Houtgast T. A physical method for measuring speech-transmission quality. J Acoust Soc Am 1980;67(1):318–326

Stewart M, Foley L, Lehman M, Gerlach A. Risks faced by recreational firearm users. Audiol Today 2011; 23(2):38–48

Subramaniam M, Campo P, Henderson D. The effect of exposure level on the development of progressive resistance to noise. Hear Res 1991a;52:181–188

Subramaniam M, Campo P, Henderson D. Development of resistance to hearing loss from high frequency noise. Hear Res 1991b;56(1–2):65–68

Subramaniam M, Henderson D, Campo P, Spongr V. The effect of "conditioning" on hearing loss from a high frequency traumatic exposure. Hear Res 1992;58(1):57–62

Suter AH. OSHA's Hearing Conservation Amendment and the audiologist. ASHA 1984;26(6):39–43

Suter AH. Speech recognition in noise by individuals with mild hearing impairments. J Acoust Soc Am 1985;78(3):887–900

Suter AH. Noise sources and effects—a new look. Sound Vibrat 1992a;26(1):18–38

Suter AH. 1992b. The Relationship of the Exchange Rate to Noise-Induced Hearing Loss. NTIS No. PB93-118610. Cincinnati, OH: Alice Suter & Assoc

Suter AH. 1993. Hearing Conservation Manual, 3rd ed. Milwaukee, WI: Council for Accreditation in Occupational Hearing Conservation

Suter AH, von Gierke HE. Noise and public policy. Ear Hear 1987;8(4):188–191

Taylor W, Pearson J, Mair A, Burns W. Study of noise and hearing in jute weavers. J Acoust Soc Am 1965;38: 113–120

Timmerman NS. Wind turbine noise. Acoustics Today 2013;9(3):22–29

Torre P III. Young adults' use and output level settings of personal music systems. Ear Hear 2008;29(5): 791–799

Towne RM. An acoustical checklist for multi-family housing units. Sound Vibrat 1994;28(7):28–32

Van Gerven PWM, Vos H, Van Boxtel MPJ, Janssen SA, Miedema HMC. Annoyance from environmental noise across the lifespan. J Acoust Soc Am 2009;126(1): 187–194

Virkkunen H, Kauppinen T, Tenkanen L. Long-term effect of occupational noise on the risk of coronary heart disease. Scand J Work Environ Health 2005;31(4): 291–299

Vogel I, Verschuure H, van der Ploeg CPB, Brug J, Raat H. Adolescents and MP3 players: too many risks, too few precautions. Pediatrics 2009;123(6):e953–e958

Ward WD. The role of intermittence in PTS. J Acoust Soc Am 1991;90(1):164–169

Webster JC. 1969. Effect of noise on speech intelligibility. In: Ward WD, Fricke JE, eds. Noise as a Public Health Hazard. ASHA report no. 4. Rockville, MD: ASHA; 49–73

Webster JC. 1978. Speech interference aspects of noise. In: Lipscomb DM, ed. Noise and Audiology. Baltimore, MD: University Park Press; 193–228

Williams W. Noise exposure levels from personal stereo use. Int J Audiol 2005;44(4):231–236

Willich SN, Wegscheider K, Stallmann M, Keil T. Noise burden and the risk of myocardial infarction. Eur Heart J 2006;27(3):276–282

Zhan W, Cruickshanks KJ, Klein BE, et al. Modifiable determinants of hearing impairment in adults. Prev Med 2011;53(4-5):338–342

Appendixes

Appendix A

This appendix gives examples of how to combine octave-band levels (OBLs) in dB into overall sound pressure level (dB SPL) and A-weighted sound level (dBA). Correction values for A-weighted OBLs are in **Table 1.7**. The same procedures can be used with third-octave-band levels except that an appropriate (different) set of A-weightings would have to be used. The OBLs of the noise being used in these examples are as follows:

Frequency (Hz)	OBLs
31.5	85
63	80
125	77
250	76
500	74
1000	68
2000	60
4000	57
8000	55

Combining OBLs into dB SPL: Simplified Method

The octave band levels are listed from highest to lowest to simplify the procedure. Then they are combined in successive pairs based on the increments given in **Table 1.3**.

Combining OBLs into dB SPL: Formula Method

The OBLs are summed logarithmically according to the formula

$$L = 10 \ log \ \sum_{i=1}^{n} 10^{Li/10}$$

where L is the overall (combined) level in dB SPL, n is the number of bands, i is the ith band, and Li is the OBL of the ith band. The formula calls for calculating $10^{Li/10}$ for each octave-band level:

Frequency (Hz)	OBLs	$10^{Li/10}$
31.5	85	316,227,766.0
63.0	80	100,000,000.0
125.0	77	50,118,723.36
250.0	76	39,810,717.06
500.0	74	25,118,864.32
1000.0	68	6,309,573.445
2000.0	60	1,000,000.0
4000.0	57	501,187.2336
8000.0	55	316,227.766

Next, the values of 10Li/10 are added, and their sum (Σ) is found to be: 539,403,059.2. At this point the formula says

$$L = 10 \ log \ 539,403,059.2.$$

The logarithm of 539,403,059.2 is 8.731913405, so that we now have

$$L = 10 \ x \ 8.731913405.$$

Hence the overall level of this sound is

$$L = 87.3 \ dB \ SPL.$$

Combining OBLs into dBA: Simplified Method

The corrected A-weighted OBLs are obtained from **Table 1.4**.

Frequency (Hz)	OBLs	dBA Corrections	Corrected OBLs
31.5	85	−39.4	45.6
63	80	−26.2	53.8
125	77	−16.1	60.9
250	76	−8.6	67.4
500	74	−3.2	70.8
1000	68	0.0	68.0
2000	60	1.2	61.2
4000	57	1.1	58.1
8000	55	−1.1	53.9

The A-weighted corrected OBLs are listed from highest to lowest to simplify the procedure. Then they are combined in successive pairs based on the increments given in **Table 1.3**. (For simplicity, the corrected OBLs shown here have been rounded to the nearest whole number.)

Combining OBLs into dBA: Formula Method

The OBLs are summed logarithmically according to the formula:

$$L_A = 10 \ log \sum_{i=1}^{n} 10^{Li+ki/10}$$

where L_A is the overall (combined) level in dBA, n is the number of bands, i is the ith band, Li is the OBL of the ith band, and ki is the dBA correction value for each OBL. The correction is accomplished by adding the correction factor to the OBL (Li + ki). Adding a negative correction value is the same as subtracting.

The corrected A-weighted OBLs are obtained from **Table 1.4**: The formula calls for calculating $10^{(Li+ki)/10}$ for each octave band level.

Frequency (Hz)	OBLs	dBA Corrections	Corrected OBLs	$10^{(Li+ki)/10}$
31.5	85	−39.4	45.6	36,307.80548
63	80	−26.2	53.8	239,883.2919
125	77	−16.1	60.9	1,230,268.771
250	76	−8.6	67.4	5,495,408.739
500	74	−3.2	70.8	12,022,644.35
1000	68	0.0	69.0	6,309,573.445
2000	60	1.2	61.2	1,318,256.739
4000	57	1.1	58.1	645,654.229
8000	55	−1.1	53.9	245,470.8916

Next, the values of $10^{(Li+ki)/10}$ are added, and their sum (Σ) is found to be: 27,543,468.26. At this point the formula says

$$L_A = 10 \ log \ 27,543,468.26.$$

The logarithm of 27,543,468.26 is 7.440018625, so that we now have

$$L_A = 10 \ x \ 7.440018625.$$

Hence the overall sound level is

$$L_A = 74.4 \ dBA.$$

■ Appendix B

Alphabetical Listing of Spondaic Words Commonly Used in Clinical Practice

Spondee word	CID W-1[a]	ASHA[b]	ASHA ½-list[c]	Streamlined list/ adults[d]	Children's picture list[e]
airplane*[f]	CID	ASHA	A		Child/picture
armchair*	CID	ASHA	B		
backbone*		ASHA	B		
baseball	CID	ASHA	A	Streamlined	Child/picture
bathtub					Child/picture
birthday	CID				
birthday*		ASHA	B		
blackboard*		ASHA	A		
bluebird					Child/picture
cookbook*		ASHA	B		
cowboy	CID	ASHA	A		Child/picture
cupcake					Child/picture
daybreak	CID				
doormat	CID				
doormat*		ASHA	B	Streamlined	
drawbridge	CID	ASHA	A	Streamlined	
duckpond*	CID	ASHA	A		
eardrum	CID	ASHA	A	Streamlined	
earthquake*		ASHA	B		
eyebrow*		ASHA	B		
farewell	CID				
firetruck					Child/picture
flashlight					Child/picture
football					Child/picture
grandson	CID			Streamlined	
greyhound*	CID	ASHA	B		
hardware	CID	ASHA	B		
headlight	CID	ASHA	B		
horseshoe*	CID	ASHA	A		
hotdog	CID	ASHA	A		Child/picture
hothouse	CID				
iceberg	CID				
icecream		ASHA	A		Child/picture
inkwell	CID	ASHA	B	Streamlined	
mailman					Child/picture
mousetrap*	CID	ASHA	A	Streamlined	
mushroom	CID	ASHA	B		
northwest*	CID	ASHA	A	Streamlined	
nutmeg		ASHA	B		

(Continued on page 500)

Alphabetical Listing of Spondaic Words Commonly Used in Clinical Practice *(Continued)*

Spondee word	CID W-1[a]	ASHA[b]	ASHA ½-list[c]	Streamlined list/ adults[d]	Children's picture list[e]
oatmeal*	CID	ASHA	A		
outside		ASHA	B		
padlock*	CID	ASHA	B	Streamlined	
pancake	CID	ASHA	A		
playground	CID	ASHA	A	Streamlined	
popcorn					Child/picture
railroad*	CID	ASHA	A	Streamlined	
reindeer					Child/picture
sailboat					Child/picture
schoolboy	CID				
seesaw					Child/picture
shoelace					Child/picture
sidewalk	CID			Streamlined	
snowman					Child/picture
stairway*	CID	ASHA	B		
sunset	CID	ASHA	A		
toothbrush*	CID	ASHA	B	Streamlined	Child/picture
toothpaste					Child/picture
whitewash*	CID	ASHA	A		
woodwork	CID	ASHA	B	Streamlined	
workshop	CID			Streamlined	

[a]Words in the original CID W-1 spondee lists (Hirsh et al 1952) are identified by "CID" in this column.

[b]Words in the ASHA spondee list, a revision of the CID W-1 list emphasizing the word selection criteria of dissimilarity and homogeneous audibility (ASHA 1979, 1988), are identified by "ASHA" in this column .

[c]The ASHA spondee list is divided into half-lists A and B. Words included in these half-lists are indicated by an "A" or a "B" in this column (ASHA 1979, 1988).

[d]Words in the Streamlined Spondaic Word List for Adults (Young et al 1982; ASHA 1988) are identified by "Streamlined" in this column.

[e]Words in the Children's Picture Spondaic Word List (Frank 1980; ASHA 1988) are identified by "Child/picture" in this column.

[f]Asterisks identify the 20 spondaic words found to have the most similar audibility when presented by both recorded and monitored live voice (Rourke-Cullen et al 1995).

References

American Speech-Language-Hearing Association (ASHA). Guidelines for determining the threshold level for speech. ASHA 1979;20:297–301

American Speech-Language-Hearing Association (ASHA). Guidelines for determining threshold level for speech. ASHA 1988;30:85–89

Frank T. Clinical significance of the relative intelligibility of pictorally represented spondee words. Ear Hear 1980;1:46–49

Hirsh IJ, Davis H, Silverman SR, Reynolds EG, Eldert E, Benson RW. Development of materials for speech audiometry. J Speech Hear Dis 1952;17:321–337

Rourke-Cullen T, Ninya RL, Nerbonne MA. Relative intelligibility of the revised CID W-1s as presented via MLV and Auditec recordings. J Am Acad Audiol 1995;6:183–186

Young LL, Dudley B, Gunter MB. Thresholds and psychometric functions of individual spondaic words. J Speech Hear Res 1982;25:586–593

■ Appendix C

CID Auditory Test W-22: Word Lists 1–4 (Randomization A)[a]

List 1A	List 2A	List 3A	List 4A
1. an	1. yore	1. bill	1. all
2. yard	2. bin	2. add	2. wood
3. carve	3. way	3. west	3. at
4. us	4. chest	4. cute	4. where
5. day	5. then	5. start	5. chin
6. toe	6. ease	6. ears	6. they
7. felt	7. smart	7. tan	7. dolls
8. stove	8. gave	8. nest	8. so
9. hunt	9. pew	9. say	9. nuts
10. ran	10. ice	10. is	10. ought
11. knees	11. odd	11. out	11. in
12. not	12. knee	12. lie	12. net
13. mew	13. move	13. three	13. my
14. low	14. now	14. oil	14. leave
15. owl	15. jaw	15. king	15. of
16. it	16. one	16. pie	16. hang
17. she	17. hit	17. he	17. save
18. high	18. send	18. smooth	18. ear
19. there	19. else	19. farm	19. tea
20. earn	20. tare	20. this	20. cook
21. twins	21. does	21. done	21. tin
22. could	22. too	22. use	22. bread
23. what	23. cap	23. camp	23. why
24. bathe	24. with	24. wool	24. arm
25. ace	25. air	25. are	25. yet
26. you	26. and	26. aim	26. darn (dawn)
27. as	27. young	27. when	27. art
28. wet	28. cars	28. book	28. will
29. chew	29. tree	29. tie	29. dust
30. see	30. dumb	30. do	30. toy
31. deaf	31. that	31. hand	31. aid
32. them	32. die	32. end	32. than
33. give	33. show	33. shove	33. eyes
34. true	34. hurt	34. have	34. shoe
35. isle	35. own	35. owes	35. his
36. or	36. key	36. jar	36. our
37. law	37. oak	37. no	37. men
38. me	38. new	38. may	38. near
39. none	39. live	39. knit	39. few
40. jam	40. off	40. on	40. jump
41. poor	41. ill	41. if	41. pale
42. him	42. rooms	42. raw	42. go
43. skin	43. ham	43. glove	43. stiff
44. east	44. star	44. ten	44. can
45. thing	45. eat	45. dull	45. through
46. dad	46. thin	46. though	46. clothes
47. up	47. flat	47. chair	47. who
48. bells	48. well	48. we	48. bee
49. wire	49. by	49. ate	49. yes
50. ache	50. ail	50. year	50. am

[a] Adapted from: Department of Defense Hearing Center of Excellence. n.d. VA CD Speech Recognition and Identification Materials. Disc 4.0: Score Sheets. Accessed March 5, 2015, at http://hearing.health.mil/EducationAdvocacy/VACDs/VA_CD_Score_Sheets.aspx

■ Appendix D

Northwestern University Auditory Test No. 6 (Alphabetical Order)[a]

List 1	List 2	List 3	List 4
bean	bite	bar	back
boat	book	base	bath
burn	bought	beg	bone
chalk	calm	cab	came
choice	chair	cause	chain
death	chief	chat	check
dime	dab	cheek	dip
door	dead	cool	dog
fall	deep	date	doll
fat	fail	ditch	fit
gap	far	dodge	food
goose	gaze	five	gas
hash	gin	germ	get
home	goal	good	hall
hurl	hate	gun	have
jail	haze	half	hole
jar	hush	hire	join
keen	juice	hit	judge
king	keep	jug	kick
kite	keg	late	kill
knock	learn	lid	lean
laud	live	life	lease
limb	loaf	luck	long
lot	lore	mess	lose
love	match	mop	make

List 1	List 2	List 3	List 4
met	merge	mouse	mob
mode	mill	name	mood
moon	nice	note	near
nag	numb	pain	neat
page	pad	pearl	pass
pool	pick	phone	peg
puff	pike	pole	perch
rag	rain	rat	red
raid	read	ring	ripe
raise	room	road	rose
reach	rot	rush	rough
sell	said	search	sail
shout	shack	seize	shirt
size	shawl	shall	should
sub	soap	sheep	sour
sure	south	soup	such
take	thought	talk	tape
third	ton	team	thumb
tip	tool	tell	time
tough	turn	thin	tire
vine	voice	void	vote
week	wag	walk	wash
which	white	when	wheat
whip	witch	wire	wife
yes	young	youth	yearn

[a]From Tillman and Carhart (1966) with permission.

Reference

Tillman TW, Carhart R. 1966. An Expanded Test for Speech Discrimination Utilizing CNC Monosyllabic Words. Northwestern University Auditory Test No. 6. Tech Report SAM-TR-66-55. Brooks AFB, TX: USAF School of Aerospace Medicine

■ Appendix E

Spanish Bisyllabic Words for Speech Recognition Testing (Alphabetical)[a]

List 1	List 2	List 3	List 4
agua (water)	Abril (April)	actriz (actress)	algo (some)
baile (dance)	alma (soul)	ambos (both)	aqui (here)
blusa (blouse)	astro (star)	ayer (yesterday)	banco (bank)
boca (mouth)	barca (boat)	barba (beard)	blanco (white)
bosque (forest)	bolsa (bag)	beso (kill)	boda (wedding)
broma (joke)	bravo (brave)	brazo (arm)	breve (short)
brusco (rough)	calle (street)	brisa (breeze)	buscan (search)
burro (donkey)	camas (beds)	cabra (goat)	calor (heat)
carta (letter)	casa (house)	calma (calm)	casta (breed)
caso (case)	centro (center)	campo (field)	chiste (joke)
cestos (baskets)	claro (clear)	casi (almost)	cita (appointment)
cinco (five)	contra (against)	cesta (basket)	compra (purchase)
clima (weather)	donde (where)	choclo (galosh)	cristal (crystal)
costa (coast)	fecha (date)	clavo (nail)	dentro (inside)
culpa (guilt)	flete (freight)	corta (short)	dolor (pain)
doce (twelve)	funda (cover)	dicha (happiness)	edad (age)
finca (farm)	ganga (bargain)	filtro (filter)	falta (missing)
frente (front)	gastar (spend)	fonda (inn)	fruta (fruit)
galgo (greyhound)	golpe (blow)	fusil (rifle)	gancho (hook)
granja (farm)	grifos (faucets)	ganso (geese)	grasa (grease)
guerra (war)	hilo (thread)	gasto (spent)	gratas (pleasant)
hambre (hunger)	horno (oven)	guante (glove)	gustar (like)
hombro (shoulder)	igual (same)	gusto (taste)	hijo (son)
huevo (egg)	kilo (kilo)	hombre (man)	hora (hour)
joven (young)	leal (loyal)	hueso (bone)	jardin (garden)
lado (side)	lila (lilac)	isla (isle)	jugo (juice)
lengua (tongue)	madre (mother)	leche (milk)	libros (books)
luna (moon)	marca (brand)	lugar (place)	lunes (monday)
mano (hand)	mismo (same)	malo (bad)	manta (blanket)
mesa (table)	motor (engine)	Martes (Tuesday)	metal (metal)
modo (way)	nariz (nose)	mitad (half)	mosca (fly)
multa (fine)	nombre (name)	mucho (much)	mundo (world)

(Continued on page 504)

Spanish Bisyllabic Words for Speech Recognition Testing (Alphabetical)[a] *(Continued)*

List 1	List 2	List 3	List 4
once (eleven)	oro (gold)	nido (nest)	orden (order)
ostras (oysters)	pais (country)	ocho (eight)	noche (night)
pasta (paste)	peso (weight)	osos (bears)	padre (father)
pipas (pipes)	plato (plate)	papel (paper)	pelo (hair)
queso (cheese)	rama (branch)	queja (complaint)	pisos (floors)
rancho (ranch)	rico (rich)	ranas (frogs)	quince (fifteen)
regla (ruler)	roncar (snore)	ropa (clothes)	rasgos (features)
rosca (thread)	rostro (face)	rumor (rumor)	resto (rest)
salsa (salsa)	salud (health)	sangre (blood)	rosa (rose)
sano (healthy)	sastre (tailor)	siglo (century)	saltar (jump)
sombra (shadow)	sordo (deaf)	tanto (much)	santo (saint)
tanque (tank)	techo (ceiling))	tela (fabric)	sopa (soup)
tema (theme)	templo (temple)	tinta (ink)	tasa (cup)
trampa (trap)	torta (cake)	total (total)	temor (fear)
tretas (tricks)	trece (thirteen)	trenza (plait)	toro (bull)
turno (turn)	tronco (trunk)	vapor (steam)	vaca (cow)
veinte (twenty)	valor (price)	verbo (verb)	venta (sale)
verdad (truth)	visa (visa)	visto (seen)	vino (wine)

[a] With permission of Auditec of St. Louis.

■ Appendix F

Boothroyd Isophonemic Word Lists (Alphabetical Order)

a. Relatively Equivalent Lists[a]

List 1[b]	List 2[b]	List 4[b]	List 5[b]
both	bone	choose	fib
cheek	cheese	comb	goes
dice	duck	fun	heel
fan	fish	guess	June
haze	hive	hide	rake
jot	log	job	shop
move	path (patch)[d]	shape	sum
rug	race	vat	thatch
ship	tomb	will	vet
well	wedge	wreath	wide

List 8[b]	List 9[b]	List 10[b]	List 11[b]
bath	chime	beep	chose
dig	dope	faith	cough
five	fake	hem	gun
hum	gas	jug	hip
joke	hush	latch	math
noose	jet	rod	ride
pot	lose	shoes	shoot
reach	rob	sign	siege
shell	thin	vote	veil
ways	weave	wick	web

List 12[b]	List 13[b]	List 14[b]	List 15[b]
buff	buzz	bike	ban
den	dodge	Dutch	chief
have	gate	fog	cove
jays	hash	heath	dish
mice	kiss	jam	hug
poach	moon	laze	loose
rule	pole	pet	moth
shock	thieve	rove	pies
teeth	wife	soon	rage
wig	wretch	wish	wet

List 17[c]	List 18[c]	List 19[c]	List 20[c]
cash	dog	cab	booth
chop	fetch	death	cave
give	height	fig	fuss
hole	jazz	hope	guide
jade	pool	lodge	home
rub	robe	nice	jell
set	shave	rush	pin
thief	suck	teach	rash
wine	theme	vase	tease
zoom	win	womb	watch

b. Relatively Easier Lists[a]

List 3[b]	List 6[b]	List 7[b]	List 16[c]
bomb	bed	badge	beach
food	catch	foam	chef
hen	fill	goose	dime
jail	got	hutch	hop
shows	heap	kill	love
teak	juice	not	rag
thug	rave	reap	suit
vice	shown	shed	thick
witch	thumb	thighs	wage
wrap	wise	wave	zone

Source: Boothroyd (2008). Courtesy of Dr. Arthur Boothroyd.
[a]Based on the findings of Mackersie, Boothroyd, and Minniear (2001).
[b]Lists 1–15 also may found in Boothroyd (1984, 2006, 2008) and Mackersie et al (2001).
[c]Lists 16–20 also may be found in Boothroyd (2006, 2008) and Mackersie et al (2001)
[d]"Patch" in Boothroyd (1984).

References

Boothroyd A. Auditory perception of speech contrasts by subjects with sensorineural hearing loss. J Speech Hear Res 1984;27:134–144

Boothroyd A. 2006. Computer-Assisted Speech Perception Assessment CASPA 5.0 Software. San Diego, CA: A. Boothroyd

Boothroyd A. 2008. Computer-Assisted Speech Perception Assessment CASPA 5.0 Manual. San Diego, CA: A. Boothroyd

Mackersie CL, Boothroyd A, Minniear D. Evaluation of the Computer-Assisted Speech Perception Assessment Test (CASPA). J Am Acad Audiol 2001;12:390–396

■ Appendix G

An Example of the AzBio Sentence Lists
(Spahr & Dorman 2004; Spahr, Dorman, Litvak, et al 2012)

List 2 Sentences	Words Scored
She had a sly way of introducing insults.	8
She was not looking forward to meeting his acquaintance.	9
They found a beak in the Thanksgiving turkey.	8
That is a great piece of information.	7
Her parents wanted to pay.	5
He did not like smoky bars.	6
I think I need a nap.	6
I just need a little air.	6
Take a big wild guess.	5
The engagement was not official yet.	6
The nasty weather caused severe flooding.	6
Your place really turned out great.	6
Why did the dog have to die in the end?	10
Why do you try to manipulate the system?	8
There is something suspicious afoot.	5
We celebrate African American culture.	5
He is completing his apprenticeship at the funeral home.	9
It became quite apparent that he had been drinking.	9
The blatant display of favoritism was shocking to the class.	10
She did not require an escort up the stairs.	9
Total	143

Source: From *The AzBio Sentence Lists.* ©2006 Arizona State University. Auditory Potential, LLC. Used with permission of Dr. Anthony J. Spahr.

References

Spahr AJ, Dorman MF. Performance of subjects fit with the Advanced Bionics CII and Nucleus 3G cochlear implant devices. Arch Otolaryngol—Head Neck Surg 2004;130:624–628

Spahr AJ, Dorman MF, Litvak LM, Van Wie S, Gifford RH, Loizou PC, Loiselle LM, Oakes T, Cook S. Development and validation of the AzBio sentence lists. Ear Hear 2012;33:112–117

■ Appendix H

Lists 1 and 2 of the *Basic English Lexicon (BEL) Sentences.* (Calandruccio & Smiljanic 2012a,b)

Key words are underlined.

List 1

The park opens in eleven months.
The thirsty kid drinks juice.
These brown mushrooms taste amazing.
The train is fast and very dangerous.
The annoying student asks many questions.
The performer wears colorful dresses.
A lazy worker rests often.
My doctor works in that busy hospital.
He lost his white hat today.
The city school is large and crowded.
The weak plant is barely alive.
The kids enjoyed the holiday parade.
The red vegetables grow in the garden.
The eggs need more salt.
The old men missed home.
The girl loves sweet candy.
The milk and cheese smelled horrible.
My grandmother baked a chocolate cake.
The bright sun warms the ground
His sister plays with beautiful toys.
The party game was really easy.
Our cat hates taking a bath.
The gray mouse ate the cheese.
The bar sells beer on the weekend.
My strong father carried my brother.

List 2

The twins live with their grandparents.
Some people drink black coffee.
The woman met her favorite actor.
That bright light seems far away.
The glass dish broke in the kitchen.
My cousin owned a silver car.
The young performer learned to sing.
The professors write simple problems.
The brown bears eat fruit.
The couple kissed after dinner.
The excited teenager was really noisy.
The players forgot to bring lunch again.
The weird noise upset the baby.
The lady walked down the street.
The lost dog was hungry and thirsty.
The scary monkey chased the child.
Our shy neighbors avoid people.
The fruit and salad taste fresh.
Her loud cough sounded horrible.
Her grandparents are serious and sometimes cruel.
The five students were late for class.
The private university is not cheap.
The plane will land in ten minutes.
Our father works in a large office.
The tourist traveled many places.

Source: Basic English Lexicon (BEL) Sentences. © Calandruccio & Smiljanic (2012b). Used with permission of Dr. Lauren Calandruccio.

References

Calandruccio L, Smiljanic R. New sentence recognition materials developed using a basic non-native English lexicon. J Speech Lang Hear Res 2012a;55:1342–1355

Calandruccio, L, Smiljanic R. 2012b. Basic English Lexicon (BEL) Sentences. Compact Disk. Chapel Hill, NC: Lauren Calandruccio

■ Appendix I

Lexical Neighborhood Test (LNT) [a]

List 1 (Easy Words)	List 1 (Hard Words)	List 2 (Easy Words)	List 2 (Hard Words)
juice	thumb	down	ear
good	pie	truck	hand
drive	wet	mouth	dry
time	fight	pig	zoo
hard	toe	give	goat
gray	cut	school	toy
foot	pink	boy	call
orange	hi	put	sing
count	song	three	cut
brown	fun	farm	wrong
home	use	fish	bed
old	mine	green	fat
watch	ball	catch	man
need	kick	break	run
food	tea	house	hot
dance	book	sit	read (/rid/)
live (/llv/)	bone	friend	grow
stand	work	jump	bag
six	dad	bird	cake
cold	game	swim	seat
push	lost	hold	nine
stop	cook	want	sun
girl	gum	snake	bath
hurt	cap	more	ten
cow	meat	white	ride

[a]© Indiana University. Reproduced by permission of the authors and Indiana University. (Test recording available from Auditec of St. Louis.)

Reference

Kirk KI, Pisoni DB, Osberger MJ. Lexical effects on spoken word recognition by pediatric cochlear implant users. Ear Hear 1995;16:470–481

■ Appendix J

Multisyllabic Lexical Neighborhood Test (MLNT) [a]

List 1 (Easy Words)	List 1 (Hard Words)	List 2 (Easy Words)	List 2 (Hard Words)
children	butter	water	puppy
animal	lion	banana	pickle
monkey	money	glasses	button
finger	jelly	airplane	summer
pocket	yellow	window	bottom
apple	purple	tiger	finish
morning	hello	cookie	bunny
sugar	carry	again	belly
alright	corner	another	couple
about	heaven	almost	under
because	measles	broken	naughty
crazy	ocean	china	really

[a]© Indiana University. Reproduced by permission of the authors and Indiana University. (Test recording available from Auditec of St. Louis.)

Reference

Kirk KI, Pisoni DB, Osberger MJ. Lexical effects on spoken word recognition by pediatric cochlear implant users. Ear Hear 1995;16:470–481

■ Appendix K

PBK-50 (PB Kindergarten) Words Lists in Alphabetical Order[a]

List 1	List 2	List 3	List 4	List 1	List 2	List 3	List 4
are	and	all	ache	need	look	knife	most
bad	ask	as	air	no	ma	laugh	nest
bath	ball	ax	black	own	new	lip	nuts
bead	barn	bee	blind	pants	night	loud	pass
beef	best	bet	bounce	pinch	off	next	press
box	calf	bless	bug	pink	pick	on	purse
bus	chew	bud	bush	please	pig	page	quick
cart	closed	cage	cab	pond	reach	park	raw
class	cloud	camp	case	put	rest	paste	rich
did	crack	cat	choose	rag	rode	path	room
dish	day	crab	clown	rat	rope	peg	seed
end	dime	darn	cost	ride	shoe	plow	sell
fed	each	fair	dad	scab	sick	race	set
few	feel	falls	drop	shop	slide	rose	sheep
five	flag	fat	else	sled	south	sack	ship
fold	food	feed	fit	slice	this	sing	that
great	forth	find	frog	slip	thread	splash	them
hit	front	freeze	grade	smile	three	suit	thick
hot	glove	fresh	had	such	toe	tray	those
hunt	good	got	hurt	take	tongue	turn	tire
is	guess	grab	if	teach	trade	wait	true
lay	gun	gray	jay	thank	wake	waste	vase
me	hook	grew	leave	tree	wash	weed	white
mouth	kept	his	low	use	wave	wreck	wide
neck	left	knee	may	ways	wood	yes	you

[a]From Haskins (1949) with permission.

Reference

Haskins, H. 1949. A phonetically balanced test of speech discrimination for children. Unpublished master's thesis. Evanston, IL: Northwestern University

■ Appendix L

Word Intelligibility by Picture Idenitification (WIPI) Test Word Lists[a]

List 1	List 2	List 3	List 4
school	broom	moon	spoon
ball	bowl	bell	bow
smoke	coat	coke	goat
floor	door	corn	horn
fox	socks	box	block
hat	flag	bag	black
pan	fan	can	man
bread	red	thread	bed
neck	desk	nest	dress
stair	bear	chair	pear
eye	pie	fly	tie
knee	tea	key	bee
street	meat	feet	teeth
wing	string	spring	ring
mouse	clown	crown	mouth
shirt	church	dirt	skirt
gun	thumb	sun	gum
bus	rug	cup	bug
train	cake	snake	plane
arm	barn	car	star
chick	stick	dish	fish
crib	ship	bib	lip
wheel	seal	queen	green
straw	dog	saw	frog
pail	nail	ail	tail

[a]From Ross and Lerman (1971), with permission.

Reference

Ross M, Lerman J. 1971. Word Intelligibility by Picture Identification: WIPI. Pittsburgh, PA: Stanwix House

■ Appendix M

Northwestern University Children's Perception of Speech (NU-CHIPS) Test Word Lists (Alphabetical Order)[a]

ball	horse
bear	house
bike	juice
bird	light
boat	man
bus	meat
cake	milk
clock	mouth
coat	nose
comb	purse
cup	school
dog	shirt
door	shoe
dress	sink
duck	smile
food	snake
foot	soap
frog	spoon
girl	teeth
gum	tongue
gun	train
hair	tree
ham	truck
hand	watch
head	witch

[a]From Elliott and Katz (1980), with permission.

Reference

Elliot L, Katz D. 1980. Northwestern University Children's Perception of Speech (NU-CHIPS). St. Louis, MO: Auditec

■ Appendix N

Selected Resources for Auditory-Visual Training

Adaptive Listening and Communication Enhancement (LACE)
Authors: RW Sweetow & JH Sabes (2006)
Neurotone
2317 Broadway
Redwood City, CA 94063
www.neurotone.com

Auditory Enhancement Guide
Authors: D Shea and the Clarke School Staff (1992)
AG Bell Association for the Deaf and Hard of Hearing
3417 Volta Place
Washington, DC 20007
www.agbell.org

Auditory Training
Author: NP Erber (1982)
AG Bell Association for the Deaf and Hard of Hearing
3417 Volta Place
Washington, DC 20007
www.agbell.org

Bringing Sound to Life: Principles and Practices of Cochlear Implant Rehabilitation
Author: M Koch (1999)
York Press
PO Box 504
Timonium, MD 21094.
www.yorkpress.com

CHATS: The Miami Cochlear Implant, Auditory and Tactile Skills Curriculum
Authors: KC Vergara & LW Miskiel (1994)
Intelligent Hearing Systems
6860 SW 81st St
Miami, FL 33143
www.ihsys.com/public_html/CHATS.asp

Cochlear Implant Auditory Training Guide
Author: D Sindrey (1997)
Wordplay Publications
PO Box 8048
London, Ontario N6G 4X1
www.wordplay.ca

Communication Training for Hearing-Impaired Children and Teenagers
Author: N Tye-Murray (1993)
PRO-ED
8700 Shoal Creek Blvd
Austin, TX 78757
www.proedinc.com

Contrasts for Auditory and Speech Training (CAST)
Author: DJ Ertmer (2003)
Linguisystems
3100 4th Ave
East Moline, IL 61244
www.linguisystems.com/custom.php

Developmental Approach to Successful Listening II
Authors: G Stout & J Windle (1992)
Resource Point
61 Inverness Drive East
Englewood, CO 80112

Guide for Optimizing Auditory Learning Skills (GOALS)
Authors: J Firszt & R Reeder (1996)
AG Bell Association for the Deaf and Hard of Hearing
3417 Volta Place
Washington, DC 20007
www.agbell.org

Listen, Learn, and Talk
Author: Cochlear Americas Corp (n.d.)
Cochlear Americas
61 Inverness Drive East
Englewood, CO 80112
www.cochlearamericas.com

Listening Games for Littles
Author: D Sindrey (1997)
Wordplay Publications
PO Box 8048
London, Ontario N6G 4X1
www.wordplay.ca

Seeing and Hearing Speech
Author: Sensimetrics (2002)
Sensimetrics
48 Grove Street
Somerville, MA 02144
www.sens.com

Sound and Beyond
Author: Cochlear Americas Corp (n.d.)
Cochlear Americas
61 Inverness Drive East
Englewood, CO 80112

Speech and the Hearing-Impaired Child: Theory and Practice, 2nd ed.
Author: D Ling (2002)
AG Bell Association for the Deaf and Hard of Hearing
3417 Volta Place
Washington, DC 20007
www.agbell.org

Speech Perception Instructional Curriculum Evaluation (SPICE)
Authors: J Moog, J Biedenstein, & L Davidson (1995)
Central Institute for the Deaf
4560 Clayton Ave
St. Louis, MO 63110
www.cid.wustl.edu

The SKI-HI Curriculum: Family-Centered Programming for Infants and Young Children with Hearing Loss
Author: S Watkins (2004)
Hope Publishing
1856 North 1200 East
North Logan, UT 84321
www.hopepubl.com

Subject Index

Note: Page numbers followed by f and t indicate figures and tables, respectively.

Author Index

Note: Numbers in italics indicate figure or table references.